PUBLIC
AND
COMMUNITY HEALTH
NURSE'S CONSULTANT

A HEALTH PROMOTION GUIDE

PUBLIC AND COMMUNITY HEALTH NURSE'S CONSULTANT

A HEALTH PROMOTION GUIDE

MARCIA STANHOPE, RN, DSN, FAAN
Associate Dean and Professor
College of Nursing
University of Kentucky
Lexington, Kentucky

RUTH N. KNOLLMUELLER, RN, PhD
Associate Professor and Director
Nursing Programs at the Center for Rural Health
College of Nursing
University of Kentucky
Lexington, Kentucky

with 90 illustrations

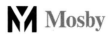

St. Louis Baltimore Boston Carlsbad Chicago Naples New York
Philadelphia Portland London Madrid Mexico City Singapore
Sydney Tokyo Toronto Wiesbaden

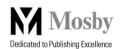

Mosby

Dedicated to Publishing Excellence

A Times Mirror Company

Vice President and Publisher: Nancy L. Coon
Editor: Loren S. Wilson
Developmental Editor: Brian Dennison
Project Manager: Mark Spann
Production Editor: Beth Hayes
Designer: Judi Lang
Manufacturing Manager: Betty Richmond
Cover Art: Sue White
Copyediting and Production: Graphic World Publishing Services

Printed in the United States of America
Composition by Graphic World, Inc.
Lithography/film by Graphic World, Inc.
Printing/binding by R. R. Donnelley & Sons, Inc.

Mosby-Year Book, Inc.
11830 Westline Industrial Drive
St. Louis, Missouri 63146

ISBN: 0-8151-9003-4

98 99 00 01 / 9 8 7 6 5 4 3 2

♻ Preface

The health care system in the United States is a paradox. As a country, we spend nearly 14% of the gross national product on health care. Yet, only three cents of each health care dollar spent goes toward the preventive services estimated to influence 50% of all disease, disability, and mortality in the country. Populations such as the homeless, minorities, children, elderly, uninsured, and underinsured fair poorly, although they represent more than 30% of the country's population.

The growing sense of urgency to resolve the health care crisis has turned policy makers' attention to alternative approaches that would decrease the need for institutionalized health care. Policy makers have begun looking at community-wide and community-coalition–based approaches that emphasize disease prevention, health promotion and protection, and community-based interventions. Such initiatives as President Clinton's emphasis on national health care reform (1993); legislation requiring health care reform in eight states; the PEW Health Professions Committee Reports (1991-1995) on the state of health care delivery, health professionals, and education; and the latest IOM (1994) study of the changing face of primary care have underscored the need for new approaches to solving the nation's health care problems.

As a result, the American health care system is experiencing its most dramatic transformation in history (PEW, 1995) with emphasis on transformation of organizations and financing, health alliances, integrated networks, and public and private sector partnerships. Major transformations will not only be demanded of health care professionals but also of educational programs that prepare students to meet the demands of the changing system.

The PEW Commission (1995) indicates that health professionals of the future will need to be competent in a number of skills, including caring for the community's health, expanding access to care, coordinating care in the integrated network, practicing prevention, promoting healthy lifestyles, managing information, and participating in a racially and culturally diverse society. These competencies are all emphasized in public and community health nursing education and are needed by practicing nurses in the community.

As the nation and its states move health care delivery toward community-based practice, a greater need for public and community health nurses will arise. Data indicate the long-standing existence of a shortage of nurses prepared in this area. This book will assist nurses in preparing themselves for community-based practice by serving as a ready resource for the many questions and situations they may encounter in their practice.

Public and Community Health Nurse's Consultant: A Health Promotion Guide is a compilation of instruments, guides, hints, charts, graphs, and forms to provide public health and community health nurses cues that will aid in caring for clients: communities, families, and individuals. The information contained herein will also assist faculty and students in providing structure for the students' synthesis of knowledge related to all parameters of public health and community health nursing practice. In addition, researchers may find resources for application to the study of problems encountered in the community.

The cues contained in this book will assist nurses in assessing, planning, and evaluating community-based nursing practice. The works in this book should not be considered exhaustive of the resources available to nurses, but sources that may be used as appropriate to job responsibilities or that may serve as a catalyst for searching the literature for related cues to complete the task of promoting the health of the community or population served. This work is a ready reference for the nurse to use while intervening with clients to promote their health and well being. These cues are also beneficial in evaluating client outcomes.

Public and Community Health Nurses's Consultant: A Health Promotion Guide is organized into four parts. The first part supplies information that nurses in the community can use daily such as sources of HIV information; health-related, world-wide web sites; resources for culturally diverse populations; and common epidemiologic rates. The second part furnishes assessment tools for a variety of client populations and settings, including community, home and industry, family, individual, and nutritional to provide an extensive assemblage of data collection instruments. The third part points to indicators of risk that help predict potential health problems such as substance or physical abuse, depression and mental illness, and communicable disease; this part also guides the nurse's intervention. The fourth part offers teaching tools to assist the nurse in providing clients with guidance on self-examination for cancer, good nutrition, living with AIDS, caring for newborns, and other health promotion topics.

We wish to thank those who have permitted their work to be shared and acknowledge the expertise and the contributions they have made to preventing disease and promoting the health of communities, families, and individuals. A special thanks to Kerrie Schnapf and Peg Teachey for their assistance in completing this work.

Marcia Stanhope
Ruth N. Knollmueller

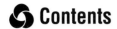 Contents

Part One: Resource Data

Part Two: Assessment

Family Assessment

Individual Assessment

Nutritional Assessment

Part Three: Indicators of Risk

Abuse

Mental Health

Life Style

Poisons

Accidents

Communicable and Infectious Diseases

Disabilities

Part Four: Teaching Techniques & Anticipatory Guidance

Educational Techniques

Screening Tools, Techniques, and Diagnostic Criteria

Nutritional Guidelines

Acquired Immune Deficiency Syndrome

Pregnancy, Infancy, Postnatal Care, and Childhood

PART ONE

RESOURCE DATA

Resource Information—Client

Resources for reference and referral are an essential part of the nurse's repetoire. Assisting clients in seeking needed information is central to public/community health nursing practice. The following is a selected group of resources to help the nurse in working with clients, families, and communities.

Community Resources—United States

The following is a list of resources on many different health-related topics, from alcoholism to water safety. The list includes names and addresses that can be used to obtain further information. It is not by any means a complete list but is meant to serve as a starting point. Because telephone numbers may change, please contact directory assistance for proper listings.

Acquired Immunodeficiency Syndrome (AIDS)

National Gay Task Force Crisisline
(212) 807-6016 (in NY, AK, and HI)

Public Health Service AIDS Information Hotline
(800) 342-AIDS
(202) 245-6867 (in AK, HI only)

National AIDS Hotline
c/o American Social Health Association
PO Box 13827
Research Triangle Park, NC 27709
(800) 342-AIDS (2437) or
(800) 342-7514

Advocacy

American Civil Liberties Union
132 W 43rd St
New York, NY 10036
(212) 944-9800

1

Occupational Safety and Health Administration (OSHA)
Office of Public and Consumer Affairs
US Department of Labor, Room N3637
200 Constitution Ave NW
Washington, DC 20210
(202) 523-8148

Alcohol and Drug Abuse

AL-ANON Family Group Headquarters, Inc
PO Box 182
Madison Square Station
New York, NY 10010

Alcohol and Drug Problems Association of North America, Inc.
1101 15th St NW
Suite 204
Washington, DC 20005

Alcoholics Anonymous
Call local chapters (see White Pages of phone directory)

Drug Information Association, Inc
1050 George St
Suite 5-L
New Brunswick, NJ 08901

Friday Nite Live
c/o Sacramento County Office of Education
9738 Lincoln Village Dr
Sacramento, CA 95827

International Commission for Prevention of Alcoholism
6830 Laurel St NW
Washington, DC 20012

MADD—Mothers Against Drunk Driving
National Headquarters
669 Airport Freeway
Suite 310
Hurst, TX 76053
(817) 268-6233 or
311 Main St
Suite C
Roseville, CA 95678
(800) 443-6233

National Association on Drug Abuse Problems, Inc
355 Lexington Ave
New York, NY 10017

National Clearinghouse for Alcohol Information
PO Box 2345
Rockville, MD 20852
(301) 468-2600

National Clearinghouse for Drug Abuse Information
PO Box 416
Kensington, MD 20795

National Cocaine Hotline
(800) COCAINE

National Committee for the Prevention of Alcoholism and Drug Dependency
6830 Laurel St NW
Washington, DC 20012

National Council on Alcoholism, Inc
733 3rd Ave
New York, NY 10017

National Council on Drug Abuse
571 W Jackson Blvd
Chicago, IL 60606

SADD—Students Against Driving Drunk
PO Box 800
Marlboro, MA 01752
(617) 481-3568 or
(state office in CA)
505 N Tustin Ave
Santa Ana, CA 92705
(714) 542-8155
(Also chapters in high schools)

Synanon Foundation, Inc
PO Box 786
Marshall, CA 94940

Volunteers and Victim Assistance (VIVA)
5716 J St
Sacramento, CA 95819
(916) 457-VIVA

Alzheimer's Disease

Alzheimer's Disease and Related Disorders Association, Inc
700 E Lake St
Chicago, IL 60601
(312) 853-3060;
(800) 621-0379;
(800) 572-6037 (in IL only)

Alzheimer's Disease Education and Referral Center (ADEAR)
(800) 438-4380

Arthritis and Collagen Disorders

American Juvenile Arthritis Organization
1314 Spring St NW
Atlanta, GA 30309
(404) 872-7100

Arthritis Foundation
1314 Spring St NW
Atlanta, GA 30309
(404) 812-0531

Arthritis Information Clearinghouse
PO Box 9782
Arlington, VA 22209
(703) 558-8250

Arthritis Information Clearinghouse
PO Box 34427
Bethesda, MD 20034
(301) 881-9411

Scleroderma Research Foundation
(800) 637-4005

United Scleroderma Foundation, Inc
(800) 722-HOPE

Asthma and Allergies

Association for the Care of Asthma, Inc
Spring Valley Rd
Ossining, NY 10562

Asthma and Allergy Foundation of America
19 W 44th St
New York, NY 10036

Asthma-Allergy Hotline
(414) 272-1004 (in WI only)

Bereavement*

Bereavement Outreach Network
127 Arundel Rd
Pasadena, MD 21122

The Candlelighters Foundation
2025 I St NW
Washington, DC 20006

---

*From Gifford B, Cleary B: Supporting the bereaved, *Am J Nurs* 90(2), 1990.

The Compassionate Friends
PO Box 3696
Oakbrook, IL 60522-3696

Growing Through Grief
PO Box 1664
Annapolis, MD 21404

Pregnancy and Infant Loss Center
1415 E Wayzata Blvd
Suite 22
Wayzata, MN 55391

SHARE
St Johns Hospital
800 E Carpenter
Springfield, IL 62702

Survivors of Suicide (SOS): Directory of Survivor Groups, American Association of Suicidology
2459 S Ash St
Denver, CO 80222

Widowed Persons Service, AARP
1909 K St NW
Washington, DC 20049

Widow to Widow Program
58 Fernwood Rd
Boston, MA 02115

Blindness

American Council of the Blind
1010 Vermont Ave NW
Suite 1100
Washington, DC 20005

American Foundation for the Blind, Inc
15 W 16th St
New York, NY 10011
(212) 620-2000

Association for Education of the Visually Handicapped
919 Walnut St
4th Floor
Philadelphia, PA 19107

Braille Institute
741 N Vermont Ave
Los Angeles, CA 90029

Guide Dogs for the Blind
PO Box 1200
San Rafael, CA 94915
(415) 479-4000

Guide Dog Users, Inc.
57 Grandview Ave
Watertown, MA 02172
(617) 926-9198

Guiding Eyes for the Blind
Yorktown Heights, NY 10598
(914) 245-4024

The Library of Congress
Division of the Blind and
Physically Handicapped
1291 Taylor St NW
Washington, DC 20542
(202) 287-5100

National Association for Visually Handicapped
22 W 21st St
New York, NY 10010
(212) 889-3141

National Eye Institute
Information Officer
Building 31, Room 6A32
Bethesda, MD 20205

National Retinitis Pigmentosa Foundation
(800) 638-2300
(301) 655-1011 (in MD only)

National Society to Prevent Blindness
500 E Remington Rd
Schaumburg, IL 60173

Recording for the Blind, Inc
20 Roszel Rd
Princeton, NJ 08540
(609) 452-0606

Burns

American Burn Association
c/o William Curreri, MD
New York Hospital
Cornell Medical Center
New York, NY 10021

National Burn Federation
3737 5th Ave
Suite 206
San Diego, CA 92103

Cancer

AMC Cancer Information
(800) 525-3777

American Cancer Society
1599 Clifford Rd NE
Atlanta, GA 30329
(800) 227-2345

Cancer Information Service (CIS)
(800) 4-CANCER
(800) 638-6070 (in AK only);
(202) 636-5700 (in DC area only);
(808) 524-1234 (in Oahu, HI—neighbor islands)

Encore (discussion and exercise program for women who have had breast cancer surgery)
National Board, YWCA
726 Broadway
New York, NY 10003
(212) 614-2700

Ever Forward Foundation, Inc (children who have cancer)
1101 SW Washington
Suite 101
Portland, OR 97205-9694
(800) 869-2995 or
(503) 224-9207 (fax)

Federation for Children with Special Needs
95 Berkley St
Boston, MA 02116
(800) 331-0688 (voice or telecommunications device for the deaf) or
(617) 482-2915

International Association Cancer Victors and Friends, Inc
7740 W Manchester Ave
Suite 110
Playa del Rey, CA 90291
(213) 822-5032

Johanna's On Call to Mend Esteem
Cancer Rehabilitation Nurse Consultants
199 New Scotland Ave
Albany, NY 12208
(518) 482-4178

Leukemia Society of America, Inc
733 3rd Ave
New York, NY 10017
(212) 573-8484

Make A Wish Foundation of America
2600 N Central Ave
Suite 936
Phoenix, AZ 85004
(602) 722-9474

Make Today Count (for persons with cancer or other life-threatening illnesses)
101½ S Union St
Alexandra, VA 22314-3323
(703) 548-9674

Medical Insurance Claims, Inc (assistance in handling insurance claims)
Kinnelon Professional Complex
170 Kennelon Rd
Suite 10
Kinnelon, NJ 07405

National Association of Meal Programs (referrals)
204 E St, NE
Washington, DC 20002
(202) 547-6157

National Cancer Information Clearinghouse
Office of Communications
National Cancer Institute,
Room 10A18
9000 Rockville Pike
Bethesda, MD 20205
(301) 496-4070
(800) 4-CANCER

National Cancer Institute
Department of Health and
Human Services
Public Inquiries Section
Office of Cancer
Communications
Building 31
Room 10A-18
9000 Rockville Pike
Bethesda, MD 20892
(301) 496-5583

National Coalition for Cancer Survivorship
323 8th St, SW
Albuquerque, NM 87102
(505) 764-9956

National Lymphedema Network
2211 Post St, Suite 404
San Francisco, CA 94115
(800) 541-3259

National Neurofibromatosis Foundation, Inc.
141 5th Ave
Suite 7-S
New York, NY 10010
(800) 323-7938 or
(212) 460-8980

Oley Foundation (home parenteral and/or enteral nutrition therapy)
214 Hun Memorial
Albany Medical Center
Albany, NY 12208
(518) 445-5079

SKIP—Sick Kids Need Involved People
990 2nd Ave
2nd Floor
New York, NY 10022
(212) 421-9160

Spirit and Breath Association (to assist those with lung cancer)
8210 Elmwood Ave
Suite 209
Skokie, IL 60077
(708) 673-1384

Y-Me National Organization for Breast Cancer Information and Support, Inc
18220 Harwood
Homewood, IL 60430
(800) 221-2141 (Patient hot-line, 9-5, CT, weekdays);
(708) 799-8338 (General Information);
(708) 799-8228 (Patient 24-hour hot-line)

Child Abuse

Child Abuse Listening Mediation, Inc
PO Box 718
Santa Barbara, CA 93102

Child Help USA
(800) 422-4453

Children's Defense Fund
122 C St NW,
Suite 400
Washington, DC 20036
(800) 222-2000

Clearinghouse on Child Abuse
and Neglect Information
PO Box 1182
Washington, DC 20013
(301) 251-5157

Children

American Association for
Maternal and Child Health,
Inc
PO Box 965
Los Altos, CA 94022

American Pediatric Society
PO Box 14871
St Louis, MO 63178

Child Health Associate
Program
4200 E 9th Ave
Box C219
Denver, CO 80262

National Sudden Infant Death
Syndrome Foundation
310 S Michigan Ave
Chicago, IL 60604

National Tay-Sachs and Allied
Disease Association
122 E 42nd St
New York, NY 10017

Pediatric Pulmonary
Association of America
150 N Pond Way
Roswell, GA 30076

Shriners Hospital Referral
Line
(800) 237-5055;
(800) 282-9161 (in FL only)

The Children's Foundation
1420 New York Ave NW
8th Floor
Washington, DC 20005

Diabetes

American Association of
Diabetes Educators
500 N Michigan Ave
Suite 1400
Chicago, IL 60611
(312) 661-1700

American Diabetes
Association
505 8th Ave
New York, NY 10018
(212) 947-9707

American Diabetes
Association Camp Directory
ADA National Center
1660 Duke St
Alexandria, VA 22314
(800) 232-3472

Juvenile Diabetes Foundation
International Hotline
432 Park Ave S
New York, NY 10016
(800) 223-1138;
(212) 889-7575 (in NY only)

National Diabetes Information
Clearinghouse
Box NDIC
Bethesda, MD 20205

The Juvenile Diabetes
Foundation
23 E 26th St
New York, NY 10010

Disability Services

Clearinghouse on Disability
Information
US Department of Education
Switzer Building
Room 3132
Washington, DC 20202
(202) 731-1241

Independent Living for the Handicapped
1301 Belmont St NW
Washington, DC 20009
(202) 797-9803

Information Center for Individuals with Disabilities
Fort Point Place
1st floor
27-43 Wormwood St
Boston, MA 02210-1606
(617) 727-5540

Library of Congress National Library Service for the Blind and Physically Handicapped
1291 Taylor St NW
Washington, DC 20542
(202) 707-5100 or
(800) 424-9100
(202) 707-0744 (TDD)

Mainstream Inc
1030 15th St NW
Suite 1010
Washington, DC 20005
(202) 898-0202

National Council on Disability
800 Independence Ave SW
Suite 808
Washington, DC 20591
(202) 267-3846
TDD: (202) 267-3232

National Easter Seal Society
70 E Lake St
Chicago, IL 60601
(800) 221-6827

National Foundation March of Dimes
1275 Mamaroneck Ave
White Plains, NY 10605
(914) 428-7100

National Rehabilitation Information Center
8455 Colesville Rd
Suite 935
Silver Springs, MD 20910-3319
(800) 346-2742 or
(301) 588-9284

President's Committee on Employment of the Handicapped
111 20th St NW
Room 636
Washington, DC 20036
(202) 653-5044

Down Syndrome

National Association for Down's Syndrome
PO Box 63
Oak Park, IL 60303

National Down Syndrome Society Hotline
(800) 221-4602;
(212) 764-3070 (in NY only)

Educational Resources

ABLEDATA
Adaptive Equipment Center
Newington Children's Hospital
181 E Cedar St
Newington, CT 06111
(203) 667-5405 or
(800) 344-5405

American Pain Society
5700 Old Orchard Rd
1st Floor
Skokie, IL 60077
(708) 966-5595

CancerFax
NCI International Cancer
Information Service
9030 Old Georgetown Rd
Building 82
Room 219
Bethesda, MD 20892
(301) 402-5874 (on fax machine
handset);
(301) 496-8880 (for technical
assistance)

Elder Abuse Agencies and Resource Groups*

Bureau of Maine's Elderly
Station 11
State House
Augusta, ME 04333
(207) 289-2561
NOTE: (Maine has a mandatory
reporting law for elder abuse)

Center on Aging
University of Massachusetts
Medical Center
55 Lake Ave N
Worcester, MA 01605

**Consortium for Elder Abuse
Prevention**
Mt Zion Hospital and Medical
Center
PO Box 7921
San Francisco, CA 94102
(415) 885-7850

Court Investigation Unit
City Hall
Room 416
San Francisco, CA 94102

*From Ebersole P, Hess P: *Toward
healthy aging: human needs and nursing
response,* ed 3, St Louis, 1990, Mosby.

Institute of Gerontology
Wayne State University
205 Library Ct
Detroit, MI 48202
(313) 577-2297

Harborview Medical Center
Social Work Department
325 9th Ave
Seattle, WA 98104
(206) 223-3331

Elderly—Care Organizations

**American College of Nursing
Home Administrators**
4650 East-West Highway
Washington, DC 20014

**Council of Nursing Home
Nurses**
American Nurses' Association
2420 Pershing Rd
Kansas City, MO 64108

Eldercare Locator
(800) 677-1116

**National Association for Home
Care**
519 C St NE
Washington, DC 20002
(202) 547-7424

**National Association of Adult
Day Care**
180 E 4050 S
Murray, UT 84107
(801) 262-9167 or
(801) 359-3077

**National Association of Home
Health Agencies**
426 C St NE
Suite 200
Washington, DC 20002
(202) 547-1717

**National Citizen's Coalition
for Nursing Home Reform**
1424 16th St NW
Suite 204
Washington, DC 20036
(202) 797-8227

National HomeCaring Council
235 Park Ave S
New York, NY 10003

**National Hospice
Organization**
1910 N Fort Meyer Dr
Suite 307
Arlington, VA 22209
(703) 243-5900

**National Institute on Adult
Day Care**
National Council on the Aging
600 Maryland Ave SW
Washington, DC 20024
(202) 479-1200

Elderly—General

Administration on Aging
330 Independence Ave SW
Washington, DC 20201
(202) 245-0724

**American Association for
Geriatric Psychiatry**
PO Box 376A
Greenbelt, MD 20770
(301) 220-0952

**American Association of
Retired Persons**
1909 K St NW
Washington, DC 20049
(202) 872-4700

American Geriatrics Society
770 Lexington Ave
Suite 400
New York, NY 10021
(212) 308-1414

**American Psychological
Association**
Division of Adult Development
and Aging
1200 17th St NW
Washington, DC 20036

**American Public Health
Association**
Section of Gerontological
Health
1015 15th St NW
Washington, DC 20005
(202) 789-5600

**American Society for
Geriatric Dentistry**
211 E Chicago Ave
Chicago, IL 60611
(312) 353-6547 or
(312) 664-8270

American Society on Aging
833 Market St
Suite 512
San Francisco, CA 94103
(415) 543-2617

**Association for Gerontology in
Higher Education**
600 Maryland Ave SW
West Wing 204
Washington, DC 20024
(202) 484-7505

**The Association for
Humanistic Gerontology**
1711 Solano Ave
Berkeley, CA 94707

**Gerontological Society of
America**
1411 K St NW
Suite 300
Washington, DC 20005
(202) 393-1411

The Institute of Retired Professionals
The New School of Social Research
60 W 12th St
New York, NY 10011

The International Federation on Aging
1909 K St NW
Washington, DC 20006

International Senior Citizens Association, Inc
11753 Wilshire Blvd
Los Angeles, CA 90025

National Association for Spanish Speaking Elderly
2025 I St NW
Suite 219
Washington, DC 20006
(202) 293-9329

National Caucus of the Black Aged
1424 K St NW
Suite 500
Washington, DC 20005

National Council of Senior Citizens
925 15th St NW
Washington, DC 20005

National Council on Aging
600 Maryland Ave SW
West Wing 100
Washington, DC 20024
(202) 479-1200

National Geriatrics Society
212 W Wisconsin Ave
3rd Floor
Milwaukee, WI 53203
(414) 272-4130

National Gerontological Nursing Association
1818 Newton St NW
Washington, DC 20010

National Indian Council on Aging
PO Box 2088
Albuquerque, NM 87103

National Institute of Mental Health
Mental Disorders of the Aging
Research Branch, DCR
5600 Fishers Ln
Room 11C-03
Rockville, MD 20857
(301) 443-1185

National Institute on Aging
National Institutes of Health
9000 Rockville Pike
Building 31
Room 5C27
Bethesda, MD 20105
(301) 496-1752

National Senior Citizens Law Center
1302 18th St NW
Suite 701
Washington, DC 20036

Older Womens' League (OWL)
National Office
1325 G St NW
Lower Level-B
Washington, DC 20005

Elderly—Services

American Association of Homes for the Aging
1129 20th St NW
Suite 400
Washington, DC 20036
(202) 296-5960

Design for Aging
American Institute of Architects
1735 New York Ave NW
Washington, DC 20006

Gray Panthers
311 S Juniper St
Suite 601
Philadelphia, PA 19107
(215) 545-6555

National Association of Meal Programs
204 E St NE
Washington, DC 20002
(202) 547-6157

National Institute on Aging
National Institutes of Health
31 Center Dr MSC 2292
Building 31
Room SC27
Bethesda, MD 20892-2292
(301) 496-1752;
(800) 222-2225 (publications);
(800) 438-4380 (Alzheimer's)

Epilepsy

American Epilepsy Society
38238 Glenn Ave
Willoughby, OH 44094

Epilepsy Foundation of America
4351 Garden City Dr
Suite 500
Landover, MD 20785
(301) 459-3700
or (800) 332-1000

Epilepsy Information Line
(206) 323-8174

Family Planning/Pregnancy

Abortion Information Service
(800) 321-0575;
(800) 362-1205 (in OH only)

American Fertility Society
1608 13th Ave
Suite 101
Birmingham, AL 35205

American Genetic Association
818 18th St NW
Washington, DC 20006

Bethany Lifeline
(800) 238-4269

The Edna Gladney Home
(800) 433-2922;
(817) 772-2740 (in TX only)

International Childbirth Education Association, Inc
8635 Fremont Ave S
Minneapolis, MN 55420

La Leche League International, Inc
9616 Minneapolis Ave
Franklin Park, IL 60131

Maternity Center Association
48 E 92nd St
New York, NY 10028

National Abortion Federation
(800) 772-9100 (hotline);
(202) 546-9060 (in DC area only)

National Clearinghouse for Family Planning Information
PO Box 2225
Rockville, MD 20852
(301) 251-5153

National Maternal and Child Health Clearinghouse
3520 Prospect St NW
Suite 1
Washington, DC 20057
(202) 625-8410

National Pregnancy Hotline
(800) 344-7211 or
(800) 831-5881

Planned Parenthood Federation of America, Inc
810 7th Ave
New York, NY 10019

Pregnancy Crisis Center
(800) 492-5530 (pregnancy
crisis hotline)

Southwest Maternity Center
(800) 255-9612;
(800) 292-7021 (in TX only)
(512) 696-7021 (in TX for
adoption information)

Food (See also Nutrition.)

**Food and Drug
Administration**
Office of Consumer Affairs
5600 Fishers Ln
Rockville, MD 20857
(301) 443-3170

**Food and Nutrition
Information Center**
National Agricultural
Library Building
Room 304
Beltsville, MD 20705
(301) 344-3719

Gastrointestinal Disorders

**International Association for
Enterostomal Therapy, Inc**
2081 Business Circle Dr
Suite 290
Irvine, CA 92715

**National Digestive Diseases
Education and Information
Clearinghouse**
1555 Wilson Blvd
Suite 600
Rosslyn, VA 22209
(301) 496-9707

**National Foundation for Ileitis
and Colitis**
444 Park Ave S
New York, NY 10016
(212) 685-3440

United Ostomy Association
36 Executive Park
Suite 120
Irvine, CA 92714
(714) 660-8624

General Public Information

**Consumer Information Center
US General Services
Administration**
Consumer Information
Center-2D
PO Box 100
Pueblo, CO 81002

**Food and Drug
Administration**
Office of Consumer Affairs
HFE-88
5600 Fishers Ln
Rockville, MD 20857
(301) 443-3170

**US Department of Health and
Human Services Public Health
Service**
Agency for Health Care Policy
and Research
2101 E Jefferson St
Suite 501
Rockville, MD 20852
(800) 952-7664

**US Department of Labor
Occupational Safety and
Health Administration
(OSHA)**
Directorate of Technical
Support
200 Constitution Ave NW
Washington, DC 20210
(202) 523-7047

Handicaps

**Architectural and
Transportation Barriers
Compliance Board**
330 C St SW
Room 1010
Washington, DC 20202

**Association for Children with
Learning Disabilities**
4156 Library Rd
Pittsburgh, PA 15234

**Association for Children with
Retarded Mental
Development, Inc**
902 Broadway
5th Floor
New York, NY 10010

Boy Scouts of America
Scouting for the Handicapped
Division
New Brunswick, NJ 08902

**Clearinghouse on Disability
Information**
Department of Education
330 C St SW
Room 3132
Washington, DC 20202-2524
(202) 732-1723

**Council of World
Organizations Interested in
the Handicapped**
432 Park Ave S
New York, NY 10016

**Directory of National
Information Sources on
Handicapping Conditions and
Related Services**
c/o Office of Handicapped
Individuals
Hubert H Humphrey Building
Washington, DC 20201

**Directory of Organizations
Interested in the Handicapped**
c/o People-to-People Programs
Connecticut Ave and L St
LaSalle Building
Suite 610
Washington, DC 20036

**Disability Rights
Center—Center for Law and
Social Policy**
1616 P St NW
Suite 435
Washington, DC 20036

**Farmers (services and devices
for handicapped farmers)**
FARM (Easter Seal Society of
Iowa, Inc)
PO Box 4002
Des Moines, IA 50333

**Income tax services for people
with disability Federal
Internal Revenue Service**
(for TDD users)
(800) 428-4732;
(800) 382-4059 (in IN only)

**Independent Living for the
Handicapped**
Department of Housing and
Urban Development
HUD Building
Washington, DC 20410
(202) 755-5720

**Information Center for
Individuals with Disabilities**
20 Park Plaza
Room 330
Boston, MA 02116
(617) 727-5540

**Library of Congress National
Library Services for the Blind
and Physically Handicapped**
(800) 424-8567;
(202) 287-5100 (in DC area
only)

National Amputation Foundation
12-45 150th St
Whitestone, NY 11357
(718) 767-0596

National Association of Councils of Stutterers
Catholic University
Speech and Hearing Center
O'Boyle Hall
Room 100
Washington, DC 20064

National Association of Retarded Citizens
2709 Ave E East
Arlington, TX 76011

National Association of the Physically Handicapped, Inc
76 Elm St
London, OH 43140

National Congress of Organizations of the Physically Handicapped
16630 Beverly
Tinley Park, IL 60477

National Easter Seal Society
2023 W Ogden Ave
Chicago, IL 60612

National Foundation March of Dimes
1275 Mamaroneck Ave
White Plains, NY 10605
(914) 428-7100

National Head Injury Foundation
333 Turnpike Rd
Southborough, MA 01772
(617) 431-7032

National Information Center for Handicapped Children and Youth
PO Box 1492
Washington, DC 20013

National Society for Autistic Children
1234 Massachusetts Ave NW
Suite 1017
Washington, DC 20005

Stroke Club International
805 12th St
Galveston, TX 77550
(409) 762-1022

United Cerebral Palsy Association, Inc
66 E 34th St
New York, NY 10016
(212) 481-6300

Health

The Aerobics and Fitness Foundation
(800) 233-4886

American Association for Vital Records and Public Health Statistics
c/o Utah Dept of Health
PO Box 2500
Salt Lake City, UT 84110

American Health Care Association
1200 15th St NW
Washington, DC 20005
(202) 833-2050

American Health Foundation
320 E 43rd St
New York, NY 10018

American Holistic Nurses' Association
205 St Luis St
#506
Springfield, MO 65806-1317

American Hospital Association Center for Health Promotion
840 N Lake Shore Dr
Chicago, IL 60611
(312) 280-6000

American Medical Radio News
(800) 621-8094

American Nurse's Association
600 Maryland Ave SW
Washington, DC 20024-2571
(202) 651-7000

American Physical Fitness Research Institute
824 Moraga Dr
Los Angeles, CA 90049

American Public Health Association
1015 15th St NW
Washington, DC 20005
(202) 789-5600

Center for Health Promotion and Education Centers for Disease Control
1600 Clifton Rd NE,
Building 1 South
Room SSB249
Atlanta, GA 30333
(404) 329-3492
(404) 329-3698

Center for Public Representation
121 S Pinckney St
Madison, WI 53703
(800) 369-0388

Clearinghouse on Health Indexes
National Center for
Health Statistics,
Division of Epidemiology and
Health Promotion
3700 East-West Highway
Room 2-27
Hyattsville, MD 20782
(301) 436-7035

Health and Education Resources
4733 Bethesda Ave
Suite 735
Bethesda, MD 20014

Health Sciences Communications Association
2343 N 115th St
Wauwatosa, WI 53226

Healthright, Inc
41 Union Square
Room 206-8
New York, NY 10003

Healthy America, National Coalition for Health Promotion and Disease Prevention
1015 15th St NW
Suite 424
Washington, DC 20005

International Council on Health, Physical Education and Recreation
1201 16th St NW
Room 417
Washington, DC 20036

National Council on Health Care Services
1200 15th St NW
Suite 601
Washington, DC 20005

National Health Council, Inc
1740 Broadway
New York, NY 10019

National Health Federation
PO Box 688
Monrovia, CA 91016

National Health Information Clearinghouse
PO Box 1133
Washington, DC 20013-1133
(800) 336-4797;
(703) 522-2590 (in VA only)

National Indian Health Board, Inc
1602 S Parker Rd
Suite 200
Denver, CO 80231

National Institutes of Health
9000 Rockville Pike
Bethesda, MD 20814
(301) 496-4000

National League of Nursing
350 Hudson St
New York, NY 10014
(212) 989-9393
(800) 669-9656

**National Wellness Association/
National Wellness Institute**
University of Wisconsin-
Stevens Point Foundation
South Hall
Stevens Point, WI 54481
(715) 346-2172

**US Department of Health and
Human Services**
Office of Disease Prevention
and Health Promotion
Washington, DC 20201
(202) 245-7611

Health—Dental

American Dental Association
211 E Chicago Ave
Chicago, IL 60611

Health—Eyes

**American Optometric
Association**
243 N Lindbergh Blvd
St Louis, MO 63141
(314) 991-4100

Health—Mental

**American Art Therapy
Association**
PO Box 11604
Pittsburgh, PA 15228

**American Mental Health
Foundation, Inc**
2 E 86th St
New York, NY 10028

**American Psychiatric
Association**
1400 K St NW
Washington, DC 20005
(202) 682-6000

**American Psychological
Association**
1200 17th St NW
Washington, DC 20036
(202) 955-7600

**Mental Health Association,
National Headquarters**
1800 N Kent St
Arlington, VA 22209

**National Clearinghouse for
Mental Health Information**
National Institute of Mental
Health
5600 Fishers Ln
Room 11A33
Rockville, MD 20857
(301) 443-4517

Hearing and Speech

**Alexander Graham Bell
Association for the Deaf**
3417 Volta Pl NW
Washington, DC 20007
(202) 337-5220

**American Deafness and
Rehabilitation Association**
Box 55369
Little, Rock, AR 55369

**American Speech, Language,
and Hearing Association**
10801 Rockville Pike
Rockville, MD 20852
(301) 897-5700

AT&T Communications
Reston, VA
(800) 222-4474;
(800) 833-3232 (TDD);
(800) 233-1222 (voice only)

Better Hearing Institute
Box 1840
Washington, DC 20013
(703) 642-0580 or
(800) 424-8576

National Association for Hearing and Speech Action Line
(800) 638-8255;
(301) 897-8682 (in HI, AK, and MD only)

National Center for Stuttering
(800) 221-2483;
(212) 532-1460 (NY only)

National Hearing Aid Helpline
(800) 521-5247;
(313) 478-2610 (in MI only)

National Hearing Aid Society
20361 Middlebelt Rd
Livonia, MI 48152

Self-Help for Hard of Hearing People
7910 Woodmont Ave
Suite 200
Bethesda, MD 20814
(301) 657-2248;
(301) 657-2249 (TTY)

Telecommunications for the Deaf
814 Thayer Ave
Silver Springs, MD 20785
(301) 589-3006

Heart

American Heart Association
7320 Greenville Ave
Dallas, TX 75231
(214) 373-6300

Amyotrophic Lateral Sclerosis Association
15300 Ventura Blvd
Suite 315
Sherman Oaks, CA 91403
(818) 990-2151

Association of Heart Patients
(800) 241-6993;
(800) 282-3119 (in GA only)

Council on Arteriosclerosis of the American Heart Association
7320 Greenville Ave
Dallas, TX 75231

Mended Hearts, Inc
7320 Greenville Ave
Dallas, TX 75231
(214) 706-1442

Hospital Care

Association for the Care of Children in Hospitals
3615 Wisconsin Ave NW
Washington, DC 20016

Hill-Burton Hospital Free Care
(800) 638-0742;
(800) 492-0359 (in MD only)

Huntington's Disease

Huntington's Disease Society of America, Inc
140 W 22nd St
New York, NY 10011-2420
(212) 242-1968

Hypertension

High Blood Pressure Information Center
National Institutes of Health
Bethesda, MD 20205
(301) 496-1809

Incontinence

Continence Restored, Inc.
407 Strawberry Hill
Stamford, CT 06905
(212) 879-3131 (day);
(203) 348-0601 (evening)

Help for Incontinent People (HIP)
PO Box 544
Union, SC 29379

The Simon Foundation for Continence
PO Box 815
Wilmette, IL 60091
(800) 23-SIMON

Kidney Disease

American Kidney Fund
(800) 638-8299;
(800) 492-8361 (in DC only)

National Kidney Foundation
2 Park Ave
Room 908
New York, NY 10016

Lung

American Lung Association
1740 Broadway
New York, NY 10019
(212) 315-8700

National Asthma Center
National Jewish Hospital and
Research Center
(800) 222-5864;
(303) 398-1477 (in CO only)

National Jewish Center for Immunology and Respiratory Medicine
1400 Jackson St
Denver, CO 80206
(303) 388-4461

Medicare/Medicaid

DHHS Inspector General's Hotline
(800) 368-5779;
(301) 597-0724 (in MD only)

Multiple Sclerosis

National Multiple Sclerosis Society
205 E 42nd St
New York, NY 10017
(212) 986-3240

Muscular Dystrophy

Muscular Dystrophy Association, Inc
810 7th Ave
New York, NY 10019
(212) 586-0808

Myasthenia Gravis

Myasthenia Gravis Foundation, Inc
53 W Jackson Blvd
Suite 909
Chicago, IL 60604

Nutrition (See also Food)

American Dietetic Association (ADA)
Journal of the American
Dietetic Association
430 N Michigan Ave
Chicago, IL 60611
(312) 899-0046;
(800) 366-1655 (toll-free hotline)

Center for Adolescent Obesity
Balboa Publishing Corporation
101 Larkspur Landing
Larkspur, CA 94939
(415) 461-8884

Consumer Information Center
Pueblo, CO 81009
(303) 544-5277, ext 370

Human Nutrition Center SEA
Room 421A
US Department of Agriculture
Washington, DC 20250
(202) 447-7854

National Dairy Council
Rosemont, IL 60018-4233

Office of Consumer Communications (HFG-10)
Food and Drug Administration
5600 Fishers Ln
Room 15B32
Parklawn Building
Rockville, MD 20857

Osteoporosis

National Osteoporosis Foundation
1150 17th St NW, Suite 500
Washington, DC 20036
(202) 223-2226
(202) 223-2237 (fax)

Organ Donors

Organ Donor Hotline
(800) 24-DONOR

The Living Bank International
PO Box 6725
Houston, TX 77265
(800) 528-2971;
(713) 528-2971 (in TX only)

Pain

National Committee on Treatment of Intractable Pain
PO Box 9553
Friendship Station
Washington, DC 20016-1553
(202) 944-8140

Parkinson's Disease

American Parkinson Disease Association
116 John St
Suite 417
New York, NY 10038
(212) 732-9550

National Parkinson Foundation
(800) 327-4545;
(800) 433-7022 (in FL only);
(305) 547-6666 (in Miami area only)

Parkinson's Disease Foundation
Columbia University Medical Center
William Black Medical Research Building
650 W 168th St
New York, NY 10032
(212) 923-4700

Personal Care Resources

About Faces Permanent Cosmetics
1001 Bridgeway Blvd
Suite 432
Sausalito, CA 94965
(415)331-0663

Airway
3960 Rosslyn Dr
Cincinnati, OH 45209
(800) 888-0458

Alkin Hair Company
254 W 40th St
New York, NY 10018
(212) 719-3070

Caring Touch Division International Hairgoods, Inc
(distributes cranial hair prostheses)
6811 Flying Cloud Dr
Eden Prairie, MN 55344
(800) 424-7567

Department of Health and Human Services
Public Health Service,
Agency for Health Care Policy and Research
Executive Office Center
2101 E Jefferson St
Suite 501
Rockville, MD 20852
(800) 952-7664

Designs for Comfort, Inc (a combination cap and hair piece called the *Headliner* as an alternative to wigs)
PO Box 8229
Northfield, IL 60093
(800) 443-9226

Fair's OPS, Inc (ostomy prosthesis)
PO Box 5760
Greenway Station
Glendale, AZ 85306
(602) 978-4435

Holly Cosmetics/Medical Image Products (corrective cosmetics)
4947 Brownsboro Rd
Louisville, KY 40220
(800) 222-3964

Intimacies by Alice (for women who have had breast surgery)
3 Hudson Watch Dr
Ossining, NY 10562
(914) 923-2010

Jodee (mastectomy products)
5085 W Park Rd
Hollywood, FL 33021
(800) 821-2767 or
(305) 987-7274

Mary Catherine's (A boutique for women who have had breast surgery)
1914 NE 42nd Ave
Portland, OR 97213
(800) 843-3215

National Cancer Institute
Bethesda, MD 20205
(301) 496-7403

Nearly Me (breast prostheses, mastectomy swimwear, and accesories)
316 W Florence Ave
Inglewood, CA 90301
(310) 330-7500 (Los Angeles);
(800) 421-2322

Office of Cancer Communications
NCI Building 31
Room 10A16
Bethesda, MD 20892
(301) 496-5583

University of Texas MD Anderson Cancer Center
ATTN: Patient Education Clearinghouse
Patient Education Office
1515 Holcombe
Box 21
Houston, TX 77030
(713) 792-7128

Worldwide Home Health Center, Inc. (a distributor for health care products and services)
926 E Tallmadge Ave
Akron, OH 44310
(800) 223-5938 (in OH);
(800) 621-5938
(800) 223-5938

Poison/Toxic Substances

National Pesticide Information Clearinghouse
(800) 858-7378

Poison Control Branch
Food and Drug Administration
5600 Fishers Ln
Parklawn Building
Room 15B-23
Rockville, MD 20857
(301) 443-6260

Toxic Substances Control Act Hotline
(800) 424-9065;
(202) 554-1404 (in DC area only)

Pregnancy (See Family Planning/Pregnancy.)

Product Safety

Consumer Product Safety Commission
Washington, DC 20207
(800) 638-CPSC;
(800) 638-8270 (TDD);
(800) 492-8104 (TDD in MD only)

Professional Organizations and Resources—Cancer

American Association of Cancer Education
Educational Research and Development
University of Alabama at Birmingham
401 CHSD University St
Birmingham, AL 35294

American Pain Society
5700 Old Orchard Rd
1st Floor
Skokie, IL 60077
(708) 966-5595

American Society of Clinical Oncology
435 N Michigan Ave
Suite 1717
Chicago, IL 60611
(312) 644-0828

Association of Community Cancer Centers
11600 Nebel St
Suite 201
Rockville, MD 20852
(301) 984-9496

Association of Pediatric Oncology Nurses
6728 Old McLean Village Dr
McLean, VA 22101
(703) 556-9222

International Society of Nurses in Cancer Care
Adelphi University School of Nursing
Box 516
Garden City, NY 11530
(516) 663-1001

Intravenous Nurses Society
2 Brighton St
Belmont, MA 02178
(617) 489-5205

Oncology Nursing Society
1016 Greentree Rd
Pittsburgh, PA 15220-3125
(412) 912-7373

Rape

National Center for the Prevention and Control of Rape
5600 Fishers Ln
Parklawn Building
Room 6C-12
Rockville, MD 20857

Rehabilitation

National Rehabilitation Information Center
Catholic University of America
4407 8th St NE
Washington, DC 20017-2299
(202) 635-5826;
(202) 635-5884 (TDD)

Rehabilitation International
22 E 21st St
New York, NY 10010
(212) 420-1500

**Rehabilitation Services
Administration**
Department of Education,
Office of Special Education and
Rehabilitative Services
330 C St SW
Room 3431
Washington, DC 20202
(202) 723-1282

**Society for the Rehabilitation
of the Facially Disfigured**
550 1st Ave
New York, NY 10016
(212) 340-5400

Safety

**Clearinghouse for
Occupational Safety and
Health Information**
Technical Information Branch
4676 Columbia Pkw
Cincinnati, OH 45226

HUD User (Housing)
PO Box 280
Germantown, MD 20874
(301) 251-5154

**Medic Alert Foundation
International**
PO Box 1009
Turlock, CA 95380

**National Highway Traffic
Safety Administration**
NTS-11, US Department of
Transportation
400 7th St SW
Washington, DC 20590
(202) 426-9294;
(800) 424-9393 (auto hotline);
(202) 426-0123 (in DC area
only)

**National Injury Information
Clearinghouse**
5401 Westbard Ave
Room 625
Washington, DC 20207
(301) 492-6424

**United States Coast Guard,
2nd District**
(800) 325-7376;
(800) 392-7780 (in MO only)

Sexually Transmitted Diseases

**American Venereal Disease
Association**
Box 385
University of Virginia Hospital
Charlottesville, VA 22908

**Sex Information and
Education Council of the US**
32 Washington Pl
New York, NY 10003
(212) 673-3850

Sexually Transmitted Diseases
(800) 227-8922

Smoking

Office on Smoking and Health
Technical Information Center
5600 Fishers Ln
Park Building
Room 1-16
Rockville, MD 20857
(301) 443-1690

Spinal Cord

**National Spinal Cord Injury
Association**
545 Concord Ave
Suite 29
Cambridge, MA 02138
(800) 962-9629 or
(617) 441-8500

National Spinal Cord Injury Foundation
369 Elliot St
Newton Upper Falls, MA 02169

National Spinal Cord Injury Hotline
(800) 526-3456;
(800) 688-1733 (in MD)

Paralyzed Veterans of America
7315 Wisconsin Ave
Suite 301-W
Washington, DC 20014

Paraplegia News
5201 N 19th Ave
Suite 108
Phoenix, AZ 85015

Spina Bifida

Spina Bifida Information and Referral
(800) 621-3141;
(312) 663-1562 (in IL only)

Surgery

National Second Surgical Opinion Program Hotline
(800) 638-6833;
(800) 492-6603 (in MD only)

Community Resources—Canada

AboutFace
99 Crowns Ln
3rd Floor
Toronto, ON M5R 3P4
(416) 944-3223;
(416) 944-2488 (fax)

Aboriginal Nurses Association of Canada
55 Murray St
3rd Floor
Ottawa, ON K1N 5M3
(613) 241-1864;
(613) 241-1542 (fax)

Acoustic Neuroma Association of Canada
PO Box 369
Edmonton, AB T5J 2J6
(800) 261-2622 or
(403) 428-3384

Active Living Canada
1600 James Naismith Dr
Suite 601
Gloucester, ON K1B 5N4
(613) 748-5743;
(613) 748-5734 (fax)

Advanced Coronary Treatment Foundation of Canada (ACT)
379 Holland Ave
Suite 2
Ottawa, ON K1Y 0Y9
(613) 729-3455;
(613) 729-5837 (fax)

From Directory of national organizations and associations involved in health promotion: *Health promotion in Canada,* Summer 1995, Health Canada, Ottawa, Ontario.

Al-Anon Family Groups (Canada)
376 Churchill Ave
Room 106
Ottawa, ON K1Z 5C3
(613) 722-1830;
(613) 761-7768 (fax)

Alcoholics Anonymous
234 Eglinton Ave E
Suite 202
Toronto, ON M4P 1K5
(416) 487-5591
(416) 487-5855 (fax)

Allergy/Asthma Information Association
30 Eglinton Ave W
Suite 750
Mississauga, ON L5R 3E7
(905) 712-2242
(905) 712-2245 (fax)

Allergy Foundation of Canada
PO Box 1904
Saskatoon, SK S7K 3S5
(306) 373-7591

Alliance for Children in Television
344 Dupont St
Suite 205
Toronto, ON M5R 1V9
(416) 515-0466;
(416) 515-0467 (fax)

Alzheimer Society of Canada
1320 Yonge St
Suite 201
Toronto, ON M4T 1X2
(416) 925-3552;
(416) 925-1649 (fax)

Amyotrophic Lateral Sclerosis Society of Canada
6 Adelaide St E
Suite 220
Toronto, ON M5C 1H6
(416) 362-0269;
(416) 362-0414 (fax)

Aplastic Anaemia Family Association of Canada
22 Aikenhead Rd
Etobicoke, ON M9R 2Z3
(416) 235-0468;
(416) 864-9929 (fax)

Arthritis Society
250 Bloor St E
Suite 901
Toronto, ON M4W 3P2
(416) 967-1414;
(416) 967-7171 (fax)

Arthritis Society
920 Yonge St
Suite 420
Toronto, Canada M4W 3J7

Asthma Society of Canada
130 Bridgeland Ave
North York, ON M6A 1Z4
(416) 787-4050;
(416) 787-5807 (fax)

Atlantic Health Promotion Research Centre
Dalhousie University
5200 Dentistry Building
5981 University Ave
Halifax, NS B3H 3J5
(902) 494-2240;
(902) 494-3594 (fax)

Autism Society Canada
129 Yorkville Ave
Unit 202
Toronto, ON M5R 1C4
(416) 922-0302;
(416) 922-1032 (fax)

Back Association of Canada
83 Cottingham St
Toronto, ON M4V 1B9
(416) 967-4670;
(416) 967-0945 (fax)

Big Brothers of Canada
5230 S Service Rd
Burlington, ON L7L 5K2
(800) 263-9133 or
(905) 639-0461;
(905) 639-0124 (fax)

Big Sisters of Canada
270 Yorkland Blvd
Suite 101
North York, ON M2J 5C9
(416) 490-0249;
(416) 490-0920 (fax)

Boys and Girls Clubs of Canada
7030 Woodbine Ave
Suite 703
Markham, ON L3R 6G2
(905) 477-7272;
(905) 477-2056 (fax)

British Columbia Consortium for Health Promotion Research
University of British Columbia,
Institute of Health Promotion Research
Library Processing Centre
2206 East Mall 3rd Floor
Vancouver, BC V6T 1Z3
(604) 822-2258;
(604) 822-9588 (fax)

Bulimia Anorexia Nervosa Association
3640 Wells Ave
Windsor, ON N9C 1T9
(519) 253-7545;
(519) 253-7421 (hotline);
(519) 258-0488 (fax)

Canada Safety Council
1020 Thomas Spratt Pl
Ottawa, ON K1G 5L5
(613) 739-1535;
(613) 739-1566 (fax)

Canadian Academy of Sport Medicine
1600 James Naismith Dr
Suite 502
Gloucester, ON K1B 5N4
(613) 748-5671;
(613) 748-5729 (fax)

Canadian AIDS Hotline/AIDS Clearinghouse
(613)725-3769 (Ottawa)
(416)392-AIDS (Toronto)

Canadian AIDS Society
100 Sparks St
Suite 400
Ottawa, ON K1P 5B7
(613) 230-3580;
(613) 563-4998 (fax)

Canadian Apheresis Study Group
435 St Laurent Blvd
Suite 206
Ottawa, ON K1K 2Z8
(613) 748-9613;
(613) 748-6392 (fax)

Canadian Art Therapy Association
216 St Clair Ave W
Toronto, ON M4V 1R2
(416) 924-6221;
(416) 924-0156 (fax)

Canadian Association for Children of Alcoholics
164 Eglinton Ave E
Suite 304
Toronto, ON M4P 1G4
(416) 813-5629;
(416) 813-5619 (fax)

Canadian Association for Community Living
Kinsmen Building
4700 Keele St
Downsview, ON M3J 1P3
(416) 661-9611;
(416) 661-5701 (fax)

Canadian Association for Health, Physical Education and Recreation
1600 James Naismith Dr
Suite 809
Gloucester, ON K1B 5N4
(613) 748-5622
(613) 748-5737 (fax)

Canadian Association for School Health
2835 Country Woods Dr
Surrey, BC V4A 9P9
(604) 535-7664
(604) 531-6454 (fax)

Canadian Association for Treatment and Study of the Family
University of Western Ontario
Department of Social Work
King's College
266 Epworth Ave
London, ON N6A 2M3
(519) 433-3491 (ext. 339);
(519) 433-2227 (fax)

Canadian Association of Friedreich's Ataxia
5620 CA Jobin St
Saint-Leonard, PQ H1P 1H8
(514) 321-8684;
(514) 321-9257 (fax)

Canadian Association on Gerontology
1306 Wellington St
Suite 500
Ottawa, ON K1Y 3B2
(613) 728-9347
(613) 728-8913 (fax)

Canadian Association of Health-Care Auxiliaries
17 York St
Suite 100
Ottawa, ON K1N 9J6
(613) 241-8005 (ext. 209);
(613) 241-5055 (fax)

Canadian Association of Occupational Therapists
110 Eglinton Ave W
3rd Floor
Toronto, ON M4R 1A3
(416) 487-5404;
(416) 487-0480 (fax)

Canadian Association of Optometrists
1785 Alta Vista Dr
Suite 301
Ottawa, ON K1G 3Y6
(613) 738-4412
(613) 738-7161 (fax)

Canadian Association of Practical Nurses and Nursing Assistants
10604 170th St
Edmonton, AB T5S 1P3
(403) 484-8886
(403) 484-9069 (fax)

Canadian Association of Schools of Social Work
30 Rosemount Ave
Suite 100B
Ottawa, ON K1Y 1P4
(613) 722-2974;
(613) 722-5661 (fax)

Canadian Association of Social Workers
383 Parkdale Ave
Suite 402
Ottawa, ON K1Y 4R4
(613) 729-6668
(613) 729-9608 (fax)

Canadian Association of Speech-Language Pathologists and Audiologists
130 Albert St
Suite 2006
Ottawa, ON K1P 5G4
(613) 567-9968
(613) 567-2859 (fax)

Canadian Association of the Deaf
2435 Holly Ln
Suite 205
Ottawa, ON K1V 7P2
(613) 526-4785;
(613) 526-4785 (TTY/TDD);
(613) 526-4718 (fax)

Canadian Association of Volunteer Bureaux and Centres
2 Dunbloor Rd
Suite 203
Etobicoke, ON M9A 2E4
(416) 236-0588
(416) 236-0590 (fax)

Canadian Bike Helmet Coalition
c/o Canadian Institute of Child Health
885 Meadowlands Dr E
Suite 512
Ottawa, ON K2C 3N2
(613) 224-4144
(613) 224-4145 (fax)

Canadian Breast Cancer Foundation
790 Bay St
Suite 1000
Toronto, ON M5G 1N8
(800) 387-9816 or
(416) 596-6773;
(416) 596-7857 (fax)

Canadian Cancer Society
10 Alcorn Ave
Suite 200
Toronto, ON M4V 3B1
(416) 961-7223;
(416) 961-4189 (fax)

Canadian Cardiovascular Society
360 Victoria Ave
Suite 401
Westmount, PQ H3Z 2N4
(514) 482-3407;
(514) 482-6574 (fax)

Canadian Celiac Association
6519B Mississauga Rd
Mississauga, ON L5N 1A6
(800) 363-7296 or
(905) 567-7195;
(905) 567-0710 (fax)

Canadian Centre for Occupational Health and Safety
250 Main St E
Hamilton, ON L8N 1H6
(800) 668-4284 or
(416) 572-2981;
(905) 527-2206 (fax)

Canadian Centre on Substance Abuse
75 Albert St
Suite 300
Ottawa, ON K1P 5E7
(613) 235-4048;
(613) 235-8101 (fax)

Canadian Child Day Care Federation
120 Holland Ave
Suite 306
Ottawa, ON K1Y 0X6
(613) 729-5289;
(613) 729-3159 (fax)

Canadian Children's Safety Network
20 Queen St W
Suite 200
Toronto, ON M5H 3V7
(416) 979-4012;
(416) 977-3538 (fax)

Canadian Chiropractic Association
1396 Eglinton Ave W
Toronto, ON M6C 2E4
(416) 781-5656,
(416) 781-7344 (fax)

Canadian Coalition for the Prevention of Developmental Disabilities
c/o Canadian Institute of Child Health
885 Meadowlands Dr
Suite 512
Ottawa, ON K2C 3N2
(613) 224-4144;
(613) 224-4145 (fax)

Canadian Coalition on Depo Provera
c/o Winnipeg Women's Health Clinic
419 Graham Ave
3rd Floor
Winnipeg, MB R3C 0M3
(204) 947-1517;
(204) 943-3844 (fax)

Canadian Coalition on Medication Use and Seniors
350 Sparks St
Suite 1005
Ottawa, ON K1R 7S8
(613) 238-7624;
(613) 235-9744 (fax)

Canadian Coalition on Organ Donor Awareness
c/o Pharmaceutical Manufacturers' Association of Canada
1111 Prince of Wales Dr
Suite 302
Ottawa, ON K2C 3T2
(613) 727-1380;
(613) 727-1407 (fax)

Canadian Council for Multicultural Health
1017 Wilson Ave
Suite 400
Downsview, ON M3K 1Z1
(416) 630-8835;
(416) 638-6076 (fax)

Canadian College of Health Service Executives
350 Sparks St
Suite 402
Ottawa, ON K1R 7S8
(613) 235-7218;
(613) 235-5451 (fax)

Canadian Council of the Blind
396 Cooper St
Suite 405
Ottawa, ON K2P 2H7
(613) 567-0311;
(613) 567-2728 (fax)

Canadian Council on Rehabilitation and Work
167 Lombard Ave
Suite 410
Winnipeg, MB R3B 0T6
(204) 942-4862;
(204) 944-0341 (TTY/TDD);
(204) 944-0753 (fax)

Canadian Council on Social Development
441 MacLaren St
4th Floor
Ottawa, ON K2P 2H3
(613) 236-8977;
(613) 236-2750 (fax)

Canadian Council on Smoking and Health
170 Laurier Ave W
Suite 1202
Ottawa, ON K1P 5V5
(613) 567-3050;
(613) 567-2730 (fax)

Canadian Cultural Society of the Deaf Inc.
11337 61st Ave
Suite 144
Edmonton, AB T6H 1M3
(403) 436-2599 (TTY/TDD);
(403) 430-9489 (fax)

Canadian Cystic Fibrosis Foundation
2221 Yonge St
Suite 601
Toronto, ON M4S 2B4
(416) 485-9149;
(416) 485-0960 (fax)

Canadian Deaf-Blind and Rubella Association
747 2nd Ave
Owen Sound, ON N4K 2G9
(519) 372-1333;
(519) 372-1334 (fax)

Canadian Dental Association
1815 Alta Vista Dr
Ottawa, ON K1G 3Y6
(613) 523-1770;
(613) 523-7736 (fax)

Canadian Dental Hygienists Association
96 Centrepointe Dr
Nepean, ON K2G 6B1
(613) 224-5515;
(613) 224-7283 (fax)

Canadian Dermatology Foundation
450 Central Ave
Suite 308
London, ON N6B 2E8
(519) 432-3968

Canadian Diabetes Association
15 Toronto St
Suite 1001
Toronto, ON M5C 2E3
(416) 363-3373;
(416) 363-3393 (fax)

Canadian Dietetic Association
480 University Ave
Suite 601
Toronto, ON M5G 1V2
(416) 596-0857
(416) 596-0603 (fax)

Canadian Down Syndrome Society
12837 76th Ave
Suite 206
Surrey, BC V3W 2V3
(604) 599-6009;
(604) 599-6165 (fax)

Canadian Fire Safety Association
2175 Sheppard Ave E
Suite 310
Willowdale, ON M2J 1W8
(416) 492-9417;
(416) 491-1670 (fax)

Canadian Fitness and Lifestyle Research Institute
185 Somerset St W
Suite 201
Ottawa, ON K2P 0J2
(613) 233-5528;
(613) 233-5536 (fax)

Canadian Foundation for the Study of Infant Deaths
586 Eglinton Ave E
Suite 308
Toronto, ON M4P 1P2
(416) 488-3260;
(416) 488-3864 (fax)

Canadian Group B Strep Association
343 Watson Ave
Windsor, ON N8S 3S3
(519) 948-6324

Canadian Guidance and Counselling Association
220 Laurier Ave W
Suite 600
Ottawa, ON K1P 5Z9
(613) 230-4236;
(613) 230-5884 (fax)

Canadian Hard of Hearing Association
2435 Holly Ln
Suite 205
Ottawa, ON K1V 7P2
(613) 526-1584
(613) 526-2692 (TTY/TDD);
(613) 526-4718 (fax)

Canadian Hearing Society
271 Spadina Rd
Toronto, ON M5R 2V3
(416) 964-9595;
(416) 964-0023 (TTY/TDD);
(416) 964-2066 (fax)

Canadian Hemochromatosis Society
PO Box 94303
Richmond, BC V6Y 2A6

Canadian Hemophilia Society
1450 City Councillors St
Suite 840
Montreal, PQ H3A 2E6
(514) 848-0503;
(514) 848-9661 (fax)

Canadian Holistic Medical Association
491 Eglinton Ave W
Suite 407
Toronto, ON M5N 1A8
(416) 485-3071;
(416) 485-3076 (fax)

Canadian Holistic Nurses Association
c/o 268 Beech St
Apt 26
New Glasgow, NS B2H 1A1
(902) 755-1137;
(902) 928-0297 (fax)

Canadian Home Economics Association
151 Slater St
Suite 901
Ottawa, ON K1P 5H3
(613) 238-8817;
(613) 238-1677 (fax)

Canadian Hospital Association
17 York St
Suite 100
Ottawa, ON K1N 9J6
(613) 241-8005;
(613) 241-5005 (fax)

Canadian Institute for Health Information
377 Dalhousie St
Suite 200
Ottawa, ON K1N 9N8
(613) 241-7860;
(613) 241-8120 (fax)

Canadian Institute of Child Health
885 Meadowlands Dr E
Suite 512
Ottawa, ON K2C 3N2
(613) 224-4144;
(613) 224-4145 (fax)

Canadian Institute of Public Health Inspectors
PO Box 5367
Station F
Ottawa, ON K2C 3J1
(613) 224-7568;
(613) 224-6055 (fax)

Canadian Institute of Stress
1235 Bay St
Suite 500
Toronto, ON M5R 3K4
(416) 961-8575;
(905) 660-2458 (fax)

Canadian Liver Foundation
1320 Yonge St
Suite 301
Toronto, ON M4T 1X2
(416) 964-1953;
(416) 964-0024 (fax)

Canadian Long Term Care Association
17 York St
Suite 301
Ottawa, ON K1N 9J6
(613) 241-7510;
(613) 241-4588 (fax)

Canadian Marfan Association
Central Plaza Postal Outlet
128 Queen St S
PO Box 42257
Mississauga, ON L5M 4Z0
(905) 826-3223;
(905) 826-2125 (fax)

Canadian Medical Association
1867 Alta Vista Dr
Ottawa, ON K1G 3Y6
(613) 731-9331;
(613) 731-9013 (fax)

Canadian Medic Alert Foundation
250 Ferrand Dr
Suite 301
Don Mills, ON M3C 2T9
(800) 668-1507 or
(416) 696-0267;
(416) 696-0156 (fax)

Canadian Mental Health Association
2160 Yonge St
3rd Floor
Toronto, ON M4S 2Z3
(416) 484-7750;
(416) 484-4617 (fax)

Canadian Mothercraft Society
32 Heath St W
Toronto, ON M4V 1T3
(416) 920-3515;
(416) 920-5983 (fax)

Canadian National Institute for the Blind
1929 Bayview Ave
Toronto, ON M4G 3E8
(416) 480-7580;
(416) 480-7677 (fax)

Canadian Nurses Association
50 The Driveway
Ottawa, ON K2P 1E2
(613) 237-2133;
(613) 237-3520 (fax)

Canadian Organization for Advancement of Computers in Health
10458 Mayfield Rd
Suite 216
Edmonton, AB T5P 4P4
(403) 489-4553;
(403) 489-3290 (fax)

Canadian Orthopaedic Association
1440 St Catherine St W
Suite 421
Montreal, PQ H3G 1R8
(514) 874-9003;
(514) 874-0464 (fax)

Canadian Osteogenesis Imperfecta Society
c/o 128 Thornhill Crescent
Chatham, ON N7L 4M3
(519) 436-0025;
(519) 627-0557 (fax)

Canadian Osteopathic Association
575 Waterloo St
London, ON N6B 2R2
(519) 439-5521;
(519) 439-2616 (fax)

Canadian Paediatric Society
c/o Children's Hospital of Eastern Ontario
401 Smyth Rd
Ottawa, ON K1H 8L1
(613) 737-2728;
(613) 737-2794 (fax)

Canadian Paraplegic Association
1101 Prince of Wales Dr
Suite 320
Ottawa, ON K2C 3W7
(613) 723-1033;
(613) 723-1060 (fax)

Canadian Parks/Recreation Association
1600 James Naismith Dr
Suite 306
Gloucester, ON K1B 5N4
(613) 748-5651;
(613) 748-5854 (fax)

Canadian Pelvic Inflammatory Disease (PID) Society
PO Box 33804, Station D
Vancouver, BC V6J 4L6
(604) 684-5704

Canadian Pharmaceutical Association
1785 Alta Vista Dr
Ottawa, ON K1G 3Y6
(613) 523-7877;
(613) 523-0445 (fax)

Canadian Physiotherapy Association
890 Yonge St
9th Floor
Toronto, ON M4W 3P4
(416) 924-5312;
(416) 924-7335 (fax)

Canadian Porphyria Foundation
PO Box 1206
Neepawa, MB R0J 1H0
(204) 476-2800

Canadian Psoriasis Foundation
1306 Wellington St
Suite 500A
Ottawa, ON K1Y 3B2
(800) 265-0926 or
(613) 728-4000;
(613) 728-8913 (fax)

Canadian Psychiatric Association
237 Argyle Ave
Suite 200
Ottawa, ON K2P 1B8
(613) 234-2815;
(613) 234-9857 (fax)

Canadian Psychiatric Research Foundation
60 Bloor St W
Suite 307
Toronto, ON M4W 3B8
(416) 975-9891;
(416) 975-4070 (fax)

Canadian Psychological Association
151 Slater St
Suite 205
Ottawa, ON K1P 5H3
(613) 237-2144;
(613) 237-1674 (fax)

Canadian Public Health Association
1565 Carling Ave
Suite 400
Ottawa, ON K1Z 8R1
(613) 725-3769;
(613) 725-9826 (fax)

Canadian Red Cross Society
1800 Alta Vista Dr
Ottawa, ON K1G 4J5
(613) 739-3000;
(613) 731-1411 (fax)

Canadian Rehabilitation Council for the Disabled
45 Sheppard Ave E
Suite 801
Toronto, ON M2N 5W9
(416) 250-7490;
(416) 229-1371 (fax)

Canadian Rett Syndrome Association
c/o Eugene Bradley
555 Fairway Rd
Suite 301
Kitchener, ON N2C 1X4
(416) 494-1954;
(519) 893-1169 (fax)

Canadian Society for International Health
170 Laurier Ave W
Suite 902
Ottawa, ON K1P 5V5
(613) 230-2654;
(613) 230-8401 (fax)

Canadian Society for Mucopolysaccaride and Related Diseases
3025 12th St NE
Suite 175
Calgary, AB T2E 7J2
(403) 250-8013;
(403) 250-7507 (fax)

Canadian Society for the Prevention of Cruelty to Children
PO Box 700
356 1st St
Midland, ON L4R 4P4
(705) 526-5647;
(705) 526-0214 (fax)

Canadian Society of Safety Engineering
330 Bay St
Suite 602
Toronto, ON M5H 2S8
(416) 368-2230;
(416) 368-8429 (fax)

Canadians for Health Research
PO Box 126
Westmount, PQ H3Z 2T1
(514) 398-7478;
(514) 398-8361 (fax)

Catholic Health Association of Canada
1247 Kilborn Pl
Ottawa, ON K1H 6K9
(613) 731-7148;
(613) 731-7797 (fax)

Centre for Health Promotion
University of Toronto
Banting Institute
100 College St
Suite 207
Toronto, ON M5G 1L5
(416) 978-1809;
(416) 971-1365 (fax)

Centre de recherche en promotion de la santé de Montréal
Université de Montréal
2375 Côte Ste-Catherine Rd
Suite 7100
Montréal, PQ H3C 3J7
(514) 343-6111 (ext 8621);
(514) 343-2207 (fax)

CMT International Association
(Charcot-Marie-Tooth Disease)
1 Springbank Dr
St Catharines, ON L2S 2K1
(905) 687-3630

College of Family Physicians of Canada
2630 Skymark Ave
Mississauga, ON L4W 5A4
(905) 629-0900;
(905) 629-0893 (fax)

Community Health Nurses Association of Canada
c/o Lee Fredeen-Kohlert
PO Box 281
Millet, AB T0C 1Z0
(403) 387-4264

Concerns Canada
4500 Sheppard Ave E
Suite 112H
Agincourt, ON M1S 3R6
(416) 293-3400;
(416) 293-1142 (fax)

Consumer Health Association of Canada
250 Sheppard Ave E
Suite 205
Willowdale, ON M2N 6M9
(416) 222-6517;
(416) 225-1243 (fax)

Consumers' Association of Canada
307 Gilmour St
Ottawa, ON K2P 0P7
(613) 238-2533;
(613) 563-2254 (fax)

Council of Canadians with Disabilities
294 Portage Ave
Suite 926
Winnipeg, MB R3C 0B9
(204) 947-0303;
(204) 942-4625 (fax)

Council on Drug Abuse
16 Scarlett Rd
Toronto, ON M6N 4K1
(416) 763-1491;
(416) 767-5343 (fax)

Crohn's and Colitis Foundation of Canada
21 St Clair Ave E
Suite 301
Toronto, ON M4T 1L9
(800) 387-1479 or
(416) 920-5035;
(416) 929-0364 (fax)

DAWN Canada (DisAbled Women's Network)
3637 Cambie St
Suite 408
Vancouver, BC V5Z 2X3
(604) 873-1564 (tel/fax)

DES Action Canada
5890 Monkland Ave
Suite 203
Montreal, PQ H4A 1G2
(514) 482-3204;
(514) 482-1445 (fax)

Disability Information Services of Canada
501 18th Ave SW
Suite 304
Calgary, AB T2S 0C7
(403) 244-2836;
(403) 299-2177 (TTY/TDD);
(403) 229-1878 (fax)

Dying with Dignity: Canadian Society Concerned with the Quality of Dying
188 Eglinton Ave E
Suite 706
Toronto, ON M4P 1P3
(416) 486-3998;
(416) 489-9010 (fax)

Endometriosis Association of Canada
74 Plateau Crescent
Don Mills, ON M3C 1M8
(800) 426-2363 or
(416) 651-2419;
(416) 447-4384 (fax)

Epilepsy Canada
1470 Peel St
Suite 745
Montreal, PQ H3A 1T1
(514) 845-7855;
(514) 845-7866 (fax)

Family Life Education Council
223 12th Ave SW
Calgary, AB T2R 0G9
(403) 262-1117;
(403) 265-6404 (fax)

Family Service Canada
220 Laurier Ave W
Suite 600
Ottawa, ON K1P 5Z9
(613) 230-9960;
(613) 230-5884 (fax)

Heart and Stroke Foundation of Canada
160 George St
Suite 200
Ottawa, ON K1N 9M2
(613) 241-4361;
(613) 241-3278 (fax)

Histiocytosis Association of Canada
c/o 634 Sydenham Ave
Westmount, PQ H3Y 2Z4

HomeSupport Canada
119 Ross Ave
Suite 104
Ottawa, ON K1Y 0N6
(613) 761-8609;
(613) 728-6101 (fax)

Huntington Society of Canada
PO Box 1269
13 Water St N
Suite 3
Cambridge, ON N1R 7G6
(519) 622-1002;
(519) 622-7370 (fax)

Infertility Awareness Association of Canada
774 Echo Dr
Suite 523
Ottawa, ON K1S 5N8
(800) 263-2929 or
(613) 730-1322;
(613) 730-1323 (fax)

International Social Service Canada
151 Slater St
Suite 714
Ottawa, ON K1P 5H3
(613) 236-6161;
(613) 233-7306 (fax)

Interstitial Cystitis Association of Canada
PO Box 5814
Station A
Toronto, ON M5W 1P2
(416) 920-8986;
(416) 968-9081 (fax)

Juvenile Diabetes Foundation Canada
89 Granton Dr
Richmond Hill, ON L4B 2N5
(800) 668-0274 or
(905) 889-4171;
(905) 889-4209 (fax)

Kidney Foundation of Canada
5160 Decarie Blvd
Suite 780
Montreal, PQ H3X 2H9
(514) 369-4806;
(514) 369-2472 (fax)

La Leche League Canada
PO Box 29
18C Industrial Dr
Chesterville, ON K0C 1H0
(613) 448-1842;
(613) 448-1845 (fax)

Learning Disabilities Association of Canada
323 Chapel St
Suite 200
Ottawa, ON K1N 7Z2
(613) 238-5721;
(613) 235-5391 (fax)

Lions-Quest Canada
515 Dotzert Ct
Unit 7
Waterloo, ON N2L 6A7
(800) 265-2680 or
(519) 725-1170;
(519) 725-3118 (fax)

Lung Association—National Office
1900 City Park Dr
Suite 508
Gloucester ON K1J 1A3
(613) 747-6776;
(613) 747-7430 (fax)

Lupus Canada
635 6th Ave SW
Room 040
Calgary, AB T2P 0T5
(800) 661-1468;
(403) 265-4613 (fax)

**McMaster Research Centre
for the Promotion of Women's
Health**
McMaster University
Kenneth Taylor Hall
1280 Main St W
Room 226a/233
Hamilton, ON L8S 4M4
(905) 525-9140 (ext 23316);
(905) 524-2522 (fax)

ME Association of Canada
(Myalgic
Encephalomyelitis—Chronic
Fatigue Syndrome)
246 Queen St
Suite 400
Ottawa, ON K1P 5E4
(613) 563-1565;
(613) 567-0614 (fax)

Migraine Foundation
120 Carlton St
Suite 210
Toronto, ON M5A 4K2
(800) 663-3557 or
(416) 920-4916;
(416) 920-3677 (fax)

**Mission Air Transportation
Network**
10 Alcorn Ave
Suite 200
Toronto, ON M4V 3B1
(416) 924-9333;
(416) 924-5685 (fax)

**Multiple Sclerosis Society of
Canada**
250 Bloor St E
Suite 1000
Toronto, ON M4W 3P9
(416) 922-6065;
(416) 922-7538 (fax)

**Muscular Dystrophy
Association of Canada**
2345 Yonge St
Suite 900
Toronto, ON M4P 2E5
(416) 488-0030;
(416) 488-7523 (fax)

National AIDS Clearinghouse
c/o Canadian Public Health
Association
1565 Carling Ave
Suite 400
Ottawa, ON K1Z 8R1
(613) 725-3769;
(613) 725-9826 (fax)

**National Anti-Poverty
Organization**
256 King Edward St
Suite 316
Ottawa, ON K1N 7M1
(613) 789-0096;
(613) 789-0141 (fax)

**National Cancer Institute of
Canada**
10 Alcorn Ave
Suite 200
Toronto, ON M4V 3B1
(416) 961-7223;
(416) 961-4189 (fax)

**National Eating Disorder
Information Centre**
CW 1-211
200 Elizabeth St
Toronto, ON M5G 2C4
(416) 340-4156;
(416) 340-3430 (fax)

National Institute of Nutrition
265 Carling Ave
Suite 302
Ottawa, ON K1S 2E1
(613) 235-3355;
(613) 235-7032 (fax)

Non-Smokers' Rights Association
120 Spadina Ave
Suite 221
Toronto, ON M5S 2T9
(416) 928-2900;
(416) 928-1860 (fax)

North American Chronic Pain Association of Canada
150 Central Park Dr
Suite 105
Brampton, ON L6T 2T9
(416) 793-5230;
(416) 793-8781 (fax)

One Parent Families Association of Canada
6979 Yonge St
Suite 203
Willowdale, ON M2M 3X9
(416) 226-0062

Organization for Nutrition Education
PO Box 25
Guelph, ON N1H 8H6
(519) 438-9456 (tel/fax)

Osteoporosis Society of Canada
33 Laird Dr
Toronto, ON M4G 3S9
(416) 696-2663;
(416) 696-2673 (fax)

Parkinson Foundation of Canada
390 Bay St
Suite 710
Toronto, ON M5H 2Y2
(416) 366-0099;
(416) 366-9190 (fax)

ParticipACTION
40 Dundas St W
Suite 220
Toronto, ON M5G 2C2
(416) 954-1212;
(416) 954-4949 (fax)

Patients' Rights Association
170 Merton St
Toronto, ON M4S 1A1
(416) 487-6287

Physicians for a Smoke-Free Canada
170 Laurier Ave W
Suite 1202
Ottawa, ON K1P 5V5
(613) 233-4878;
(613) 567-2730 (fax)

Planned Parenthood Federation of Canada
1 Nicholas St
Suite 430
Ottawa, ON K1N 7B7
(613) 241-4474;
(613) 241-7550 (fax)

Prairie Region Health Promotion Research Centre
University of Saskatchewan,
Department of Community
Health and Epidemiology
Saskatoon, SK S7N 0W0
(306) 966-7932 or
(306) 966-7939;
(306) 966-7920 (fax)

PRIDE (Parent Resources Institute for Drug Education) Canada
University of Saskatchewan
College of Pharmacy
Saskatoon, SK S7N 0W0
(800) 667-3747 or
(306) 975-3755

Psoriasis Society of Canada
PO Box 25015
Halifax, NS B3M 4H4
(902) 443-8680;
(902) 457-1664 (fax)

Psychiatric Nurses Association of Canada
509 Pandora Ave W
Winnipeg, MB R2C 1M8
(204) 222-6984 (tel/fax)

Regional Centre for Health Promotion and Community Studies
University of Lethbridge
4401 University Dr
Room TH324
Lethbridge, AB T1K 3M4
(403) 382-7152;
(403) 329-2668 (fax)

Reye's Syndrome Foundation of Canada
c/o Alan Gee
RR #2
Kerwood, ON N0M 2B0
(519) 652-3888 or
(519) 247-3694;
(519) 652-1126 (fax)

St John Ambulance
312 Laurier Ave E
Ottawa, ON K1N 6P6
(613) 236-7461;
(613) 236-2425 (fax)

Schizophrenia Society of Canada
75 The Donway W
Suite 814
Don Mills, ON M3C 2E9
(800) 809-4673 or
(416) 445-8204;
(416) 445-2270 (fax)

Self Help Canada
PO Box 64094
1620 Scott St
Ottawa, ON K1Y 4V1

Serena Canada
151 Holland Ave
Ottawa, ON K1Y 0Y2
(613) 728-6536

Sleep/Wake Disorders Canada
3089 Bathurst St
Suite 304
Toronto, ON M6A 2A4
(800) 387-9253 or
(416) 787-5374;
(416) 787-4431 (fax)

Smoking and Health Action Foundation
120 Spadina Ave
Suite 22
Toronto, ON M5S 2T9
(416) 928-2900;
(416) 928-1860 (fax)

Spina Bifida Association of Canada
388 Donald St
Suite 220
Winnipeg, MB R3B 2J4
(800) 565-9488 or
(204) 957-1784;
(204) 957-1794 (fax)

Spinal Cord Society Canada
120 Newkirk Rd
Unit 32
Richmond Hill, ON L4C 9S7
(905) 508-4000;
(905) 508-4002 (fax)

Stay Alert . . . Stay Safe Organization
2190 Yonge St
6th Floor
Toronto, ON M4P 2V8
(416) 480-8225;
(416) 487-6524 (fax)

Sturge-Weber Foundation (Canada) Inc
1960 Prairie Ave
Port Coquitlam, BC V3B 1V4
(604) 942-9209;
(604) 942-6429 (fax)

Thyroid Foundation of Canada
1040 Gardiners Rd
Suite C
Kingston, ON K7P 1R7
(613) 634-3426;
(613) 634-3483 (fax)

**Tourette Syndrome
Foundation of Canada**
PO Box 343
238 Davenport Rd
North York, ON M5R 1J6
(416) 351-7757;
(416) 351-9267 (fax)

**Tracheo Esophageal Fistula
Parent Network**
c/o 42 Saskatoon Dr
Etobicoke, ON M9P 2E9
(416) 249-8710

**Traffic Injury Research
Foundation of Canada**
171 Nepean St
Suite 200
Ottawa, ON K2P 0B4
(613) 238-5235;
(613) 238-5292 (fax)

Turner's Syndrome Society
7777 Keele St
2nd Floor
Concord, ON L4K 1Y7
(800) 465-6744 or
(905) 660-7766;
(905) 660-7450 (fax)

United Way Canada
56 Sparks St
Suite 404
Ottawa, ON K1P 5A9
(613) 236-7041;
(613) 236-3087 (fax)

Vanier Institute of the Family
120 Holland Ave
Suite 300
Ottawa, ON K1Y 0X6
(613) 722-4007;
(613) 729-5249 (fax)

**Victoria Order of Nurses for
Canada**
5 Blackburn Ave
Ottawa, ON K1N 8A2
(613) 233-5694;
(613) 230-4376 (fax)

Women's Health Interaction
c/o Inter Pares
58 Arthur St
Ottawa, ON K1R 7B9
(613) 563-4801;
(613) 594-4704 (fax)

**World Food Day Association
of Canada**
176 Gloucester St
Suite 400
Ottawa, ON K2P 0A6
(613) 233-9002;
(613) 238-8839 (fax)

YMCA Canada
2160 Yonge St
2nd Floor
Toronto, ON M4S 2A9
(416) 485-9447;
(416) 485-8228 (fax) or
80 Gerrard St E
Toronto, ON M5B 1G6
(416) 593-9886;
(416) 971-8084 (fax)

Travel Resources for the Disabled

California

**Anglo-California Travel
Service**
San Jose
(408) 257-2257

Encino Travel
Encino
(818) 343-6339

State list from Simmons J, ed: *The next step,* Atlanta, 1990, Glasrock Home Health.

New Directions
Santa Barbara
(805) 967-2841

Visual Adventures
Mill Valley
(415) 383-6610

Wheels on Tour
Canoga Park
(818) 882-0441

Nautilus Tours
Tarzana
(818) 343-6339

Colorado

Destinations Travel
Denver
(303) 832-8810

Florida

Florida Wheelchair TPN
Orlando
(407) 352-1280

Unique Reservations
Indian Rocks Beach
(813) 596-7604

Wheelchair Wagon Tours
Kissimmee
(407) 846-7175

Massachusetts

New Horizons
Belmont

Maryland

Catholic Travel Office
Chevy Chase
(301) 657-9762

Michigan

Adventure Travel Service
Detroit
(313) 961-8550

Bee Kalt Travel Service
Royal Oak
(313) 549-6733

Minnesota

Flying Wheels Travel Service
Owatonna
(800) 722-9351 (MN);
(800) 657-4446 (Nat)

Missouri

Action Travel
Creve Coeur
(314) 576-9736

New Jersey

Doral Travel
Brick
(201) 840-0084

The Travel World
Shrewsbury
(201) 842-1000

Whole Person Tours
Bayonne
(201) 858-3400

New York

Access Tours
Mount Kisko
(914) 241-1700

Newlife
New York
(212) 557-5540

People Inc
Buffalo
(716) 631-8223

Preferred Travel
Yonkers
(914) 237-4108

Sprout
New York
(212) 431-1265

Take a Guide
New York
(212) 628-4823

Bonaparte's Access Adventures
East Rochester
(716) 385-6050

Oregon

Emmett Travel
Portland
(503) 233-3190

Sundial Special Vacations
Seaside
(503) 738-3324

Pennsylvania

Accessible Journeys
Ridley Park
(610) 521-0339

LM World Travel Services
Chester Springs
(215) 469-6676

The Guided Tour
Elkins Park
(215) 782-1370

Utah

Wonderland Travel
Salt Lake City
(801) 487-1731

Washington

Evergreen Travel Service
Lynnwood
(800) 562-9298 (WA);
(800) 435-2288 (Nat)

Redmont Travel
Redmont
(206) 885-2210

Organizations

World Federation of Hemophilia
Publishes *Passport,* a guide to national and international treatment centers.
1310 Green Ave
Montreal, Quebec, Canada
H3Z 2B2
(514) 933-7944

International Dialysis Organization
Publishes *Eurodial,* a guide to dialysis centers worldwide. Information may also be available from local dialysis centers.
153 rue du Pont, 69390
Vernaison, France
(33) 72 30 12 30

Medic Alert
Provides medical identification; has a 24-hour telephone information number.
PO Box 1009
Turlock, CA 95381-1009
(800) 344-3226

Reading Material*

Traveling Healthy
It costs $29 a year, $49 for two[1] years; back issues are $4
108-48 70th Rd
Forest Hills, NY 11375
(718) 268-7290

Handicapped Travel Newsletter
The cost is $10 a year (six issues)
PO Box Drawer 269
Athens, TX 75751

---

*NOTE: Quoted costs may be subject to change.

The Diabetic Traveler
The newsletter costs $18.95 for four issues; it provides detailed information on travel for those with diabetes; send a stamped self-addressed envelope for an "Insulin Adjustment" card (coping with jet lag) and "Management of Diabetes During Intercontinental Travel" (both free)
Box 8223 RW
Stamford, CT 06905
(203) 327-5832

Directory of Travel Agencies for the Disabled
Available for $19.95, $2 shipping and handling
The Disability Bookshop
PO Box 129
Vancouver, WA 98666
(800) 637-2256

Wheels and Waves: A Cruise, Ferry, River and Canal Barge Guide for the Physically Handicapped
$19.95 for the hard cover; $13.95 for the paperback, postage included.
The Aroyans' Company
Wheels Aweigh
17105 San Carlos Blvd
Suite A-6107
Fort Myers Beach, Fla 33931

Travel Agent Guide to Wheelchair Cruise Travel
The cost is $19.95 plus $2 shipping
Bill Cushing
TAG Publishing
PO Box 1046
Camarillo, Calif 93011

Resources For Culturally Diverse Populations

Multiple Populations

American Academy of Child and Adolescent Psychiatry
Committee on Ethnic and Cultural Issues
3615 Wisconsin Ave NW
Washington, DC 20016-3007
(202) 966-7300

American Academy of Family Physicians
Committee on Minority Health Affairs
8880 Ward Pkwy
Kansas City, Mo 64114-2797
(816) 333-9700 or
(800) 274-2237

American Psychological Association
Office of Ethnic Minority Affairs
750 1st St NE
Washington, DC 20002
(202) 336-5500

Bureau of Primary Health Care
Parklawn Building, Room 7-34
5600 Fishers Ln
US Department of Health and Human Services
Rockville, MD 20857
(301) 443-2403

Association of State and Territorial Health Officials
415 2nd St NE
Suite 200
Washington, DC 20002
(202) 546-5400

Center for Substance Abuse Prevention
US Department of Health and Human Services
Alcohol, Drug Abuse & Mental Health Administration
5600 Fishers Ln
Rockville, MD 20857
(800) 729-6686 (clearinghouse)

Maternal and Child Health Bureau
Parklawn Building
5600 Fishers Ln
Room 9-48
Rockville, MD 20857
(301) 443-2170

Minority Cultural Initiative Project
Research and Training Center on Family Support and Children's Mental Health
Portland State University
PO Box 751
Portland, OR 97207-0751
(503) 725-4040

National Center for Youth with Disabilities
University of Minnesota
420 Delaware
PO Box 721
Minneapolis, MN 55455
(800) 333-6293

National Migrant Resource Program
1515 Capital of Texas Highway S
Suite 220
Austin, TX 78746
(512) 328-7682

National Minority AIDS Council
300 I St NE
Suite 400
Washington, DC 20002
(202) 544-1076

National Minority Health Association
PO Box 11876
Harrisburg, PA 17108-1876
(717) 763-1323

Office of Disease Prevention and Health Promotion
National Health Information Center
PO Box 1133
Washington, DC 20013-1133

Office of Minority Health Resource Center
PO Box 37-337
Washington, DC 20013-7337
(800) 444-MHRC (ext 6472)

People of Color Leadership Institute
714 G St SE
Suite A
Washington, DC 20003
(202) 544-3144

African-American Population

National Black Child Development Institute
1463 Rhode Island Ave NW
Washington, DC 20005
(202) 387-1281

National Black Nurses' Association, Inc.
1012 10th St NW
Washington, DC 20001-4492
(202) 393-6870 or
(202) 347-1895

National Medical Association
1012 10th St NW
Washington, DC 20001
(202) 347-1895

National Urban League, Inc.
500 E 62nd St
New York, NY 10021
(212) 310-9000

Asian/Pacific Islander Population

Asian and Pacific Islander American Health Forum
116 New Montgomery
Suite 531
San Francisco, CA 94105
(415) 541-0866

Hispanic American/Latino/ Latina Population

National Coalition of Hispanic Health and Human Services Organizations (COSSMHO)
1030 15th St NW
Tenth Floor
Washington, DC 20005
(202) 371-2100

National Council of La Raza
810 1st St NE
Suite 300
Washington, DC 20002
(202) 289-1380

Native American Population

American Indian Health Care Association
245 E 6th St
Suite 499
St Paul, MN 55101
(612) 293-0233

US Indian Health Service
US Department of Health and
Human Services
Public Health Service
5600 Fishers Ln
Bethesda, MD 20852
(301) 443-1083

United National Indian Tribal Youth, Inc
PO Box 25042
Oklahoma City, OK 73125
(405) 424-3010

Sources of HIV Information

General Information
English: (800) 342-AIDS
(ext 2437)
Spanish: (800) 344-7432
TDD service for the deaf: (800) 243-7889

General Information for Health Care Providers
HIV telephone consultation
service: (800) 933-3413

State Hotlines
For information about HIV-specific resources and

counseling and testing services,
call your state AIDS hotline:

Alabama	(800) 228-0469
Alaska	(800) 478-2437
Arizona	(800) 548-4695
Arkansas	(501) 661-2133
California (No.)	(800) 367-2437
California (So.)	(800) 922-2437
Colorado	(800) 252-2437
Connecticut	(800) 342-2437
Delaware	(800) 422-0429
District of Columbia	(202) 332-2437
Florida	(800) 352-2437
Georgia	(800) 551-2728
Hawaii	(800) 922-1313

From USDHHS/PHS, Rockville, Md, AHCPR 94-0573, 1994.

Idaho ....(208) 345-2277	North Carolina ...(800) 733-7301
Illinois ....(800) 243-2437	North Dakota .....(800) 472-2180
Indiana...............(800) 848-2437	Ohio...................(800) 332-2437
Iowa...................(800) 445-2437	Oklahoma...........(800) 535-2437
Kansas ....(800) 232-0040	Oregon................(800) 777-2437
Kentucky ....(800) 654-2437	Pennsylvania ......(800) 662-6080
Louisiana............(800) 922-4379	Puerto Rico ....(800) 765-1010
Maine ....(800) 851-2437	Rhode Island ......(800) 726-3010
Maryland............(800) 638-6252	South Carolina ...(800) 322-2437
Massachusetts ....(800) 235-2331	South Dakota .....(800) 592-1861
Michigan ....(800) 827-2437	Tennessee ....(800) 525-2437
Minnesota...........(800) 248-2437	Texas ....(800) 299-2437
Mississippi ....(800) 537-0851	Utah...................(800) 366-2437
Missouri ....(800) 533-2437	Vermont..............(800) 882-2437
Montana ....(800) 233-6668	Virginia ....(800) 533-4148
Nebraska ....(800) 782-2437	Virgin Islands.....(809) 773-2437
Nevada ....(800) 842-2437	Washington.........(800) 272-2437
New Hampshire .(800) 324-2437	West Virginia .....(800) 642-8244
New Jersey.........(800) 624-2377	Wisconsin...........(800) 334-2437
New Mexico ......(800) 545-2437	Wyoming............(800) 327-3577
New York ....(800) 541-2437	

Directory of State Legislative Service

The following reference guide lists the names and telephone numbers of each state's legislative service. These offices can provide photocopies of legislation upon request. Contact these offices directly for information on ordering procedures and cost.

Alabama
Legislative Reference Service
State Capitol
Montgomery, AL 36130
House: (205) 242-7627
Senate: (205) 242-7826

Alaska
Pouch Y, State Capitol
Juneau, AK 99811
(907) 465-3737

Arizona
Capitol West Wing
1700 Washington
Phoenix, AZ 85007
(602) 225-4900

Arkansas
Office of the Legislative
Council
Room 315
State Capitol
Little Rock, AR 72201
(501) 375-1937

California
State Capitol Building
Sacramento, CA 95814
(916) 445-2323

From *State Nursing Legislature Quarterly,* Spring, 1990.

Colorado
State Capitol Building
200 Colfax
Denver, CO 80203
(303) 866-3055

Connecticut
Connecticut State Library
231 Capitol Ave
Hartford, CT 06106
(860) 566-5736

Delaware
Office of the Legislative
Council
Legislative Hall
Dover, DE 19901
(302) 736-4114

Florida
House: 513 Capitol
Tallahassee, FL 32301
(904) 488-7475
Senate: 404 State Capitol
Tallahassee, FL 32301
(904) 487-5285

Georgia
Clerk's Office
Legislative Documents
309 State Capitol
Atlanta, GA 30334
House: (404) 656-5015
Senate: (404) 656-5040

Hawaii
Chief Clerk's Office
State Capitol Building
Honolulu, HI 96813
(808) 548-7843

Idaho
Legislative Information Center
State House
Boise, ID 83720
(208) 334-2300

Illinois
State House
Springfield, IL 62706
House: (217) 782-5799
Senate: (217) 782-4517

Indiana
Legislative Services Agency
Room 302
State House
Indianapolis, IN 46204
(317) 232-9856

Iowa
State Capitol
Des Moines, IA 50319
(515) 281-5129

Kansas
Document Office
State House
Topeka, KS 66612
(913) 296-4096

Kentucky
State Capitol Building
Frankfort, KY 40601
(502) 564-8100

Louisiana
State Capitol Building
Baton Rouge, LA 70804
(504) 342-7259

Maine
Clerk of the House, State House
Augusta, ME 04330
(207) 289-1408

Maryland
Legislative Services Building
90 State Circle
Annapolis, MD 21401
(301) 841-3810

Massachusetts
State House
Boston, MA 02133
(617) 722-2860

Michigan
Legislative Services Bureau
State Capitol Building
Lansing, MI 48909
(517) 373-0169

Minnesota
Room 117
University Ave
St Paul, MN 55155
(612) 296-2314

Mississippi
New Capitol Building
Jackson, MS 39205
(601) 359-3358

Missouri
State Capitol Building
Jefferson City, MO 65101
House: (314) 451-3968
Senate: (314) 751-2966

Montana
State Capitol Building
Helena, MT 59620
House: (406) 444-3482
Senate: (406) 444-2508

Nebraska
Clerk of the Legislature
2018 State Capitol
Lincoln, NE 68509
(402) 471-2271

Nevada
Legislative Counsel Bureau
Legislative Building, Capitol
Complex
Carson City, NV 89710
(702) 687-6835

New Hampshire
Secretary of State
Room 204
State House
Concord, NH 03301
(603) 271-3315

New Jersey
State House
Trenton, NJ 08625
(609) 292-6395

New Mexico
Legislative Council Service
State Capitol
Santa Fe, NM 87503
(505) 984-9350

New York
State Capitol
Albany, NY 12248
Assembly: (518) 455-5164
Senate: (518) 455-2311

North Carolina
Office of Legislative Services
State Legislative Building
Raleigh, NC 27611
(919) 733-5648

North Dakota
State Capitol
Bismarck, ND 58505
(701) 224-3248

Ohio
Legislative Document Office
State House
Columbus, OH 43215
House: (614) 466-8207
Senate: (614) 466-7168

Oklahoma
200 NE 18th St
Oklahoma City, OK 73105
House: (405) 521-2498
Senate: (405) 521-5515

Oregon
State Capitol
Salem, OR 97310
(503) 378-8891

Pennsylvania
Capitol Building
Harrisburg, PA 17120
House: (717) 787-5320
Senate: (717) 787-6732

Rhode Island
State House
Providence, RI 02903
(410) 277-2473

South Carolina
State House, PO Box 11414
Columbia, SC 29211
(803) 734-2333

South Dakota
State Capitol
Pierre, SD 57501
(605) 773-3842

Tennessee
G 20 War Memorial Building
Nashville, TN 37243-0058
(615) 741-0945

Texas
State Capitol
PO Box 12068
Austin, TX 78711
House: (512) 463-1155
Senate: (512) 463-0252

Utah
State Capitol
Salt Lake City, UT 84114
House: (801) 538-1029
Senate: (801) 538-1588

Vermont
State Capitol Building
115 State St
Montpelier, VT 05602
(802) 828-2231

Virginia
House of Delegates
PO Box 406
Richmond, VA 23203
(804) 786-6530

Washington
Legislative Building
Olympia, WA 98504
(206) 786-7573

West Virginia
State Capitol
Charleston, WV 25305
House: (304) 357-3200
Senate: (304) 357-7800

Wisconsin
State Offices
1 E Maine
Madison, WI 53702
(608) 266-2400

Wyoming
State Capitol
Cheyenne, WY 82001
(307) 777-7648

Nurses' Resources

State Nurses Associations

Alabama State Nurses Association
360 N Hull St
Montgomery, AL 36104-3658
(205) 262-8321
(205) 262-8578 (fax)

Alaska Nurses Association
237 E 3rd Ave
Anchorage, AK 99501
(907) 274-0827
or (907) 264-1706
(907) 272-0292 (fax)

Arizona Nurses Association
1850 E Southern Ave
Suite 1
Tempe, AZ 85282
(602) 831-0404
(602) 839-4780 (fax)

Arkansas Nurses Association
117 S Cedar St
Little Rock, AR
(501) 664-5853
(501) 664-5859 (fax)

California Nurses Association
1145 Market St
Suite 1100
San Francisco, CA 94103
(415) 864-4141
(415) 252-9083 (fax)

Colorado Nurses Association
5453 E Evans Pl
Denver, CO 80222
(303) 757-7483 (ext. 13)
(303) 757-2679 (fax)

**Connecticut Nurses
Association**
Meritech Business Park
377 Research Pkwy
Suite 2D
Meriden, CT 06450
(203) 238-1207
(203) 238-3437 (fax)

Delaware Nurses Association
2634 Capitol Trail
Suite A
Newark, DE 19711
(302) 368-2333
(302) 366-1775 (fax)

**District of Columbia Nurses
Association, Inc.**
5100 Wisconsin Ave NW
Suite 306
Washington, DC 20016
(202) 244-2705
(202) 362-8285 (fax)

Florida Nurses Association
PO Box 536985
Orlando, FL 32853-6985
(407) 896-3261
(407) 896-9042 (fax)

Georgia Nurses Association
1362 W Peachtree St NW
Atlanta, GA 30339
(404) 876-4624
(404) 876-4621 (fax)

Guam Nurses Association
PO Box 3134
Agana, Guam 96910
011-671-565-2590

Hawaii Nurses Association
677 Ala Moana Blvd
Suite 301
Honolulu, HI 96813
(808) 521-8361
(808) 524-2760 (fax)

Idaho Nurses Association
200 N 4th St
Suite 20
Boise, ID 83702-6001
(208) 345-0500
(208) 345-1163 (fax)

Illinois Nurses Association
300 S Wacker Dr
Suite 2200
Chicago, IL 60606
(312) 360-2300
(312) 360-9380 (fax)

**Indiana State Nurses
Association**
2915 N High School Rd
Indianapolis, IN 46224
(317) 299-4575
(317) 297-3525 (fax)

Iowa Nurses Association
1501 42nd St
Suite 471
West Des Moines, IA 50266
(515) 255-0495
(515) 255-2201 (fax)

**Kansas State Nurses
Association**
700 SW Jackson
Suite 601
Topeka, KS 66603
(913) 233-8638
(913) 233-5222 (fax)

Kentucky Nurses Association
1400 S 1st St
PO Box 2616
Louisville, KY 40201
(502) 637-2546/2547
(502) 637-8236 (fax)

**Louisiana State Nurses
Association**
712 Transcontinental Dr
Metairie, LA 70001
(504) 889-1030
(504) 888-1158 (fax)

**Maine State Nurses
Association**
PO Box 2240
Augusta, ME 04330
(207) 622-1057
(207) 623-4072 (fax)

**Maryland Nurses Association,
Inc.**
849 International Dr
Airport Square 21
Suite 255
Linthicum, MD 21090
(410) 859-3000
(410) 859-3001 (fax)

**Massachusetts Nurses
Association**
340 Turnpike St
Canton, MA 02021
(617) 821-4625
(617) 821-4445 (fax)

Michigan Nurses Association
2310 Jolly Oak Rd
Okemos, MI 48864-4599
(517) 349-5640
(517) 349-5818 (fax)

Minnesota Nurses Association
1295 Bandana Blvd N
Suite 140
St Paul, MN 55108-5115
(612) 646-4807 or (800) 536-4662
(612) 646-4807 (ext 82—fax)

Mississippi Nurses Association
135 Bounds St
Suite 100
Jackson, MS 39206
(601) 982-9182
(601) 982-9183 (fax)

Missouri Nurses Association
206 E Dunklin St
Box 325
Jefferson City, MO 65101
(573) 636-4623
(573) 636-9576 (fax)

Montana Nurses Association
104 Broadway
Suite G-2
PO Box 5718
Helena, MT 59601
(406) 442-6710
(406) 442-6738 (fax)

Nebraska Nurses Association
941 O St
Suite 707-711
Lincoln, NE 68508
(402) 475-3859
(402) 475-3961 (fax)

Nevada Nurses Association
3660 Baker Ln
Suite 104
Reno, NV 89509
(702) 825-3555
(702) 825-3555 (fax)

**New Hampshire Nurses
Association**
48 West St
Concord, NH 03301
(603) 225-3783
(603) 226-4550 (fax)

**New Jersey State Nurses
Association**
320 W State St
Trenton, NJ 08618
(609) 392-4884/2031
(609) 396-2330 (fax)

**New Mexico Nurses
Association**
909 Virginia NE
Suite 101
Albuquerque, NM 87108
(505) 268-7744
(505) 260-1919 (fax)

**New York State Nurses
Association**
2113 Western Ave
Guilderland, NY 12084
(518) 456-5371
(518) 456-0697 (fax)

**North Carolina Nurses
Association**
103 Enterprise St
Box 12025
Raleigh, NC 27605
(919) 821-4250
(919) 829-5807 (fax)

**North Dakota Nurses
Association**
212 N 4th St
Bismarck, ND 58501
(701) 223-1385
(701) 223-0575 (fax)

Ohio Nurses Association
4000 E Main St
Columbus, OH 43213-2950
(614) 237-5414
(614) 237-6074 (fax)

Oklahoma Nurses Association
6414 N Santa Fe
Suite A
Oklahoma City, OK 73116
(405) 840-3476
(405) 840-3013 (fax)

Oregon Nurses Association
9600 SW Oak
Suite 550
Portland, OR 97223
(503) 293-0011
(503) 293-0013 (fax)

**Pennsylvania Nurses
Association**
2578 Interstate Dr
PO Box 68525
Harrisburg, PA 17106-8525
(717) 657-1222
(717) 657-3796 (fax)

**Rhode Island State Nurses
Association**
300 Ray Dr
Suite 5
Providence, RI 02906-4861
(401) 421-9703
(401) 421-6793 (fax)

**South Carolina Nurses
Association**
1821 Gadsden St
Columbia, SC 29201
(803) 252-4781
(803) 779-3870 (fax)

**South Dakota Nurses
Association**
1505 S Minnesota Ave
Suite 6
Sioux Falls, SD 57105
(605) 338-1401

Tennessee Nurses Association
545 Mainstream Dr
Suite 405
Nashville, TN 37228-1201
(615) 254-0350
(615) 254-0303 (fax)

Texas Nurses Association
7600 Burnet Rd
Suite 440
Austin, TX 78757-1292
(512) 452-0645
(512) 452-0648 (fax)

Utah Nurses Association
455 E 400 S
Suite 402
Salt Lake City, UT 84111
(801) 322-3439
(801) 322-3430 (fax)

**Vermont State Nurses
Association**
Box 26 Champlain Mill
1 Main St
Winooski, VT 05404-2230
(802) 655-7123
(802) 655-7187 (fax)

Virgin Islands State Nurses Association
3011 Golden Rock
St Croix, VI 00820-4355
(809) 773-2323 (ext. 119/116)
(809) 776-0610 (fax)

Virginia Nurses Association
7113 Three Chopt Rd
Richmond, VA 23226
(804) 282-1808
(804) 282-4916 (fax)

Washington State Nurses Association
2505 2nd Ave
Suite 500
Seattle, WA 98121
(206) 443-9762
(206) 728-2074 (fax)

West Virginia Nurses Association
101 Dee Dr
PO Box 1946
Charleston, WV 25327
(304) 342-1169
(304) 345-1538 (fax)

Wisconsin Nurses Association
6117 Monona Dr
Madison, WI 53716
(608) 221-0383
(608) 221-2788 (fax)

Wyoming Nurses Association
Majestic Building
Room 305
1603 Capitol Ave
Cheyenne, WY 82001
(307) 635-3955
(307) 635-6744 (fax)

State Boards of Nursing

Alabama Board of Nursing
RSA Plaza
Suite 250
770 Washington Ave
Montgomery, AL 36130-3900
(205) 242-4060
(205) 242-4360 (fax)

Alaska Board of Nursing Licensing
Department of Commerce and Economic Development
Division of Occupational Licensing
PO Box 110806
Juneau, AK 99811-0806
(907) 465-2544

Arizona Board of Nursing
2001 W Camelback Rd
Suite 350
Phoenix, AZ 85015
(602) 255-5092

Arkansas State Board of Nursing
University Tower Building
1123 S University Ave
Suite 800
Little Rock, AR 72204
(501) 686-2700
(501) 686-2714 (fax)

California Board of Registered Nursing
PO Box 944210
400 R St
Suite 4030
Sacramento, CA 95814
(916) 322-3350

Colorado Board of Nursing
1650 Broadway
Suite 670
Denver, CO 80202
(303) 894-2430

Connecticut Board of Examiners for Nursing
150 Washington St
Hartford, CT 06106
(860) 566-1041

Delaware Board of Nursing
Margaret O'Neill Building
Federal and Court Sts
PO Box 1401
Dover, DE 19903-1401
(302) 739-4522

District of Columbia Board of Nursing
Department of Consumer and Regulatory Affairs
614 H St NW
Room 904
PO Box 37200
Washington, DC 20001
(202) 727-7461

Florida State Board of Nursing
111 E Coastline Dr
Suite 516
Jacksonville, FL 32202
(904) 359-6331

Georgia Board of Nursing Registered Nurses
166 Pryor St SW
Suite 400
Atlanta, GA 30303
(404) 656-3943

Guam Board of Nurse Examiners
PO Box 2816
Agana, GU 96910
001-671-477-8766 (or-8517)
011-671-734-2066 (fax)

State of Hawaii Board of Nursing
PO Box 3469
Honolulu, HI 96801
(808) 548-3086

Idaho Board of Nursing
280 N 8th St
Suite 210
Boise, ID 83720
(208) 334-3110

Illinois Department of Professional Regulation
320 W Washington St
3rd floor
Springfield, IL 62786
(217) 785-0800

Indiana State Board of Nursing
Health Professions Service Bureau
402 W Washington St
Room 041
Indianapolis, IN 46204
(317) 232-2960

Iowa Board of Nursing
1223 E Court
Des Moines, IA 50319
(515) 281-3255

Kansas Board of Nursing
Landon State Office Building
900 SW Jackson
Room 551
Topeka, KS 66612-1230
(913) 296-4929
(913) 296-3929 (fax)

Kentucky Board of Nursing
312 Whittington Pkwy
Suite 300
Louisville, KY 40222-5172
(502) 329-7000
(502) 329-7011 (fax)

Louisiana State Board of Nursing
150 Baronne St
Room 912
New Orleans, LA 70112
(504) 568-5464
(504) 568-5467 (fax)

Maine State Board of Nursing
State House Station
PO Box 158
Augusta, ME 04433-0158
(207) 624-5275

Maryland Board of Nursing
Metro Executive Center
4201 Patterson Ave
Baltimore, MD 21215-2299
(410) 764-4747

Massachusetts Board of Registration in Nursing
100 Cambridge St
Suite 1519
Boston, MA 02202
(617) 727-9961

Michigan Board of Nursing
PO Box 30018
Lansing, MI 48909
(517) 373-1600

Minnesota Board of Nursing
2700 University Ave W
Suite 108
St Paul, MN 55114
(612) 642-0567

Mississippi Board of Nursing
239 N Lamar
Suite 401
Jackson, MS 39201
(601) 359-6170

Missouri State Board of Nursing
3605 Missouri Blvd
PO Box 656
Jefferson City, MO 65102
(573) 751-0681

Montana State Board of Nursing
Department of Commerce
Arcade Building
Lower Level
111 N Jackson
PO Box 200513
Helena, MT 59620-0513
(406) 444-4279

Nebraska Board of Nursing
State House Station
PO Box 95007
Lincoln, NE 68509-5007
(402) 471-2115

Nevada State Board of Nursing
1281 Terminal Way
Suite 116
Reno, NV 89502
(702) 786-2778

New Hampshire Board of Nursing
Division of Public Health Services
Health and Welfare Building
#6 Hazen Dr
Concord, NH 03301-2657
(603) 271-2323

New Jersey Board of Nursing
124 Halsey St
6th floor
PO Box 45010
Newark, NJ 07101
(201) 504-6493

New Mexico Board of Nursing
4253 Montgomery NE
Suite 130
Albuquerque, NM 87109
(505) 841-8340

New York Board of Nursing
State Education Department
Cultural Education Center
Albany, NY 12230
(518) 474-3843

North Carolina Board of Nursing
PO Box 2129
Raleigh, NC 27602-2129
(919) 782-3211

North Dakota Board of Nursing
919 S 7th St
Suite 504
Bismarck, ND 58504-5881
(701) 224-2974

Ohio Board of Nursing
77 S High St
17th floor
Columbus, OH 43266-0316
(614) 466-3947

**Oklahoma Board of Nursing
Registration and Nursing
Education**
2915 N Classen Blvd
Suite 524
Oklahoma City, OK 73106
(405) 525-2076

**Oregon State Board of
Nursing**
800 NE Oregon St #25
Suite 465
Portland, OR 97232
(503) 731-4745

**Pennsylvania State Board of
Nursing**
PO Box 2649
Harrisburg, PA 17105-2649
(717) 783-7142

**Colegio de Professionales de
la Enfermeria de Puerto Rico**
Board of Nurse Examiners
Call Box 10200
Santurce, PR 00908-0200
(809) 725-8161 (ext. 234/235)

**Rhode Island Board of
Nursing Registration and
Nursing Education**
Cannon Health Building
Room 104
#3 Capitol Hill
Providence, RI 02908
(401) 277-2827

**State Board of Nursing for
South Carolina**
220 Executive Center Dr
Suite 220
Columbia, SC 29210
(803) 731-1648

**South Dakota Board of
Nursing**
3307 S Lincoln Ave
Sioux Falls, SD 57105-5224
(605) 335-4973

**Tennessee State Board of
Nursing**
283 Plus Park Blvd
Nashville, TN 37427-1010
(615) 367-6232

**Board of Nurse Examiners for
the State of Texas**
9101 Burnet Rd
Suite 104
PO Box 140466
Austin, TX 78714-0466
(512) 835-4880

Utah State Board of Nursing
Division of Occupational and
Professional Licensing
Heber M. Wells Building
160 E 300 St
4th floor
PO Box 45802
Salt Lake City, UT 84145-0801
(801) 530-6628

**Vermont State Board of
Nursing**
109 State St
Montpelier, VT 05609-1106
(802) 828-2396

**Virgin Island Board of Nurse
Licensor**
Kongens Gade #3
PO Box 4247
St Thomas, VI 00803
(809) 776-7397
(809) 779-6368 (fax)

**Virginia State Board of
Nursing**
6606 W Broad St
4th floor
Richmond, VA 23230-1717
(804) 662-9909

Washington State Board of Nursing
Division of Professional Licensing
PO Box 47864
Olympia, WA 98504-7864
(206) 453-2686

West Virginia Board of Examiners for Registered Nurses
101 Dee Dr
Charleston, WV 25311-1620
(304) 558-3692 (or 3728)

Wisconsin Board of Nursing
Room 174
PO Box 8935
Madison, WI 53708-8935
(608) 266-0145

Wyoming State Board of Nursing
Barrett Building
2nd floor
2301 Central Ave
Cheyenne, WY 82002
(307) 777-7601

Health-Related World Wide Web Sites

Source	Site
CDC home page	http://www.cdc.gov/
Morbidity & Mortality Weekly Report	http://www.crawford.com/cdc/mmwr/mmwr.html/
Office of Disease Prevention/ Health Promotion	http://nhic-nt.health.org/
Public health, other	http.//amber.medlib.arizona.edu/ph-other.html/
National Library of Medicine (NLM)	http://www.nlm.nih.gov/
World Health Organization home page	http://www.who.ch/
National Clearinghouse for Alcohol and Drug Information	http://www.health.org/
US Department of Health and Human Services	http://www.os.dhhs.gov/
TRDEV-L home page	http://www.iconode.ca/trdev/
American Demographics/ Marketing Tools	http://www.marketingtools.com/
Yahoo: Health	http://www.yahoo.com/Health/
Dole Five a Day	http:www.dole4aday.com/
K-12 sources-curriculum plans	http:execpc.com/-dboals/K-12.html/
Health Hitlist: Health (education)	http:www.ec.ac.uk/-dregis/healthy.html/
Columbia Healthwise home page	http://www.columbia.ed/cu/healthwise/
Journal of Technology Eduction	http:scholar.lib.vt.edu/ejournals/JTE/jte.html/

Resource Information—Nurse

Professional resources serve to assist the nurse in defining scope of practice and in assessing health risks for individual clients and the community. New nurses to the specialty will want to be oriented to their practice, and the nurse manager can use a standard procedure for providing this orientation. The following is a selected group of resources that will provide direction for this.

ANA Standards of Community Health Nursing Practice

Standard I—Theory: The nurse applies theoretical concepts as a basis for decisions in practice.

Standard II—Data collection: The nurse systematically collects data that are comprehensive and accurate.

Standard III—Diagnosis: The nurse analyzes data collected about the community, family, and individual to determine diagnoses.

Standard IV—Planning: At each level of prevention, the nurse develops plans that specify nursing actions unique to client needs.

Standard V—Intervention: The nurse, guided by the plan, intervenes to promote, maintain, or restore health; to prevent illness; and to effect rehabilitation.

Standard VI—Evaluation: The nurse evaluates responses of the community, family, and individual to interventions in order to determine progress toward goal achievement and to revise the data base, diagnoses, and plan.

Standard VII—Quality assurance and professional development: The nurse participates in peer review and other means of evaluation to assure quality of nursing practice; the nurse assumes responsibility for professional development and contributes to the professional growth of others.

Standard VIII—Interdisciplinary collaboration: The nurse collaborates with other health care providers, professionals, and community representatives in assessing, planning, implementing, and evaluating programs for community health.

Standard IX—Research: The nurse contributes to theory and practice in community health nursing through research.

From American Nurses' Association: *Standards of community health nursing practice,* Kansas City, 1986. The Association. Reprinted with the permission of ANA.

NOTE: Currently in revision.

ANA Standards of Home Health Nursing Practice

Standard I—Organization of home health services: All home health services are planned, organized, and directed by a master's-prepared professional nurse with experience in community health and administration.

Standard II—Theory: The nurse applies theoretical concepts as a basis for decisions in practice.

Standard III—Data collection: The nurse continuously collects and records data that are comprehensive, accurate, and systematic.

Standard IV—Diagnosis: The nurse uses health assessment data to determine nursing diagnoses.

Standard V—Planning: The nurse develops care plans that establish goals. The care plan is based on nursing diagnoses and incorporates therapeutic, preventive, and rehabilitative nursing actions.

Standard VI—Intervention: The nurse, guided by the care plan, intervenes to provide comfort, to restore, improve, and promote health, to prevent complications and sequelae of illness, and to effect rehabilitation.

Standard VII—Evaluation: The nurse continually evaluates the client's and family's responses to interventions in order to determine progress toward goal attainment and to revise the data base, nursing diagnoses, and plan of care.

Standard VIII—Continuity of care: The nurse is responsible for the client's appropriate and uninterrupted care along the health care continuum, and therefore uses discharge planning, case management, and coordination of community resources.

Standard IX—Interdisciplinary collaboration: The nurse initiates and maintains a liaison relationship with all appropriate health care providers to ensure that all efforts effectively complement one another.

Standard X—Professional development: The nurse assumes responsibility for professional development and contributes to the professional growth of others.

Standard XI—Research: The nurse participates in research activities that contribute to the profession's continuing development of knowledge of home health care.

NOTE: Currently in revision.

Standard XII—Ethics: The nurse uses the code for nurses established by the American Nurses' Association as a guide for ethical decision making in practice.

Inspection List for OSHA

Use this list as a guide for making plant inspections. Details on requirements are found in the OSHA *General Industry Standards*. Keep records of what you see and the action taken!

Walking—working surfaces
Slippery
Damaged
Clear
Openings
Egress

Electrical
Disconnects
Defective
Exposed
Controls

Housekeeping/general plant environment
Clean
Debris
Ventilation
Sanitation

Vehicles
Authorized use
Defective
Rules and regulations
Adequate safeguards
Charging areas
Preventive maintenance and tag-out procedure

Cranes and hoisting equipment
Defective
Capacity
Controls
Authorized use

Powered tools
Defective
Guards
Use
Storage

Personal protective equipment
Eye protection
Hearing protection
Body protection
Emergency equipment
Sanitation and storage

Fire hazards
Flammable materials
Access
Areas identified
Storage

Compressed air and gases
Storage
Secured
Use

Machinery and equipment
Defective
Lock-out
Use
Guarding
Controls
Safety devices
Pinch points

Reprinted with permission from MacLeod I: *Health and safety: what every UAW representative should know,* 1980, United Auto Workers International Union, p 19.

Material handling and storage
Hazardous material
Proper use
Identification
Containment
Proper location

Hazardous materials
Chemicals

Fumes
Noise
Dusts

Safe job procedures
Job safety analysis conducted
Proper training
Job procedures

Laboratory Values of Clinical Importance

$$mmol/L = \frac{mg/dl \times 10}{atomic\ weight}$$

$$mg/dl = \frac{mmol/L \times atomic\ weight}{10}$$

Body Fluids and Other Mass Data
Body fluid, total volume: 50% (in obese) to 70% (lean) body weight
    Intracellular: 30-40% body weight
    Extracellular: 20-30% body weight
Blood:
    Total volume:
      Males: 69 ml/kg body weight
      Females: 65 ml/kg body weight
    Plasma volume:
      Males: 39 ml/kg body weight
      Females: 40 ml/kg body weight
    RBC volume:
      Males: 30 ml/kg body weight (1.15-1.21 L/M^2 body surface area)
      Females: 25 ml/kg body weight (0.95-1.00 L/m^2 body surface area)

$$Body\ surface\ area\ (m^2) = \frac{(wt\ in\ kg)^{0.425} \times (ht\ in\ cm)^{0.725}}{139.315}$$

CSF
Glucose: 2.2-3.9 mmol/L (40-70 mg/dl)
Total protein: 0.2-0.5 g/L (20-50 mg/dl)
CSF pressure: 50-180 mm H_2O

From Harrison: *Principles of internal medicine,* ed 13, New York, 1995, McGraw-Hill.

Leukocytes:
  Total: < 4 per mm^3
  Differential:
      Lymphocytes: 60-70%
      Monocytes: 30-50%
      Neutrophils: None

Chemical Constituents of Blood

Albumin, serum: 35-55 g/l (3.5-5.5 g/dl)
Aldolase: 0-100 nkat/L (0-6 U/L)
Aminotransferases, serum:
    Aspartate (AST, SGOT): 0-0.58 µkat/L (0-35 U/L)
    Alanine (ALT, SGPT): 0-0.58 µkat/L (0-35 U/L)
Ammonia, whole blood, venous: 47-65 µmol/L (80-110 µg/dl)
Amylase, serum: 0.8-3.2 µkat/L (60-180 U/L)
Arterial blood gases:
    [HCO$_3$]: 21-28 mmol/L
    P$_{CO_2}$: 4.7-6.0 kPa (35-45 mm Hg)
    pH: 7.38-7.44
    P$_{O_2}$: 11-13 kPa (80-100 mm Hg)
Bilirubin, total, serum (Malloy-Evelyn): 5.1-17 µmol/L (0.3-1.0 mg/dl)
    Direct, serum: 1.7-5.1 µmol/L (0.1-0.3 mg/dl)
    Indirect, serum: 3.4-12 µmol/L (0.2-0.7 mg/dl)
Calcium, ionized: 1.1-1.4 mmol/L (4.5-5.6 mg/dl)
Calcium, plasma: 2.2-2.6 mmol/L (9-10.5 mg/dl)
Carbon dioxide content, plasma (sea level): 21-30 mmol/L
Carbon dioxide tension (P$_{CO_2}$), arterial blood (sea level): 4.7-6.0 kPa (35-45 mm Hg)
Chloride, serum: 98-106 mmol/L
Cholesterol, plasma: <5.20 mmol/L (<200 mg/dl)
Complement, serum:
    C3: 0.55-1.20 g/L (55-120 mg/dl)
    C4: 0.20-0.50 g/L (20-50 mg/dl)
Creatine phosphokinase, serum (total):
    Females: 0.17-1.17 µkat/L (10-70 U/L)
    Males: 0.42-1.50 µkat/L (25-90 U/L)
    Isoenzymes, serum: fraction 2 (MB) <5% of total
Creatinine, serum: <133 µmol/L (<1.5 mg/dl)
Digoxin, serum:
    Therapeutic level: 0.6-2.8 nmol/L (0.5-2.2 ng/ml)
    Toxic level: >3.1 nmol/L (>2.4 ng/ml)
Ethanol, plasma:
    Moderate intoxication: 17-43 mmol/L (80-200 mg/dl)

Marked intoxication: 54-87 mmol/L (250-400 mg/dl)
Severe intoxication: >87 mmol/L (>400 mg/dl)
Ferritin, serum:
Females: 10-200 µg/L (10-200 ng/ml)
Males: 15-400 µg/L (15-400 ng/ml)
Glucose (fasting), plasma:
Normal: 4.2-6.4 mmol/L (75-115 mg/dl)
Diabetes mellitus: >7.8 mmol/L (>140 mg/dl) (on more than one occasion)
Glucose, 2-hour postprandial, plasma:
Normal: <7.8 mmol/L (<140 mg/dl)
Impaired glucose tolerance: 7.8-11.1 mmol/L (140-200 mg/dl)
Diabetes mellitus: >11.1 mmol/L (>200 mg/dl) (on more than one occasion)
Hemoglobin, blood (sea level):
Males: 140-180 g/L (14-18 g/dl)
Females: 120-160 g/L (12-16 g/dl)
Hemoglobin A_{1c}: Up to 6% of total hemoglobin
Immunoglobins, serum:
IgA: 0.9-3.2 g/L (90-325 mg/dl)
IgD: 0-0.08 g/L (0-8 mg/dl)
IgE: <0.00025 g/L (<0.025 mg/dl)
IgG: 8.0-15.0 g/L (800-1500 mg/dl)
IgM: 0.45-1.5 g/L (45-150 mg/dl)
Iron, serum: 9.0-26.9 µmol/L (50-150 µg/dl)
Iron-binding capacity, serum: 45-66 µmol/L (250-370 µg/dl)
Saturation: 20-45%
Lactate dehydrogenase, serum:
200-450 U/ml (Wrobleski)
60-100 U/ml (Wacker)
0.4-1.7 µkat/L (25-100 U/L)
Lipoproteins, plasma (desirable):
LDL cholesterol: <3.36-4.14 mmol/L (<130 mg/dl)
HDL cholesterol: >1.8 mmol/L (>70 mg/dl)
Magnesium, serum: 0.8-1.2 mmol/L (2-3 mg/dl)
Osmolality, plasma: 285-295 mosmol/kg of serum water
Phenytoin, plasma:
Therapeutic range: 40-80 µmol/L (10-20 mg/L)
Toxic level: >120 µmol/L (>30 mg/L)
Phosphatase, acid, serum: 0.90 nkat/L (0-5.5 U/L)
Phosphatase, alkaline, serum: 0.5-2.0 µkat/L (30-120 U/L)
Phosphorus, inorg., serum: 1.0-1.4 mmol/L (3-4.5 mg/dl)
Potassium, serum: 3.5-5.0 mmol/L
Proteins, total, serum: 55-80 g/L (5.5-8.0 g/dl)

Protein fractions, serum:
  Albumin: 35-55 g/L (3.5-5.0 g/dl) (50-60%)
  Globulin: 20-35 g/L (2.0-3.5 g/dl) (40-50%)
  Alpha$_1$: 2-4 g/L (0.2-0.4 g/dl) 4.2-7.2%)
  Alpha$_2$: 5-9 g/L (0.5-0.9 g/dl) (6.8-12%)
  Beta: 6-11 g/L (0.6-1.1 g/dl) (9.3-15%)
  Gamma: 7-17 g/L (0.7-1.7 g/dl) (13-23%)
Sodium, serum: 136-145 mmol/L
Triglycerides, plasma: 1.8 mmol/L (<160 mg/dl)
Urea nitrogen, serum: 3.6-7.1 mmol/L (10-20 mg/dl)
Uric acid, serum:
  Males: 0.15-0.48 mmol/L (2.5-8.0 mg/dl)
  Females: 0.09-0.36 mmol/L (1.5-6.0 mg/dl)

Function Tests
Circulation

Cardiac output (Fick): 2.5-3.6 L/m^2 body surface area per min
Ejection fraction, stroke volume/end-diastolic volume (SV/EDV):
Normal range: 0.55-0.78, average 0.67
Pulmonary vascular resistance: 2-12 kPa·s/L (20-120 [dyn·s]/cm^5)
Systemic vascular resistance: 77-150 (dyn·s)/cm^5 (770-1500 [kPa·s]/L)

Gastrointestinal

D-Xylose absorption test: After an overnight fast, 25 g xylose is given PO in aqueous solution; urine collected for the following 5 hours should contain 33-53 mmol (5-8 g) (or >20% of ingested dose); serum xylose should be 1.7-2.7 mmol/L (25-40 mg per 100 ml) 1 hour after the oral dose.
Gastric juice:
  Volume:
    24 hours: 2-3L
    Nocturnal: 600-700 ml
    Basal, fasting: 30-70 ml/h
  pH: 1.6-1.8
  Acid output:
    Basal:
      Females (mean ± 1 SD): 0.6 ± 0.5 µmol/s (2.0 ± 1.8 meq/h)
      Males (mean ± 1 SD): 0.8 ± 0.6 µmol/s (3.0 ± 2.0 meq/h)
    Maximal (after subcutaneous histamine acid phosphate 0.004 mg/kg and preceded by 50 mg promethazine; or after betazole 1.7 mg/kg or pentagastrin 6 µg/kg):
    Females: 4.4 ± 1.4 µmol/s (16 ± 5 meq/h)
    Males: 6.4 ± 1.4 µmol/s (23 ± 5 meq/h)

Secretin test (pancreatic exocrine function: 1 U/kg body weight, IV):
  Volume (pancreatic juice): >2.0 ml/kg in 80 min
  Bicarbonate concentration: >80 mmol/L
  Bicarbonate output: >10 mmol in 30 min

Metabolic and endocrine

Adrenal steroids, plasma:
  Cortisol:
  8 AM 140-690 nmol/L (5-25 µg/dl)
  4 PM 80-330 nmol/L (3-12 µg/dl)
Adrenal steroids, urinary excretion:
  Aldosterone: 14-53 nmol/day (5-19 µg/day)
  Cortisol, free: 55-275 nmol/day (20-100 µg/day)
  17-Hydroxycorticosteroids: 5.5-28 µmol/d (2-10 mg/d)
  17-Kelosteroids:
    Males: 24-88 µmol/day (7-25 mg/day)
    Females: 14-52 µmol/day (4-15 mg/day)
Estradiol:
  Females: 70-220 pmol/L (20-60 pg/ml), higher at ovulation
  Males: <180 pmol/L (<50 pg/ml)
Progesterone:
  Males, prepubertal females, preovulatory females, and postmeno-
    pausal females: <6 nmol/L (2 ng/ml)
  Females, luteal, peak: >16 nmol/L (>5 ng/ml)
Testosterone:
  Females: <3.5 nmol/L (<1 ng/ml)
  Males: 10-35 nmol/L (3-10 ng/ml)
  Prepubertal boys and girls: 0.17-0.7 nmol/L (0.05-0.2 ng/ml)
Thyroid function tests:
  Radioactive iodine uptake, 24 hours: 5-30% (range varies in
  different areas due to variations in iodine intake)
  Resin T_3 uptake: 25-35% (varies among laboratories)
  Thyroid-stimulating hormone (TSH): <5 mU/L (<5 µU/ml)
  Thyroxine (T_4), serum radioimmunoassay: 64-154 nmol/L (5-
  12 µg/dl)
  Triiodothyronine (T_3), plasma: 1.1-2.9 nmol/L (70-190 ng/dl)

Renal

Clearances (corrected to 1.72 m^2 body surface area):
  Insulin clearance (mean ± 1 SD):
    Males: 2.1 ± 0.4 ml/s (124 ± 25.8 ml/min)
    Females: 2.0 ± 0.2 ml/s (119 ± 12.8 ml/min)
  Endogenous creatinine clearance: 1.5-2.2 ml/s (91-130 ml/min)

Concentration and dilution test:
  Specific gravity of urine:
    After 12-hour fluid restriction: 1.025 or more
    After 12-hour deliberate water intake: 1.003 or less

Hematologic Examinations
(See also "Chemical Constituents of Blood")

Carboxyhemoglobin:
  Nonsmoker: 0-2.3%
  Smoker: 2.1-4.2%
Haptoglobin, serum: 0.5-2.2 g/L (50-220 mg/dl)
Hemoglobin, adults:
  Females: 14 ± 2.0 g/dl
  Males: 16.0 ± 2.0 g/dl
Leukocytes, total, adults: 4500-11,000 cells/µl

Differential count	Approx. % of total
Segmented neutrophils	40-74
Bands	0-4
Lymphocytes	16-45
Monocytes	4-10
Eosinophils	0-7
Basophils	0-2

Platelets and coagulation parameters:
  Fibrinogen: 2-4 g/L (200-400 mg/dl)
  Fibrin split products: <10 mg/L (<10 µg/ml)
  Platelets: 130,000-400,000/mm^3
Sedimentation rate:
  Westergren, <50 years of age:
    Males: 0-15 mm/hour
    Females: 0-20 mm/hour
  Westergren, >50 years of age:
    Males: 0-20 mm/hour
    Females: 0-30 mm/hour

URINE
Creatinine: 8.8-14 mmol/d (1.0-1.6 g/day)
Protein: <0.15 g/d (<150 mg/day)
Potassium: 25-100 mmol/day (varies with intake)
Sodium: 100-260 mmol/day (varies with intake)

Common Epidemiologic Rates

General Mortality Rates

Crude mortality rate

$$\frac{\text{Number of deaths occurring during 1 year}}{\text{Midyear population}} \times 100,000$$

Cause-specific mortality rate

$$\frac{\text{Number of deaths from a stated cause during 1 year}}{\text{Midyear population}} \times 100,000$$

Case-fatality rate

$$\frac{\text{Number of deaths from a specific disease}}{\text{Number of cases of the same disease}} \times 100$$

Proportional mortality ratio

$$\frac{\text{Number of deaths from a specific cause within a given time period}}{\text{Total deaths in the same time period}} \times 100$$

Age-specific mortality rate

$$\frac{\text{Number of persons in a specific age group dying during 1 year}}{\text{Midyear population of the specific age group}} \times 100,000$$

Maternal and Infant Indices

Crude birth rate

$$\frac{\text{Number of live births during 1 year}}{\text{Midyear population}} \times 1000$$

General fertility rate

$$\frac{\text{Number of live births during 1 year}}{\text{Number of females aged 15-44 at midyear}} \times 1000$$

Maternal mortality rate

$$\frac{\text{Number of deaths from puerperal causes during 1 year}}{\text{Number of live births during same year}} \times 100,000$$

Infant mortality rate

$$\frac{\text{Number of deaths of children under 1 year of age during 1 year}}{\text{Number of live births during same year}} \times 1000$$

Perinatal mortality rate

$$\frac{\text{Number of fetal deaths plus infant deaths under 7 days of age during 1 year}}{\text{Number of live births plus fetal deaths during same year}} \times 1000$$

From Harkness GA: *Epidemiology in nursing practice,* St. Louis, 1994, Mosby.

Neonatal mortality rate

$$\frac{\text{Number of deaths of children under 28 days of age during 1 year}}{\text{Number of live births during same year}} \times 1000$$

Fetal mortality rate

$$\frac{\text{Number of fetal deaths during 1 year}}{\text{Number of live births plus fetal deaths during same year}} \times 1000$$

Orientation of New Nurse to Community Health

A model skills list for community health nursing can guide individual agencies in tailoring orientation programs to their respective needs. Because every agency is different, lists may vary from one to another, and nurse managers will have to determine specific standards for baseline competence and time lines for achievement according to the agencies' needs.

Nursing process skills

I. Obtains initial nursing data for the client in the family context

A. Sociocultural assessment

	Initial hire	3 mo.	6 mo.
1. Family composition			
2. Family function			
3. Internal/external support systems			
4. Spiritual beliefs			
5. Cultural/ethnic factors			
6. Health care resources/behaviors			
7. Marital status			
8. Finances			
9. Education			
10. Communication			
11. Abuse and neglect			
12. Bonding and affiliation			

Sample key: N/A = not performed, not observed, or unable to evaluate at this date

1 = unsatisfactory performance

2 = performs adequately but inconsistently OR consistent but needs improvement

3 = performance is consistently competent

4 = outstanding performance

Hefty L, et al: "Model skills list," *Public Health Nurs* 9(4), 1992.

B. Environmental assessment

  1. Individual and family

    a. Home safety
    b. Use of space
    c. Basic needs—housing, water, heat, sanitation
    d. Equipment needs, environmental modifications

  2. Community context

    a. Neighborhood safety
    b. Isolation, neighborhood relationships
    c. Resources to meet family needs
    d. Transportation, mobility

C. Psychophysiologic assessment

  1. General physiologic assessments that apply across the life span
    a. General appearance
    b. Vital signs
    c. Review of systems
      (1) Head, neck
      (2) Cardiopulmonary
      (3) Respiratory
      (4) Vascular—circulatory, BP
      (5) Gastrointestinal
      (6) Genitourinary
      (7) Neuromuscular
      (8) Musculoskeletal
      (9) Metabolic/endocrine
      (10) Integumentary
    d. Sleep
    e. Pain
    f. Age- and situation-appropriate immunizations
    g. Nutrition
    h. Elimination
    i. Weight—gain, loss, maintenance
    j. Medications—prescription, OTC

2. General psychosocial
   assessment

   a. Cognitive functioning
   b. Learning abilities
   c. Coping abilities
   d. Mood
   e. Drug, alcohol use
   f. Body image
   g. Activities of daily living,
      self-care ability

3. Developmental assessments

   a. Antepartum

      (1) Vitamins, iron
      (2) Prenatal care, health
          history
      (3) Delivery plans—
          hospital, help at home,
          labor and delivery sup-
          port
      (4) Infant care and equip-
          ment preparation, health
          care plans for infant
      (5) Normal course,
          complications of
          pregnancy
      (6) Family planning

   b. Postpartum

      (1) Prenatal, health history
      (2) Labor, delivery course
      (3) Incisions
          (a) Cesarean section
          (b) Episiotomy
      (4) Lochia
      (5) Breasts
      (6) Vitamins, iron
      (7) Assistance at home
      (8) Family planning

   c. Neonate

      (1) Measurements—weight,
          length, OFC
      (2) Cord
      (3) Circumcision
      (4) PKU

(5) Sleep patterns, integration with family sleep habits

(6) Family interactions with infant, responses to cues

(7) NCAST assessments (Barnard, 1978)

d. Infant and child

(1) Measurements, growth curve/growth norms

(2) Language development

(3) Sibling relationships

(4) Parent-child relationships

(5) DDST

(6) NCAST assessments

(7) Accident prevention

(8) Education; school plans, school relationships

e. Adolescent

(1) Measurements, growth curve/growth norms

(2) Maturation

(3) Accident risk/prevention

(4) Suicide risk

f. Geriatric

(1) Mobility

(2) Accident risk, prevention

(3) Suicide risk

II. Planning

A. Identification of client, family, and community strengths/problems

B. Establishing a nursing diagnosis

C. Establishing short-term goals with client

1. Client-centered goals

2. Nurse goals

3. Agency requirements

III. Interventions

A. Procedural skills

1. Measurements

   a. Head (OFC)
   b. Weight
   c. Length/height
   d. Fontanelles
   e. Vital signs, BP

2. Aiding/assessing mobility, mobility aids

   a. Transfer techniques
   b. Range of motion
   c. Use of walker
   d. Use of cane
   e. Use of crutches
   f. Use of Hoyer lift

3. Wound care

   a. Packing
   b. Debridement
   c. Suture, staple removal

4. Dressing changes

   a. Sterile
   b. Clean
   c. Wet-to-dry
   d. Duoderm

5. Intravenous therapy

   a. Inserting IV
   b. Monitoring IV therapy
   c. Care of Hickman/Broviac catheter
   d. Care of epidural catheter

6. Injections

   a. Intradermal
   b. Subcutaneous
   c. Intramuscular
   d. Z-track

7. Nasogastric tube care

   a. Insertion
   b. Care
   c. Feedings, medications
   d. Suction

8. Gastrostomy tube care

  a. Change

  b. Care

  c. Feedings, medications

9. Enema administration

  a. Rectal

  b. Colostomy

10. Ostomy care

  a. Colostomy

  b. Ileostomy

  c. Nephrostomy

11. Urinary catheter care

  a. Indwelling catheter

    (1) Transurethral

    (2) Suprapubic

  b. External appliances

  c. I/O catheter for specimen collection

12. Tracheostomy care

13. Ventilator care

14. Oxygen management in the home

15. Handling/care of hazardous waste

16. Specimen collection

  a. Blood

  b. Wound secretions

  c. Sputum

  d. Urine

17. CPR

B. Teaching skills

  1. Principles of teaching/learning

    a. Adult learning

    b. Adolescent learning

    c. Infant, preschooler, school-age child learning

    d. Learning in the elderly

  2. Adaptation of teaching to home/classroom environments

    3. Evaluation of teachability

    4. Evaluation of learning

    5. Content areas

       a. Parenting

       b. Growth, development

       c. Home safety

       d. Nutrition

       e. Medications

       f. Problem solving

       g. Access to resources and
          agencies

IV. Evaluation

    A. Interpretation of findings

       1. Use of nursing diagnosis consistent with findings

       2. Intervention strategies appropriate to diagnosis

       3. Care plan reflects health promotion concepts/practice

    B. Goal achievement

       1. Measurement of short-term goals realistic

       2. Measurement of long-term goals realistic

    C. Continuing assessment

       1. Reassessments reflect changes in clients' condition, environment

       2. Nursing care plan reflects changes in clients' condition, environment

       3. Nursing care plan reflects long-term care

Professional skills

I. Communication skills

    A. Employee/co-workers

       1. Communicates with co-workers in a courteous, nonjudgmental, and helpful manner

       2. Identifies problems in communications, facilitates improvement

B. Employee/agency

   1. Uses appropriate lines of communication within organization

   2. Responds to requests for information in timely manner

   3. Recognizes/uses supervisory role appropriately

   4. Documents work accurately, within agency guidelines

C. Employee/individual

   1. Communicates in courteous, nonjudgmental, helpful, and sensitive manner

   2. Returns phone calls in timely manner

   3. Ensures confidentiality of written/verbal information

   4. Evaluates communication within families

II. Coordination/collaboration

   A. Communicates with other agencies regarding clients' needs, condition

   B. Communicates with other health care professionals regarding clients' needs, condition

   C. Demonstrates interdisciplinary case management through an interdisciplinary nursing care plan

   D. Demonstrates a working knowledge of community resources

   E. Can access community resources to the benefit of clients

III. Ethical/legal considerations

   A. Knows current legislation affecting practice

   B. Practices confidentiality

   C. Follows agency policies regarding clients' rights

IV. Advocacy

   A. Advocates for clients' rights/well-being within the family, within the agency, in the community

V. Personal/professional growth

A. Identifies own learning needs
B. Participates in staff development activities, continuing education
C. Manages time/tasks efficiently, setting appropriate priorities
D. Independently seeks to improve learning/performance
E. Participates in nursing audit process and/or quality assurance activities
F. Promotes others' learning

Handwashing Technique

1. Use a sink with warm running water, soap, and paper towels.
2. Push wristwatch and long uniform sleeves up above wrists. Remove jewelry, except a plain band, from fingers and arms.
3. Keep fingernails short and filed.
4. Inspect the surface of the hands and fingers for breaks or cuts in the skin and cuticles. Report such lesions when caring for highly susceptible clients.
5. Stand in front of the sink, keeping hands and uniform away from the sink surface. (If hands touch the sink during handwashing, repeat the process.) Use a sink where it is comfortable to reach the faucet.
6. Turn on the water. Turn on hand-operated faucets by covering the faucet with a paper towel.
7. Avoid splashing water against your uniform or clothes.
8. Regulate flow of water so the temperature is warm.
9. Wet hands and lower arms thoroughly under running water. Keep the hands and forearms lower than the elbows during washing.
10. Apply 1 ml of regular or 3 ml of antiseptic liquid soap to the hands, lathering thoroughly. If bar soap is used, hold it throughout the lathering period. Soap granules and leaflet preparations may be used.
11. Wash the hands, using plenty of lather and friction for at least 10 to 15 seconds. Interlace the fingers and rub the palms and back of hands with a circular motion at least 5 times each.

Modified from Potter PA, Perry AG: *Fundamentals of nursing: concepts, process, and practice,* ed 3, St. Louis, 1993, Mosby.

12. If areas underlying fingernails are soiled, clean them with fingernails of the other hand and additional soap or a clean orangewood stick. Do not tear or cut the skin under or around the nail.
13. Rinse hands and wrists thoroughly, keeping hands down and elbows up.
14. Repeat steps 10 through 12 but extend the actual period of washing for 1-, 2-, and 3-minute hand washings.
15. Dry the hands thoroughly from the fingers up to the wrists and forearms.
16. Discard paper towel in proper receptacle.
17. To turn off a hand faucet, use a clean, dry paper towel.

Remember to treat the inside of your "black bag" as clean. Always wash hands before removing supplies and equipment from bag or putting clean supplies in the bag. Carry soap and paper towels in outside packets of your bag or at inner top.

Reportable Diseases

The Center for Disease Control requires states, agencies, and health providers to provide information about specific diseases. Furthermore, states and localities also often have such requirements related to specific disease states within communities. Following is a listing of the national reportable diseases and an example of one state's reportable diseases. The user may obtain updated information from the state health department.

National Reportable Diseases

Acquired immune deficiency syndrome (AIDS)
Amebiasis
Anthrax
Aseptic meningitis
Botulism
Brucellosis
Campylobacteriosis
Cholera
Diptheria
Encephalitis
Gonorrhea
Hepatitis A-D
Influenza activity
Legionellosis/Legionnaire's Disease
Leprosy
Leptospirosis
Listeriosis
Lyme disease
Malaria
Measles
Meningococcal infections
Mumps
Pertussis
Plague
Poliomyelitis
Psittacosis
Rabies
Reye's syndrome
Rheumatic fever
Rocky Mountain spotted fever
Rubella
Salmonellosis
Shigellosis
Syphilis
Tetanus
Toxic shock syndrome
Trichinosis
Tuberculosis
Tularemia
Typhoid fever
Typhus fever
Varicella (chickenpox)
Yellow fever

From Centers for Disease Control: Annual summary 1992: reported morbidity and mortality in the United States, *MMWR Morb Mortal Wkly Rep* 33(54), 1992.

State Reportable Diseases

Category I

Report immediately by telephone to the Department of Health Services and to your patient's local health department the occurrence or suspicion of any of the diseases listed below. Also mail a communicable disease report within 24 hours.

Animal bite
Anthrax
Botulism (other than infant botulism)
Campylobacteriosis
Cholera
Diphtheria
Encephalitis
Gonococcal infections (all suspected or confirmed antibiotic-resistant strains)
Hepatitis (viral)
Measles
Meningitis (and other invasive disease caused by *Haemophilus influenzae* type B)
Meningitis caused by *Neisseria meningitidis*

Meningococcemia
Pertussis (whooping cough)
Plague
Poliomyelitis
Rabies (human)
Rubella (including congenital rubella syndrome)
Salmonellosis
Shigellosis
Syphilis (primary, secondary, congenital, or early latent)
Trichinosis
Tuberculosis*
Typhoid fever
Yellow fever
Yersiniosis
A suspected epidemic of any disease

Category II

Complete and mail a Communicable Disease Report within 7 days of diagnosis.

Acquired immune deficiency syndrome (AIDS)
Amebiasis
Botulism
Brucellosis
Chancroid
Chlamydia infections
Cryptococcosis
Ehrlichiosis (human)
Giardiasis

Gonococcal infections (other than antibiotic-resistant strains)
Granuloma inguinale
Herpes simplex infections (genital)
Histoplasmosis
Human immunodeficiency virus infection
Kaposi's sarcoma

---

*Report directly to the local health department or to the Tuberculosis Control Program.

Kawasaki syndrome
Legionellosis
Leprosy
Leptospirosis
Lyme disease
Lymphogranuloma venereum
Malaria
Mumps
Mycobacterium avium-
   intracellulare infection
Pneumocystis carinii pneumonia
Positive tuberculin skin tests (in
   children 6 years of age or less)

Psittacosis
Q fever
Reye's syndrome
Rocky Mountain spotted fever
Syphilis (all stages other than
   those listed previously)
Tetanus
Toxic-shock syndrome
Toxoplasmosis
Tularemia
Typhus
Varicella (chickenpox—adult)

Report the number of cases of chickenpox on a weekly basis.

Category III

Reporting required within 3 months:

Asbestosis
Coal worker's pneumoconiosis

Mesothelioma
Silicosis

PART TWO

ASSESSMENT

Community Assessment

Caring for the community has been an important part of practice for the public and community health nurse. In order to be knowledgeable about relevant care to individuals and family members, it is essential to know the community where they live, to identify resources that may participate in care, and to learn about deficits that might be strengthened through public and community health nursing practice.

Windshield Survey: A Micro Approach

This tool is designed to assist the nurse traveling around the community in identifying objective data which will help define the community, the trends, stability, and changes that will affect the health of the population.

Boundaries

To what extent do the identified boundaries of the catchment reflect the boundaries (such as a river or a different terrain), constructed (such as a highway or railroad) or economic (such as a difference in real estate or the presence of industrial or commercial units along with residential ones)? Does the neighborhood have an identity or a name? Is it displayed? Are there unofficial names? Are there subcommunities within the area?

Housing and Zoning

How old are the houses? What style are they and of what materials are they constructed? Are all the neighborhood houses similar? If not, how would you characterize the differences? Are there single or

Modified from Mizrahi TM: School of Social Work, Richmond, VA, Virginia Commonwealth University, September, 1992.

multifamily homes? What size are the lots? Are there signs of disrepair (such as broken doors, steps, or windows)? Are there vacant houses?

Signs of Decay

Is the neighborhood on the way up or down? Is it "alive"? How would you decide? Is there trash, abandoned cars, boarded-up buildings, rubble, dilapidated sheds, rubble-filled vacant lots, poor drainage, disease vector harborage, or the like?

Parks and Recreational Areas

Are there parks and recreational areas in the neighborhood? Is the open space public or private? Who uses it?

"Commons"

What are the neighborhood hangouts? For what groups, and at what hours (e.g., school year, candy store, bar, restaurant, park)? Does the "commons" have a sense of territoriality, or is it open to strangers?

Stores

What supermarkets or neighborhood stores are available? How do residents travel to the store? Are there drug stores, laundries, or dry cleaners?

Transportation

How do people get in and out of the neighborhood? What is the condition of the streets? Is there a major highway near the neighborhood? Whom does it serve? Is public transportation available?

Service Centers

Are there social agencies, clinics, recreation centers, or schools? Are there doctors, dentists, or other health care providers? Is there a hospital in the area?

Street People

If you are traveling during the day, who is on the streets (women, children, teenagers, community health nurses, collection agents, salesmen, etc.)? How are they dressed? What animals do you see (strays, pets, watchdogs, or livestock)?

Protective Services

Is there evidence of police and fire protection in the area?

Race

Of what ethnicity are the residents (black, white, Asian)? How are the different racial groups residentially located? Is the area integrated?

Ethnicity

Are there indicies of ethnicity—food stores, restaurants, churches, private schools, language information other than in English?

Religion

What churches and church-operated schools are in the neighborhood? How many are there?

Class

How would you categorize the residents: I, upper class; II, upper-middle class; III, middle class; IV, working class; V, lower class? On what do you base this judgment?

Health and Morbidity

Are there evidences of acute or chronic diseases or conditions, of accidents, communicable diseases, alcoholism, drug abuse, or mental illness? On what do you base this judgment?

Politics

Do you see any political campaign posters? Is there a party headquarters? Is there any evidence of a predominant party affiliation?

Community Assessment: A Macro Approach

The following questions have been designed to assist personnel in analyzing the data collected relative to the communities. The list is not exhaustive but is designed to stimulate thinking as providers residing within their communities begin to determine health needs. Analysis of the data is one step of the nursing process. The data analysis may best be done by those most familiar with the community, in preference to analysis performed by those less familiar with the community (that is, the state agency).

I. **Subjective**
  A. Impressions/perceived problems are probably of most value. Where possible, see if objective data confirm them.

Modified from the Colorado State Health Department, Denver, CO, September, 1982.

B. Are identified gaps "needs" or "wants"?

C. Are "needs" clearly health service areas, or do they belong to other agencies such as Social Services, Education?

D. Are "needs" such that they could be met by existing or new resources? If so, how?

II. Objective

A. Spatial

1. Does the size of the county/city present travel problems?

   Are the people in isolated pockets rather than spread throughout the area?

   Are there mountain passes?

   Is this a desirable area for health professionals, or is the turnover high?

   Are there accidents related to terrain?

   Are there land areas that contribute to vector problems?

2. Do roads criss-cross the area or are certain communities isolated?

   How near (accessible) is emergency/illness/preventive health care?

   Do residents have the ability to easily "escape" home for a while?

   Are highways and bridges safe and maintained? Does the maintenance collaborate with the highway safety department?

   Is ambulance service adequate and accessible to all?

   Are there any other high accident rates caused by the number of snowmobiles, dirt bikes, motorcycles?

3. Are there employers of large numbers of workers in or near the area?

   Does the type of industry have particular health hazards associated with it?

4. Is the area sparsely populated? Is it congested?

   Are sanitary conditions (density/plumbing) comparable to/better than/worse than that of the state?

   Are residents year-round, migratory, recreational?

   How will communication abilities affect securing health services?

5. Is an adequate water supply available for home use? For agriculture? Is it fluoridated? Is it polluted with items such as nitrates or bacteria?

6. Is air pollution a major problem? If so, what is the source?

7. What is the effect of land usage in industry? In recreation? In travel?

B. Demographic
  1. Is the population growing? Is it decreasing? Is this putting a stress on local resources?
  2. Does the area have a particularly high/low number of people in specific age groups?
     Is this proportion likely to change based on current migratory trends?
     Have health programs developed that are directed at large age groups?
  3. Is there a significant number of ethnic minorities? If so, which group?
     What effect will a preponderance of a particular minority have on vital statistics data when compared to the state?
     What health programs exist that are directed at significant minority groups?
  4. How will the level of education affect the type of health services offered?
     Is a low educational level indicative of a whole cycle of poverty?
  5. Do health providers accept Medicare? Do they accept Medicaid patients?
     Are there persons eligible for food stamps who are not using the program? Can they afford to buy stamps?
     Do health services have sliding fee scales?
  6. How large a segment of the population is at poverty-level income?
     What health programs exist for these people?
  7. Have large numbers of unemployed persons resulted in the need for additional mental health services?
     Are there child care services available for working mothers?
  8. Is the pattern of communicable disease significantly different from what is happening elsewhere? If so, why?
     Has one or more diseases become more prevalent? If so, why?
  9. Is the birth rate high or low? If high, is it attributable to age makeup of the population? Is it associated with ethnic behaviors? Is it attributable to environmental or other community-specific factors?
     Are there factors within the community that contribute to a rising divorce rate?
  10. Is the death rate different from that of the state? If so, what are the probable causes?

Is a preponderance of elderly in the community affecting the death rate?

Has there been a recent significant increase in one or more causes of death?

Are lifestyles affecting the causes of death?

11. Family planning—do women in need use it? If not, why not (availability, religious reasons, etc)?

12. Is the community adequately immunized?

C. Public service

1. Is there money available locally to support health services? Do people save money?

Is lack of money generally a problem?

2. Will lack of utility services have a direct effect on health conditions?

3. What official persons need to be involved in planning for and providing health services?

Is local government making decisions in the best interest of the general population? Are government officials active, strong, knowledgeable? Are lobbying efforts for health issues possible or effective?

4. Are local law enforcement services available on a 24-hour basis?

How are law enforcement agencies involved in the health arena? How could they be?

5. What effects do fire protection or lack thereof have in planning safety measures or in community education?

6. Are services staffed volunteers or by full-time employees?

D. Health services

1. Are institutional beds available? If not, where do people go for these services? Can/should patterns of use be changed?

2. Are there adequate resources to meet the needs? What resources are missing in the community?

3. Are emergency personnel adequately trained?

Are services available on a 24-hour basis?

4. Are there adequate resources? What resources are missing in the community?

Do community health agencies work together effectively? Is there a network to cover the entire area?

5. How does the ratio compare to the state as a whole? How does it compare to other surrounding comparable areas? What changes in the program would occur if the nurse-to-population ratio were improved?

6. Are there sufficient numbers of primary care providers?

Where are specialty services secured if not available locally?

How does a lack of specialty services affect the level of health in the community?

7. What is the physician-to-population ratio? Is it adequate? Where can data be secured?

   Are dental services available in the schools? Are the residents willing or able to afford dental services?

E. Community services

1. What types of school health services are available? What health education means are available? What means are used?

   What is the nurse-to-pupil ratio?

   Is the library a clearinghouse for community education?

2. What effect will the presence or lack of such facilities have on the health of the community?

3. What activities, organizations, etc., are available to young-sters, teens, adults, and elderly for enjoyment? Are they crowded? Are they safe? Are they adequate? Who uses the facilities?

4. Is the church a social center for the community?

   Does the church provide a support system for families and individuals?

   Do religious beliefs have an effect on the use of health services?

   Is child abuse a problem?

5. Is there a local communication network that could help in disseminating health information?

   Is the communication available on a local, regional, state, or national level?

Data-Gathering Sources and Strategies

The table on pages 89–91 provides a list of sources of information that may be helpful in completing the community assessment. This list is not exhaustive. Others may be added as appropriate to a specific community. The nurse may use maps, aerial photos, community photos, government reports, newspaper articles, census data, local

Modified from Stanhope M, Lancaster J: *Community health nursing: process and practice for promoting health,* ed 3, St Louis, 1992, Mosby; Connor O: *Understanding your community,* ed 2, Ontario, 1969, Development Press; Anderson E, McFarlane J: *Community as partner,* ed. 2, Philadelphia, 1995, JB Lippincott.

books, health department vital statistics, agency annual reports, participant observation, windshield survey, key informant interviews (government, school, church, health care system), citizen and consumer interviews, community forums of interested persons, diaries, checklists, community self-surveys, and sketch maps as strategies to collect data for each of the components of the categories described.

Data gathering sources and strategies

Categories/Components	History	Boundaries	Resources	Technology	Norms and values	Roles and positions	Power structures
Family	Ethnic origin Traditions Extended family	Migration patterns Strength Land and home use Community interaction	Census data Income Education Home Recreation	Nutrition Shelter Hygiene Health Education	Diary Family stories Celebrations Family functions	Family assessment Individual interview Observation	Family influence in community Family involvement in groups
Education	Growth of schools Curricula trends Reports Diary Survey	School districts School sites Number of schools Survey administrators	Board of education Census data Annual reports Interviews with parents, teachers, school nurses	PTO/PTA Teachers Administrators Student surveys Windshield survey	Interviews Budget Active PTO Type of curriculum Attendance Absenteeism	Number of elected and appointed positions Policies on relationships	Key figures Tenure policy PTO influence
Government	Historical society Newspaper columns Reports Books Library Key informants Observation	Maps Aerial photographs Census tracts Population density Voting districts	Key informants Tax structure Budget Population trends Trained personnel Eligible voters	Government structure Government departments Services offered Tax networks Government planning office	Citizen attendance Elected party Expansion laws	Sketch map List of office holders Government duties Services offered	Key figures Stability of office Number of community factions
Economy Family finances Industrial finances Community finances	Changes in median household and per capita incomes Welfare records Population trends Past/present industry	Intra/interstate use of products Geographic distribution of labor force Local/national financing	Census data Land use Number in labor force Banks Unemployment rate	City planner interviews City commissioner interviews Plant facilities and equipment State welfare records	Stability Windshield survey Employee interviews "Good worker" standard Income adequacy	Job descriptions Employer and employee surveys	Formal leaders Informal leaders Windshield survey Unions

Continued.

Data gathering sources and strategies—cont'd

Categories/ Components	History	Boundaries	Resources	Technology	Norms and values	Roles and positions	Power structures
Religion	Library Historical society Church libraries Newspaper archives	Types of churches Number of churches Population served Number of participants Geographic distribution of members	Budgets Size of congregation National affiliations	Organizational structures Number of new members Religious practices of church and citizens	Rituals Church size Programs of church Citizen commitment Social changes Intergroup activities	Windshield survey Lay participation in church Ministers' behaviors	Turnover of leaders Stability of leaders Lay leaders
Recreation and safety	Trends Popular support Key personalities	Area served Facilities Types of activities Schedules	City planner Fire, police departments Water department Sewage treatment plants	Professional or volunteer workers Equipment	Traditional vs new practices Personnel interviews Organized or informal services	Stability Turnover Key Informants	Personal interviews Organizational structure
Social issues	Library Historical society Ethnic origins Trends in distribution	Geography Social structure Types of people moving in and out	Census data Income Land use Number in educational levels Occupations		Citizen interviews Citizen participation with groups Subcultures	Sketch map of citizen associations and communications	Informal leaders Styles Ranking of classes
Communication networks and transportation	Growth trends Library Chamber of commerce	Population and housing census data Transportation authorities State highway departments TV and newspaper	Number of TV/ radio stations and newspapers Local airports and bus terminals Telephone services	Media sources Transportation sources	Windshield survey Resident interviews Community survey Types of news	Sketch map Use of transportation Public attention to media	Censorship Community opinion Types of editorials Transportation service distribution

Health and illness	Statistical trends Health planning agency reports Agency annual reports Census data Health department vital statistics Epidemics	Number of like agencies Health planning agency Agency service area Location of services	Phone directory Community resource book Annual reports Budgets Services offered	Treatment patterns Preventive services Diagnostic aids	Folk vs scientific medicine Self-care activities Cost of care Quality of life	Key leaders Job descriptions Practice laws and patterns	Participant observation Key informants Employee interview Consumer interview
Agriculture	Maps Aerial photos Census data Chamber of commerce	Distribution size	Census data Crops Income Laborers State agricultural department	Individual Family farms Coop farms Machines Farm labor	Farm support Prices Federal subsidy	Windshield survey Personal interviews	Citizen interviews Community participation by farmers
Industry	Department of labor and statistics Chamber of commerce Census data	Organizational charts Policies Size and number of plants	Census data Union records Employee support services	Small industry White collar vs blue collar industry Large firms	Employee demographics Policies Work space and size Support services Recreation facilities Company social activities	Job descriptions Organizational structure Types of jobs	Key informants Influential members serving community Commitment to community

Public Health Capacity-Building

Public Health Practices

Assessment Practices

1. **Assess the health needs of the community** by establishing a systematic needs assessment process that periodically provides information on the health status and health needs of the community.
2. **Investigate the occurrence of adverse health effects and health hazards in the community** by conducting timely investigations that identify the magnitude of health problems, duration, trends, location, and populations at risk.
3. **Analyze the determinants of identified health needs** in order to identify etiologic and contributing factors that place certain segments of the population at risk for adverse health outcomes.

Policy Development Practices

4. **Advocate for public health, build constituencies, and identify resources in the community** by generating supportive and collaborative relationships with public and private agencies and constituent groups for the effective planning, implementation, and management of public health activities.
5. **Set priorities among health needs** based on the size and seriousness of the problems, the acceptability, economic feasibility, and effectiveness of interventions.
6. **Develop plans and policies to address priority health needs** by establishing goals and objectives to be achieved through a systematic course of action that focuses on local community needs and equitable distribution of resources and involves the participation of constituents and other related governmental agencies.

From Turnock B et al: *Journal of Public Health Management and Practice,* 1(3):50-58, 1995.

Assurance Practices

7. **Manage resources and develop organizational structure** through the acquisition, allocation, and control of human, physical, and fiscal resources; maximize the operational functions of the local public health system through coordination of community agencies' efforts and avoidance of duplication of services.

8. **Implement programs** and other arrangements ensuring or providing direct services for priority health needs identified in the community by taking actions that translate plans and policies into services.

9. **Evaluate programs and provide quality assurance** in accordance with applicable professional and regulatory standards to ensure that programs are consistent with plans and policies; provide feedback on inadequacies and changes needed to redirect programs and resources.

10. **Inform and educate the public** on public health issues of concern in the community, promoting an awareness about public health services availability and health education initiatives that contribute to individual and collective changes in health knowledge, attitudes, and practices toward a healthier community.

Perfomance Measure—Local Health Department Assessment practices

Assess

1. Reviews health status and needs of entire jurisdiction
2. Includes community input and participation
3. Includes mortality and morbidity information from vital records
4. Includes information from behavioral risk factor surveys

Investigate

5. Monitors all outbreak and adverse health effects

Analyze

6. For determinants of health problems
7. For population groups at risk
8. For adequacy of existing health resources

Policy development practices

Advocate

9. Meets with health-related organizations
10. Reports on issues disseminated to the community
11. Regularly informs media
12. Publicly reviews mission and role

Prioritize

13. Based on consequences of health problems
14. Based on acceptability, economic feasibility, and effectiveness of interventions

Plan

15. Community health action plan addresses priority health needs
16. Incorporates public participation
17. Agency strategic plan is linked to community health action plan

Assurance Practices

Manage
18. Organizational self-assessment completed
19. Job descriptions and minimum qualifications updated
20. Strategy for securing funding in place

Implement
21. Mandated programs are addressed
22. Agency providing or ensuring services for each priority health need

Evaluate
23. Compliance with professional and regulatory standards
24. Program goals and objectives monitored
25. Program changes made on basis of evaluation and quality assurance activities

Inform and educate
26. Public information and education

Methods of Community Involvement

	Phase of involvement					
	Preparation of providers	Outreach and recruitment	Preparation of community	Obtaining community input	Using community input	Follow-up
Goal	To enable providers to be receptive to community input	To identify and select representatives of the community to participate in COPC* program	To increase community members' ability to participate in COPC	To obtain information from individuals and groups that will contribute to COPC	To incorporate information from the community into the program	To report back to the community on the results of their input and to obtain their reaction to how it was used

Methods					
Orientation to community involvement Training on: Group process Board roles Cross-cultural awareness Community organizing	Appointment (by the clinic or a community organization) Election (by the clinic or community) Self-selection Random method	Orientation to health program and COPC Education on health care system Training on: Group process Board roles Cross-cultural awareness Community organizing	For obtaining information from groups: Brainstorming Nominal group Role play Gaming simulation For making group decisions: Autocratic Democratic Consensus Default For obtaining information from individuals: Interviews in person or by telephone Written questionnaires	Select an articulate community member to present info to the clinic Select an influential clinic member to present info Write a formal report to the clinic staff or board Write informal memo	Individual acknowledgments Report formally to participating organizations Public information campaigns

*COPC, Community-oriented primary care.

From Overall N, Williamson J, editors: *Community oriented primary care in action: a practice manual for primary care settings*, USDA's, PHS, HRSA, Contract no 240-84-0124.

Community Functional Health Pattern Assessment— a Nursing Diagnosis Approach

Suggested Use

The community functional health pattern approach is a typology of assessment categories of basic information to be evaluated in a sequence of behaviors across time. There are 11 pattern areas that describe actual or potential needs, patterns of behavior, and goals of communities based on Gordon's functional health pattern assessment for nursing diagnosis of clients. Assessment parameters are provided for each pattern area.

Community Functional Health Patterns and Assessment Parameters

Health perception—health management pattern

Describes the patterns of health and well-being as well as how health is managed. Includes the community's perception of its health status and its relevance to current activities and future planning. Also includes the availability of health-care resources and usage rates.

Assessment parameters. Health facilities, prevention programs, usage rates, perceived health problems, perceived level of wellness, and the availability of health professionals.

Nutrition-metabolic pattern

Describes the patterns of food and fluid consumption relative to metabolic need and indicators of nutrient supply. Includes the community's patterns of food and fluid consumption, the type and quantity of foods and fluids available, particular food preferences, and the availability and use of food supplement programs. Also includes fuel availability and usage in relation to climate.

Assessment parameters.   Food supplement programs, the availability of natural resources (fish, game, gardens, farms), income rates, the availability of stores, water supply and quality, water usage rate and restrictions, growth patterns of the community, and climate.

Elimination pattern

Describes the patterns of waste production and disposal. Also includes the actual and perceived ability to handle waste disposal.

From Gikow FF and Kucharski PM: A new look at the community: functional health pattern assessment, *Community Health Nurs* 1(4):21-27, 1987.

Assessment parameters. Types of waste, sewage system, waste disposal, recycling programs, pest control, and the community's perception of problems.

Activity-exercise pattern

Describes the patterns of activity, exercise, leisure, and recreation. Includes sites for work, housing, recreation, shopping, and so forth. The emphasis is on activities of high importance to the community.

Assessment parameters. Employment opportunities, transportation, community centers, communication systems, housing types and location, recreation facilities, clubs, organizations, and shopping centers.

Sleep-rest pattern

Describes the patterns of sleep, rest, and relaxation. Includes community's patterns of rest, relaxation, and sleep during a 24-hour period. Also includes the community's perceptions of quality and quantity of sleep and rest.

Assessment parameters. Usual business hours, activity levels, noise levels, quiet and busy areas.

Cognitive-perceptual pattern

Describes the community's sensoriperceptual and cognitive patterns. Includes the community's perception of problems, decision-making structures, education levels of the population, education facilities, and the predominant languages.

Assessment parameters. Opportunities for education within the community, education levels of the population, achievement testing results, language prevalence, school system, truancy rates, and the effects of the outside system on the community (such as laws and rules).

Self-perception—self-concept pattern

Describes the community's sensoriperceptual and cognitive patterns. Includes the community's perception of problems, decision-making structures, education levels of the population, education facilities, and the predominant languages.

Assessment parameters. Community history, age levels, ethnic and racial composition, pride indicators, mechanism for self-evaluation, and published descriptions of the community.

Role-relationship pattern

Describes the patterns of role engagements and relationships. Includes the community's perception of major roles and responsibilities in current situations. Also includes disturbances in legal, governmental, or social relationships with other communities and the responsibilities related to these.

Assessment parameters.   Fire and safety programs, highway and public works programs, inspection programs, contracts with other communities, civil defense program, leadership and management style, budget, the perception of problem-solving ability, informal relationships with other communities, and power bases.

Sexuality-reproductive pattern

Describes the patterns of satisfaction or dissatisfaction with sexual mores and reproductive patterns. Includes birth and death rates, family size and type, and any perceived problems.

Assessment   parameters.   Male-female   ratio,   population changes, fertility rates, family size and type, maternal age, neonatality rate, laws governing pornography, and the prevalence of prostitution.

Coping—stress-tolerance pattern

Describes the community's general coping patterns and the effectiveness of the patterns in terms of stress tolerance. Includes the capacity to resist challenges to self-integrity, modes of handling stress, support systems, and the perceived ability to control and manage situations.

Assessment parameters.   Delinquency, drug abuse, crime, divorce, alcoholism and suicide rates; the presence of phone-help lines; the poverty level; incidence of psychiatric illness; support groups; child, spouse, and elder abuse; and occupational stress.

Value—belief pattern

Describes the community's pattern of values, goals, and beliefs (including spiritual) that guides choices or decisions. Includes what is perceived important to the community and perceived conflicts in community values, beliefs, and expectations that are health related.

Assessment parameters.   The priority of health issues to the community, community-identified health problems, community expectations of health, religious denominations, churches, cults, limits of acceptable behavior, housing values, zoning laws, political issues, ethnic groups, philosophies, goals, and social issues.

A Lifespan Community Assessment— a Developmental Approach

Suggested Use

The lifespan perspective of human development has the potential for providing a comprehensive model for community health nursing practice. The community can be viewed from this lifespan perspective. The nurse can observe the dynamic relations between a developing community and its changing context. The sources of data and data collection methods that are appropriate for this type of assessment are similar to those used in other community analyses. What is important is the concept of time. The nurse should gather information over several points of time to offer a true feel for the life and health of a community.

Community Assessment Instrument

I. Population.
    A. Total population.
    B. Age distribution.
        1. List by age groups of 5 years (0-4, 5-9, etc.).
        2. Give actual numbers and percentages for each group.
    C. Sex distribution. Actual numbers and percentages.
    D. Race distribution. As above.
    E. Ethnicity. As above.
    F. Religion
        1. As above.
        2. Separate "other," separating persons in nonmajor denominations from actual nonbelievers.
    G. Education. As above.
    H. Socioeconomic status.
        1. Incomes of families. As above, in increments of $10,000 until $40,000 and above.
        2. Categories of occupations.
        3. Unemployment levels.
II. Environment.
    A. Geography.
        1. Topography.
        2. Location.
        3. Boundaries.

From McCool, Susman: Life span perspective of community health, *Public Health Nurs* 7(1), 1990.

B. Climate.

C. Sanitation.
1. Water supply source.
2. Sewage disposal.
3. Trash and garbage.

D. Protection.
1. Fire. Describe services.
2. Police. Describe services.

E. Housing.
1. Ownership. Give numbers and percentages; describe.
2. Rental. As above.

F. Pollution-safety hazards.
1. Air.
2. Water.
3. Land.

III. Organization.

A. Government.
1. Type.
2. Leaders.

B. History. Include major changes (such as shifts in industry, highway development, urban renewal, regionalization).

C. Economics. List primary sources of government and private income.

D. Recreation.
1. Parks (public and private).
2. Entertainment.
a. Theaters.
b. Museums.
c. Amateur/professional sporting teams.
3. Social organizations.

E. Education. Levels, types, and number of schools.

F. Religion.
1. Churches. Number and size.
2. Religious organizations.

G. Power structure.
1. Community leaders.
2. Decision makers.

IV. Technology/business.

A. Leading industries.
1. Name.
2. Type.
3. Number of employees.

B. Utilities.
   1. Energy sources (such as electricity, oil, gas, coal, solar).
   2. Telephone services.
C. Transportation.
   1. Highways.
   2. Train.
   3. Bus.
   4. Air.
D. Business organizations.
E. Basic services.
   1. Food. Sources, major stores.
   2. Clothing. As above.
V. Communication.
   A. Newspapers.
      1. Name.
      2. Publication schedule.
      3. Circulation.
   B. Radio stations.
      1. Name.
      2. Format style and content.
      3. Frequencies.
   C. Television.
      1. Name.
      2. Commercial/public.
   D. Informal networking.
VI. Health.
   A. Vital statistics.
      1. Live births.
      2. Mortality.
         a. Leading causes of death, including number and rate.
         b. Neonatal, infant, and maternal deaths, including number and rate.
      3. Morbidity. Chronic diseases, number and rate.
   B. Hospitals.
      1. Name.
      2. Ownership.
      3. Number of beds.
      4. Types of service.
      5. Average length of stay.
   C. Nursing homes.
      1. Name.
      2. Ownership.

    3. Bed capacity/bed numbers.

    4. Services offered.

D. Ambulatory services/clinics.

    1. Name.

    2. Public/private ownership.

    3. Services offered.

E. Mental health facilities.

    1. Name.

    2. Ownership.

    3. Number of beds.

    4. Services offered.

F. Emergency services.

    1. Name.

    2. Ownership.

    3. Personnel involved.

    4. Availability.

G. Social/health services.

    1. Occupational.

    2. School.

    3. Voluntary agencies.

    4. Comprehensive health centers/clinics.

    5. Prepaid group health plans.

    6. Health councils.

    7. Social service agencies.

H. Health care personnel.

    1. Physicians.

    2. Registered nurses.

    3. Dentists.

    4. Social workers.

    5. Chiropractors.

    6. Others.

⟳ Environmental Assessment: Home and Industry

Assessment of the environment where individuals and families live and work is an integral aspect of community health nursing practice. These tools will assist the nurse in establishing a baseline for evaluating that environment and for teaching and planning appropriate interventions.

Assessment Survey: Housing for the Disabled

Entry

__ Ramp
    __ 1 foot rise per 12 feet length
    __ 4 feet wide
    __ Nonslip surface
    __ Handrail extended 18 inches beyond top and bottom step
    __ 5 feet flat platform at top
    __ 6 feet clearance at bottom
__ Elevator
__ Steps
__ Lighting
__ Sidewalks
__ Surface level
__ Parking
__ Carport has 13-14 inches clearance space

Living Area

__ Floors nonslip
__ Floors same level
__ Doorways 36 inches wide with 5 foot square turning area
__ Doors have push handles
__ Mirrors are correct height
__ Telephone at bedside
__ Controls and electrical switches 36 inches from floor
__ Cords out of traffic pattern
__ Windows 36 inches from floor
__ Carpet secure—no scatter rugs
__ Linoleum free of holes, dips

From Stanhope M, Lancaster J: *Community health nursing: process and practice for promoting health,* ed 2, St Louis, 1988, Mosby.

__ Furniture sturdy, arranged for free movement
__ Lighting
__ Heating—location of vents and radiators

Kitchen

__ Stove, burner controls safe
__ Pots and pans—check weight
__ Potholders, mitts of sufficient thickness
__ Dishes accessible
__ Counter space—check height
__ Faucets accessible and easy to turn on/off
__ Table top equipment free from clutter

Bathroom

__ Tub rails 3 to 4 inches out from wall
__ Toilet—transfer space
__ Toilet—height of seat
__ Mirror height
__ Sink—check height, handles
__ Doorway 36 inches wide
__ Floor surface nonslip
__ Tub surface nonslip
__ Medicine chest—check height
__ Linen storage—check height
__ Lighting

Bedroom

__ Space
__ Floor surface, nonslip
__ Doorway 36 inches wide
__ Closet accessible
__ Lighting
__ Bed, ancillary equipment (e.g., side rails, trapeze)
__ Emergency call mechanism

General description

Hazards identified

Inconveniences identified

Recommendations

Family Members
Names, ages, and relationships

Source of income

Source for medical costs coverage/payments

Caretaker
    Schedule of care

    Contingency plans

Assessment of Immediate Living Environment

Client's name _____

Date _____

Parameters	Assessment	Recommendations
Neighborhood	Adequate __ Inadequate __	
Amount of physical space	Adequate __ Inadequate __	
Cleanliness	Adequate __ Inadequate __	
Convenient toilet facilities	Adequate __ Inadequate __	
Useable and accessible telephone	Adequate __ Inadequate __	
Adequate and safe heating	Adequate __ Inadequate __	
Stairway and halls	Adequate __ Inadequate __	
Cooking facilities	Adequate __ Inadequate __	
Tub, shower, hot water	Adequate __ Inadequate __	
Laundry facilities	Adequate __ Inadequate __	
Physical barriers in home	Present __ Absent __	
Physical barriers to exits from home	Present __ Absent __	
Physical hazards	Present __ Absent __	
Home accessible to care-givers	Yes __ No __	
Use of alcohol or drugs by patient or care-giver	Yes __ No __	
Client mobility	Adequate __ Inadequate __	
Client safety	Adequate __ Inadequate __	
Escort necessary	Yes __ No __	
Pets	Yes __ No __	

Strengths of physical environment: _____

_____

Areas of concern: _____

_____

_____

_____

From Skelly AH: Physical disabilities and rehabilitation: the role of the nurse in the community. In Bullough B, Bullough V, editors: *Nursing in the community,* St Louis, 1990, Mosby.

Tools for Living for the Aged and Disabled

The following items are suggested for use in the home to assist the elderly and disabled in self help.

Location/activity	Equipment
Kitchen	
Meal preparation	Pots and pans with large-diameter handles
	Extended faucets for finger or wrist force
	Lazy Susans and Ferris wheel-type holders for cans and spices in cabinet
	Side-by-side refrigerator
	Microwave and crock pots
	Electric can opener
	Lid removers
	Rocker knives
	Put food in small packages
	Label packages
	Provide braille labels for visually impaired
Eating	Rocker knife for single hand function
	Scoop dish with plate guard
	Electric self-feeder
	Utensils with built-up handles
	Long straws
	Mugs
	ADL/Universal cuff, c-clip holder
Doors	Lever-type action doorknob
	Vertical bar door openers to push with hand, foot, wheelchair footrest
	Electric power doors
Floors	Nonskid linoleum
	Easy to clean floors
Stairs	Small chairlift
	Small elevator
Walls	Waist-level electric outlet bars

Continued.

Modified from Brody S and Ruff G: *Aging and rehabilitation,* Springer, New York, 1990. Springer: Thistle H, D'Amico D, and Prowler C: *Preparing the physical environment.*

Tools for living for the aged and disabled—cont'd

Location/activity	Equipment
Bathroom	
Bathing, toileting	Grab bars for tubs, showers, toilets
	Elevated toilet seat
	Bathtub bench
	Nonskid mats
	Long-handled sponge
	Suction nail
	Soap-on-a-rope
	Wash mitt
	Raised-faucet letters for visually impaired
	Digital readout temperature faucets
Hygiene—other	
Hair	Long-handled brush or comb
	C-clip holder
	Built-up handles
Brushing teeth	Built-up handle toothbrush
	Suction denture brush
	Electric toothbrush
Shaving	Electric shaver
	Electric razor
	Shaving cream dispenser with handle
Bedroom	Ceiling poles near bed to help get in or out of bed
	Bedrails
	Pressure mattress
	Dynamic rocking bed
	Electric bed
	Bedside light and appliance control
Communication	Large button telephones
	Amplified receivers
	Ringing light for hearing impaired
	Remote controlled TV, recorders, stereos
	Low-mounted telephone
	Telephone shoulder rest
	Dialing stick
	Automatic dialer
	Portable telephone

Tools for living for the aged and disabled—cont'd

Location/activity	Equipment
Dressing	Button loops
	Velcro closures for buttons, shoes, bra
	Long shoe horn
	Slip-in shoes
	Dressing stick
	Stocking aid
	Trouser pull
	Leg lifter
	Zipper pull
Mobility	Canes and walkers
	Large handgrips on above
	Large rubber tips on above
	Cut canes so that when the tip is on the floor, the arm is slightly flexed
	Have wheelchair seats fitted to client
	Adjust wheelchair arm and footrests
	Three-wheeled power chair
	Van with lift or ramp
	Wheelchair drive controls (hand, breath, chin)
Security	System to monitor client activity in home (such as Lifecall)
	Small transmitter for wrist or neck attached to security
Recreation	Talking books
	Page turners
	Keys attached to tape recorders for ease of turning on
	Stationary cycle for ambulatory clients
	Taped ministries from church
	Elevated gardens for wheelchair clients

Life Skills and Community Living

Safe and accessible housing, transportation, vocational rehabilitation, disability management in the workplace, educational programs, adaptive equipment to facilitate community living, support services

From McCourt A, editor: *The specialty of rehabilitation nursing: a core curriculum,* ed 3, Skokie, IL 1993. *The rehabilitation nursing foundation of the association of rehabilitation nurses.*

and advocacy groups, and community resources are essential for the maximum functioning of the disabled person. These are issues to consider.

I. Housing: selection and assessment
   A. Factors and alternatives to consider in selecting housing
      1. Be aware that many alternatives are available depending upon the client's functional ability, support systems, needs, and goals
      2. Secure an appropriately adapted residence; if necessary, make adaptations
         a. Build access ramp(s)
         b. Widen doors
         c. Modify the kitchen and bathroom so that all facilities and appliances are easily accessible
         d. Make parking available
      3. Consider moving client into congregate housing with or without attendant services
      4. Encourage client to join an independent living program that allows people with disabilities to remain in their own dwellings while offering, but not managing, provision of support services
         a. Support services related to ADLs
            (1) Training in communication techniques
            (2) Communal meals
            (3) Training in homemaking skills
            (4) Supervision of and guidance in transportation skills
            (5) Recreational opportunities
            (6) Emergency procedures
            (7) Housing options
         b. Support services related to personal health management
            (1) Training in communication techniques
            (2) Counseling regarding sexuality and family relationships
            (3) Management of attendants
         c. Support services related to counseling assistance
            (1) Advocacy services
            (2) Peer counseling
            (3) Consumer and legal information
            (4) Personal business management
      5. Be aware of laws governing housing availability and accessibility

    a. The Housing Act of 1959: Provided funding for mortgage loans to developers to build housing for the elderly and the handicapped

    b. The Architectural Barriers Act of 1968: Mandated physical accessibility to any federally-funded building being constructed

    c. The Rehabilitation Act of 1973: Prohibited discrimination against the disabled when they rented or purchased federally subsidized property

    d. The Housing and Community Development Act of 1974: Subsidized rent payments to low-income families

    e. The Rehabilitation, Comprehensive Services, and Developmental Disabilities Amendment of 1978: Issued grants for housing

    f. The Americans with Disabilities Act of 1990: Established new laws, governing physical access to the community, which need to be evaluated in relation to access to services and ways to implement them in communities in order to ensure access

6. Consider alternative housing situations for clients who are unable to remain in their previous residence

    a. Independent living programs (see I.A.4.)

    b. Residential living—an arrangement in which a group of people with disabilities live in the same building or geographic area and share support services—can involve several challenges

       (1) Finding accessible housing

       (2) Securing attendant assistance

       (3) Providing accessible transportation

       (4) Obtaining rent subsidies

    c. Extended-care facilities such as subacute rehabilitation or neurobehavioral programs or skilled care facilities

B. Factors to consider in assessing a home

1. Availability of occupational therapy, physical therapy, and nursing evaluations to assist in determining safety, access, interventions, and the patient's ability to function in his or her own environment

2. Definition of the type of living quarters; design of the building

3. Lighting of the residence and its entrance, heating, running water, electrical outlets, and toilet facilities

4. Access to the residence and the need for wider doors, assistance with door opening, and handrails; bathroom and kitchen modifications
5. Assistive devices needed to facilitate mobility and safe participation in community environments
6. Availability of support systems to assist with mobility
7. Patient's level of independence regarding transfers, homemaking skills, personal care, food procurement and preparation, and household maintenance
8. Availability and adequacy of communications devices
9. Clutter in the environment—for example, scatter rugs, cords, carpets, toys, animals that might pose safety risks
10. Presence and accessibility of an elevator, availability of adaptive equipment such as braille buttons, an elevator bell to indicate floor for visually impaired; automatic door timing for opening and closing
11. Furniture—arrangement, functionality, client's ability to use it safely, the need for adaptive equipment such as chair with a seat lift
12. Type of floor surface and ability to maneuver assistive device(s) on it
13. Storage of a vehicle and access to residence from the storage area
14. Ability to hear the telephone, fire alarms, doorbells, and availability of required adaptive equipment

II. Transportation
   A. Legislative mandates for public transportation systems and buildings—designed to guarantee all persons two basic rights
      1. Equal access to public transportation
      2. Completion of required modifications of airplanes, terminals, buses, subways, and public railroad systems
         a. Space to accommodate wheelchairs
         b. Wider doors and aisles, shorter or tiered steps
         c. Ramp or lift systems, elevators
   B. Issues related to modifications for vehicles for people with disabilities
      1. Hand controls, lifts, seating, and transfer mechanisms
      2. Funding for vehicle modification
      3. Travel programs and clubs for the disabled
   C. Adapted driver education and evaluation procedures
   D. Considerations regarding public transportation for those with disabilities
      1. Transportation services should be contacted prior to use

to ensure that assistive services and accommodations are available

    a. The chamber of commerce in many cities can provide booklets with information regarding community accessibility

    b. The U.S. Department of Transportation has information regarding highways and airports

2. It is vital that people with disabilities have access to the workplace, medical services, shopping, support services, recreational facilities, churches, public buildings, banks, clinics, post offices, grocery stores, and clothing stores, among other places, in order to increase independence in self-care and community participation

3. Other transportation factors to be considered for people with disabilities

    a. Distance from residence to public transportation

    b. Cost of both public transportation and privately owned, specially adapted vehicles

    c. Availability of assistance

    d. Amount of assistance required

III. Vocational rehabilitation

  A. Federal law mandates that each state have a public agency that provides vocational rehabilitation (Office of Vocational Rehabilitation [OVR])

  B. Funding is provided for various aspects of vocational rehabilitation to facilitate a return to competitive work or supported employment

    1. Vehicle and home modifications

    2. Work-hardening programs, assessment of work capacities

    3. Assessment of training facilities, equipment, and transportation

    4. Determination of each individual's vocational limitations

    5. Identification of vocational interests, previous work experience, and current abilities

    6. Assessment of the job market

    7. Employer education and development

    8. Matching the disabled person's functional, cognitive, and emotional abilities with job placement options

        a. Job training

        b. Job modification

        c. Job placement

  C. Supported employment integrates people with disabilities into work settings

1. History
   a. Rehabilitation Act Amendments of 1986: Describe the content of supported employment programs
   b. Traditional vocational rehabilitation programs have served individuals with disabilities primarily in sheltered environments
2. Foci of supported employment settings
   a. Providing services to the severely disabled is a priority
   b. Workers are paid
   c. Work settings are integrated—persons with disabilities work in settings with able-bodied workers
   d. Ongoing support is provided
      (1) Supervision
      (2) Job adaptations
      (3) Personal care
      (4) Money management
      (5) Social skills
      (6) Transportation

IV. Disability management programs in the workplace
   A. Emphasize early identification of disabled workers and focus on prevention of work-related injuries
   B. Identify conditions in the work environment that result in worker disability
   C. Provide evaluations to identify the medical, social, and psychological assistance that would enable the worker to return to work
   D. Provide case management services in the form of job analysis, job modifications, and job placement
   E. Monitor services to address problems that arise after job placement occurs
   F. Motivate businesses to develop these programs due to the cost of worker disabilities and subsequent healthcare costs
   G. Develop work-hardening programs
   H. May result in favorable outcomes
      1. Lower workers' compensation costs
      2. Reduced absenteeism
      3. Reduced costs of rehabilitation services
      4. Reduced medical costs
      5. Employee retention

V. Educational program considerations
   A. Availability of institutions offering programs for the disabled such as residential schools for hearing-impaired, blind, or head-injured persons

B. Special services offered for the disabled to facilitate access to educational services
   1. Services related to the learning process
      a. Adaptation of educational materials such as talking books, braille books, textbook recordings, cognitive software, computer-assisted learning programs
      b. Equipment such as reading machines, audiology services, communication augmentation devices, voice-activated computers
      c. Tutors, interpreters, or note-takers
   2. Other access issues—access to
      a. Classrooms, including parking
      b. Cafeteria, library, bookstore, dorms, chapel
      c. Social activities
      d. Entertainment, recreation, or sports activities
      e. Adapted bathrooms and shower facilities
C. Availability of support services
   1. Financial assistance
   2. Attendant services for students residing on campus
   3. Healthcare services
   4. Career planning and placement services
   5. Accessibility of programs for persons with disabilities
   6. Programs that take into consideration each individual's functional and cognitive abilities
   7. Vocational or guidance counseling
D. Adapted driver evaluation and education—modification of existing driver education program within the school system or referral to a rehabilitation facility for adapted driver training (for example, a teenager with a spinal cord injury who has never driven)
VI. Adaptive equipment to facilitate community reintegration—considerations
A. Devices for ADLs and mobility
   1. Specific type needed for physical mobility, such as a wheelchair, walker, crutches, commode, braces, scooter, or sliding board
   2. Adaptive equipment needed for independent functioning (personal hygiene, dressing, cooking)
      a. Need for and availability of amplification systems, assistive listening devices, telecommunication devices, vibrator for alarm clock, visual alert systems, telephone amplifiers
      b. Provision of round-the-clock relay services by tele-

phone companies that is mandated by the Americans with Disabilities Act of 1990 (effective as of June 26, 1993) for individuals who have telecommunication devices for the deaf (TDDs) so they can communicate with those who do not

    c. Communication boards, speech synthesizers

    d. Hearing-ear dogs for the hearing-impaired, guide dogs for the visually impaired, independence dogs

  3. Devices needed to prevent medical sequelae after a disability—for example, a wheelchair cushion or equipment for self-catheterization

B. Funding needed for equipment or devices

C. Availability of vendor and repair contracts

D. Client and family education regarding use, repair, and replacement of equipment

VII. Support and advocacy groups

  A. Associations established and composed of individuals with disabilities such as the National Head Injury Foundation or the Paralyzed Veterans of America

  B. Self-help organizations that assist the disabled by providing a variety of services, such as the Easter Seal Society or Variety Clubs

    1. Offer mutual assistance

    2. Assist with development of coping strategies

    3. Foster abilities and skills to combat isolation and alienation

    4. Develop information networks and counseling

  C. National Institute on Disability and Rehabilitation Research

    1. Oversees comprehensive rehabilitation service programs under the supervision and auspices of the U.S. Department of Education

    2. Participates in research and data collection, provides research grants

    3. Emphasizes community reentry

Occupational/Environmental Health History

Occupational/Environmental Health History—Adapted to Neuman's Systems Model

Identifying Data: Medical Record #:

Name:
Address:
Telephone:
Social Security #:
Sex (circle): Male   Female
Age: _____ Date of Birth: _____

Stressors Perceived by the Client:
I. Chief complaint:

This statement is to be in the patient's own words. It should reflect the reason why the client is currently seeking health care information or services.

Key questions:

1. Describe the health problem or injury you are currently experiencing.
2. Does any other member of your family experience this problem? Any co-worker? Any acquaintance?
3. Do you smoke (packs per day, length of time in years)? Use chewing tobacco? Consume alcohol (how much)?
4. Do you smoke while on the job? At home? Do your co-workers smoke while on the job? Do your family members smoke while you are in the room?
5. Have you missed work within the past 6 weeks? When did these symptoms begin? Have you been forced to stay in bed since the onset of this problem? Are you distressed by this level of disability?
6. Have you ever worked at a job or hobby that caused you to have this problem before? If so, describe the pattern of illness or difficulty. Have you ever found yourself short of breath, lightheaded, dizzy, with a cough, or wheezing while at work or after work? At the beginning of a work week? At the end of a work week? During the weekend?

From Bomar P, editor: *Nurses and family health promotion: concepts, assessment, and interventions,* ed 2, Philadelphia, 1996, WB Saunders.

7. Have you ever changed jobs, homes, hobbies due to a health condition?
8. Have you ever experienced musculoskeletal difficulties, such as back pain, fractures, or muscle strain related to work, home, or play?
9. Name the chemicals and compounds you work with and the frequency of contact with each.
10. Describe your neighborhood. Map out the location of industrial areas, waste disposal sites, water sources, and waste disposal.
11. Are there any community environmental problems that have evolved in recent time? Toxic spills, sewage breakage, smog changes, NIOSH/OSHA investigations pertinent to the patient's condition?
12. Do you use pesticides, cleaning solutions, glues, solvents, heavy metals, or poisons within the home?
13. Type of heating and cooling within the home (electric, natural gas, other) and its impact on the (temporal) illness pattern.

II. Lifestyle patterns:

Note changes in previously stated patterns. It's important to note changes within the physical living environment, occupational setting (of client or other family members), and recreational environment.

Power and authority: Who makes decisions for the family? Is there a struggle for power within the family unit? Does this illness evidence possibly impact on power distribution within family?

Allocation of role and division of labor: Are roles perceived as appropriate by the client? Do the roles meet the client's needs? How are family chores and responsibilities divided among family members? Does the client perceive that this issue will affect the distribution of labor in any particular fashion?

Financial resources: Note the income and major outflow stressors. Will this illness cause any change within the home (physical) environment or location? Will this stressor cause perceived changes within the occupational and recreational spheres?

Spiritual beliefs: What are the spiritual beliefs of this family? Do such beliefs have bearing on the physical environment?

Activities of daily living: Include information about dietary habits, transportation method and patterns, housekeeping patterns and products, care of ill and infirm family members, sleep and rest patterns. Does the client perceive any of these areas to be of major concern?

Process characteristics: Note atmosphere within the home, methods of communication, developmental tasks, and use of extended family network. How does the family process information from the physical environment? How does the family or individual respond to adverse conditions within the occupational, recreational, or general environment? Are they able to act when the physical environment appears dangerous? When given advice about issues within their physical environment, are they able to process the information and make changes that diminish stressors?

Coping patterns: What makes the symptom or problem diminish or go away? Temporal sequence—map out the correlation of symptoms with work time, play time, home time, and recreational habits of the patient and individuals within the family.

Availability of resources: What resources are available from personal, local government, or national government assets to treat this environmental stressor? Is the family able to act independently on advice to use services within the health care or general community, or must a professional assist? Is this stressor occupationally induced or exacerbated? If so, what resources are available through the employer to deal with this stressor?

Client goals and perceived assets: What does the client perceive as his or her sphere of influence on this problem? Health beliefs and attitudes—observable wellness activities, fatalism, use of emergency rooms or clinics. Does the client show evidence of a primary provider of health care services or use of informal nonprofessional network of health care providers?

Stressors as perceived by the caregiver:

List the major problems or stressors as perceived by the provider.

Do these observations differ from the client's perceptions? If so, how so?

How have previous problems or stressors paralleled this situation? How did the client treat the problem? What was the outcome?

What resources does the client possess? What resources are missing? What available resources need augmentation?

What do you perceive the client expects from the health care provider? What role will you play in their illness and recovery?

Impressions:
1. Intrapersonal factors
   a. Physical factors
   b. Psychosociocultural
   c. Developmental
2. Interpersonal factors—summarize the resources of immediate and extended family, work environment, and recreational environment.
3. Extrapersonal factors—summarize community resources, occupational, and federal and state programs that may facilitate resolution of this problem.

4. Problem statement—use nursing diagnosis to formulate your problem statement. Note target dates for reassessment, and state changes in stressors, intra-, inter-, and extrapersonal stressors when reassessing a problem.

Taking an Exposure History

This section provides two examples of environmental and occupational history-taking forms that could be used by nurses in a variety of practice settings. The first form, *Comprehensive Occupational and Environmental History,* was created for a faculty development workshop on Environmental and Occupational Health offered by the University of Maryland at Baltimore (June 1993); the second, *Occupational and Environmental Health History Form,* is reprinted with permission from Alyce B. Tarcher's *Principles and Practice of Environmental Medicine* (Plenum Publishing Co., 1992). Both forms enable nurses and other health professionals to assess individual risk and the need for prevention, to diagnose and treat occupational and environmental illnesses, and to develop a sensitivity to the environmental conditions in a community that may contribute to ill health. Taking an exposure history also provides an opportunity for nurses to enhance their relationship with patients by learning more about an individual's workplace, home, and community environments.

Comprehensive Occupational and Environmental History

Work History

1. List your current and past longest held jobs, including the military:

Company	Dates employed	Job title	Known exposure
_____	_____	_____	_____
_____	_____	_____	_____
_____	_____	_____	_____

From Institute of Medicine: *Nursing, Health, and Environment,* Washington, 1995, National Academy Press.

From Pope A, Snyder M, Mood L, editors: *Nursing, health and the environment,* 1995, Institute of Medicine, National Academy Press, Washington, D.C..

Comprehensive Occupational and Environmental History—cont'd

2. Do you work full-time? NO ____ YES ____ How many hours per week? ____

3. Do you work part-time? NO ____ YES ____ How many hours per week?____

4. Please describe any health problems or injuries that you have experienced in connection with your present or past jobs:

5. Have you ever had to change jobs due to health problems or injuries? YES ____ NO ____
   If so, describe:

   Did any of your co-workers experience similar problems?

6. In what type of business do you currently work?

7. Describe your work (what do you actually do):

Continued.

Comprehensive Occupational and Environmental History—cont'd

Work History

8. Have you had any current or past exposure (through breathing or touching) to any of the following?

__ acids
__ alcohols
__ alkalies
__ ammonia
__ arsenic
__ asbestos
__ benzene
__ beryllium
__ cadmium
__ carbon tetrachloride
__ chlorinated napthalenes
__ chloroform
__ chloroprene
__ chromates
__ coal dust
__ cold (severe)
__ dichlorobenzene
__ ethylene dibromide
__ ethylene dichloride
__ fiberglass
__ halothane
__ heat (severe)
__ isocyanates
__ ketones

__ lead
__ manganese
__ mercury
__ methylene chloride
__ nickel
__ noise (loud)
__ PBBs
__ PCBs
__ perchloroethylene
__ pesticides
__ phenol
__ phosgene
__ radiation
__ rock dust
__ silica powder
__ solvents
__ styrene
__ toluene
__ TDI or MDI
__ trichloroethylene
__ trinitrotoluene (TNT)
__ vibration
__ vinyl chloride
__ welding fumes
__ x-rays
__ talc

9. Did you receive any safety training about these agents?   YES ____   NO ____
Explain:

Comprehensive Occupational and Environmental History—cont'd

10. Are you involved in any work processes such as grinding, welding, soldering, or polishing that create dust, mists, or fumes?   YES___   NO___   (If yes, describe):

11. Did you use any of the following personal protective equipment when exposed?

    ___ boots   ___ respirator
    ___ coveralls   ___ safety shoes
    ___ earplugs/muffs   ___ shield
    ___ glasses/goggles   ___ sleeves
    ___ gloves   ___ welding mask

12. Is your work environment generally clean? If not, describe:

13. What ventilation systems are used in your workplace?

14. Do they seem to work? Are you aware of any chemical odors in your environment (if so, explain)?

15. Where do you eat, smoke, and take your breaks when you are on the job?

16. Do you use a uniform or have clothing that you wear only to work?

17. How is your work clothing laundered (at home, by employer, other)?

18. How often do you wash your hands at work and how do you wash them (running water, special soaps, other)?

Continued.

Comprehensive Occupational and Environmental History—cont'd

---

19. Do you shower before leaving the worksite?

20. Do you have any physical symptoms associated with work? If yes, describe:

21. Are other workers similarly affected?

Home Exposures

1. Which of the following do you have in your home?

__ air conditioner   __ woodstove
__ air purifier   __ central heating (gas)
__ electric stove   __ central heating (oil)
__ fireplace

2. In approximately what year was your home built?

3. Have there been any recent renovations? If yes, describe:

4. Have you recently installed new carpet, bought new furniture, or refinished existing furniture? If yes, explain:

5. Do you use pesticides around your home or garden? If yes, describe:

6. What household cleaners do you use? (List most common and any new products you use.)

Comprehensive Occupational and Environmental History—cont'd

7. List all hobbies done at your home:

   Are any of the agents listed earlier for work exposures encountered in hobbies or recreational activities?

   Is any special protective equipment or ventilation used during hobbies? Explain:

8. What are the occupations of other household members?

9. Do other household members have contact with any form of chemicals at work or during leisure activities? If so, explain:

10. Is anyone else in your home environment having symptoms similar to yours?
    If yes, explain briefly:

Community Exposures

1. Are any of the following located in your community?

___ industrial plant   ___ toxic spill
___ landfill   ___ waste site
___ major source of   ___ other (specify: _____)
    air pollution

2. What is your source of drinking water?

___ private well   ___ other (specify: _____)
___ public water source

3. Are neighbors experiencing any health problems similar to yours? If yes, explain.

Key Occupational and Environmental Health Questions to Be Asked with All Histories

1. What are your current and past longest-held jobs?

2. Have you been exposed to any radiation or chemical liquids, dusts, mists, or fumes?

3. Is there any relationship between current symptoms and activities at work or at home?

Occupational and environmental health history form

I. Identification

Name _____

Address _____

_____ Zip _____

Telephone: home _____ work _____

Soc. Sec. ____ - ____ - ____

Sex: M ___ F ___

Birthday _____

II. Occupational history

Fill in the table below listing all jobs at which you have worked, including short-term, seasonal, and part-time employment. Start with your present job and go back to the first. Use additional paper if necessary.

Workplace (employer's name and address or city)	Dates worked		Type of industry (describe)	Your job duties (describe)	Health hazards in workplace (gases, dust, metals, solvents, radiation, infectious agents, etc.)	Protective equipment used (describe)	Health problems related to work (describe)
	From	To					

Occupational exposure

1. Describe any health problems or injuries related to present or past jobs.

2. Have you or your co-workers had health problems or injuries?
3. Do you believe you have health problems related to your present or past work?
4. Have you been absent from work because of a work-related illness or injury? If so, describe:

5. Have you worked with a substance that caused a skin rash? What was the substance? Describe your reaction:

6. Have you had trouble with breathing, coughing, or wheezing while at work? If so, describe:

7. Do you have any allergies? If so, describe:

8. Have you had difficulty conceiving a child?
9. Do you have any children who were born with abnormalities?
10. Do you smoke or have you ever smoked cigarettes, cigars, or pipes? For how long and how many per day?

11. Do you smoke on the job?

12. Have you ever worked at a job or hobby in which you came into direct contact with any of the following substances through breathing, touching, or direct exposure? If so, please place a checkmark beside the substance.

__ acids	__ manganese
__ alcohols (industrial)	__ mercury
__ alkalis	__ methylene chloride
__ ammonia	__ nickel
__ arsenic	__ noise (loud)
__ asbestos	__ PBBs
__ benzene	__ PCBs
__ beryllium	__ perchloroethylene
__ cadmium	__ pesticides
__ carbon tetrachloride	__ phenols
__ chlorinated napthalenes	__ phosgene
__ chloroform	__ radiation
__ chloroprene	__ rock dust
__ chromates	__ silica powder
__ coal dust	__ solvents
__ cold (severe)	__ styrene
__ dichlorobenzene	__ talc
__ ethylene dibromide	__ toluene
__ ethylene dichloride	__ TDI or MDI
__ fiberglass	__ trichloroethylene
__ halothane	__ trinitrotoluene (TNT)
__ heat (severe)	__ vibration
__ isocyanates	__ vinyl chloride
__ ketones	__ welding fumes
__ lead	__ x-rays

If you have answered "yes" to any of the above, please describe your exposure on a separate sheet of paper.

Environmental exposure

1. Do you live in the central city or in a rural, urban, or suburban area?
2. Have you ever changed your residence or home because of a health problem? If so, describe:

3. Do you live in the immediate vicinity of a refinery, smelter, factory, battery recycling plant, hazardous waste site, or other potential pollution source?

4. Do you (and your child) live in or regularly visit a building with peeling or chipped lead paint (such as those built before 1960)? Has there been recent, ongoing, or planned renovation or remodeling of this structure(s)?

5. Do any members of your household have contact with dusts or chemicals in the workplace that are then brought into the home?

6. Do you have a hobby that you do at home? If so, describe:

7. Do you fumigate your home or use pesticides in and around your home and on a pet? Do you use mothballs?

8. What cleaning agents and solvents are used in your home?

9. Is there evidence of mold in your home?

10. Which of the following do you use in your home?

  __ air conditioner   __ humidifier
  __ electric stove   __ wood stove
  __ air purifier   __ gas stove
  __ fireplace   __ unvented kerosene or gas heater

11. What is your source of drinking water?

   __ community water system   __ bottled water
   __ private well

Agency for Toxic Substances and Disease Registry 1993 Priority List of Rank-Ordered Top 10 Hazardous Substances

Hazardous agents	Sources	Exposure pathways	Systems affected
Lead	Storage batteries Manufacture of paint, enamel, ink, glass, rubber, ceramics, chemicals	Ingestion Inhalation	Hematologic Renal Neuromuscular GI, CNS
Arsenic	Manufacture of pigments, glass, pharmaceuticals, insecticides, fungicides, rodenticides Tanning	Ingestion Inhalation	Neuromuscular Skin GI
Metallic mercury	Electronics Paints Metal and textile production Chemical manufacturing Pharmaceutical production	Inhalation Percutaneous and GI absorption	Pulmonary CNS Renal
Benzene	Manufacture of organic chemicals, detergents, pesticides, solvents, paint removers	Inhalation Percutaneous absorption	CNS Hematopoietic

Continued

NOTE: CNS, central nervous system; GI, gastrointestinal.

From Pope A, Snyder M, Mood L editors: *Nursing, health and the environment*, Washington, DC, 1995, Institute of Medicine, National Academy Press.

Agency for Toxic Substances and Disease Registry 1993 Priority List of Rank-Ordered Top 10 Hazardous Substances—cont'd

Hazardous agents	Sources	Exposure pathways	Systems affected
Vinyl chloride	Production of polyvinyl chloride and other plastics Chlorinated compounds Used as a refrigerant	Inhalation Ingestion	Hepatic Neurologic Pulmonary
Cadmium	Electroplating Solder	Inhalation	Pulmonary Renal
Polychlorinated biphenyls	Formerly used in electrical equipment	Inhalation Ingestion	Skin Eyes Hepatic
Benzo(a)pyrene*	Emissions from refuse burning and autos Used as laboratory reagent Found in charcoal-grilled meats and in cigarette smoke	Inhalation Ingestion Percutaneous absorption	Pulmonary Skin Eyes
Chloroform	Aerosol propellants Fluorinated resins produced during chlorination of water Used as a refrigerant	Inhalation Percutaneous absorption Ingestion	CNS Renal Hepatic Mucous membrane Cardiac
Benzo(b)-fluoranthene	Cigarette smoke	Inhalation	Pulmonary

*BAP is a probable human carcinogen.

Selected Work-Related Health Risks

Diseases, disorders, and conditions associated with various agents, industries, or occupations: infections, malignant neoplasms, and hematological, cardiovascular, pulmonary, neurological, and miscellaneous disorders

Diseases, disorders, and conditions	Industry or occupation	Agent
Infections		
Anthrax	Shepherds, farmers, butchers, handlers of imported hides or fibers, veterinarians, veterinarian pathologists, weavers	*Bacillus anthracis*
Brucellosis	Farmers, shepherds, veterinarians, lab and slaughterhouse workers	*Brucella abortus, B. suis*
Plague	Shepherds, farmers, ranchers, hunters, field geologists	*Yersinia pestis*
Hepatitis A	Day-care center, orphanage, and mental retardation institution staff, medical personnel	Hepatitis A virus
Hepatitis B	Nurses and aides, anesthesiologists, orphanage and mental institution staffs, medical lab workers, general dentists, oral surgeons, physicians	Hepatitis B virus
Hepatitis C (formerly included in non-A, non-B)	Same as hepatitis A and B	Hepatitis C virus
Ornithosis	Psittacine bird breeders, pet shop and zoo workers, poultry producers, veterinarians	*Chlamydia psittaci*
Rabies	Veterinarians, game wardens, lab workers, farmers, ranchers, trappers	Rabies virus
Rubella	Medical personnel	Rubella virus
Tetanus	Farmers, ranchers	*Clostridium tetani*

Continued.

From Tarcher AB, editor: *Principles and practice of environmental medicine,* 1992, Plenum Publishing.

Selected work-related health risks—cont'd

Diseases, disorders, and conditions	Industry or occupation	Agent
Infections—cont'd		
Tuberculosis (pulmonary)	Physicians, medical personnel, medical lab workers	*Mycobacterium tuberculosis*
Tubercuolosis (silicotuberculosis)	Quarrymen, sandblasters, silica processors, miners, foundry workers, ceramic industry workers	Silicon dixoide (silica), *M. tuberculosis*
Tularemia	Hunters, fur handlers, sheep industry workers, cooks, veterinarians, ranchers, veterinarian pathologists	*Francisella tularensis*
Malignant neoplasms		
Bladder	Rubber and dye workers	Benzidine, 1- and 2-naphthylamine, auramine, magenta, 4-aminobiphenyl, 4-nitrophenyl
Bone	Dial painters, radium chemists and processors	Radium
Kidney and other urinary tract organs	Coke oven workers	Coke oven emissions
Liver	Vinyl chloride polymerization industry workers	Vinyl chloride monomer
Liver hemangiosarcoma	Vintners	Arsenical pesticides
Lung, bronchial, tracheal	Asbestos industry workers, asbestos users	Asbestos
	Topside coke oven workers	Coke oven emissions
	Uranium and fluorspar miners	Radon daughters
	Chromium producers, processors, users	Chromates
	Smelters	Arsenic
	Mustard gas formulators	Mustard gas
	Ion-exchange resin makers, chemists	Bis(chloro-methyl)-ether, chloromethyl, methyl ether

Selected work-related health risks—cont'd

Diseases, disorders, and conditions	Industry or occupation	Agent
Nasal cavity	Woodworkers, furniture makers	Hardwood dusts
	Boot and shoe industry workers	Unknown
	Radium chemists and processors, dial painters	Radium
	Chromium producers, processors, users	Chromates
	Nickel smelting and refining workers	Nickel Asbestos
Peritoneal, pleural mesothelioma	Asbestos industry workers, asbestos users	Asbestos
Scrotal	Automatic lathe operators, metalworkers	Mineral, cutting oils
	Coke oven workers, petroleum refiners, tar distillers	Soots and tars, tar distillates
Hematologic disorders		
Agranulocytosis or neutropenia	Workers exposed to benzene	Benzene
	Explosives, pesticide industry workers	Phosphorus
	Pesticide, pigment, pharmaceutical industry workers	Inorganic arsenic
Anemia (aplastic)	Explosives manufacturing	TNT
	Workers exposed to benzene	Benzene
	Radiologists, radium chemists, dial painters	Ionizing radiation
Anemia (hemolytic, nonautoimmune)	Whitewashing and leather industry workers	Copper sulfate
	Electrolytic processes, arsenical ore smelting	Arsines
	Plastics industry workers	Trimellitic anhydride
	Dye, celluloid, and resin industry workers	Naphthalene
Leukemia (acute lymphoid)	Rubber industry workers	Unknown
	Radiologists	Ionizing radiation
Leukemia (acute myeloid)	Workers exposed to benzene	Benzene
	Radiologists	Ionizing radiation

Continued.

Selected work-related health risks—cont'd

Diseases, disorders, and conditions	Industry or occupation	Agent
Hematologic Disorders—cont'd		
Leukemia (erythroleukemia)	Workers exposed to benzene	Benzene
Methemoglobinemia	Explosives, dye industry workers	Aromatic amino and nitro compounds (such as aniline, TNT, nitroglycerin)
Cardiovascular disorders		
Angina	Auto mechanics, foundry workers, wood finishers, traffic control, driving in heavy traffic	Carbon monoxide
Arrhythmias	Metal cleaning, solvent use, refrigerator maintenance	Solvents, fluorocarbons
Raynaud's phenomenon	Lumberjacks, chain sawyers, grinders, chippers	Whole-body or segmental vibration
(Secondary)	Vinyl chloride polymerization industry workers	Vinyl chloride monomer
Pulmonary disorders		
Alveolitis (extrinsic, allergic)	Farmers (farmer's lung bagassosis), bird breeders (bird-breeder's lung), cook handlers (suberosis), brewery and distillery workers (maltworker's lung); mushroom workers (mushroom worker's lung); maple bark disease, cheese makers (cheese makers, cheese-washer's lung) coffee workers (coffee-worker's lung), fish meal workers (fish-meal-worker's lung), furriers (furrier's lung); logging and sawmill workers (sequoiosis); woodworkers (woodworker's lung); mill workers (miller's lung)	Various agents

Selected work-related health risks—cont'd

Diseases, disorders, and conditions	Industry or occupation	Agent
Asbestosis	Asbestos industry workers, asbestos users	Asbestos
Asthma (extrinsic)	Jewelry, alloy, catalyst makers	Platinum
	Polyurethane, adhesive, paint workers	Isocyanates
	Alloy, catalyst, refinery workers	Chromium, cobalt
	Solderers	Aluminum soldering flux
	Plastic, dye, insecticide makers	Phthalic anhydride
	Foam workers, latex makers, biologists	Formaldehyde
	Printing industry	Gum arabic
	Nickel platers	Nickel sulfate
	Bakers	Flour
	Plastics industry workers	Trimellitic anhydride
	Woodworkers, furniture makers	Red cedar, wood dusts
	Detergent formulators	Bacillus-derived exoenzymes
	Animal handlers	Animal dander
Beryllium disease (chronic)	Beryllium alloy, ceramic, cathode-ray tube, nuclear reactor workers	Beryllium
Bronchitis, pneumonitis, pulmonary edema (acute)	Refrigeration, fertilizer, oil-refining industry workers	Ammonia
	Alkali, beach industry workers	Chlorine
	Silo fillers, arc welders, nitric acid workers	Nitrogen oxides
	Paper, refrigeration, oil-refining industry workers	Sulfur dioxide
	Cadmium smelters, processors	Cadmium
	Plastics industry workers	Trimellitic anhydride
Byssinosis	Cotton industry workers	Cotton, flax, hemp, cotton-synthetic dusts

Continued.

Selected work-related health risks—cont'd

Diseases, disorders, and conditions	Industry or occupation	Agent
Pulmonary Disorders—cont'd		
Pneumoconiosis	Coal miners, bauxite workers	Coal dust, bauxite fumes
Silicosis	Mining, metal, and ceramic industry workers, quarrymen, sand blasters, silica processors	Silica
Talcosis	Talc processors	Talc
Neurological disorders		
Cerebellar ataxia	Chemical industry	Toluene
	Electrolytic chlorine production workers, battery manufacturing workers, fungicide formulators	Organic mercury
Encephalitis (toxic)	Battery, smelter, foundry workers	Lead
	Electrolytic chlorine production workers, battery manufacturing workers, fungicide formulators	Organic, inorganic mercury
Neuropathy (toxic and inflammatory)	Pesticide, pigment, pharmaceutical industry workers	Arsenic, arsenic compounds
	Furniture refinishers, degreasers	Hexane
	Plastic-coated-fabric workers	Methyl butyl ketone
	Explosives industry workers	TNT
	Rayon manufacturing workers	Carbon disulfide
	Plastics, hydraulics, coke industry workers	Tri-*o*-cresyl phosphate
	Battery, smelter, foundry workers	Inorganic lead
	Dentists, chloralkali workers	Inorganic mercury
	Chloralkali, fungicide, battery workers	Organic mercury
	Plastics, paper manufacturing workers	Acrylamide

Selected work-related health risks—cont'd

Diseases, disorders, and conditions	Industry or occupation	Agent
Parkinson's disease (secondary)	Manganese processors, battery manufacturing workers, welders	Manganese
	Internal combustion engine industry workers	Carbon monoxide
Miscellaneous		
Abdominal pain	Battery manufacturing workers, enamelers, smelter, painters, ceramics workers, plumbers, welders	Lead
Cataract	Microwave, radar technicians	Microwaves
	Explosive industry workers	TNT
	Radiologists	Ionizing radiation
	Blacksmiths, glass blowers, bakers	Infrared radiation
	Moth repellent formulators, fumigators	Naphthalene
	Explosives, dye, herbicide, pesticide industry workers	Dinitrophenol, dinitro-*o*-cresol
Dermatitis (contact, allergic)	Adhesives, sealants, and plastics industry workers, leather tanning workers, poultry dressing workers, fish packing workers, boat building and repair workers, electroplating workers, metal cleaning workers, machining, housekeeping	Irritants (cutting oils, solvents, phenols, acids, alkalies, detergents, fibrous glass), allergens (nickel, epoxy resins, chromates, formaldehyde, dyes, rubber products)
Headache	Firefighters, foundry workers, wood finishers, dry cleaners, traffic control workers, driving in heavy traffic	Carbon monoxide, solvents

Continued.

Selected work-related health risks—cont'd

Diseases, disorders, and conditions	Industry or occupation	Agent
Miscellaneous—cont'd		
Hepatitis (toxic)	Solvent users, dry cleaners, plastics industry workers	Carbon tetrachloride, chloroform, tetrachlorethane, trichloroethylene
	Explosives and dye industries	Phosphorus, TNT
	Fire and waterproofing additive formulators	Chloronaphthalene
	Plastics formulators	4,4-Methylenedianiline
	Fumigators, gasoline and fire-extinguisher formulators	Ethylene dibromide
	Disinfectant, fumigant, synthetic resin formulators	Cresol
Inner ear damage	Various	Excessive noise
Infertility (male)	Formulators	Kepone
	Producers, formulators, applicators	1,2-Dibromo-3-chloropropane
Psychosis (acute)	Gasoline, seed, and fungicide workers, wood preservation, rayon manufacturing	Lead (especially organic), mercury, carbon disulfide
Renal failure (acute, chronic)	Battery manufacturing, plumbers, solderers	Inorganic lead
	Electrolytic processes, arsenical ore smelting	Arsine
	Battery manufacturing, jewelers, dentists	Inorganic mercury
	Fluorocarbon, fire-extinguisher formulators	Carbon tetrachloride
	Antifreeze manufacturing	Ethylene glycol

Selected Job Categories, Exposures, and Associated Work-Related Diseases and Conditions

Job categories	Exposures	Work-related diseases and conditions
Agricultural workers	Pesticides, infectious agents, gases, sunlight	Pesticide poisoning, farmer's lung, skin cancer
Anesthetists	Anesthetic gases	Reproductive effects, cancer
Animal handlers	Infectious agents, allergens	Asthma
Automobile workers	Asbestos, plastics, lead, solvents	Asbestosis, dermatitis
Bakers	Flour	Asthma
Battery makers	Lead, arsenic	Lead poisoning, cancer
Butchers	Vinyl plastic fumes	Meat wrappers' asthma
Caisson workers	Pressurized work environments	Nitrogen narcosis (Caisson disease, the bends)
Carpenters	Wood dust, wood preservatives, adhesives	Nasopharyngeal cancer, dermatitis
Cement workers	Cement dust, metals	Dermatitis, bronchitis
Ceramic workers	Talc, clays	Pneumoconiosis
Demolition workers	Asbestos, wood dust	Asbestosis
Drug manufacturers	Hormones, nitroglycerin, etc.	Reproductive effects
Dry cleaners	Solvents	Liver disease, dermatitis
Dye workers	Dyestuffs, metals, solvents	Bladder cancer, dermatitis
Embalmers	Formaldehyde, infectious agents	Dermatitis
Felt makers	Mercury, polycyclic hydrocarbons	Mercuralism
Foundry workers	Silica, molten metals	Silicosis
Glass workers	Heat, solvents, metal powders	Cataracts

Continued.

Selected job categories, exposures, and associated work-related diseases and conditions—cont'd

Job categories	Exposures	Work-related diseases and conditions
Hospital workers	Infectious agents, cleansers, radiation	Infections, accidents
Insulators	Asbestos, fibrous glass	Asbestosis, lung cancer, mesothelioma
Jack hammer operators	Vibration	Raynaud's phenomenon
Lathe operators	Metal dusts, cutting oils	Lung disease, cancer
Laundry workers	Bleaches, soaps, alkalies	Dermatitis
Lead burners	Lead	Lead poisoning
Miners (coal, hard rock, metals, etc.)	Talc, radiation, metals, coal dust, silica	Pneumoconiosis, lung cancer
Natural gas workers	Polycyclic hydrocarbons	Lung cancer
Nuclear workers	Radiation, plutonium	Metal poisoning, cancer
Office workers	Poor lighting, poorly designed equipment	Joint problems, eye problems
Painters	Paints, solvents, spackling compounds	Neurologic problems
Paper makers	Acids, alkalies, solvents, metals	Lung disorders, dermatitis
Petroleum workers	Polycyclic hydrocarbons, catalysts, zeolites	Cancer, pneumoconiosis
Plumbers	Lead, solvents, asbestos	Lead poisoning
Railroad workers	Creosote, sunlight, oils, solvents	Cancer, dermatitis
Seamen	Sunlight, asbestos	Cancer, accidents
Smelter workers	Metals, heat, sulfur dioxide, arsenic	Cancer
Steel workers	Heat, metals, silica	Cataracts, heat stroke
Stone cutters	Silica	Silicosis
Textile workers	Cotton dust, fabrics, finishers, dyes, carbon disulfide	Byssinosis, dermatitis, psychosis
Varnish makers	Solvents, waxes	Dermatitis
Vineyard workers	Arsenic, pesticides	Cancer, dermatitis
Welders	Fumes, nonionizing radiation	Lead poisoning, cataracts

Building Accessibility Checklist

The following checklist can be used as a guide to comply with the American National Standards Institute and Uniform Federal Accessibility Standards for making buildings accessible to the physically handicapped. The following checklist is based on both the ANSI and UFAS standards. In some places where UFAS differs from ANSI, both specifications are included. This is done particularly in the use of technical terms.

Type of Building or Project
1. A new construction?
2. An addition?
3. An alteration?
4. A historic preservation building?
5. A leased building?
6. A housing or dwelling unit?

Building Site, Exterior, Route
1. Does the grading of the building site allow the approaches to the building to be substantially level?
2. Is there parking within 200 feet of the building entrance?
3. Is any of the parking reserved for the handicapped?
4. Are any parking spaces open on one side to allow easy access for wheelchairs and for people who use braces to get in and out of the automobile?
5. Are the parking spaces on level ground?
6. Are there ramps or level spaces to allow people to enter the building without crossing a curb?
7. How many accessible parking spaces are there?
8. Is there an accessible route connecting buildings, facilities, other architectural elements and spaces on the same site?
9. Is there an accessible route within the site from transportation stops, accessible parking spaces, passenger loading zones, and public streets and sidewalks?
10. Are ground and floor surfaces free of protruding objects and otherwise accessible?

Walkways
1. Are walks at least 48 inches wide?
2. Is the gradient not greater than a 1-foot rise in 20 feet (5 percent)?

From Mumma CM, editor: *Rehabilitation nursing: concepts and practice, a core curriculum,* Skokie, Ill., 1987, Rehabilitation Nursing Foundation.

3. Are walks without interruption (i.e., steps or abrupt changes in level)?
4. If the walks cross a driveway, parking lot or other walks, do they blend into a common, level surface?
5. On elevated walks, is there at least a 5 × 5 foot platform if a door swings out onto the platform or 3 × 5 foot platform if the door swings in?
6. Do walks have nonslip or slip-resistant surfaces?

Buildings: Ramps

1. Do ramps have a slope no greater than a 1-foot rise in 12 feet (8.33 percent)?
2. If ramps are steeper than a 5 percent gradient rise (a rise of 6 inches) or have a horizontal projection of more than 72 inches, are handrails provided?
3. If there are handrails, are they at least 32 inches above ramp surface?
4. Are there handrails on both sides?
5. Are the ramp surfaces smooth?
6. Is the clear width of the ramp at least 36 inches (3 feet)?
7. Do the handrails extend 1 foot beyond the top and bottom of the ramp?
8. Are the ramp surfaces nonslip or slip-resistant?
9. Do ramps have a level 6-foot clearance at the bottom?
10. Do ramps with a gradient steeper than 5 percent have level spaces (a minimum of 3 feet in length) at 30-foot intervals?
11. Are these level rest areas at least 5 feet wide (to provide for turns)?
12. Is the cross slope 1:50 or less?
13. Are edges protected to preclude slipping off?
14. Will water accumulate on outdoor ramp or approach to it?

Buildings: Entrances and Exits

1. Is at least one entrance to the building accessible to people in wheelchairs?
2. Is at least one entrance accessible to wheelchairs on a level that would make the elevators accessible?
3. Is the accessible entrance on an accessible route?
4. Is the service entrance the only accessible entrance?

Buildings: Doors and Doorways

1. Do doors have a clear opening at least 32 inches wide?
2. Can doors be opened in a single effort? Can handles, pulls, latches, locks be grasped and operated with one hand?

3. Is the floor of the doorway level within 5 feet from the door in the direction it swings?
4. Does this level space extend 1 foot beyond each side of the door?
5. Does it extend 3 feet in the direction opposite to the door swing?
6. Do thresholds exceed ½ inch (¾ inches for exterior sliding doors)?
7. Is the speed of door closers at least 3 seconds?
8. Does the door require more than 5 pounds of pressure to open?
9. Where there are hinged or pivoted doors in a series, are they at least 48 inches plus the width of the swinging inward door path?

Buildings: Stairs and Steps

1. Do the steps avoid protruding lips and abrupt nosings at the edge of each step?
2. Do stairs have handrails at least 32 inches above step level?
3. Will water accumulate on outdoor stairs and approaches?
4. Are tread heights and risers uniform?
5. How many accessible stairs and sets of stairs are there?
6. Do stairs have handrails on both sides that extend at least 12 inches beyond the top and at least 19 inches from the bottom step?
7. Do steps have risers 7 inches or less?

Buildings: Floors

1. Do floors have nonslip or slip-resistant surface?
2. Are floors on each story at a common level or connected by a ramp?
3. Is carpet (or carpet tile) securely attached?
4. Do grates have a maximum opening of ½ inch?

Buildings: Restrooms

1. How many toilets for either sex are there on each floor with facilities for the physically handicapped?
2. Can physically handicapped persons, particularly those in wheelchairs, enter the restroom?
3. Do toilet rooms have turning space 60 × 60 inches to allow traffic of individuals in wheelchairs?
4. Do toilet rooms have at least one toilet stall that:
   - Is three feet wide?
   - Is at least 4 feet, 8 inches deep?
   - Has a door that is 32 inches wide and swings out?
   - Has a handrail on each side, 33 inches high and parallel to floor, 1½ inches in diameter, with 1½ inches clearance between rail and wall, fastened securely to wall at the ends and center?
   - Has a toilet seat of 17-19 inches from stand?

5. Do toilet rooms have wash basins with narrow aprons, which when mounted at standard height are no greater than 34 inches at the top, and which have a clearance underneath of 29 inches?
6. Are drainpipes and hot water pipes covered or insulated?
7. Is one mirror as low as possible and no higher than 40 inches above the floor?
8. Is one shelf at a height within range and reach of a person in a wheelchair and no lower than 15 inches above the floor?
9. Do toilet rooms for men have wall-mounted urinals with the opening of the basin 19 inches (17 inches under UFAS standards) from the floor, or have floor-mounted urinals that are level with the main floor of the toilet rooms?
10. Are flush controls automatic or hand-operated? Are they 44 inches or less from the floor?
11. Do toilet rooms have controls, coat hooks, towel racks, and towel dispensers mounted no lower than 15 inches from the floor and otherwise within reach?
12. Are disposal units mounted no higher than 40 inches from the floor?
13. Are towel racks, towel dispensers and other appropriate disposal units located to the side rather than above the basins?
14. Is there a shower or bathtub with an accessible seat, grab bars, controls, and proper spacing?

Buildings: Water Fountains

1. How many drinking fountains for use by physically handicapped persons are there on each floor?
2. Can persons in wheelchairs wheel up to fountain?
3. Do water fountains have up-front spouts and controls?
4. Are they hand-operated?
5. If coolers are wall-mounted, are they hand-operated? Are basins 36 inches or less from the floor?

Buildings: Public Telephones

1. How many public telephones in each bank of phones are accessible to the physically handicapped?
2. Is the height of the dial 48 inches or less from the floor?
3. Is the coin slot located 48 inches or less from floor?
4. Is there a clear space of at least 30×40 inches to allow forward or parallel approach?
5. Are these telephones equipped for persons with hearing disabilities? Are those telephones identified as such?
6. Are telephone books (if provided) 48 inches or less from the floor?
7. Are push-button controls (if available) provided?

Buildings: Elevators/Lifts

1. If more than a one-story building, how many elevators are available for the physically handicapped?
2. Can physically handicapped persons, particularly those in wheelchairs, enter elevator?
3. Are outside call buttons centered 48 inches (42 inches under UFAS standards) or less from the floor? Do they have visual signals?
4. Are control buttons inside at least ¾ inches raised? Are they located 48 inches or less from floor?
5. Are the buttons labeled with raised or indented letters beside them?
6. Are they touch-sensitive and easy to push?
7. Is the elevator cab at least 5 × 5 feet?
8. Are visual and audible signals provided at each elevator group to indicate which car is answering the call?
9. Do jambs of each elevator have raised floor designations on both sides?
10. Does the elevator door remain open at least 3 seconds?
11. Can a person in a wheelchair facing the rear see floor numbers, either by mirror or floor identification at rear of car?
12. Are floors announced orally by recorded devices for the benefit of the blind?
13. Are there platform lifts with operable controls, adequate clearances, and appropriate surfaces?

Building: Controls

1. Are light switches no more than 48 inches above the floor?
2. Are controls for heating, cooling, and ventilation no more than 48 inches above the floor?
3. Are controls for fire alarms and other warning devices no more than 48 inches from floor?
4. Are other frequently used controls, such as drapery pulls, no more than 48 inches from floor?
5. Is the force needed to operate the controls no more than 5 pounds?
6. Is there clear space to allow a forward or parallel approach by a person in a wheelchair?

Building: Identification

1. Are raised or recessed letters or numbers used to identify rooms or offices?
2. Is identification placed on wall, either to right or left of door?
3. Is it at a height between 4 feet, 6 inches and 5 feet, 6 inches (measured from floor)?

4. Are doors that might prove dangerous to a blind person if he or she were to enter or exit through them made quickly identifiable to the touch?

Buildings: Warning Signals/Alarms

1. Are audible warning signals accompanied by simultaneous visual signals for the benefit of those with hearing and sight disabilities? Are they set at a level not to exceed 120 decibels?
2. Are visual alarms flashing at less than 5 hertz (hz)?

Buildings: Hazards, Tactile Warnings, Protruding Objects

1. When hazards such as open manhole covers, panels and excavation exits are present, are barricades placed on all open sides at least 8 feet from the hazard? Are warning devices installed?
2. Are there low-hanging door closers that remain within opening of doorways which might protrude dangerously or are more than 2 inches into regular corridors or traffic ways?
3. Are there low-hanging signs, ceiling lights, fixtures or similar objects that protrude more than 4 inches into regular corridors or traffic ways?
4. Is lighting on ramps adequate?
5. Are exit signs easily identifiable to all disabled persons?
6. Are there tactile warnings on doors to hazardous areas?
7. Are there at least 80 inches of clear head room in walls, halls, corridors, aisles, passageways, and circulation spaces?

The following items are not contained in the ANSI standards, but are included in the UFAS document.

Dwelling Units

1. How many units are accessible?
2. How many units are adaptable?
3. Has consumer information about adaptability been provided to the owner or occupant of the dwelling?
4. Has consumer information been provided to the parties who will be responsible for making adaptations?
5. Does the kitchen have at least 40-inch clearances for cabinets, countertops, appliances and walls (U-shaped kitchens: 60 inches)?
6. Is there at least a 30 × 48-inch clear floor space in the kitchen?
7. Are all controls in the kitchen within reach of a person in a wheelchair?

8. In the kitchen is there at least one 30-inch work surface not more than 34 inches above the ground and at least 2 inches thick?
9. Is the maximum height of the sink 34 inches? Is the sink and counter width a maximum of 30 inches?
10. Are ranges and cooktops and their controls insulated or otherwise protected to prevent burns, abrasions, or shocks?
11. Is there a maximum 48-inch height for at least one shelf of all cabinets and storage shelves above work counters?
12. Are ovens self-cleaning with controls on front panels?
13. Are refrigerator and freezers side-by-side or over-and-under types?
14. Are dishwater racks accessbile from the front of the machine?
15. Are laundry facilities on an accessible route? Are the controls within reach?

Food Service Areas (Restaurant or Cafeteria)

1. Is at least 5 percent of all fixed seating or tables 27 inches high, 30 inches wide, and 19 inches deep for knee clearance? Is the tabletop 28-34 inches from the floor?
2. Are there accessible aisles?
3. Where there are mezzanine levels, loggias, or raised platforms, are the same services and decorative character provided on accessible routes?
4. Do food service lines have a minimum clear width of 35 inches?
5. Are tray slides mounted no higher than 34 inches?
6. Are vending machines within reach and easily operable by persons in wheelchairs?
7. Are tableware, dishes, condiments, foods, and beverages displayed and dispensed within reach of a person in a wheelchair, bearing in mind width, turning space, and clearances?

Health Care

1. Is there an accessible entrance to the facility that is protected from the weather by canopy or roof overhang?
2. Does the accessible entrance have an accessible passenger loading zone?
3. Do patient rooms have adequate clear floor and turning space as well as an accessible toilet?

Libraries

1. Is at least 5 percent (minimum 1) of fixed seating, tables, and study carrels accessible in terms of having seating and work surfaces and allowing passage and use by persons in wheelchairs?

2. Is there at least one lane (including any traffic control, security gate, or turnstile) at each checkout area that is accessible?

3. Is the clear aisle space at card catalogs, magazine displays, and reference stacks at least 35 inches?

4. Is the clear aisle width in the stacks 42 inches if possible (36 inches minimum)?

5. Are all public areas accessible?

Home Environment Assessment Guide

General Information

Family Name: _____ Date: _____

Address: _____

_____

Phone: _____

Directions: _____

_____

Type of living quarters:
    Single room: __   Apartment: __   Home: __

If a room or apartment:
    Floor: __   Rent: __   Own: __

Method for gaining access into home:
    Front door: __   Back door: __
    Other: __   Elevator: __   Stairs: __

Family prefers that nurse:
    Call ahead: __   Ring bell: __   Knock: __

A. Outside access has adequate:
Room for entry: __   Lighting: __

_____

Facilities for handicapped or needed equipment and appliances: __

_____

Environmental conditions can be controlled (ice, mud, etc.): _____

_____

Security measures/personnel: _____

_____

_____

From Keating S, Kilmer G: *Home health care nursing concepts and practices,* Philadelphia, 1988, Lippincott.

B. Surrounding grounds provide opportunities for change of scene, recreation, exercise. Neighborhood is safe and secure. Sidewalks, shopping, and public transportation are available. Describe briefly:

_____

_____

_____

C. Living quarters have adequate utilities:
   Telephone: __   Heat: __   Lighting: __
      Garbage disposal: __   (if applicable)
   Hot and cold water from safe supply: __
      Sewage disposal: __   (if applicable)
   Food storage and preparation: __
      Bathing facilities: __   (if applicable)
   Furniture: __   Sleeping room: __   (if applicable)
   Study and leisure time facilities: _____
   Other: _____

   _____

D. The ill client's room or care providing site has space for:
   Equipment and supplies: _____
   Storage facilities: _____
   Ambulation and mobility: _____
   Privacy: _____
      adequate:
   Access to water and disposal of wastes: _____
   Lighting: _____
   Summary of assessment data: _____

   _____

   _____

Diagnostic Cluster: Environment: Safety Patterns

Problem list of actual or potential environmental hazards:

1.
2.

Nursing diagnoses:
   Coping, ineffective, family
   Family processes, alterations in
   Health maintenance, alterations in
   Home maintenance management, impaired
   Infection, potential for
   Injury, potential for
   Knowledge deficit
   Mobility, impaired, physical
   Self-care deficit, total or partial

Related to which problems:

1.
2.

Long-term goals (outcomes):

1.
2.

Short-term goals (objectives) for each long-term goal:

1. Specific outcome desired
2. Measurable action verb
3. Extent of expectations
4. By whom
5. Time frame

Nursing care plan:

1. What is to be done
2. By whom
3. When and how often
4. Where
5. Method(s)
6. Documentation

Evaluation

Progress as measured by meeting objectives:
Outcome as measured by meeting long-term goal(s):
Diagnosis #: Resolved on date _____
Problems not resolved: Reasons _____

_____

Signed _____, RN

_____

Client/family member

Summary of Steps in Formulating an Environmental Health Nursing Diagnosis

Part	Function	Question to answer
1	Identify target group or community aggregate (e.g., children or residents within 1 mile of site contamination)	Who in the community is at highest risk?
2	Identify potential (or actual) unhealthful response or potential for injury	Is there a significant potential for injury or has an actual injury occurred?
3	Identify related host and environmental factors	Host: What characteristics of the target group influence the potential for injury? Environment: What characteristics of the environment influence the potential for injury?
4	Identify any existing data that may substantiate the nursing diagnosis	Do any epidemiologic or other health outcome data correlate potential for injury with environmental contamination?

From Neufer L: The role of the community health nurse in environmental health, *PublicHealth Nurs* 11(3):155.

A Model Assessment Guide for Nursing in Industry

Components	Questions to ask
The company	
Historic development	How, why, and by whom was the company founded?
Organization chart	What is the formal order of the system, and to whom are the health providers responsible?
Company Policies	Is there a policy manual? Are the workers aware of existence of the manual?
Length of the work week	How many days a week does the industry operate?
Length of the work time	Are there several shifts? How many breaks? Is there paid vacation?

Continued.

Adapted from Serafini P: Nursing assessment in industry: a model. *Am J Public Health* 66(8):755-760, 1976. In Anderson E, McFarlane: *Community as partner: theory and practice in nursing,* ed 2, Philadelphia, 1996, Lippincott.

A model assessment guide for nursing in industry—cont'd

Components	Questions to ask
Sick leave	Is there a clear policy? Do the workers know it?
Safety and fire provisions	Is management aware of situations or substances in the plant that represent a potential danger? Are there organized fire drills? (The *Federal Register* is the source of information for federal standards and serves as a helpful guide.)
Support services (benefits)	
Insurance programs	Is there a system for health insurance and life insurance, and is it compulsory? Does the company pay all or part? Who fills out the necessary forms?
Retirement program	Are the benefits realistic?
Educational support	Can the workers further their education? Will the company help financially?
Safety committee	If there is no committee, do certain people routinely handle emergencies? The Red Cross First Aid Course through programmed instruction is excellent (for information, consult your local Red Cross).
Recreation committee	Do the workers have any communication with or interest in each other outside the work setting?
Employee relations	Are there problems in employee relations? (This is difficult information to get, but it is important to get a sense of employees generally feelings about management and vice versa.)
The plant	
General physical setting	What is the overall appearance?
The construction	What is the size and general condition of buildings and grounds?
Parking facilities and public transportation stops	How far does the worker have to walk to get inside?
Entrances and exits	How many people must use them? How accessible are they?
Physical environment	What conditions exist in the physical environment? (Comment on heating, air-conditioning, lighting, glare, drafts, etc.)
Communication facilities	Are there bulletin boards and newsletters?

A model assessment guide for nursing in industry—cont'd

Components	Questions to ask
Housekeeping	Is the physical setting maintained adequately?
Interior decoration	Are the surroundings conducive to work? Are they pleasing?
Work areas	
Space	Are workers isolated or crowded?
Heights: workplace and supply areas	Is there a chance of workers falling or being injured by falling objects? (Falls and falling objects are dangerous and costly to industry.)
Stimulation	Is the worker too bored to pay attention?
Safety signs and markings	Are dangerous areas well marked?
Standing and sitting facilities	Are chairs safe and comfortable? Are there platforms to stand on, especially for wet processes?
Safety equipment	Do the workers make use of hard hats, safety glasses, face masks, radiation badges, and so forth? Do they know the safety devices that the OSHA regulations require?
Nonwork areas	
Lockers	If the work is dirty, workers should be able to change clothes. Are they accidentally carrying toxic substances home on their clothes?
Hand-washing facilities	If facilities and supplies are available, do workers know how and when to wash their hands?
Rest rooms	How accessible are they, and what condition are they in?
Drinking water	Can workers leave their jobs long enough to get a drink of water when they want to?
Recreation and rest facilities	Can a worker who is not feeling well lie down? Do workers feel free to use the facilities?
Telephones	Can a worker receive or make a call? Does a working mother have to stay home for a call because she can't be reached at work?
Ashtrays	Are people allowed to smoke in designated areas? Are they safe areas?

Continued.

A model assessment guide for nursing in industry—cont'd

Components	Questions to ask
The working population*	
General characteristics	(Be as accurate as possible, but estimate when necessary.)
Total number of employees	(Usually, if an employer has 500 or more employees, full-time nursing services are necessary.)
General appearance	Are there records of heights, weights, cleanliness, and so forth? Ask to see them.
Age and sex distribution	What are the proportions of the different groups? (Certain screening programs are specific for young adults, whereas others are more for the elderly. Some programs are more for women, and others are more for men.) Is there any difference between day and evening shift populations? Are the problems of the minority sex unattended?
Race distribution	Does one race predominate? How does this compare with the general community?
Socioeconomic distribution	Are there great differences in worker salaries? (This can sometimes cause problems.)
Religious distribution	Does one religion predominate? Are religious holidays observed?
Ethnic distribution	Is there a language barrier?
Marital status	What proportion of the workers are widowed, singles, or divorced? (These groups often have different needs.)
Education backgrounds	Can all teaching be done at approximately the same level?
Lifestyles practiced	Is there disapproval of certain lifestyles?
Types of employment offered	
Background necessary	What educational level is required? Skilled versus unskilled?
Work demands on physical condition	What level of strength is needed? Is the work sedentary or active?
Work status	How many employees work full-time? Part-time? Is there overtime?
Absenteeism	Is there a record kept? By whom? Why?
causes	What are the five most common reasons for absence?

*Include worker and management, but separate data for comparison.

A model assessment guide for nursing in industry—cont'd

Components	Questions to ask
Length	What are the patterns of absences? (Absenteeism is costly to the employer. There is some difference between one 10-day absence and 10 one-day absences by the same person.)
Physically handicapped	Does the company have a policy about hiring the handicapped?
Number employed	Where do they work? What do they do?
Extent of handicaps	Are they specially trained? Are they in a special program? Do they use prosthetic devices?
Personnel on medication	What medication does each of these employees take? Where does each person work?
Personnel with chronic illness	At what stage of illness is the employee? Where does the employee work? Will he or she be able to continue at this job?

The industrial process: what does the company produce and how?

Equipment used	Is the equipment portable or fixed? Light or heavy?
General description of placement	Ask to have each piece of large equipment marked on a scale map.
Type of equipment	Fans, blowers, fast moving, wet, or dry?
Nature of the operation	Ask for a brief description of each stage of the process so that you can compare the needs and abilities of the worker with the needs of the job.
Raw materials used	What are they and how dangerous are they? Are they properly stored? (Check the *Federal Register* for guidelines on storage.)
Nature of the final product	Can the workers take pride in the final product, or do they just "make parts"?
Description of the jobs	Who does what? Where? (Label the map.)
Waste products produced	What is the system for waste disposal? Are the pollution-control devices in place and functioning?
Exposure to toxic substances	To which toxins are the workers exposed? What is the extent of exposure? (Include physical and emotional hazards. Remember that chronic effects of industrial exposure are subtle; a person often gets used to having mild symptoms and won't report them. The *Federal Register* contains specifications for exposure to toxins, and some states issue state standards.)

Continued.

A model assessment guide for nursing in industry—cont'd

Components	Questions to ask
The health program*	
Existing policies	Are there informal, unwritten policies?
Objectives of the program	Are they clear?
Preemployment physicals	Are they required? Are they paid for by the company? Is the information used to select?
First aid facilities	What is available? What is not available?
Standing orders	Is there a company physician who is responsible for first aid or emergency policy? (If so, work closely with him or her in planning nursing services.)
Job descriptions for health personnel	Are they in writing? (If there are no guidelines to be followed, write some.)
Existing facilities and resources:	Sometimes an industry that denies having a health program has more of a system than it realizes.
Trained personnel	Who responds in an emergency?
Space	Where is the sick worker taken? Where is the emergency equipment kept?
Supplies	What are they? Where are they kept? (Make a list and describe the condition of each item.)
Records and reports	What exists? (The OSHA requires that employers keep three types of records: a log of occupational injuries and illnesses, a supplemental record of certain illnesses or injuries, and an annual summary [forms 100, 101, and 102 are provided under the act]. Good records provide data for good planning.)
Services rendered in the past year:	Describe as specifically as possible.
Care needed	Chronic or acute? Why?
Screening done	Where? By whom? Why?
Referrals made	By whom? To whom? Why?
Counseling done	Formal or informal? (Often informal counseling goes unnoticed.)
Health education	What individual or group education was offered by the company?

---

*Outline what is actually in existence as well as what employees perceive to be in existence.

A model assessment guide for nursing in industry—cont'd

Components	Questions to ask
Accidents in the past year	During working hours? After hours? (Include those that occur after work hours; some may be directly or indirectly work related.)
Reasons why employees sought health care	What are the five major reasons?
Stressors	
As identified by employees	What pressures are felt on the job?
As identified by health providers	What problems do they perceive?

Self-Assessment of Environmental Health

Primary Prevention
Occupational

1. Do I work with substances my employer, my doctor, official agencies, or I consider potentially hazardous to my health? Frequency? Duration?
2. Am I asked to use safety/personal protective devices while I work? Why? When? Where? Who else?
3. Do I use the safety/personal protective devices my employer requires me to use while performing my job? If not, why not? If yes, when? Where? With whom?
4. Do I notice any patterns of illness in my working peers or family members? What specifically? Does anyone consider this a problem? Family? Company?
5. In describing my workplace, is/are there clutter, vapors, liquids, dust, fumes, heat, or vibration?
6. Do I feel that my work or workplace presents physical dangers such as falls, slips, or falling objects?

From Bomar P: *Nurses and family health promotion,* ed 2, Philadelphia, 1996, WB Saunders.

Home

1. What hobbies do I or family members participate in while in our home? What products are used? Are warning or special use labels present on any of these products?

2. Do we undergo regular checkups with our primary health care provider or doctor? Frequency? Has our health care provider advised us to change any personal or environmental factors present within our lives? If so, what?

3. Are all family members up to date on their immunization status?

4. What cleaning, home-maintenance, or home-repair products are used or stored within our home? Do package directions indicate proper use and storage? How are they used and stored? Does this comply with directions?

5. What type of insulation is used in my home? Are there known health hazards with this type of home insulation?

6. What type of heating is used in my home? Are there health hazards associated with this type of heating?

7. What source of water is used for my home (ground, surface, reclaimed, desalinated, or rain)? Are there any problems known to be associated with this water resource? Is water purified, filtered, and/or chlorinated prior to entering my home?

Recreational

1. List all playtime activities. List frequency and duration of the activity.

2. Are there any known dangers associated with these recreational activities?

3. Are there any substances or chemicals required to perform the recreational pastime? If so, what? Are directions for use and storage present? Do we/I follow them precisely?

4. Is safety equipment recommended for the recreational activity? If so, is it used? If recommended and not used, why not?

Environmental

1. Draw a map of known greenbelts, industries, dumps, housing patterns, and bodies of water.

2. Is my community targeted as a "high-risk" area for any toxic waste or radiation? If so, where? Do family members have any contact with resources from this area?

3. Are environmental problems suspected within my immediate neighborhood? If yes, what?

4. List your immediate concern when you think of environmental problems within your community.

Personal

1. Do I or other family members smoke?
2. How much alcohol consumption occurs during one week for each family member? Has alcohol ever been a problem in daily life (i.e., driving, business, school)?
3. Do I or other family members use recreational/illicit drugs? If so, which ones and how frequently?
4. How many sexual partners do individuals within family encounter within a month? A year? Can you/they describe "safe sex" practices? Do they/you use safe sex practices?

Do any of the above risk factors combine to increase the risk of disease (e.g., tobacco smoking and asbestos mining)?

Secondary Prevention
Occupational

1. Have I experienced any changes in my health, possibly related to my job, that caused me or my family to worry during the last week, month, or year?
2. Describe a typical work week.
   a. Do I feel better on the first day of my work week or the last day?
   b. Is there any change between the way I feel on weekends and during the work week?
   c. Are my coworkers showing signs of illness? If so, what signs?
   d. How much sick leave have I used this quarter? How many sick-leave days are spent in bed due to illness or poor health? How many days are spent off work and not in bed? When did I last see a doctor during a sick-leave period? What information did the doctor give me about my illness?
   e. Do I think I need to see a physician or health care provider soon? If so, who? Why?
   f. During the performance of my work, am I at risk for physical injury or disease?

Home

1. If I work or play at home, have I become exposed to substances that cause detectable illness?
2. Are there any illnesses that have been experienced within the home by more than one family member? If yes, what disease or symptoms? Is there any pattern of association common to all members?
3. Are family members acutely or chronically ill? If so, what diseases or conditions? Are they transmittable? Are they detectable through screening tests (e.g., tuberculosis)?

Recreational

1. Have I experienced any injuries related to my playtime activities in recent months or years? If so, what? Do these injuries indicate a need to seek screening for disease or chronic injury (e.g., neurologic compromise due to falls or moving vehicle accidents)?
2. Do any recreational activities aggravate preexisting diseases or injuries?

Environmental

1. Is my community or neighborhood targeted for any screening for disease or disability?
2. Do any environmental conditions exist (historical or current) that would alarm health officials or family members and indicate need for screening for disease? If so, what conditions? What exposures (e.g., radiation, infectious disease, and so on)?

Personal

1. Are family members at high risk for AIDS or other sexually transmitted diseases (homosexual males, IV drug abusers, multiple sex partners, sexual partners of the aforementioned)? Do I have single or multiple sex partners? Do I or my partners practice safe sex? Is HIV screening and treatment available within my community? Am I/family member in a risk group that indicates the need for screening and early diagnosis?
2. Do I or family members have habits that may put me or them at risk for diseases (e.g., IV drug abuse, illicit substance abuse, alcohol abuse)? Are they wishing screening and treatment? What services are available for screening and treatment within our community? What is the price to be paid for screening and treatment?
3. Is a family member a smoker with recent unexplained weight loss? When was last physical examination? When was last chest x-ray?
4. Is there any personal history of exposure that might indicate a need for periodic screening (e.g., radiation exposure)?
5. Is there any endemic disease I should be regularly tested for due to lifestyle or location (e.g., tuberculosis)?

Do any of the above risk factors combine to increase the risk of disease (e.g., tobacco smoking and asbestos mining)?

Tertiary Prevention
Occupational

1. Do I feel better or worse when I am in my normal work environment? What circumstances or activities make me feel worse? Which make me feel better?

2. Does my condition require that my employer accommodate the activities and circumstances that make me feel better? Are the accommodations made? Do the accommodations impose hardship on coworkers?
3. Can adjustments of the environment or equipment be made to allow me to work? Is retraining (habilitation) feasible? Do I or my family wish me to change jobs or retrain?

Home

1. How does the illness affect my role within the family and the completion of my tasks within the home?
2. Can adjustments of the environment or equipment be made so that I may better complete my activities within the home?
3. Do any home chores or activities exacerbate my illness or condition? If so, which ones? Can they be modified?

Recreational

1. Are my recreational activities limited due to illness or disability? If so, which ones? Can they be altered to accommodate the conditions without causing an increase in symptoms or exacerbation of illness?
2. Do any recreational activities worsen my condition? If so, which ones? Have they been altered or avoided to diminish physical or mental stress?

Environmental

1. Do environmental conditions exist within my community or home that exacerbate my condition (e.g., smog)? If so, are they alterable? If so, how?
2. Describe the climatic and general environmental conditions that potentiate your wellness. Can they be achieved within your current locale? If not, why not? If so, how?

Personal

1. Do my habits worsen my illness or conditions (e.g., smoking and emphysema)?
2. Is there a personal behavior I can enact that will facilitate recovery or rehabilitation? If so, what? If so, what lifestyle changes or resources will be needed? If so, are the resources available, accessible, or acceptable?

Do any of the above risk factors combine to increase the risk of disease (e.g., tobacco smoking and asbestos mining).

Summary—Environmental Assessments

Instrument title and author	Environmental attributes measured	Environmental application	Purpose—to determine	Clinical utility	Instrument development	Psychometric testing
1. The Accessibility Checklist (Goltsman et al, 1992)	Physical	Community	Accessibility of buildings and outdoor facilities	Survey checklists for a large number of physical spaces (e.g., playgrounds, retail areas) Useful in consultation with other professionals	Manual with clear instructions Based on ADA, UFAS, California Building Code	Content validity during scale construction No reliability testing
2. Assessment of Home Environments (Yarrow et al, 1975)	Social and cultural	Family	Adequacy of the infant's early developmental environment at home (ages newborn to 6 months)	Structured observations Limited instructions Useful for early intervention	Nominal data Content not justified No manual	One interrater reliability study No validity testing

3. Assessment Tool (Maltais et al, 1989)	Physical	Individual	Environmental barriers in a house, specific to functional limitations of an elderly person	Structured questionnaire Clear instructions Useful to promote independence of clients in their homes	Manual available Nominal data Norms available	One interrater reliability study One content validity study
4. Behavioral Environment Assessment Technique (Whitehead et al, 1984)	Social	Community	How adults behave in or use institutional space	Structured observations Useful for institutional planning, evaluation of environmental modifications	No manual	One reliability study One content validity study using factor analysis
5. Child Care Centre Accessibility Checklist (Metro Toronto Community Services, 1991)	Physical	Community	Barrier-free accessibility of child care centers	Direct observation and measurement of the environment Clear instructions Useful for determining physical accessibility	Manual available Nominal data Norms based on ANSI standards and Ontario building code	Reliability unknown Content validity determined based on instrument development

Continued.

NOTE: ADA, Americans With Disabilities Act; UFAS, Uniform Federal Accessibility Standards; ANSI, American National Standards Institute; ADL, activities of daily living; CMHC, Canada Mortgage and Housing Corporation; COTA, Community Occupational Therapists and Associates; UCP-OT, United Cerebral Palsy-Occupational Therapy; CSA, Canadian Standards Association.

From Letts L et al: Person-environment assessments in occupational therapy. *Am J Occup Ther* 48(7), 1994.

Summary—environmental assessments—cont'd

Instrument title and author	Environmental attributes measured	Environmental application	Purpose— to determine	Clinical utility	Instrument development	Psychometric testing
6. Classroom Environment Scale (Trickett and Moos, 1973)	Social	Individual and community	Aspects of classroom psychosocial environment salient to students and teachers	Questionnaire 3 forms, 90 items for each Useful for consultation within a classroom	Manual, with clear instructions Items selected based on theory and expert opinion Nominal data Norms available	One reliability study: internal consistency Content validity tested using factor analysis
7. Classroom Environment Index (Stern and Walker 1971)	Social and cultural	Individual and community	Student's perception of the classroom environment	Self-administered questionnaire 300 true/false statements Useful to describe classroom variables (e.g., achievement level) and student-environment fit	Manual available Item selection based on experts, literature, and testing in schools Norms available Nominal data	Internal consistency tested Factor analysis and discriminative validity tested

8. Disability Rights Guide (Goldman, 1991)	Economic and institutional	Individual and community	Problems affecting persons with disabilities in accessing their community	Self-report questionnaires address institutional barriers to accessibility Useful for community planning, advocacy	Questionnaires are contained within textbook Content based on ADA Nominal data	Unknown reliability Content validity based on instrument development
9. Environment Assessment Index (Poresky, 1987)	Physical and social	Family	Educational and developmental quality of the home environment for children ages 3 to 11 years living in rural communities	Questionnaire Structured interview and observations Clear instructions Useful for direct service, family education, program evaluation	Manual available from author Item selection based on literature review and expert opinion Nominal data	One reliability study: internal consistency Validity: content validity with factor analysis; concurrent and predictive correlations
10. Environment Assessment Scale (Kannegieter, 1986)	Economic and institutional	Individual	Characteristics of the occupational therapy clinical environment as perceived by the psychiatric client	Structured interview Useful for individual program planning, program evaluation	Manual available from unpublished source No norms Nominal data Comprehensive item selection	Internal consistency and test-retest reliability established Criterion and content validity testing underway

Continued.

Summary—environmental assessments—cont'd

Instrument title and author	Environmental attributes measured	Environmental application	Purpose—to determine	Clinical utility	Instrument development	Psychometric testing
11. Environmental Competence Questionnaire (CMHC, 1982)	Physical and social	Individual and community	Competence of elderly persons living independently in their homes	Questionnaire Structured interview Instructions not provided Useful for direct service to adults with physical limitations	No manual Item selection appears adequate Nominal data	Unknown reliability and validity
12. Environmental Grid Description Assessment (Dunning, 1972)	Physical, social, and cultural	Individual and family	Person's relationship with environmental space, persons, and tasks	Semi-structured interview No instructions Useful as a client-centered assessment of occupational choice	No manual Item selection appears adequate	Unknown reliability and validity
13. Environment Preference Questionnaire (Kaplan, 1977)	Physical	Individual and community	Individual difference in environmental preferences	Questionnaire Respondent can complete independently Clear instructions Useful in direct service	Manual available from author Item selection based on literature review, expert opinion Ordinal data	Reliability: internal consistency Content validity based on factor analysis

14. Environmental Response Inventory (McKechnie, 1974)	Social	Individual, family, and community	Differences in the ways persons habitually interact with the environment	Questionnaire Can be completed independently Clear instructions Useful for career, lifestyle counseling, program planning	Manual available Item selection based on literature review, limited by factor analysis Ordinal data	Reliability unknown Content, construct, criterion validity established
15. Functional Requirements in the Physical Environment (United Nations, 1981)	Physical, economic, and institutional	Community, province and country	Features of the built environment for accessibility by persons with physical, sensory, or cognitive disability	Checklist Clear instructions Useful for community consultation about accessibility	Manual available from United Nations Item selection comprehensive Nominal data	Unknown reliability Content validity based on instrument development
16. Home Observation for Measurement of the Environment (Caldwell and Bradley, 1979)	Physical, social, and cultural	Family	Adequacy of a child's early developmental environment at home (ages newborn to 6 years)	Structured observation and interviews with parents Clear instructions Useful for consultation and family education	Manual available Item selection based on factor analysis Nominal data	Internal consistency and test-retest reliability tested, adequate statistical results Content and construct validity established

Continued.

Summary—environmental assessments—cont'd

Instrument title and author	Environmental attributes measured	Environmental application	Purpose— to determine	Clinical utility	Instrument development	Psychometric testing
17. Home Modification Workbook (Adaptive Environments Center, 1988)	Physical	Individual	Home safety and potential for independent function of elderly individuals' homes	Questionnaire and observations in checklist format Useful to structure modifications to home for an individual's needs	Manual available Content justified Nominal data	Unknown reliability Content validity addressed during instrument development
18. Importance, Locus, and Range of Activities Checklist (Hulicka et al, 1975)	Physical, social, and cultural	Individual	Individual's perceived latitude of choice in ADL	Interview with checklist Clear instructions Useful for client-centered program planning	No manual available Item selection process not well described Ordinal data	Test-retest reliability established Construct and content validity tested
19. Infant-Toddler Environment Rating Scale (Harms et al, 1990)	Social	Community	Quality of center-based child care for children up to 30 months of age	Structure observation Clear instructions Useful for consultation, program planning	Manual available Item selection based on other scales Ordinal data	Interrater, test-retest and internal consistency established Content and criterion validity established

20. Interpersonal Support Evaluation List (Cohen et al, 1985)	Social	Individual	Availability of social support for adults	Self-report questionnaire Clear, concise instructions Useful for direct service, consultation	Manual available from author Item selection comprehensive Nominal data	Internal consistency and test-retest reliability established Concurrent and construct validity established
21. Life Stressors and Social Resources Inventory (Moos, Fenn, & Billings, 1988)	Physical, social, and cultural	Individual, family, and community	Common life stressors and social resources that influence well-being	Semi-structured interview Clear instructions Useful for direct service, consultation and community planning	Manual available Item selection based on literature review and expert opinion Nominal data	Internal consistency established Content validity based on factor analysis
22. Modification Checklist (CMHC, 1988)	Physical	Individual and community	Accessibility barriers of a house or apartment	Checklist based on observations Clear instructions Useful for direct service	Manual available Item selection based on opinions of clinical experts, disabled persons, rehabilitation centers, architects, etc. Nominal data	Unknown reliability Content validity based on instrument development

Continued.

Summary—environmental assessments—cont'd

Instrument title and author	Environmental attributes measured	Environmental application	Purpose—to determine	Clinical utility	Instrument development	Psychometric testing
23. Multilevel Assessment Instrument (Lawton et al, 1982)	Social	Individual	Well-being and behavioral competence of elderly persons at home and in community	Structured interview Limited instructions Useful for comprehensive assessment of function in an environment	No manual Item selection based on literature review and expert opinion Nominal data	Internal consistency established Content validity established
24. Multiphasic Environmental Assessment Procedure (Moos and Lemke, 1988)	Physical, economic, institutional, and social	Community	Adequacy of sheltered care settings	Structured questionnaire in five parts Clear instructions Useful for consultation in sheltered care settings	Manual available Item selection based on theory, literature review, and experts Ordinal and interval data Norms available	Internal consistency, interrater and test-retest reliability established Content, construct validity established
25. Need Satisfaction of Activity Interview (Tickle and Yerxa, 1981)	Social	Individual	Person's preferences for activities within his or her environment	Interview Clear instructions Useful for direct service, program planning	No manual Instructions available in published paper Item selection comprehensive Descriptive data	One test-retest reliability study Content validity based on factor analysis

26. Perceived Environment Constraint Index (Wolk and Telleen, 1976)	Economic and institutional	Individual and community	Level of personal autonomy allowed in a geriatric residential setting	Self-report questionnaire Clear instructions Useful for institutional planning	Instructions available in text Item selection comprehensive Ordinal data	Unknown reliability Content validity established
27. Person-Environment Fit (Kahana, 1974)	Physical, social, cultural, economic, and institutional	Individual and community	Congruence between residential environment and elderly individual	Self-report questionnaire Limited instructions Useful for long-term care planning, consultation	No manual Item selection comprehensive Nominal data	Unknown reliability and validity
28. Person-Environment Fit Scale (Coulton, 1979)	Physical, social, cultural, economic, and institutional	Individual and community	Person-environment fit	Self-report questionnaire Clear instructions Useful for direct service, community consultation, and planning	Manual available from author Item selection based on literature review and expert opinion Ordinal data	Internal consistency established Content and construct validity established

Continued.

Summary—environmental assessments—cont'd

Instrument title and author	Environmental attributes measured	Environmental application	Purpose— to determine	Clinical utility	Instrument development	Psychometric testing
29. Planner's Guide to Barrier-Free Meetings (Russell, 1980)	Physical	Community	Barrier-free accessibility of facilities for group meetings	Checklist Clear instructions Useful for consultation about accessibility	Manual available Item selection based on ANSI standards Nominal data	Unknown reliability Content validity addressed in instrument development
30. Planning Barrier-Free Libraries (National Library Service, 1981)	Physical, economic, and institutional	Community	Barrier-free accessibility of public libraries	Checklist Clear instructions Useful for community consultation	Manual available Item selection based on ANSI standards, expert and consumer opinions Nominal data	Unknown reliability Content validity addressed in instrument development
31. Play History (Takata, 1969; Behnke and Fetkovich, 1984)	Physical, social, and cultural	Individual and family	Child's past and present play experiences and environmental opportunities	Semi-structured interview Clear instructions Useful for direct service	No manual— instructions available from authors Item selection based on literature review Ordinal data	Interrater and test-retest reliability established Content and concurrent validity tested

32. Quality of Life Interview (Lehman, 1988)	Social	Individual	Satisfaction in nine life domains	Interview Clear instructions Useful in direct, client-centered service	Manual available Item selection based on literature review Ordinal data	Internal consistency and test-retest reliability tested Construct validity established
33. Readily Achievable Checklist (Cronburg et al, 1991)	Physical	Community	Barriers to accessibility	Structured observations and measurements Useful for obtaining public accessibility	Manual available Instructions and guidelines comprehensive	Unknown reliability Content validity addressed during instrument development
34. Safety Assessment of Function and the Environment for Rehabilitation (COTA, 1991)	Physical and social	Individual	Ability of the elderly person to function safely in his or her home	Checklist using observations and interview Clear instructions Useful for community-based practice, discharge planning	Manual available from author Item selection based on literature review, clinician and consumer opinion Nominal data	Internal consistency established Content and construct validity tested

Continued.

Summary—environmental assessments—cont'd

Instrument title and author	Environmental attributes measured	Environmental application	Purpose—to determine	Clinical utility	Instrument development	Psychometric testing
35. School-Quick Checklist (Ontario Ministry of Education, 1986)	Physical	Community	Accessibility barriers of schools Modification requirements	Checklist, observations Clear instructions Useful for school consultations	Manual available Item selection based on building code standards Nominal data	Unknown reliability Content validity addressed in instrument development
36. Source Book (Kelly and Snell, 1989)	Physical	Individual	Environmental barriers in a house, specific to functional limitations of a person with physical disabilities	Structured questionnaire, observations, and guidelines Clear instructions Useful for direct service, consultation	Manual available Item selection based on literature review and expert opinion Nominal data Standards based on ANSI and CSA	No reliability testing Content validity addressed in instrument development
37. Tenant Interview (Howell, 1980)	Social	Community	Behavioral preferences of adults living in congregate housing	Structured interview Clear instructions Useful for program planning	Manual available Item selection based on literature review and expert opinion Nominal data	Unknown reliability and validity

38. Therapeutic Environment Guidelines (Chambers et al, 1988)	Economic and institutional	Community	Attributes of residential lodges for adults needing long-term care	Checklist to use with observations and unstructured interview. Clear instructions. Useful for consultation	No manual available. Item selection based on literature review and expert opinions. Ordinal data	Unknown reliability. Content validity based on instrument development
39. UCP-OT Initial Evaluation (Colvin and Korn, 1984)	Physical	Family	Physical barriers to the care of children with cerebral palsy within their own home environment	Semi-structured questionnaire using observations and interview. Clear instructions. Useful in community practice	No manual available. Item selection based on ANSI standards. Nominal data	Unknown reliability. Content validity addressed in instrument development
40. Work Environment Scale (Moos, 1981)	Social	Individual and community	Interpersonal environment of workplace as perceived by employers and staff members	Structured questionnaire. Clear instructions. Useful for direct service, workplace consultations	Manual available. Item selection based on theory, literature review, expert opinion. Nominal data	Internal consistency and test-retest reliability established. Content validity based on factor analysis

Continued.

Summary—environmental assessments—cont'd

Instrument title and author	Environmental attributes measured	Environmental application	Purpose— to determine	Clinical utility	Instrument development	Psychometric testing
41. Workplace Workbook (Mueller, 1990)	Physical	Individual	Environmental barriers in a workplace	Structured observations and measurements for barrier-free accessibility Useful for preparing the work environment for a person with a physical disability	Manual available Content justified Nominal data	Unknown reliability Content validity addressed during instrument development

NOTE: ADA, Americans With Disabilities Act; UFAS, Uniform Federal Accessibility Standards; ANSI, American National Standards Institute; ADL, activities of daily living; CMHC, Canada Mortgage and Housing Corporation; COTA, Community Occupational Therapists and Associates; UCP-OT, United Cerebral Palsy-Occupational Therapy; CSA, Canadian Standards Association.

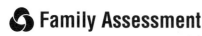 Family Assessment

Family assessment is a central part of public health and community health nursing practice. These tools will serve as cues to assist the nurse in making key observations about how families live, work and play together. It is essential to understand the structure and function of the family and the roles that each individual plays in order for the nurse to be effective in disease prevention and health promotion activities.

Family Self-Care Patterns

The following tool suggests a method for identifying family health goals and monitoring progress toward these goals.

Designed for (family name): _____
Family form: _____
Family members:

Name	Sex	Position in family	Birth date	Occupation (if employed)
_____	___	_____	_____	_____
_____	___	_____	_____	_____
_____	___	_____	_____	_____
_____	___	_____	_____	_____
_____	___	_____	_____	_____
_____	___	_____	_____	_____

Home address: _____
Home telephone number: _____
Work telephone number: _____
Cultural background: _____
Spiritual-religious orientation: _____
Major formal roles of family members: _____
_____
_____
_____
_____

From Pender NL: *Health promotion in nursing practice,* ed 2, Norwalk, Conn., 1987, Appleton & Lange.

Community affiliations of family: _____

_____

_____

_____

_____

_____

Communication patterns (verbal and nonverbal, including expression of caring and affection):

Family decision-making patterns:

Family values with highest rank:

   1. _____

   2. _____

   3. _____

   4. _____

   5. _____

Rank order of health as a value (if not listed above): _____

Value conflicts in family (if any):

Goals important to family:

                              Mutual goal or specific
                              to dyad (d) or triad (t)

_____   _____

_____   _____

_____   _____

_____   _____

Family strengths:

Major sources of stress for family and perceived ability to deal with stressors:

Current or recent family developmental or situational transitions:

Family concerns or challenges:

Family Self-Care Patterns

Current health protecting or preventive behaviors (such as immunization, self-examination, periodic screening or examination by health professionals, avoidance of toxic exposure, use of seat belts):

Current health-promoting behaviors (life style review):
  Nutritional practices:

  Physical-recreational activities:

Sleep-relaxation patterns:

Stress management:

Family sense of purpose:

Family actualization efforts:

Relationships in family and with others:

Environmental control:

Information-seeking patterns of family in relation to health promotion:

Use of health-promotion facilities or services by family:

Other behaviors:

Consistency among family values, goals, and health actions:

Family Health Goals

Goals	Family priority (1 = most important)

Areas for Improvement in Family Health

Target Health Goal:

Area of change (see categories under family self-care patterns)	Specific behavior change	Family priority (1 = most desirable)	Approaches selected to facilitate family change

Evaluation of progress toward change in family life style

Two weeks:

One month:

Three months:

Six months:

One year:

Stages of Family Development: Health Promotion and Disease Prevention

The following table presents nursing roles for families in various stages of development. This guide may be helpful in assisting families to move successfully through life stages, thereby reducing the risk of illness or crisis.

Stage	Nursing role
Couple	Counselor on sexual and marital role adjustment
	Teacher and counselor in family planning
	Teacher of parenting skills
	Coordinator for genetic counseling
	Facilitator in interpersonal relationships
Childbearing family	Monitor of prenatal care and referrer for problems of pregnancy
	Counselor on prenatal nutrition
	Counselor on prenatal maternal habits
	Supporter of amniocentesis
	Counselor on breastfeeding
	Coordinator with pediatric services
	Supervisor of immunizations
	Refer to social services
Family with preschool and school-age children	Monitor of early childhood development; refer when indicated
	Teacher in first-aid and emergency measures
	Coordinator with pediatric services
	Supervisor of immunizations
	Counselor on nutrition and exercise
	Teacher in problem-solving issues regarding health habits
	Participant in community organizations for environmental control
	Teacher of dental care hygiene
	Counselor on environmental safety in the home
	Facilitator in interpersonal relationships

From Edelman CL, Mandle CL: *Health promotion throughout the lifespan,* ed 3, St Louis, 1994, Mosby.

Stage	**Nursing role**
Family with adolescents	Teacher of risk factors to health
	Teacher in problem-solving issues regarding alcohol, smoking, diet, and exercise
	Facilitator of interpersonal skills with teenagers and parents
	Direct supporter, counselor, or referrer to mental health resources
	Counselor on family planning
	Refer for sexually transmittable disease
	Participant in community organizations on disease control
Family with young or middle-aged adults	Teacher in problem-solving issues regarding lifestyle and habits
	Participant in community organizations for environmental control
	Case finder in the home and community
	Screener for hypertension, Pap smear, breast examination, cancer signs, mental health, and dental care
	Counselor on menopausal transition for husband and wife
	Facilitator in interpersonal relationships among family members
Family with older adults	Refer for work and social activity, nutritional programs, homemakers' services, and so on
	Monitor of exercise, nutrition, preventive services, and medications
	Supervisor of immunization
	Counselor on safety in the home

Family Health Assessment Guide

Suggested Use
General instructions.   Content areas of the guide should be modified and adapted as appropriate for individual families and the circumstances of the family and community health nurse contact(s). The factors listed for many of the major family assessment areas are examples and should be added to or omitted as necessary.

Family Unit
Family composition (see table on p. 191)
Extended family (such as parents, children, and other relatives outside of household)
   Relationship
   Place of residency
   Frequency of contact
Residential history
   Length of time at present address
   Frequency of residential and geographical changes
Education of family member (present and highest level attained)
   Educational level
   Attending school/college
   Educational goal
Vocational interests of family member
   Interest
   Goal
Avocational interests of family member (hobbies, other creative endeavors)
   Interest
   Goal
Occupation of family member
   Type of work
   Hours of work
   Satisfaction with job
   Goal(s)
Financial resources
   Sources (e.g., salaries, pension, and public assistance)
   Total income

From Stanhope M, Lancaster J: *Community health nursing: process and practice for promoting health,* ed 3, St Louis 1992, Mosby.

Family member	Age	Sex	Ethnicity/ race	Family position (mother, spouse, etc.)	Special status (adopted, single, divorced, etc.)
———	——	——	———	—————	—————
———	——	——	———	—————	—————
———	——	——	———	—————	—————

Distribution of income (e.g., housing, food, clothing, health/illness care, utilities, recreation, and insurance)
Adequacy of income
Religious practices of family members
Religious preferences
Extent of involvement
Relative importance of religion in everyday life (e.g., influence on activities of daily living and relationships)
Rituals
Holidays and celebrations related to activities of daily living
Recreational interests of family members
Interests around home (alone and with family)
Interests outside home (alone and with family)
Activities with relatives
With friends
With community groups
What does the family do for "fun" around home? Outside of home?

Family Environment
Residence

Housing
Type of dwelling
Number and types of rooms
General condition
Furnishings
Condition
Adequacy
Living space
Adequate for family size
Privacy for family members
Sleeping arrangements
Where members sleep
Sharing of bed(s)
Adequacy of sleeping arrangements

Bathroom facilities
  Location
  Adequacy
  Sanitation
Food preparation arrangements
  Cleanliness
  Cooking
  Refrigeration
Eating arrangements and mealtime environment
General state of cleanliness and sanitation
Adequacy of
  Water supply and source
  Waste/garbage disposal
  Lighting
  Heating and cooling
  Ventilation
  Laundry facilities
  Telephone
Condition of yard
Pets
  Number
  Kinds
  Care
Automobile
  Number
  Conditions
Provisions for emergencies
  Smoke alarm
  Emergency numbers by telephone
Environmental stressors
  Noise
  Lack of individual territory
Environmental hazards
  Storage of medicines and household cleaners/poisons
  Sharp tools
  Fire dangers
  Unsafe toys
  Loose rugs
  Clutter
  Swimming pool
Family attitudes toward home, neighborhood, and community

Goals for Future
Neighborhood

Type
  Residential
  Semicommercial
  Urban/nonmetropolitan
Dwellings
  Single-family house
  Apartment
  Combination
Age of area
  Newly constructed
  Deteriorating
  Foliage (trees, shrubbery)
Sociocultural characteristics
  Age composition
  Ethnic groups
  Employment (or unemployment)
General condition of structures, yards, streets, alleys
Traffic patterns
Efficiency of street lighting systems
Availability of fire hydrants
Resources
  Shopping
  Transportation
  Recreational
  Educational
  Religious
  Protective services
  Health/illness
  Emergency
  Human services
  Business
  Garbage/refuse disposal
Environmental stressors
  Noise
  Crime rate
  Substance abuse
  Crowding
  Poverty
Environmental hazards
  Air pollution
  Garbage/debris

Traffic flow
Unsafe play areas
"In" and "out" migration of residents
Neighbors' attitude toward the family
Family's involvement in the neighborhood

Community

Leadership and government
Resources (essentially the same as those listed for neighborhood)
Occupations, industries, businesses
Family's involvement in the community
    Community memberships
    Interaction with social institutions
    Use of resources

Family Structure

Organization
    As a system
    Subsystems
Roles
    Roles being filled
    Satisfaction/dissatisfaction with role(s)
    Level of role functioning
    Perceptions about roles
    Acceptance of roles
    Flexibility/interchangeability of roles
Socialization processes for roles
Division of labor
    How is delegation of tasks determined?
    Who carries out which tasks?
    What is the flexibility of task responsibilities?
    What is the extent of satisfaction or dissatisfaction with task
        delegation and performance?
Authority and power
    Degree of autonomy for each family member
    Locus of authority
    Power relationships
    How authority is exercised
    How power is demonstrated
    Satisfaction or dissatisfaction with autonomy, authority, and power
        in family
Values, attitudes, and beliefs regarding family organization, roles,
    division of labor, autonomy, authority, and power

Stresses related to family organization, roles, division of labor, autonomy, authority, and power—how is it handled?

Family Processes
Communication
Patterns
  Ways used to communicate effectively
  Content of communications
  Interpretation of content
  Linguistic characteristics (cultural)
  Frequency of communications
  How do joy, love, anger, sadness, frustration get communicated?
  Communication patterns within family subsystems
  Effectiveness of communications—is understood, clear, consistent?
Satisfaction or dissatisfaction with family communication patterns
Values, attitudes, and beliefs regarding family communications
Stresses related to family communications

Decision making
How are decisions made?
  What is the process?
Who makes decisions affecting adults?
  Children?
  Entire group?
How are decisions implemented?
How are decision-making skills learned in the family?
Satisfaction or dissatisfaction with family decision-making process
Values, attitudes, and beliefs regarding family decision making
Stresses related to family decision making

Problem solving
How are problems handled?
  What is the process?
Who is involved in the problem-solving process?
  Who provides leadership in the process?
Extent to which family can deal with problem solving and for what types of problems
Flexibility in approaches to problem solving
Ability to use information from outside family in problem-solving process
Satisfaction or dissatisfaction with family's problem-solving ability and process
Values, attitudes, and beliefs regarding family's problem solving
Stresses related to family problem solving

Family Functions
Physical

How are needs (food, shelter, clothing, etc.) met?

Are physical needs being met satisfactorily? If not, what solutions have been tried by the family?

Values, attitudes, and beliefs regarding family's physical needs and functions

Stresses related to meeting family's physical needs

Emotional

Affectional relationships
  Between adults
  Between adults and children
  Between siblings

Ways of obtaining and giving emotional support: distribution of support, when given, how given, acceptance by other family member(s)

Ways in which family members do or do not assist each other in developing self-esteem, in developing autonomy

How do family members show respect for each other?

To what extent and how is intimacy expressed?
  Physical affection and companionship?

Satisfaction or dissatisfaction regarding how family's emotional needs are met

Values, attitudes, and beliefs regarding family's emotional needs and functions

Stresses related to family's emotional functions

Social

Goals for family and individual family members

Support for individual creativity, initiative, and leadership

Process for developing and supporting family and individual leadership

Process for strengthening family members' competency regarding adjustment in social organizations (such as school)

Competency regarding appropriate use of social organizations

Seeking new experiences—kind, etc.

Discipline and limit-setting practices

Individual developmental tasks (physical, affective, intellectual, language, psychosocial, sexual, moral, personality)
  Level of knowledge
  Seeks information as needed
  Provides support

Seeks support resources as needed
Adopts socialization approaches to meet individual needs and tasks
Family developmental tasks
Level of knowledge
Seeks information as needed
Intrafamily support
Uses resources as needed
Satisfaction or dissatisfaction regarding social functions
Values, attitudes, and beliefs regarding social functions
Stresses related to social functions

Coping
Conflict

To what extent and how are conflicts expressed covertly and overtly?
Frequency of conflicts? Kinds? Attributed causes?
How are conflicts avoided? How are conflicts resolved?
Satisfaction or dissatisfaction regarding conflict resolution process
Values, attitudes, and beliefs regarding conflict resolution
Stresses related to conflicts and conflict resolution

Life changes

Recent, present, and anticipated life changes
Impact of change(s) on family's functioning as a unit
Impact of change(s) on family roles and functions
Ability to cope with change(s): practices, behaviors, values, attitudes,
beliefs
Stresses associated with change(s)

Support systems

Resources within family—What are they? How are they used? When
are they used? What is their effectiveness?
External support systems—How are they used? When? What is their
effectiveness?
Significant others (e.g., extended family members and friends)
Nonprofessional organizations
Professional systems
Understand how to use—seek relevant information
Availability, accessibility, use patterns
Satisfaction or dissatisfaction with support systems
Values, attitudes, and beliefs related to using support systems

Life satisfaction

How does family feel about its quality of life?
What influences family's quality of life?

What influences the family's feelings about life?
Would the family like to change anything about its life? What?
What impedes change?
What can family do? Others do?

Health Behavior
Health history

Genetic or familial diseases (such as diabetes, heart disease)
Family history of emotional problems, suicide, etc.
Past illnesses, operations, accidents, injuries
Present illnesses or physical discomforts
Use of prescribed or over-the-counter medications
Present symptoms such as anxiety, depression, etc.
Concerns about hearing, vision, speech
Recent history regarding physical and dental examinations, immunizations, Pap smear, etc.

Health status

Family's assessment of present health status
Concerns about present health status or potential health problems
Family's perceptions of vulnerability to disease and illness
What does the family perceive as a health problem?
What present and potential health problems are identified by the family? Priorities for health problems?
What is family's belief about cause of problem(s)?
What is family's belief(s) about cure/treatment for problem(s)?

Activities of daily living

Eating patterns and foods
Personal hygiene and daily grooming
Physical activity
Sleeping behavior
Dental practices
What are family members' daily rhythms (such as morning person, night person)?
How does family describe a typical weekday? A weekend?

Risk behaviors

Inadequate nutritional behavior (overeating, undereating, irregular meals, diet high in sugar or sodium, beverages high in caffeine)
Physical inactivity
Limited sleep or irregular sleeping patterns
Smoking
Use of alcohol

Nonuse of seat belts

Excessive exposure to stress situations (family, work, social)

Health beliefs

How does family define health? Illness?

How does family define health and illness for each family member?

What value does family assign health? Health promotion? Prevention?

What are family's perceptions about cause(s) of illness?

What are family's perceptions about control over health and illness?

What are family's perceptions about how illness and disease are cured?

What are family's health goals?

How are values, attitudes, and beliefs regarding health promotion communicated to children? What is the socialization process? How does family members' involvement in the community influence family's health values, attitudes, and beliefs?

Self-care
Knowledge

Level of knowledge regarding health promotion, preventive measures, emergency care, causes and treatment of illness and diseases

How is health knowledge transmitted to family members?

What are sources of health information?

How does family assess its level of health knowledge?

What would family like to know about health promotion? Prevention? Illness care?

Practices

What does family do to protect its health (physical, emotional, social, spiritual)?

What does family do to improve its health status?

What does family do to prevent illness and disease?

What does family do to generate and support health protective behaviors in family members?

What does family do to care for health problems and illnesses in the home?

How are health and illness care responsibilities distributed in the family? Is there flexibility of family roles and tasks?

What are family's perceptions regarding ability to protect family's health?

How does family care for health problems and illnesses in the home?

What are the family's values, attitudes, and beliefs regarding self-care?

Family planning

Family's values, attitudes, and beliefs regarding family planning (such as methods, child spacing, childlessness, and appropriateness for which family members)

Decision-making process

Practices

Health care resources

Utilization practices regarding formal informal health and illness care systems (such as what the systems are and the frequency of their use)

Availability of emergency care resources

Availability, accessibility, and attractiveness of health and illness care resources

Effectiveness and efficiency with which family uses resources

How is health and illness care financed? What are other costs for family such as transportation and work time lost?

Family's knowledge about health and illness care resources

Family's perceptions of and attitudes about experiences with health and illness care resources and health care providers (such as nurses and physicians)

What are the family's feelings about the kinds of health services available to them in the community?

What kinds of health services would they like to receive?

What suggestions do they have about making any necessary changes in the delivery of services?

What are the family's feelings about health care providers?

What kind of relationship would the family like to have with health care providers?

What suggestions do they have about helping the health care providers to better meet the needs of the family?

Family's values and beliefs related to health and illness care resources and health care providers

Stresses related to use of health and illness care resources and interactions with health care providers

Community health nursing services

Knowledge about community health nursing

Attitudes toward community health nursing services

Expectations of community health nursing services

Family Health Assessment Summary

Family's sociodemographic profile

Family's environment—strengths and problems regarding home, neighborhood, and community

Family structure, processes, functions—strengths and limitations, existing or potential problems

Family's coping profile

  Conflict management—strengths and limititations

  Life changes—strengths and limitations regarding coping with changes

  Support systems—strengths and limitations

  Life satisfaction profile

Family's health behavior profile

  Health history—existing or potential problems

  Health status—existing or potential problems

  Activities of daily living—strengths and limitations or problems

  Risk profile—for family unit and family members

  Health beliefs profile of values, attitudes, and beliefs regarding health and illness

Self-care—strengths and limitations

Health care resources—adequacy of availability, accessibility, attractiveness, and use; general practices

Community health nursing services—attitudes and expectations

Suggested Areas for Assessment of Family Health-Related Lifestyle

Nutrition

1. Meals prepared in the home are generally consistent with the food guide pyramid.

2. Healthy snacks are consumed in the home.

3. Knowledge about healthy eating habits is shared among family members.

4. Mutual assistance occurs among family members for maintenance of recommended weights and avoidance of overweight and underweight.

5. Family members praise each other for healthy eating.

6. Family members encourage each other to drink 6-8 glasses of water per day.

From Pender MJ: *Health promotion in nursing practice,* ed 3, 1996, Appleton & Lange.

7. Family member base purchase decisions on nutritional labels on food.

Physical Activity

1. Many family outings consist of vigorous or moderate physical activity.
2. Exercise equipment is available within the home.
3. Use of home exercise equipment is part of "family time."
4. Family members expect each other to be physically active.
5. A family membership is held in recreational facilities or programs.
6. Time together is seldom spent watching television or playing video games.
7. Family prefers to spend as much time out-of-doors as possible.

Stess Control and Management

1. Family manages time well to minimize stressful demands on members
2. Family often relaxes, shares stories, and laughs together.
3. Emotional expression is encouraged within the family.
4. Family members share stressful experiences with each other.
5. Family members offer each other assistance with difficult tasks.
6. Family members seldom "get on each other" about their faults.
7. Periods of relaxation and sleep are considered important by the family.

Health Responsibility

1. A schedule for preventive care visits is maintained by the family.
2. Family often discusses news and articles about health topics.
3. Family members are encouraged to seek health care early if a problem develops.
4. Personal responsibility for health is encouraged by the family.
5. Family feels a sense of responsibility for the health of the family and each member.
6. Health professionals are consulted about health promotion as well as care in illness.
7. Appropriate protective behaviors are openly discussed and encouraged (abstinence, use of condoms, hearing protection, eye protection, sunscreen).

Family Resilience and Resources

1. Worship or spiritual experiences are a regular part of family activities.
2. Family members share a sense of "togetherness" despite difficult life events.

3. Family has a common sense of purpose in life.
4. Family members encourage each other to "keep going" when life is difficult.
5. Growth in positive directions is mutually encouraged within the family.
6. Health is nurtured as a positive family resource.
7. Personal strengths and capabilities are nurtured.

Family Support
1. Family has a number of friends or relatives that they see frequently.
2. Family is involved in community activities and groups.
3. Family members frequently praise each other.
4. In times of distress, the family can call on a number of other families or individuals for help.
5. Disagreements are settled through discussion rather than verbal abuse or physical violence.
6. Family members model healthy habits for each other.
7. Professional support services are sought when needed.

Stages of Family Life Cycles

Suggested Use
The life cycle of the family consists of a series of periods characterized by states of movement or change and quiescence or stability. The times of change represent an instability in the structures, and may lead to crisis or illness. The following is a guide to assist in assessing periods of family change which may affect health.

The stages of the family life cycle

Family life cycle stage	Emotional process of transition: key principles	Second order changes in family status required to proceed developmentally
1. Between families: the unattached young adult	Accepting parent off-spring separation	Differentiation of self in relation to family of origin Development of intimate peer relationships Establishment of self in work
2. The joining of families through marriage: the newly married couple	Commitment to new system	Formation of marital system Realignment of relationships with extended families and friends to include spouse
3. The family with young children	Accepting new members into the system	Adjusting marital system to make space for child(ren) Taking on parenting roles Realignment of relationships with extended family to include parenting and grand-parenting roles
4. The family with adolescents	Increasing flexibility of family boundaries to include children's independence	Shifting of parent-child relationships to permit adolescent to move in and out of system Refocus on mid-life marital and career issues Beginning shift toward concerns for older generation
5. Launching children and moving on	Accepting a multitude of exits from and entries into the family system	Renegotiation of marital system as a dyad Development of adult-to-adult relationships between grown children and their parents Realignment of relationships to include in-laws and grandchildren

6. The family in later life	Accepting the shifting of generational roles	Maintaining own or couple functioning and interests in face of physiological decline, exploration of new familial and social role options
		Support for a more central role for middle generation
		Making room in the system for the wisdom and experience of the elderly, supporting the older generation without overfunctioning for them
		Dealing with loss of spouse, siblings, and other peers and preparation for own death
		Life review and integration

Reprinted with permission from Carter E, McGoldrick M: *The family life cycle: a framework for family therapy,* New York, 1988, Gardner Press.

The Eight-Stage Family Life Cycle

Stage 1	Beginning families (also referred to as married couples or the stage of marriage)
Stage II	Childbearing families (the oldest child is an infant through 30 months)
Stage III	Families with preschool children (oldest child is 2½ to 6 years of age)
Stage IV	Families with school children (oldest child is 6 to 13 years of age)
Stage V	Families with teenagers (oldest child is 13 to 20 years of age)
Stage VI	Families launching young adults (covering the first child who has left through the last child leaving home)
Stage VII	Middle-aged parents (empty nest through retirement)
Stage VIII	Family in retirement and old age (also referred to as aging family members or retirement to death of both spouses

Adapted from Duvall E, (1977); Duvall E, Miller B: Marriage and family development, ed 6, New York, 1985, Harper & Row.

Comparison of Family Life Cycle Stages of Duvall and Miller with Carter and McGoldrick

Family therapy perspective (Carter and McGoldrick)	Sociological perspective (Duvall and Miller)
1. Between families: the unattached young adult	No stage identified here, although Duvall considers young adult to be in process of "being launched." Because there is often a considerable time period between adolescence and marriage, addition of this "between stage" is indicated.
2. The joining of families through marriage: the newly married couple	1. Beginning families or the stage of marriage.
3. Families with young children (infancy through school age)	2. Childbearing families (oldest child up to 30 months of age) 3. Families with preschool children (oldest child is 2½ to 5 years of age) 4. Families with school-aged children (oldest child is 6 to 12 years of age)
4. Families with adolescents	5. Families with teenagers (oldest child is 13 to 20 years of age)
5. Launching children and moving on	6. Families launching young adults (all children leaving home) 7. Middle-aged parents (empty nest, up to retirement)
6. Families in later life	8. Families in retirement and old age (retirement to death of both spouses)

Carter B, McGoldrick M, editors: *The changing family life cycle,* ed 2, New York, 1988, Gardner Press; Duvall E, Miller B: *Marriage and family development,* ed 6, New York, 1985, Harper and Row.

Dislocations of the Family Life Cycle by Divorce, Requiring Additional Steps to Restabilize and Proceed Developmentally

Phase	Emotional process of transition—prerequisite attitude	Developmental issues
Divorce		
1. The decision to divorce	Acceptance of inability to resolve marital tensions sufficiently to continue relationship	Acceptance of one's own part in the failure of the marriage
2. Planning the breakup of the system	Supporting viable arrangements for all parts of the system	Working cooperatively on problems of custody, visitation, and finances Dealing with extended family about the divorce
3. Separation	Willingness to continue cooperative co-parental relationship and joint financial support of children Work on resolution of attachment to spouse	Mourning loss of intact family Restructuring marital and parent-child relationships and finances, adaptation to living apart Realignment of relationships with extended family, staying connected with spouse's extended family
4. The divorce	More work on emotional divorce: overcoming hurt, anger, guilt, etc.	Mourning loss of intact family: giving up fantasies of reunion Retrieval of hopes, dreams, expectations from the marriage Staying connected with extended families

Postdivorce family

1. Single-parent (custodial household or primary residence)	Willingness to maintain financial responsibilities, continue parental contact with ex-spouse, and support contact of children with ex-spouse and his or her family	Making flexible visitation arrangements with ex-spouse and his or her family Rebuilding own financial resources Rebuilding own social network
2. Single-parent (noncustodial)	Willingness to maintain parental contact with ex-spouse and support custodial parent's relationships with children	Finding ways to continue effective parenting relationship with children Maintaining financial responsibilities to ex-spouse and children Rebuilding own social network

From Carter B, McGoldrick M, editors: *The changing family life cycle*, 2nd ed, New York, 1988, Gardner Press.

Remarried Family Formation: a Developmental Outline

Steps	Prerequisite attitude	Developmental issues
1. Entering the new relationship	Recovery from loss of first marriage (adequate "emotional divorce")	Recommitment to marriage and to forming a family with readiness to deal with the complexity and ambiguity
2. Conceptualizing and planning new marriage and family	Accepting one's own fears and those of new spouse and children about remarriage and forming a stepfamily Accepting need for time and patience for adjustment to complexity and ambiguity of 1. Multiple new roles 2. Boundaries: space, time, membership, and authority 3. Affective issues: guilt, loyalty conflicts, desire for mutuality, unresolvable past hurts	Work on openness in the new relationships to avoid pseudomutuality Plan for maintenance of cooperative financial and coparental relationships with ex-spouses Plan to help children deal with fears, loyalty conflicts, and membership in two systems Realignment of relationships with extended family to include new spouse and children Plan maintenance of connections for children with extended family of ex-spouse(s)
3. Remarriage and reconstitution of family	Final resolution of attachment to previous spouse and ideal of "intact" family; acceptance of a differnet model of family with permeable boundaries.	Restructuring family boundaries to allow for inclusion of new spouse or step-parent Realignment of relationships and financial arrangements throughout subsystems to permit interweaving of several systems Making room for relationships of all children with biological (noncustodial) parents, grandparents, and other extended family Sharing memories and histories to enhance stepfamily integration

From Carter B, McGoldrick M, editors: *The changing family life cycle,* 2nd ed, New York, 1988, Gardner Press.

Cultural Heritage Assessment Tool

1. Where was your mother born: _____
2. Where was your father born: _____
3. Where were your grandparents born: _____
   a. Your mother's mother: _____
   b. Your mother's father: _____
   c. Your father's mother: _____
   d. Your father's father: _____
4. How many brothers _____ and sisters _____ do you have?
5. What setting did you grow up in? Urban: _____
   Rural: _____   Suburban: _____
6. What country did you parents grow up in?
   Father: _____
   Mother: _____
7. How old were you when you came to the United
   States: _____
8. How old were your parents when they came to the United
   States?
   Mother: _____
   Father: _____
9. When you were growing up, who lived with you?
   Nuclear: _____ or extended: _____ family
10. Have you maintained contact with
    a. Aunts, uncles, cousins? (1) Yes: _____ (2) No: _____
    b. Brothers and sisters? (1) Yes: _____ (2) No: _____
    c. Parents   (1) Yes: _____ (2) No: _____
    d. Your own children?   (1) Yes: _____ (2) No: _____
11. Did most of your aunts, uncles, cousins live near to your
    home?
    (1) Yes: _____   (2) No: _____
12. Approximately how often did you visit your family members
    who lived outside of your home?
    (1) Daily: _____ (2) Weekly: _____ (3) Monthly: _____
    (4) Once a year or less: _____   (5) Never: _____
13. Was your original family name changed?
    (1) Yes: _____ (2) No: _____

From Spector RE: *Cultural diversity in health and illness,* ed 3, Norwalk, Conn., 1991, Appleton-Lange.

14. What is your religious preference?
   (1) Catholic: _____   (2) Jewish: _____
   (3) Protestant: _____   Denomination: _____
   (4) Other: _____   (5) None: _____
15. Is your spouse the same religion as you?
   (1) Yes: _____   (2) No: _____
16. Is your spouse the same ethnic background as you?
   (1) Yes: _____   (2) No: _____
17. What kind of school did you go to?
   (1) Public: _____   (2) Private: _____   (3) Parochial: _____
18. As an adult, do you live in a neighborhood where the neighbors are the same religion and ethnic background as yourself?
   (1) Yes: _____   (2) No: _____
19. Do you belong to a religious institution?
   (1) Yes: _____   (2) No: _____
20. Would you describe yourself as an active member?
   (1) Yes: _____   (2) No: _____
21. How often do you attend your religious institution?
   (1) More than once a week: _____   (2) Weekly: _____
   (3) Monthly: _____   (4) Special holidays only: _____
   (5) Never: _____
22. Do you practice your religion in your home?
   (1) Yes: _____   (2) No: _____ (if yes, please specify)
   (3) Praying: _____   (4) Bible reading: _____
   (5) Diet: _____   (6) Celebrating religious holidays: _____
23. Do you prepare foods of your ethnic background?
   (1) Yes: _____   (2) No: _____
24. Do you participate in ethnic activities?
   (1) Yes: _____   (2) No: _____ (if yes, please specify)
   (3) Singing: _____   (4) Holiday celebrations: _____
   (5) Dancing: _____   (6) Festivals: _____
   (7) Costumes: _____   (8) Other: _____
25. Are your friends from the same religious background as you?
   (1) Yes: _____   (2) No: _____
26. Are your friends from the same ethnic background as you?
   (1) Yes: _____   (2) No: _____
27. What is your native language: _____
28. Do you speak this language?
   (1) Prefer: _____   (2) Occasionally: _____   (3) Rarely: _____

29. Do you read your native language?
(1) Yes: ____ (2) No: ____

The greater the number of *yes* answers, the more likely the client is to strongly identify with a traditional heritage. (The one *no* answer that indicates continued heritage identity is "Was your original family name changed?")

Cultural Adaptation of the Nursing Process

Process	Action
Assessment	
Heritage consistency	Perform heritage-consistency assessment on self and client
Environmental control	Ask about the client's beliefs about the nature of the health problem and the actions being taken at home or in the community to treat and resolve it
	Ask about other health care resources being used
Biological variations	Ask about nutritional preferences
	Observe body structure, skin tone, and color
	Be aware of health problems that may be more common in that client's background
Social organizations	Conduct community activities
Communication skills	Determine the needs of the client who does not speak the dominant language and provide competent interpreters
Space	Be aware of territoriality; seek permission before intruding in the client's territory
	Be aware of touch and eye-contact expectations
Time	Understand the differences in time orientation
Nursing diagnosis	
Development of problem list	Ask about the client's interpretation of the problem and possible effective interventions
Planning	Include client, family, and community in plans as needed
Implementation	Alter usual ways of interacting to adjust to client's social interaction and etiquette
	Incorporate interventions agreeing with client's cultural heritage, educational level, and language skills
Evaluation	With client, determine whether nursing care has met expectations and needs

From Carpenito, 1992; Conley, 1990. In Wong DL: *Whaley and Wong's Nursing care of infants and children,* ed 5, St. Louis, 1995, Mosby.

Religious Beliefs that Affect Nursing Care

Beliefs about birth and death	Beliefs about diet and food practices	Beliefs regarding medical care	Comments
Adventist (Seventh-Day Adventist; Church of God)			
Birth Opposed to infant baptism Baptism in adulthood	Meat prohibited in some groups No alcohol, coffee, or tea	Some believe in divine healing and practice anointing with oil and use of prayer May desire communion or baptism when ill Believe in man's choice and God's sovereignty Some oppose hypnosis as therapy	Sabbath: Saturday for many Accept Bible literally
Baptist (27 groups)			
Birth Opposed to infant baptism Believers baptized by immersion as adults	Some groups discourage coffee, tea, and alcohol	"Laying on of hands" (some) May encounter some resistance to some therapies, such as abortion Believe God functions through physician Some believe in predestination, may respond passively to care	Fundamentalist and conservative groups accept Bible as inspired word of God
Death Counsel and prayer with clergy, family, patient			

Continued.

From Carpenito, 1992; Conley, 1990; personal communications. From Wong DL: *Whaley and Wong's nursing care of infants and children*, ed 5, St Louis, 1995, Mosby.

Religous beliefs that affect nursing care—cont'd

	Beliefs about birth and death	Beliefs about diet and food practices	Beliefs regarding medical care	Comments
Black Muslim				
Birth	No baptism	Prohibit alcohol, pork, and foods traditional among American blacks (such as corn bread, collard greens)	Faith healing unacceptable Always maintain personal habits of cleanliness	General adherence to Moslem tenets overlaid, in many instances, by antagonism to whites, especially Christians and Jews Do not indulge in activities (such as sleeping) more than is necessary to health
Death	Carefully prescribed procedure for washing and shrouding dead			
Buddhist Churches of America				
Birth	No infant baptism Infant presentation	No requirements or restrictions Some sects are strictly vegetarian Discourage use of alcohol and drugs	Illness believed to be a trial to aid development of soul, illness due to Karmic causes May be reluctant to have surgery or certain treatments on holy days Cleanliness believed to be of great importance Family may request Buddhist priest for counseling	Optimistic outlook; teach ways to overcome fears, anxieties, apprehension
Death	Last rite chanting often practiced at bedside soon after death Priest should be contacted			

Church of Christ Scientist (Christian Science)

Birth	No baptism	No requirements or restrictions	Deny the existence of health crisis, see sickness and sin as errors of mind that can be altered by prayer	Many desire services of practitioner or reader; will sometimes refuse even emergency treatment until they have consulted a reader
Death	No last rites		Oppose human intervention with drugs or other therapies; however, they accept legally required immunizations	Unlikely to donate organs for transplant
			Many adhere to belief that disease is a human mental concept that can be dispelled by "spiritual truth" to extent that they refuse all medical treatment	

Church of Jesus Christ of Latter Day Saints (Mormon)

Birth	No baptism at birth Infant is "blessed" by church official at first opportunity after birth (in church)	Prohibit tea, coffee, alcohol Some individuals avoid chocolate and other products that contain caffeine Encourage sparing use of meats	Devout adherents believe in divine healing through anointment with oil and "laying on of hands" by church officials (appointed church members)	May request Sacrament on Sunday while in hospital Financial support for sick available through well-funded welfare system Discourage use of tobacco

Continued.

Religous beliefs that affect nursing care—cont'd

	Beliefs about birth and death	Beliefs about diet and food practices	Beliefs regarding medical care	Comments
Death	Baptism by immersion at 8 years No special rites but may desire presence of church elders during any acute illness, when condition worsens, when undergoing risky or frightening tests or procedures, when feeling sick enough to die, or when dying	Fasting for 24 hours on first Sunday each month (from after evening meal Saturday until evening meal Sunday)	Medical therapy not prohibited	Married adults wear special undergarments Discourage cremation
Eastern Orthodox (Turkey, Egypt, Syria, Rumania, Bulgaria, Cyprus, Albania, etc.)				
Birth	Most believe in infant baptism by immersion 8 to 40 days after birth	Restrictions depend on specific sect	Anointment of the sick No conflict with medical science	
Death	Last rites obligatory for impending death			Discourage cremation

Episcopal (Anglican)				
Birth	Infant baptism mandatory; urgent if poor prognosis	Abstain from meat on fast days May fast on Wednesday, Friday, during Lent, and before Christmas Some fast for 6 hours before receiving Holy Communion	Some believe in spiritual healing Rite for anointing sick available but not mandatory	Religious icons very important Communion four times yearly: Christmas, Easter, June 30, and August 15; may be mandatory for some
Death	Last rites available but not mandatory			
Friends (Quakers)				
Birth	No baptism Infant's name recorded in official book	No requirements or restrictions Most practice moderation Avoid alcohol and illicit drugs	No special rites or restrictions	Believe in plain speech and dress Pacifists
Greek Orthodox				
Birth	Baptism considered important Performed 40 days after birth If not possible to baptize by sprinkling or immersion, church allows	Church-prescribed fast periods—usually occur on Wednesday, Friday, and during Lent; consist of avoiding meat and (in some cases) dairy products If health compromised, priest may be contacted to con-	Each health crisis handled by ordained priest; deacon may also serve in some cases Holy Communion administered in hospital Some may desire Sacrament of the Holy Unction performed by priest	Oppose euthanasia Believe every reasonable effort should be made to preserve life until termination by God

Continued.

Religous beliefs that affect nursing care—cont'd

Beliefs about birth and death	Beliefs about diet and food practices	Beliefs regarding medical care	Comments
child baptism "in the air" by moving child in the form of a cross as appropriate words are said	vince family to forego fasting		
Death Last rites, administration of Sacrament of Holy Communion			Discourage autopsies that may cause dismemberment Prefer burial to cremation
Should be performed while dying person is still conscious			
Hindu			
Birth No ritual			
Death Special prescribed rites	Many dietary restrictions Beef and veal not eaten Some strict vegetarians	Illness or injury believed to represent sins committed in previous life	Cremation preferred
Priest pours water into mouth of dead child, ties a thread around neck or wrist to signify blessing (should not be removed)		Accept most modern medical practices	

Family washes body and is particular about who touches body			
Islam (Muslim/Moslem)			
Birth No baptism	Prohibit all pork products and any meat that is not ritually slaughtered	Faith healing not acceptable unless psychologic conditions of patient is deteriorating; performed for morale	Older Muslims often have a fatalistic view that may interfere with compliance to therapy
Death Patient must confess sins and beg forgiveness before death; family should be present	Daylight fasting practiced during ninth month of Muhammadan year (Ramadan)	Ritual washing after prayer; prayer takes place five times daily (on rising, midday, afternoon, early evening, and before bed); during prayer, face Mecca and kneel on prayer rug	May oppose autopsy
Family washes and prepares body, then turns it to face Mecca	Strict Muslims do not use alcohol or mind-altering drugs		
Only relatives and friends may touch body			

Continued.

Religous Beliefs that Affect Nursing Care—cont'd

Beliefs about birth and death	Beliefs about diet and food practices	Beliefs regarding medical care	Comments
Jehovah's Witness			
Birth No baptism	Eat nothing to which blood has been added; can eat animal flesh that has been drained	Adherents are generally absolutely opposed to transfusions of whole blood, packed red blood cells, platelets, and fresh or frozen plasma, including banking of own blood; individuals can sometimes be persuaded in emergencies	Often possible to obtain a court order appointing a hospital official as temporary guardian to consent to a child's transfusion when parents refuse consent
Death No last rites		May be opposed to use of albumin, globulin, factor replacement (hemophilia) vaccines	Autopsy approved only as required by law
		Not opposed to non–blood plasma expanders	No restrictions on giving blood sample
Judaism (Orthodox and Conservative)			
Birth No baptism Ritual circumcision of male infants on eighth day; performed by Mohel (ritual circumciser familiar with Jew-	Numerous dietary kosher laws exist that may be influenced by local practices and family and cultural tradition Allowed only meat from animals that are vegetable eaters, are cloven hoofed, chew	May resist surgical procedures during Sabbath, which extends from sundown Friday until sundown Saturday Seriously ill and pregnant women are exempt from fasting	

ish law and aseptic technique) Reform Jews favor ritual circumcision, but not as a religious imperative	their cud, and are ritually slaughtered; fish that have scales and fins Prohibit any combination of meat and milk; milk products served first can be followed by meat in a few minutes, but milk may not be consumed for several hours after eating meat Fasting for 24 hours is part of Yom Kippur observance Matzo replaces leavened bread during Passover week	Illness is grounds for violating dietary laws (such as patient with congestive heart failure does not have to use kosher meats, which are high in sodium)	Oppose all forms of mutilation, including autopsy; body parts not donated or removed; amputated limbs, organs, or surgically removed tissues should be made available to family for burial Donation or transplantation of organs require rabbinical consent May oppose prolongation of life after irreversible brain damage
Death Remains are ritually washed by members of the Ritual Burial Society Burial should take place as soon as possible			
Lutheran *Birth* Baptize only living infants shortly after birth	No requirements or restrictions	Church or pastor notified of hospitalization Communion may be given before or after surgery or similar crisis	Accept scientific developments
Death Rite for anointing of sick optional Family or patient may request anointing if prognosis is grave			

Continued.

Religous beliefs that affect nursing care—cont'd

	Beliefs about birth and death	Beliefs about diet and food practices	Beliefs regarding medical care	Comments
Mennonite (similar to Amish)				
Birth	No baptism in infancy Baptism during early or middle teens	No requirements or restrictions	No illness rituals Deep concern for dignity and self-determination of individual that would conflict with shock treatment or medical treatment affecting personality or will	
Methodist				
Birth	No baptism at birth; performed on children or adults	No requirements or restrictions	Communion may be requested before surgery or similar crisis	
Death	No ritual			Encourage donations of body or body parts to medical science
Nazarene				
Birth	Baptism optional	No requirements or restrictions Alcohol prohibited	Church official administers communion and laying on of hands Adherents believe in divine healing but not exclusive of medical treatment	Cremation permitted
Death	No last rites			

Pentecostal (Assembly of God, Four-Square)

Birth	No baptism at birth Baptism by complete immersion after age of accountability	No restrictions regarding medical care Deliverance from sickness is provided for in atonement; may pray for divine intervention in health matters and seek God in prayer for themselves and others when ill	Some insist illness is divine punishment; most consider it an intrusion of Satan Practice glossolalia (speaking in tongues)
Death	No last rites	Abstain from alcohol, eating blood, strangled animals, or anything to which blood has been added Some individuals may resist pork	

Orthodox Presbyterian

Birth	Infant baptism by sprinkling	No requirements or restrictions	Full forgiveness granted for any illness connected with a sin
Death	Last rites not a sacramental procedure; scripture reading and prayer	Communion administered when appropriate and convenient Blood transfusion accepted when advisable Pastor or elder should be called for ill person Believe science should be used for relief of suffering	

Continued.

Religous beliefs that affect nursing care—cont'd

Beliefs about birth and death	Beliefs about diet and food practices	Beliefs regarding medical care	Comments
Roman Catholic			
Birth			
Infant baptism mandatory; especially urgent in poor prognosis, when it may be performed by anyone	Fasting (eating only one full meal and no eating between meals) and abstaining from meat mandatory on Ash Wednesday and Good Friday; fasting optional during Lent; no meat on Friday	Encourage anointing of sick, although this may be interpreted by older members of church as equivalent to old terminology "extreme unction" or "last rites"; they may require careful explanation if reluctance is associated with fear of imminent death	Family may request that major amputated limb be buried in consecrated ground
Death	days during Lent as general rule		Transplant accepted as long as loss of organ does not deprive donor of life or functional integrity of body
Rite for anointing of sick is mandatory	Children and most hospital patients exempt from fasting	Traditional church teaching does not approve of contraceptives or abortion	Autopsy acceptable
Family or patient may request anointing if prognosis is grave	Some older Catholics may adhere to older rule of no meat on Friday		Religious articles important

Russian Orthodox

Birth	Baptism by priest only	Cross necklace is important and should be removed only when necessary and replaced as soon as possible
Death	Traditionally after death arms are crossed, fingers set in a cross	No meat or dairy products on Wednesday, Friday, and during Lent
		Adherents believe in divine healing, but not exclusive of medical treatment
		Opposed to autopsy, embalming, or cremation

Unitarian Universalist

Birth	Some practice infant baptism; most consider it unnecessary	No requirements or restrictions
Death	No ritual	Most believe in general goodness of their fellow humans and appreciate expression of that goodness by visits from clergy and fellow parishioners during times of illness
		Believe in fully living this life as they know and understand it
		Cremation preferred to burial

Cultural Characteristics Related to Health Care of Children and Families

Cultural group	Health beliefs	Health practices
Asians		
Chinese	A healthy body viewed as a gift from parents and ancestors and must be cared for Health is one of the results of balance between the forces of *yin* (cold) and *yang* (hot)—energy forces that rule the world Illness caused by imbalance Believe blood is source of life and is not regenerated *Chi* is innate energy Lack of *chi* and blood results in deficiency that produces fatigue, poor constitution, and long illness	Goal of therapy is to restore balance of *yin* and *yang* Acupuncturist applies needles to appropriate meridians identified in terms of *yin* and *yang* Acupressure and *tai chi* replacing acupuncture in some areas *Moxibustion* is application of heat to skin over specific meridians Wide use of medicinal herbs procured and applied in prescribed ways Folk healers are herbalist, spiritual healer, temple healer, fortune healer Meals may or may not be planned to balance hot and cold Milk intolerance relatively common Use of condiments (such as monosodium glutamate and soy sauce) may create difficulty with some diet regimens (such as low-salt diets)
Japanese	Three major belief systems: *Shinto* religious influence Humans inherently good Evil caused by outside spirits	Believe evil removed by purification Energy restored by means of acupuncture, acupressure, massage, and moxibustion along affected meridians

From Anderson and Fenichel, 1989; Clark, 1981; DeSantis, 1988; Geissler, 1994; Giger and Davidhizar, 1991; Holland and Sweeney, 1985; Hollingsworth, Brown, and Brooten, 1980; Orgue, Bloch, and Monrroy, 1983, Randall-David, 1989. In Wong DL: *Whaley and Wong's nursing care of infants and children,* ed 5, St Louis, 1995, Mosby.

Family relationships	Communication	Comments
Extended family pattern common	Open expression of emotions unacceptable	Do not react well to painful diagnostic workup; are especially upset by drawing of blood
Strong concept of loyalty of young to old	Often smile when do not comprehend	
Respect for elders taught at early age—acceptance without questioning or talking back		Deep respect for their bodies and believe it best to die with bodies intact; therefore may refuse surgery
Children's behavior a reflection on family		Believe in reincarnation
Family and individual honor and "face" important		Older members fear hospitals; often believe hospital is a place to go to die
Self-reliance and self-restraint highly valued; self-exression repressed		Children sometimes breast-fed for up to 4 or 5 years*
Males valued more highly than females; women submissive to men in family		
Close intergenerational relationships	*Issei*—born in Japan; usually speak Japanese only	Generational categories:
Family provides anchor	*Nisei, Sansei,* and *Yonsei* have few language difficulties	*Issei*—1st generation to live in U.S.
Family tends to keep problems to self	New immigrants able to read and write	*Nisei*—2nd generation
Value self-control and self-sufficiency		

*Most Asian cultures consider the child 1 year old at the time of birth. Traditional Chinese custom adds 1 year on January 1 regardless of the birthday—a child born in December is 2 years old the next January.

Continued.

Cultural characteristics related to health care of children and families—cont'd

Cultural group	Health beliefs	Health practices
Asians—cont'd **Japanese—** **cont'd**	Illness caused by contact with polluting agents (such as blood, corpses, skin diseases) Chinese and Korean influence Health achieved through harmony and balance between self and society Disease caused by disharmony with society and not caring for body Portuguese influence Upholds germ theory of disease	*Kampō* medicine—use of natural herbs Believe in removal of diseased parts Trend is to use both Western and Oriental healing methods Care for disabled viewed as family's responsibility Take pride in child's good health Seek preventive care, medical care for illness May avoid some food combinations (such as milk and cherries, watermelon and crab) and believe pickled plums to have special properties
Vietnamese	Good health considered to be balance between *yin* and *yang* Believe person's life has been predisposed toward certain phenomena by cosmic forces Health believed to be result of harmony with existing universal order; harmony attained by pleasing good spirits and avoiding evil ones Belief in *am duc,* the amount of good deeds accumulated by ancestors Many use rituals to prevent illness Practice some restrictions to prevent incurring wrath of evil spirits	Family uses all means possible before using outside agencies for health care Fortune-tellers determine event that caused disturbance May visit temple to procure divine instruction Use astrologer to calculate cyclical changes and forces Regard health as family responsibility; outside aid sought when resources run out Certain illnesses considered only temporary (such as pustules, open wounds) and ignored Seek generalist health healers

Family relationships	Communication	Comments
Concept of *haji* (shame) imposes strong control; unacceptable behavior of children reflects on family Many adopt practices of contemporary middle class Concern for child's missing school may result in sending to school before fully recovered from illness	English better than able to speak or understand it Make significant use of nonverbal communication with subtle gestures and facial expression Tend to suppress emotions Will often wait silently	*Sansei*—3rd generation *Yonsei*—4th generation *Issei* and *Nissei*—tolerant and permissive childrearing until 5 or 6, then emphasis on emotional reserve and control Cleanliness highly valued Time considered valuable and used wisely Tendency to practice emotional control may make assessment of pain more difficult
Family is revered institution Multigenerational families Family is chief social network Children highly valued Individual needs and interests are subordinate to those of family group Father is main decision maker Women taught submission to men Parents expect respect and obedience from children	Many immigrants are not proficient in speaking and understanding English May hesitate to ask questions Questioning authority is sign of disrespect; asking questions considered impolite Use indirectness rather than forthrightness in expressing disagreement May avoid eye contact with health professionals as a sign of respect	Consider status more important than money Children taught emotional control Time concept more relaxed—consider punctuality less significant than other values (such as propriety) Place high value on social harmony

Continued.

Cultural characteristics related to health care of children and families—cont'd

Cultural group	Health beliefs	Health practices
Asians—cont'd **Vietnamese—** **cont'd**		May use special diets to prevent illness and promote health Lactose intolerance prevalent
Filipinos	Believe God's will and supernatural forces govern universe Illness, accidents, and other misfortunes are God's punishment for violations of His will Widely accept "hot" and "cold" balance and imbalance as cause of health and illness	Some use amulets as a shield from witchcraft or as good luck pieces Catholics substitute religious medals and other items
Blacks	Illness classified as: Natural—affected by forces of nature without adequate protection (such as cold air, pollution, food and water) Unnatural—evil influences (such as witchcraft, voodoo, hoodoo, hex, fix, rootwork); symptoms often associated with eating Believe serious illness sent by God as punishment (such as parents punished by illness or death of child) Believe serious illness can be avoided May resist health care because illness is "will of God"	Self-care and folk medicine very prevalent Folk therapies usually religious in origin Attempt home remedies first; poorer people do not seek help until illness serious Usually seek help from: "Old lady"—woman in community with a common knowledge of herbs; consulted regarding pediatric care Spiritualist—has received gift from God for healing incurable diseases or solving personal problems; strongly based in Christianity Priest (voodoo priest/priestess)—most powerful healer

Family relationships	Communication	Comments
Family is highly valued, with strong family ties	Immigrants and older persons may not be able to speak or understand English	Tend to have a fatalistic outlook on life
Multigenerational family structure common, often with collateral members as well		Believe time and providence will solve all
Personal interests are subordinated to family interests and needs		
Members avoid any behavior that would bring shame on the family		
Strong kinship bonds in extended family; members come to aid of others in crisis	Alert to any evidence of discrimination	High level of caution and distrust of majority group
Less likely to view illness as a burden	Place importance on nonverbal behavior	Social anxiety related to tradition of humiliation, oppression, and loss of dignity
Augmented families common (unrelated persons living in same household)	May use nonstandard English or "black English"	Will elect to retain dignity rather than seek care if values are compromised
Place strong emphasis on work and ambition	Use "testing" behaviors to assess personnel in health care situations before seeking active care	Strong sense of peoplehood
Sex-role sharing among parents	Best to use simple, direct, but caring approach	High incidence of poverty
Elderly members respected		Black minister a strong influence in black community
Maternal grandparent strong influence		Visits by family minister are sought, expected, and valued in helping to cope with illness and suffering

Cultural characteristics related to health care of children and families—cont'd

Cultural group	Health beliefs	Health practices
Blacks—cont'd		Root doctor—meets need for herbs, oils, candles, and ointments Prayer is common means for prevention and treatment
Haitians†	Illnesses have a supernatural or natural origin Supernatural illnesses are caused by angry voodoo spirits, enemies, or the dead, especially deceased ancestors Natural illnesses are based on conceptions of natural causation: Irregularities of blood volume, flow, purity, viscosity, color, or temperature (hot-cold) Gas *(gaz)* Movement and consistency of mother's milk Hot-cold imbalance in the body Bone displacement Movement of diseases Health is maintained by good dietary and hygienic habits	Health is a personal responsibility Foods have properties of "hot" or "cold" and "light" or "heavy" and must be in harmony with one's life cycle and bodily states Natural illnesses are treated by home remedies first Supernatural illness treated by healers: voodoo priest *(houngan)* or priestess *(mambo)*, midwife *(fam saj)*, and herbalist or leaf doctor *(dokte fey)* Amulets and prayer used to protect against illness due to curses or willed by evil people
Hispanics **Mexicans** **(Latinos,** **Chicanos,** **Raza-** **Latinos)**	Health beliefs have strong religious association Believe in body imbalance as a cause of illness, especially imbalance between *caliente* (hot) and *frio* (cold) or "wet" and "dry" Some maintain good health is a result of	Seek help from *curandero* or *curandera,* especially in rural areas *Curandero(a)* receives his or her position by birth, apprenticeship, or a "calling" via dream or vision Treatments involve use of herbs, rituals, and religious artifacts

†This section was written by Lydia DeSantis, RN, PhD.

Family relationships	Communication	Comments
Maintenance of family reputation is paramount	Recent immigrants and older persons may speak only Haitian creole	Will use biomedical and ethnomedical (folk) systems simultaneously
Lineal authority supreme; children in a subordinate position in family hierarchy	May prefer family or friends to act as translators and confidants	Resistant to dietary and work restrictions
Children valued for parental social security in old age and expected to contribute to family welfare at an early age	Often smile and nod in agreement when do not understand	Adherence to prescribed treatments directly related to perceived severity of illness
Children viewed as "gifts from god" and treated with indulgence and affection	Quiet and gentle communication style and lack of assertiveness lead health care providers to falsely believe they comprehend health teaching and are compliant	
	Will not ask questions if health care provider is busy or rushed	
Traditionally men considered breadwinners and key decision makers in matters outside the home; women considered homemakers	May use nonstandard English	High degree of modesty—often a deterrent to seeking medical care and open discussions of sex
Males considered big and strong *(macho)*	Some bilingual; many only speak Spanish	Youngsters often reluctant to share communal showers in schools
Strong kinship; extended families in	May have a strong preference for native language and revert to it in times of stress	Relaxed concept of time—may be late
	May shake hands or engage in introduc-	

Continued.

Cultural characteristics related to health care of children and families—cont'd

Cultural group	Health beliefs	Health practices
Hispanics—cont'd		
Mexicans—cont'd	"good luck"—a reward for good behavior Illness prevented by performing properly, eating proper foods, and working proper amount of time; accomplished through prayer, wearing religious medals or amulets, and sleeping with relics at home Illness is a punishment from God for wrongdoing, forces of nature, and the supernatural	Practice for severe illness—make promises, visit shrines, offer medals and candles, offer prayers Adhere to "hot" and "cold" food prescriptions and prohibitions for prevention and treatment of illness
Puerto Ricans	Subscribe to the "hot-cold" theory of causation of illness Believe some illness caused by evil spirits and forces	Infrequent use of health care systems Seek folk healers—use of herbs, rituals Consult spiritualist medium for mental disorders *Santeria* is system, and practitioners are called *santeros* Treatments classified as "hot" or "cold"
Cubans‡	Prevention and good nutrition are related to good health	Diligent users of the medical model Eclectic health-seeking practices, including preventive measures, and, in some instances, folk medicine of both religious and nonreligious origins; home remedies; in many in-

‡This section was written by Mercedes Sandaval, PhD.

Family relationships	Communication	Comments
clude *compadres* (godparents) established by ritual kinship Children valued highly and desired, taken everywhere with family Many homes contain shrines with statues and pictures of saints Elderly treated with respect	tory embrace Interpret prolonged eye contact as disrespectful	for appointments More concerned with present than with future and therefore may focus on immediate solutions rather than long-term goals Magicoreligious practices common May view hospital as place to go to die
Family usually large and home centered—the core of existence Father has complete authority in family—family provider and decision maker Wife and children subordinate to father Children valued—seen as a gift from God Children taught to obey and respect parents; corporal punishment to ensure obedience	May use nonstard English Spanish speaking or bilingual Strong sense of family privacy—may view questions regarding family as impudent	Relaxed sense of time Pay little attention to exact time of day Suspicious and fearful of hospitals
Strong family ties with mother and father kinships Children supported and assisted by parents long after becoming adults Elderly cared for at home	Most are bilingual (English/Spanish) except for segments of the senior population	In less than 30 years Cubans have been able to obtain a higher standard of living than other Hispanic groups in U.S. Have been able to retain many of their former social insti-

Continued.

Cultural characteristics related to health care of children and families—cont'd

Cultural group	Health beliefs	Health practices
Hispanics—cont'd **Cubans— cont'd**		stances seek assistance of santeros and spiritualists to complement medical treatment Nutrition is important; parents show overconcern with eating habits of their children and spend a considerable part of the budget on food; traditional Cuban diet is rich in meat and starch; consumption of fresh vegetables added in U.S.
Native Americans (numerous tribes)	Believe health is state of harmony with nature and universe Respect of bodies through proper management All disorders believed to have aspects of supernatural Violation of a restriction or prohibition thought to cause illness Fear of witchcraft May carry objects believed to guard against witchcraft Theology and medicine strongly interwoven	Medicine persons: Altruistic persons who must use powers in purely positive ways Persons capable of both good and evil—perform negative acts against enemies Diviner-diagnosticians—diagnose but do not have powers or skill to implement medical treatment Specialsts—use herbs and curative but nonsacred medical procedures Medicine persons—use herbs and ritual Singers—cure by the power of their song obtained from supernatural beings; effect cures by laying on of hands

Family relationships	Communication	Comments
		tutions: bilingual and private schools, clinics, social clubs, the family as an extended network of support, etc.
		Many do not feel discriminated against nor harbor feelings of inferiority with respect to Anglo-Americans or "mainstream" population
Extended family structure—usually include relatives from boths sides of family	Most continue to speak their Indian language, as well as English	Time orientation—present
Elder members assume leadership roles	Nonverbal communication	Respect for age
		Going to hospital associated with illness or disease; therefore may not seek prenatal care, since pregnancy viewed as natural process
		Tend to take time to form an opinion of professionals
		Sexual matters not openly discussed with members of opposite sex

Genogram Form

Date: _____ Completed: _____

Family name: _____

Generation 1

Generation 2

Generation 3

Adapted from: McGoldrick M, Gerson R: *Genograms in family assessment,* NY, 1985, WW Norton.

Genogram Symbols

A. Symbols to Describe Basic Family Structure

Male: □   Female: ○   Birth date — 43-75 — Death date

Death = X

Index Person (IP): ▣ ◎

Marriage (give date) (Husband on left, wife on right):

Living together relationship or liaison:

Marital separation (give date):

Divorce (give date):

Children: List in birth order, beginning with oldest on left:

Adopted or foster children:

Fraternal twins:

Identical twins:

Pregnancy:

Spontaneous abortion:

Induced abortion:

Stillbirth:

Members of current IP household (circle them):

Adapted from: McGoldrick M, Gerson R: *Genograms in family assessment,* NY, 1985, WW Norton.

B. Family Interaction Patterns—Optimal

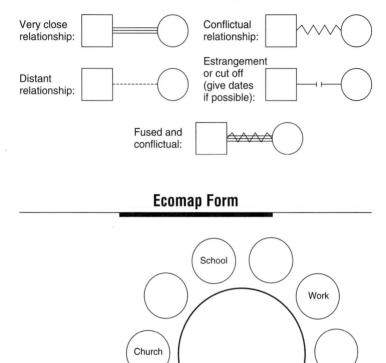

Very close
relationship:

Conflictual
relationship:

Distant
relationship:

Estrangement
or cut off
(give dates
if possible):

Fused and
conflictual:

Ecomap Form

School

Work

Church

Friends

Extended
Family

Key

≡ Strong
--- Tenuous
-///- Stressful
→ Energy flow

Adapted from Friedman MM: *Family nursing: theory and practice,* Norwalk, Conn.,
1992, Appleton & Lange.

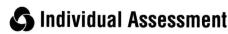 Individual Assessment

The most common intervention by a nurse is at the individual level. Planning appropriate care to persons living in the community will enhance quality of life through prevention and health-promotion initiatives.

Mental Health Status Assessment

During client contact the nurse must develop ways to assess the presence or extent of a client's mental health disability. The nurse must be constantly alert to altered behaviors, physical appearance, mood, and changes in family interactions and responses. The following instrument will assist in making this assessment.

Family Structure/Situation: Employment

Family members _____   Occupations _____

     Primary person responsible for care _____

     Role relationships/interactions/decision makers _____

     Family health status _____

     Client's history and current health status _____

     Long term/short term? _____

     Communication patterns and emotional support within

family _____

     Socioeconomic status (and health care benefits) _____

     Values, attitudes or cultural, religious influences that

impact care _____

   Available community resources _____

   Equipment/procedures/skills required for care

     Mental health assessment: If yes, check where applies: client/family member

General Appearance:

Posture: Slouched   _____

       Rigid   _____

Dress: Inappropriate for place   _____

   or weather

Grooming: Meticulous   _____

       Unkempt   _____

       Poor hygiene   _____

From Jernigan D: Mental health assessment tool, *Caring* 5(7):July, 1986.

Nonverbal Communication:

Angry facial expression   _____

Restless   _____

Agitated   _____

Lack of eye contact   _____

General Behavior:

Tense   _____

Resentful/hostile   _____

Unwilling to participate in care/   _____
   uncooperative

Mood:

Tearful   _____

Elated   _____

Sudden mood changes   _____

Flat affect   _____

Speech/Language:

Slow   _____

Monotonous tone   _____

Discusses inappropriate topics   _____

Manic—flight of ideas   _____

Incoherent or garbled   _____

Disorganized speech   _____

Rapid, nonstop talk   _____

Orientation (Level of Awareness):

Unaware of time   _____

Unaware of place   _____

Unaware of self/others/circumstances   _____

Transient confusion/unawareness   _____

State of Consciousness:

Slow movements and delayed   _____
   response to stimuli

Responds only to vigorous,   _____
   painful stimuli

No response to stimuli   _____

Memory:

No recall of recent events   _____

No recall of remote/past events   _____

Inaccurate (distorted) recall of   _____
   recent/past events

Information or Knowledge Level:

Distorted perception of cause of
 problem/illness _____

Lack of understanding of reason
 for treatment _____

Poor comprehension of required
 skills/procedures for home
 maintenance _____

Denial of a problem or need
 for treatment _____

Client's Physical Abilities:

Unable to perform ADL/self-care _____

Immobile/needs assistance for
 ADL/self-care _____

Nutritional status/general intake _____

Thought Content (A Guide for Questioning Client or Family Member Concerning Mental Health):

What do you think about at times like this? _____

Do you feel discouraged or low? _____

What do you see for yourself and your family in the future? _____

What do you see as your main problem? Need? _____

What solutions do you think would solve this problem? _____

Review of recent events (in client's own words): _____

Do you feel capable of handling your situation? _____

Do you think about something over and over? _____

Do you have any doubts or real fears? _____

Do you feel anxious inside? _____

What are your biggest obstacles? Strengths? _____

Do you feel alone; isolated? _____

Do you feel you can talk to someone; that someone
 understands? _____

Do you have trouble sleeping? _____

Do you feel like you've lost something? What? _____

How do you feel about/see yourself? _____

Can you see yourself as productive? _____

Do you feel guilt? Self-blame? Failure? _____

Has your sexual relationship with your mate changed? _____

Anything else you would like to talk about or mention? _____

*Summary of client/family coping mechanisms—functional versus
 dysfunctional:*

Current or potential problems/nursing diagnoses (prioritize):

Major strengths: *Major limitations:*

Additional comments or observations:

Teaching needs:

Mental health plans:

Short Portable Mental Status Questionnaire (SPMSQ)

Mental Assessment*

The nurse can evaluate cognitive function with a simple bedside examination such as the mini–mental state examination. This brief examination covers orientation, registration, attention, calculation, recall, and language. The test is scored with a maximum of 30 points. A score below 24 is considered abnormal. Consideration for the client's education and life experience may influence the overall score. Early in a dementing illness, mild signs and symptoms of dementia may be difficult to identify. Thus diagnosing dementia with certainty can be difficult. Detailed neuropsychologic testing may be helpful in evaluating higher cortical functions and providing a baseline for following the client over time.

Pertinent questions	Scoring
1. What is the date today (month/day/year)?	0-2 errors = intact
	3-4 errors = mild intellectual impairment
2. What day of the week is it?	
3. What is the name of this place?	5-7 errors = moderate intellectual impairment
4. What is your telephone number? (If no telephone, what is your street address?)	
	8-10 errors = severe intellectual impairment
5. How old are you?	
6. When were you born (month/day/year)?	Allow one more error if subject had no grade-school education
7. Who is the current president of the United States?	Allow one fewer error if subject has had education beyond high school
8. Who was the president just before him?	
9. What was your mother's maiden name?	
10. Subtract 3 from 20 and keep subtracting 3 from each new number all the way down.	

From Kane R, Ouslander J, Abrass I: *Essentials of clinical geriatrics,* New York, 1994, McGraw-Hill.

*From Barker E: *Neuroscience nursing,* St. Louis, 1994, Mosby.

Folstein's Mini–Mental State Examination

Maximum score	Score	
5	( )	**Orientation** What is the (year) (season) (date) (day) (month)?
5	( )	Where are we (state) (country) (town) (hospital) (floor)?
3	( )	**Registration** Name three objects: one (1) second to say each. Then ask the client all three after you have said them. Give one point for each correct answer. Then repeat them until the client learns all three. Count trials and record.
5	( )	**Attention and calculation trial** Serial 7s. Give one point for each correct. Stop after five answers. Alternatively spell "world" backwards.
3	( )	**Recall** Ask for three objects repeated above. Give one point for each correct.

Continued.

From Folstein MF, Folstein S, McHugh PR: Mini-mental state: a practical method for grading the cognitive state of patients for the clinician, *J Psychiatr Res* 12:189, 1975. In Ebersole P, Hess P: *Toward healthy aging: human needs and nursing response*, ed 4, St Louis, 1994, Mosby.

Folstein's Mini–Mental State Examination—cont'd

Maximum score	Score	
9	( )	**Language trial**
		Name a pencil and a watch (two points).
		Repeat the following: "No ifs, ands, or buts" (one point).
		Follow a three-stage command: "Take a paper in your right hand, fold it in half, and put it on the floor" (three points).
		Read and obey the following:
		"Close your eyes" (one point).
		"Write a sentence" (one point).
		"Copy design" (one point).
		Assess level of consciousness along a continuum.

Alert	Drowsy	Stupor	Coma

TOTAL ( )

Directions for Mental Status Test (Mini–Mental State)

I. Orientation (Maximum score 10)

Ask "What is today's date?" Then ask specifically for parts omitted; e.g., "Can you also tell me what season it is?"

	Points
Date (e.g., Jan. 21)	___
Year	___
Month	___
Day (e.g., Monday)	___
Season	___

Ask "Can you tell me the name of this hospital or where we are?"
"What floor are we on?" (if applicable)
"What town (or city) are we in?"
"What county are we in?"
"What state are we in?"

	Points
Hospital (home)	___
Floor	___
Town/City	___
County	___
State	___

Continued.

From Kane R, Ouslander, J, Abrass I: *Essentials of clinical geriatrics.* New York, 1994, McGraw-Hill.

Directions for mental status test (mini–mental state)—cont'd

II. Registration (Maximum score 3)

Ask the subject if you may test his or her memory, then say "ball," "flag," "tree" clearly and slowly, about 1 second for each. After you have said all three words, ask subject to repeat them. This first repetition determines the score (0 to 3) but keep saying them (up to 6 trials) until the subject can repeat all three words. If subject does not eventually learn all three, recall cannot be meaningfully tested.

"ball" .... |___|
"flag" .... |___|
"tree" .... |___|

III. Attention and calculation (Maximum score 5)

Ask the subject to begin at 100 and count backward by 7. Stop after 5 subtractions (93, 86, 79, 72, 65). Score one point for each correct number.

"93" .... |___|
"86" .... |___|
"79" .... |___|
"72" .... |___|
"65" .... |___|

or

If the subject cannot or will not perform this task, ask him or her to spell the word "world" backwards (D,L,R,O,W). The score is 1 point for each correctly placed letter, e.g., DLROW = 5, DLORW = 3. Record how the subject spelled "world" backwards: $\dfrac{\text{D L R O W}}{}$

# of correctly
placed letters .... |___|

IV. Recall (Maximum score 3)

Ask the subject to recall the three words you previously asked him or her to remember (learned in Registration)

"ball" .... |___|
"flag" .... |___|
"tree" .... |___|

V. Language (Maximum score 9)

Naming: Show the subject a wristwatch and ask "What is this?"
Repeat for pencil. Score one point for each item named correctly.

Watch .... |
Pencil .... |

Repetition: Ask the subject to repeat, "No ifs, ands, or buts." Score one point for correct repetition.

Repetition .... |

Three-Stage Command: Give the subject a piece of blank paper and say, "Take the paper in your right hand, fold it in half, and put it on the floor." Score one point for each action performed correctly.

Takes in rt. hand ...... |
Folds in half .... |
Puts on floor .... |

Reading: On a blank piece of paper, print the sentence "Close your eyes" in letters large enough for the subject to see clearly. Ask subject to read it and do what it says. Score correct only if subject actually closes his or her eyes.

Closes eyes .... |

Writing: Give the subject a blank piece of paper and ask him or her to write a sentence. It is to be written spontaneously. It must contain a subject and verb and make sense. Correct grammar and punctuation are not necessary.

Writes sentence .... |

Copying: On a clean piece of paper, draw intersecting pentagons, each side about 1 inch, and ask subject to copy it exactly as it is. All 10 angles must be present and two must intersect to score 1 point. Tremor and rotation are ignored. For example,

Draws pentagons ...... |

TOTAL SCORE _____

Flow Chart Showing Growth and Development Changes throughout the Life Cycle*

Overview of developmental changes	Prenatal →	Infancy →	Childhood →	Puberty and adolescence →	Adulthood →	Middle age →	Old age
Heart and circulatory system							
Action of heart and circulatory system is under control of autonomic nervous system. Throughout life cardiac rate is responsive to organ needs and emotional states (fear, anxiety, tension, depression)	Heart formed and begins to beat about third week	Heart grows a little more slowly than rest of body (weight doubled by 1 year, body weight tripled) Grows steadily during childhood With birth, considerable change in paths and relative volumes of blood flow, reflected in loss of certain fetal structures and changes in heart and major vessels		At puberty, heart takes part in rapid growth, reaching mature size with rest of body	Heart weight remains relatively constant after age 25 (only organ other than prostate that does not decrease in weight with age) Cardiac output decreases 30% to 40% between age 25 and 65 Cardiac power is less with age, whereas expenditure of energy is more than in youth. Capacity to increase rate and strength of beat during physical work is diminished		

Heart rate high, approximately 150 beats/min	Heart rate falls steadily throughout childhood 130 beats/min 70-80 beats/min Heart rate more variable during childhood—regular	60 beats/min in adolescence; rates differ between sexes	After maturity, women have slightly higher pulse rate than men, 65 beats/min (girls; temperature remains stationary, higher than boys'); men maintain same pulse rate in maturity (slightly lower body temperature than women)
		Not until midchildhood does peripheral blood picture become same as adult	

Urinary system

As a whole, parallels growth of body as a whole. Proportion of body water and solids follows pattern related to growth—tendency for human organism to dry out as life progresses	Young fetus is about 90% water Urinary system begins in first month	Newborn is about 70% water Urinary system does not complete full development until end of first year All renal units immature at birth; thus fluid and electrolyte	Composition of urine in healthy child (after age 2) changes little as child matures; thus renal function and urinalysis can be used as monitor of well-being	Adult is about 58% water Glomerular filtration rate decreases about 57% from age 20 to 90
				Renal mass decreases with age; renal flow decreases 53% (some researchers believe this is an adaptive change, compensating for declining cardiac output)

Continued.

*This chart indicates only general trends and directions of growth and development; it is not all-inclusive. No distinct ages, absolute values, or ranges of normal variations are intended in this flow chart.

Adapted from Sutterly D, Donneley G: *Perspectives in human development: nursing throughout the life cycle*, Philadelphia, 1973, Lippincott. In Edelman CL, Mandle CL: *Health promotion throughout the lifespan*, ed 3, St Louis, 1994, Mosby.

Flow chart showing growth and development changes throughout the life cycle—cont'd

Overview of developmental changes	Prenatal →	Infancy →	Childhood →	Puberty and adolescence →	Adulthood →	Middle age →	Old age
Urinary system—cont'd							
Function of kidneys, with other organ systems, is to help in regulation of internal environment of body.		imbalance occurs readily Kidney function adequate at birth if not subject to undue stress					
Digestive system							
As a whole grows as total body grows, although evidence suggests that various parts of gastroin	Before birth nutrients are supplied through placental circulation; digestion and absorption do not	Stomach size increases rapidly first months, then grows steadily through childhood Digestive apparatus immature at birth (food passes through rapidly, reverse peristalis common)		Spurt of growth of puberty	All actions of the GI tract (food intake, digestion, absorption, elimination) not only respond to physiologic needs but from birth to old age are sensitive to tensions and anxiety Available data suggest generalized atrophy of entire GI tract with advancing age Nutritional needs vary according to individual variation—decreasing metabolism →decreasing enzyme production →HCl →stomach volume—		

testinal system undergo separate periods of growth, maturity, and senescence.

occur in the gastrointestinal (GI) tract

tone of large intestine may become impaired

Activity of gastric juices varies over life span; low during infancy, rises in childhood; plateau about age 10, rise in puberty

Free gastric acid (HCl) more pronounced in boys

Salivary glands small at birth

Increase rapidly during first 3 mo; reach relative adult proportions by age 2

Until decrease with senescence (also diminished taste)

Special senses

Most are well developed at birth, although their association with higher centers comes about gradually

Begin early in embryonic development — 3-6 wk

Sense of touch is developed first, then hearing and vision

Vision: infant can perceive simple differences in shape but not complex patterns (greater proportion of total growth before birth); various dimensions of vision develop at various ages, eye muscles function at mature level first year, fusion begins 9 mo until 6 yr; refractive power changes over life cycle—hyperopia increases until eyeball reaches adult size (approximately 8 yr), then reverses trend toward emmetropia—postpubertal years—toward total myopia until 30—myopia decreases—hyperopia increases

Continued.

Flow chart showing growth and development changes throughout the life cycle—cont'd

Overview of developmental changes	Prenatal →	Infancy →	Childhood →	Puberty and adolescence →	Adulthood →	Middle age →	Old age
Special senses—cont'd							
during early life and diminishes with advancing age							
Adipose tissue							
Although adipose tissue varies greatly from individual to individual, overall lifetime pattern exists. Fat accumulation varies greatly with body build and constitution	Accumulates rapidly before birth; peak at seventh prenatal month	Increases rapidly during first 6 mo	Decreases from first to seventh year in both sexes	Begins to increase slowly to puberty		Typically both sexes tend to gain weight in fifties and sixties but do not maintain same body contours of earlier years at same weight (increase de-	Usually fat stores are lost after seventh decade in both sexes Sharpness in contours, increasingly prominent bony landmarks
	Premature infant may look	(Gender differences are not noted in the body shape of prepubescent children)		Fat begins to accumulate slowly and	Some girls slim down after full		

Relationship between caloric intake, amount of exercise, and utilization and accumulation of fat is not yet fully understood but is basis of much interrelated research

wrinkled and scrawny beause of lack of adipose tissue

Deposition of fat differs in body—amount decreases sharply at time of maximum growth spurt (increased

continues uninterrupted in girls, producing feminine curves; accounts for much of weight gain

After full maturation, fat accumulation begins →

maturation; many maintain about same amount of adipose as at puberty

posit on abdomen and hips)

(Continues →)

Continued.

Flow chart showing growth and development changes throughout the life cycle—cont'd

Overview of developmental changes	Prenatal →	Infancy →	Childhood →	Puberty and adolescence →	Adulthood →	Middle age →	Old age
Adipose tissue—cont'd							
				weight caused by increase in muscle mass and bones)			
Lymphoid tissue							
Lymphoid tissue is scattered widely throughout body and includes lymph nodes, tonsils, adenoids, thymus, spleen, and lymphocytes of the blood; follows unique	Begins in last month of uterine life—immunoglobulins cross placental at levels equal to mother's and continue for several months after delivery	Grows most rapidly during infancy and childhood, reaching maximum size a few years before puberty; parallels development of immunity Increased incidence of disease with increasing age of child		Atrophies and is smaller in volume at full maturity than during childhood			Thymus so small that it is difficult to locate in older people

pattern of growth, rapid in infancy and puberty			
Respiratory system			
Growth parallels that of total body growth. Respiratory apparatus is a highly organized system of organs under nervous and hormonal regulation, which functions in coordination with rest of body. Sex difference in gaseous exchange be-	Before birth, air sacs do not contain air; oxygen supplied through maternal circulation	Whem umbilical cord is cut, infant must use own breathing apparatus—breathing irregular at first both in rate and depth—fast in infancy—gradually slowing through childhood until full maturity is reached	No sex difference in respiratory rate at any time of life Basal metabolism rate declines (rate higher in men than women)

Continued.

Flow chart showing growth and development changes throughout the life cycle—cont'd

Overview of developmental changes	Prenatal →	Infancy →	Childhood →	Puberty and adolescence →	Adulthood →	Middle age →	Old age
Respiratory system—cont'd comes apparent during puberty		Respiratory exchange gradually becomes more efficient as life advances. Actual volume of air inhaled with each breath increases as lung size expands with general body growth. Vital capacity and maximum breathing capacity rise gradually in both sexes, increasing more in boys during puberty; adult men have more efficient respiratory exchange, are capable of greater feats of muscular exertion without exhaustion than women					
Skeletal system Bone growth passes through successive stages of development from connective tissue to cartilage to osseous tissue;	70% of head growth before birth;	Follows cephalocaudal law of development After first year, legs fastest growing, 66% of total increase in height; longer puberty is delayed, greater the leg length	Reserved during growth spurt		Maximum height in early twenties to thirties	Gradual decline until onset of senescence Thinning of vertebral disk beginning in middle years, most rapid in last decade	

completion of calcification indicates end of growing period and is thus useful measure of growth rate and physiologic maturity. Most growth ceases in adolescence	bones of hands and wrist laid down in cartilage	Trunk fastest growing, 60% of total increase	Length of trunk and depth of chest reach peak growth speeds last
		At birth, shafts of metacarpals are ossified (and visible by radiograph); carpal bones begin to ossify	Growth of both sexes nearly even until onset of puberty in girls first (approximately 10½ yr) Boys begin approximately 2½ yr later, but noticeably greater Peak in height comes before peak in weight	Spinal column shortens (osteoporosis) with thinning vertebrae—shortening of trunk with long extremities—reversal of growth proportions in infancy

Continued.

Flow chart showing growth and development changes throughout the life cycle—cont'd

Overview of developmental changes	Prenatal →	Infancy →	Childhood →	Puberty and adolescence →	Adulthood →	Middle age →	Old age
Muscular system							
Number of striated muscle fibers is roughly same in all human beings. Tremendous difference in size, not only from fetus to adult but among adults, is caused by ability of individual muscle fibers to increase in size. Growth potential,	Muscle formation begins early assuming final shape by end of second month	Increases rapidly during infancy but slowly during childhood Growth in both sexes is same in childhood		With onset of puberty, muscle strength is greater in boys (when muscle growth is stimulated by testosterone) Greatest increase begins in puberty; muscle size precedes muscle strength in boys	Muscle mass continues to increase gradually—maximum strength in early adulthood—then declines slight—according to use and genetic constitution Will increase in bulk and strength as used		Until onset of senescence—atrophy and loss of muscle tone

however, is influenced by genes, hormones, nutrition, exercise, and possibly other unknown factors as well

Increase in muscle size means increasing strength in children; increase in skill is more intimately related to maturation of nervous system

Nervous system

Growth and maturation of central nervous system (brain, cord, peripheral nerves, many sense organs) follow pattern reflected	Growth rapid during intrauterine development; head increases at greater rate than rest of body	Has all the brain cells of first year, which will continue to increase in size; number and complexity of axons and dendrites will continue to increase	Function continues with use	Possible decrease in size and number of brain cells in senescence (?) (subject of study)

Continued.

Flow chart showing growth and development changes throughout the life cycle—cont'd

Overview of developmental changes	Prenatal →	Infancy →	Childhood →	Puberty and adolescence →	Adulthood →	Middle age →	Old age
Nervous system—cont'd							
by changing size of the head							Decrease in myelin sheath, impulses decrease; slow down speed of action and reaction
		All neural tissues grow rapidly during infancy and early childhood		(No neural growth spurt at puberty)			
		Brain grows rapidly after birth, reaching 90% of total size by age 2	By midchildhood, almost reaches adult size	Slow increase to full maturity	Brain weight decreases with age		
		Segmented spinal nerves are mature, fully myelinated, and functioning at term (e.g., knee jerk), but acquisition of myelin in cortex, brain stem, and cord is closely correlated with observed behavior (myelinization of this tract follows cephalocaudal, proximodistal law)					
		Equipment for sense of taste and smell present at birth and perhaps most acute at that time				Taste less acute, less discrimatory with advancing age	
						Structural changes in CNS result in impaired perception	

Reproductive system

Overview	Prenatal	Birth	Childhood	Puberty	Pregnancy	Later years
Organs of reproductive system show little increase during early life but rapid development just before and coincident with puberty. Maturation and fulfillment of reproductive functions of maturity (in female) are followed by involution in later years	Genital organs form during uterine life; uterus undergoes growth spurt before birth (hormone stimulation from mother)	Female sex organs well formed but not functioning at birth (but have full quota of sensory nerves)	Quiescent during childhood →	Maturation at puberty (menstruation) →		Involution after menopause
		Uterus undergoes involution to half its birth weight	Regained size by age 10-11 →	Adult size at puberty →	Maximum increase with pregnancy →	Begin to atrophy with advancing age
		In male—testes, as with ovary, remain dormant and		Until puberty, interstitial cells of Leydig reappear and secrete testosterone; so testes and penis continue increase in size (pubic hair appears)		

Continued.

Flow chart showing growth and development changes throughout the life cycle—cont'd

Overview of developmental changes	Prenatal →	Infancy →	Childhood →	Puberty and adolescence →	Adulthood →	Middle age →	Old age
Reproductive system—cont'd							
		small, not even growing in proportion to rest of body (with sensory nerves)					
	Mammary glands develop in both sexes during fetal life	Enlargement of breasts at birth (both sexes) →	Nonsecretory during childhood until puberty →	Development rapid →	Enlarge during pregnancy, developing alveoli →		Atrophy with advanced age
	Sex hormones; until puberty girls and boys produce male hormones (androgens) and female hormones (chiefly estrogens) in small and roughly equal amounts						
Integumentary system							
Includes skin and its appendages and	Hair, skin, and sebaceous	Skin contains all its adult structures at	Matures slowly until puberty	Rapid spurt in maturation of skin and		Changes in skin most obvious sign of aging (exposure and environmental conditions)	

adnexa (nails, hair, sebaceous glands, eccrine and apocrine sweat glands). Although all skin is similar, this organ shows considerable variability in different parts of body (and from individual to individual) and varies greatly during the life span	glands fully formed in utero	birth but immature in function	(children prone to rashes)	all its structured
	Lanugo begins to decrease before birth and continues regression few weeks postnatally →		Replaced by body hair, less extensive distribution; large difference in type and distribution of hair at puberty →	
	Activity of sebaceous decreases after birth →			Increases rapidly at puberty (more prone to acne)

Decrease in regenerative and growth power decreases and skin loses elasticity

Continued.

Flow chart showing growth and development changes throughout the life cycle—cont'd

Overview of developmental changes	Prenatal →	Infancy →	Childhood →	Puberty and adolescence →	Adulthood →	Middle age →	Old age
Endocrine system							
Consists of a number of glandular structures scattered throughout the body. Although small in size, their hormones influence all growth and development of whole organism	Immaturity of entire endocrine system puts infant at disadvantage if required to adjust to wide fluctuations in concentration of water, electrolytes, glucose, amino acids. All are interrelated, but each organ develops at own rate: Thyroid—increases from midfetal life to maturity; little larger in boys than girls; growth spurt at adolescence Adrenals—after birth decreases in size and continues throughout first year, increases again during childhood (but smaller than birth); spurts at puberty, reaching maturity with rest of body; greater increase in male gonads and testes and female ovaries—are endocrine glands as well as reproductive organs; follow genital type of growth pattern Hypophysis or pituitary gland—produces or stimulates hormones that influence growth Parathyroids—produce hormones that maintain homeostasis of calcium and phosphorus Islets of Langerhans—dispersed through pancreas; produce insulin and glucagon					With age, decline occurs in all endocrine gland functions	

Erikson's Eight Stages of Human Development

Stage (approximate)	Psychosocial stages	Lasting outcomes
1. Infancy	Basic trust versus basic mistrust	Drive and hope
2. Toddlerhood	Autonomy versus shame and doubt	Self-control and willpower
3. Preschool	Initiative versus guilt	Direction and purpose
4. Middle childhood (school age)	Industry versus inferiority	Method and competence
5. Adolescence	Identity versus role confusion	Devotion and fidelity
6. Young adulthood	Intimacy versus isolation	Affiliation and love
7. Middle adulthood	Generativity versus stagnation	Production and care
8. Older adulthood	Ego integrity versus despair	Renunciation and wisdom

Adapted from Erikson EH: *Childhood and society*, New York, 1993, Norton, with permisson of WW Norton. In Edelman CL, Mandle CL: *Health promotion throughout the lifespan*, ed 3, St Louis, 1994, Mosby.

Piaget's Levels of Cognitive Development

Stage	Age	Characteristics
Sensorimotor	0-2 yr	Thought dominated by physical manipulation of objects and events
Substage 1	0-1 mo	Pure reflex adaptations
Substage 2	1-4 mo	Primary circular reactions
Substage 3	4-8 mo	Secondary circular reactions
Substage 4	8-12 mo	Coordination of secondary schemata
Substage 5	12-18 mo	Tertiary circular reactions
Substage 6	18-24 mo	Invention of new solutions through mental combinations
Preoperational	2-7 yr	Functions symbolically using language as major tool
Preconceptual	2-4 yr	Uses representational thought to recall past, represent present, and anticipate future
Intuitive	4-7 yr	Increased symbolic functioning
Concrete operations	7-11 yr	Mental reasoning processes assume logical approaches to solving concrete problems
Formal operations	11-15 yr	True logical thought and manipulation of abstract concepts emerge

Adapted from Schuster C, Ashburn S: *The process of human development: a holistic lifespan approach*, Boston, 1992, Lippincott. In Edelman CL, Mandle CL: *Health promotion throughout the lifespan*, ed 3, St Louis, 1994, Mosby.

Kohlberg's Stages of Moral Development

The responses to moral dilemmas indicate that there are distinct sequential stages of moral thinking. These stages depend greatly on cognitive development and always follow the same sequence. There are three levels of moral judgment, and each consists of two stages. These levels and stages are outlined in Table 1.

In our society progression through the successive stages of moral development generally takes place during the school-age, adolescent, and young adult years. Not everyone progresses through all stages. In fact, only a minority of adults operate in stage 6 or even stage 5. Beyond the very young adult years, a stabilization or increased consistency of thought and perhaps an increased correlation between moral judgment and moral action can occur.

Table 1

Level and stage	What is right	Reasons for doing right
Level A: preconventional		
Stage 1: punishment and obedience	Avoiding breaking rules, to obey for obedience's sake, and to avoid doing physical damage to people and property	Avoiding punishment and the superior power of authorities
Stage 2: individual instrumental purpose and exchange	Following rules when it is in someone's immediate interest	Serving one's own needs or interests in a world where one must recognize that other people have interests as well
	Using fairness, equal exchange, agreement	
Level B: conventional		
Stage 3: mutual interpersonal expectations, relationships, and conformity	Living up to what is expected by relatives and friends or what is generally expected in one's role as son, sister, friend, and so on; "being good" is important	Needing to be good in one's own eyes and those of others
		Following the "golden rule"
Stage 4: social system and conscience maintenance	Fulfilling actual duties to which one has agreed	Keeping institution going as a whole
	Laws are to be upheld unless they conflict with other fixed social duties and rights	Using self-respect or conscience to meet one's defined obligations
	Contributing to society, the group, or institution	
Level B/C: transition		Basing reasons on emotions; conscience is arbitrary and relative

Level C: postconventional and principled		
Stage 5: prior rights and social contract or utility	Being aware that people hold a variety of values and opinions, most of which are relative to one's group	Feeling obligated to obey the law because one has made a social contract to make and abide by laws for good of all; the greatest good for the greatest number
	Realizing that some nonrelative values and rights, such as life and liberty, must be upheld in any society	
Stage 6: universal ethical principles	Acting in accordance with the principle when laws violate universal ethical principles	As a rational person, seeing validity of principles and becoming committed to them
	Understanding the equality of human rights and respecting dignity of human beings as individuals	

Compiled from Kohlberg L: *The philosophy of moral development*, San Francisco, 1981, Harper & Row. From Edelman CL, Mandle CL: *Health promotion throughout the lifespan*, ed 3, St Louis, 1994, Mosby.

Support Needs Assessment

Instructions

Please look at the "map" of your family, friends, relatives, and other people who are important to you as I ask you some questions about the ways that the people you have listed may help you.

1. Does anyone give you information or advice?

Yes _____   No _____

a. If yes, who gives you information or advice?

b. Do you want more information or advice?

Yes _____   No _____

c. Do you give information or advice to others?

Yes _____   No _____

If yes, to whom do you give information or advice?

2. Can you count on others to be there for you when you need them?

Yes _____   No _____

a. If yes, who can you count on?

b. Do you want to be able to count on others more than you do?

Yes _____   No _____

c. Do you feel others can count on you?

Yes _____   No _____

If yes, who can count on you?

3. Do others help you get out of the dumps when you feel down?

Yes _____   No _____

a. If yes, who helps you?

b. Do you want more help to get out of the dumps when you feel down?

Yes _____   No _____

c. Do you help others get out of the dumps when they feel down?

Yes _____   No _____

If yes, who do you help?

4. Do others let you know that they care about you?

Yes _____   No _____

a. If yes, who lets you know they care about you?

b. Do you need more help from others in letting you know they care about you?

Yes _____   No _____

From Crawford G: Support networks and health related change in the elderly; theory based nursing strategies, *Fam Comm Health* 10(2):1987.

   c. Do you let others know you care about them?

     Yes ____   No ____

     If yes, who do you help?

5. Do others help you with everyday things such as household chores, shopping, or transportation?

   Yes ____   No ____

   a. If yes, who helps you with everyday things and how do they help?

   b. Do you need more help with everyday things?

     Yes ____   No ____

     If yes, what kinds of help do you need?

   c. Do you help others with everyday things such as household chores, shopping, or transportation?

     Yes ____   No ____

     If yes, who do you help and how?

Social Network Scales

Social network assessments are recommended as a regular part of a client health assessment because of the recognized link between social networks and morbidity and mortality. If the client is at risk, the nurse should be aware of the impact on health and progress in care. The nurse may want to consider a referral to an appropriate community agency.

Lubben Social Network Scale

Family Networks

  Q1. How many relatives do you see or hear from at least once a month? (NOTE: Include in-laws with relatives.)   Q1 ____

0 = zero	3 = three or four
1 = one	4 = five to eight
2 = two	5 = nine or more

From Lubben I: Assessing social networks among elderly populations, *Fam Comm Health* 11(3):1988.

Q2. Tell me about the relative with whom you have the most contact. How often do you see or hear from that person?   Q2 ____

    0 = <monthly   3 = weekly
    1 = monthly   4 = a few times a week
    2 = a few times   5 = daily
       a month

Q3. How many relatives do you feel close to? That is, how many of them do you feel at ease with, can talk to about private matters, or can call on for help?   Q3 ____

    0 = zero   3 = three or four
    1 = one   4 = five to eight
    2 = two   5 = nine or more

Friends Networks

Q4. Do you have any close friends? That is, do you have any friends with whom you feel at ease, can talk to about private matters, or can call on for help? If so, how many?   Q4 ____

    0 = zero   3 = three or four
    1 = one   4 = five to eight
    2 = two   5 = nine or more

Q5. How many of these friends do you see or hear from at least once a month?   Q5 ____

    0 = zero   3 = three or four
    1 = one   4 = five to eight
    2 = two   5 = nine or more

Q6. Tell me about the friend with whom you have the most contact. How often do you see or hear from that person?   Q6 ____

    0 = <monthly   3 = weekly
    1 = monthly   4 = a few times a week
    2 = a few times   5 = daily
    a month

Confidant Relationships

Q7. When you have an important decision to make, do you have someone you can talk to about it? Q7 ___

Always	Very often	Often	Sometimes	Seldom	Never
5	4	3	2	1	0

Q8. When other people you know have an important decision to make, do they talk to you about it? Q8 ___

Always	Very often	Often	Sometimes	Seldom	Never
5	4	3	2	1	0

Helping Others

Q9a. Does anybody rely on you to do something for them each day? For example: shopping, cooking dinner, doing repairs, cleaning house, providing child care, etc.

    NO— if no, go on to Q9b.

    YES— if yes, Q9 is scored "5" and skip to Q10

Q9b. Do you help anybody with things like shopping, filling out forms, doing repairs, providing child care, and so on? Q9 ___

Always	Very often	Often	Sometimes	Seldom	Never
5	4	3	2	1	0

Living Arrangements

Q10. Do you live alone or with other people? (NOTE: Include in-laws with relatives.) Q10 ___

    5   Live with spouse
    4   Live with other relatives or friends
    1   Live with other unrelated individuals (e.g., paid help)
    0   Live alone

                       TOTAL LSNS SCORE: ___

SCORING:
The total LSNS score is obtained by adding up scores from each of the 10 individual items. Thus total LSNS scores can range from 0 to 50. Scores on each item were anchored between 0 and 5 to permit equal weighting of the 10 items. It is suggested that a score below 20 indicates an extreme risk for limited social networks.

Social Assessment of the Elderly

Social assessment is an important indicator of the level of independent functioning of the elderly. It is recommended that this be a part of the comprehensive client assessment.

1. Has any of the following happened in the last year (describe if yes)?
   Death of spouse   ____
   Death of other close family member   ____
   Change in health of family member   ____
   Change in living situation   ____
   Divorce or separation   ____
   Marriage or "pairing up"   ____
   Change in financial state   ____
2. Living situation
   a. House   ____
      Apartment   ____
      Other   ____
   b. Alone   ____
      With another person or others   ____
      If so, who lives with client?
Name	Relationship
1. _____	_____
2. _____	_____
3. _____	_____
   c. Telephone
      None   ____
      Yes [phone number (____)____-_____]   ____

From Kane R, Ouslander J, Abrass I: *Essentials of clinical geriatrics,* New York, 1994, McGraw-Hill.

    d. Stairs

       No   ____

       Yes   ____

       If yes, how many? ____

       Is elevator available? No ____ Yes ____

3. a. Does client require help in any of the following? If so, who provides it?

	Help needed	Provided by
Meal preparation		
Shopping		
Light housecleaning		
Laundry		
Getting out of bed		
Getting into bed		
Dressing		
Bathing		

   b. Describe what the client ate yesterday:

Breakfast	Lunch	Dinner

4. How often in past week did client leave the house (other than this visit)?

   At least daily ____ Several times ____ Once ____ Never ____

5. How often do visitors come to client's house?

   Daily ____ Weekly ____ Less often ____ Never____

6. Whom would client call in an emergency (nonprofessional)?

_____

7. Does client have a legal guardian or durable power of attorney for health care?

   No ____ Yes ____ (If yes, list name, address and telephone number.)

_____

_____

_____

8. Is client's care covered by

   Medicaid   ____

   Supplemental private insurance (beyond Medicare) ____

9. Does the client receive
   Social Security   ____
   Supplemental Security Income (SSI) ____
   Private pension   ____
   Other income   ____
10. Does income permit purchase of needed
    Food   ____
    Clothing   ____
    Housing   ____
    Heating   ____
    Transportation ____
    Drugs   ____
    Is money a problem for the client? No ____   Yes ____
11. Does client receive services from any social agency?
    Yes ____   No ____
    Name and phone number of agency _____

Primary Changes of Aging

Skin	Wrinkling, sagging of subcutaneous support, hair loss, ↓ in sebaceous secretions, epidermal thinning, degeneration of the elastic fibers providing dermal support, ↓ in vascularity
Skeletal	↓ in bone density, shrinkage of vertebral disks, deterioration of cartilage
Muscular	↓ in muscle mass strength, and endurance, ↓ in myofibrils; impaired coordination and reflexes
Cardiovascular	↑ in blood pressure, ↓ in cardiac contractile function, ↓ in cardiac output under stress, progressive stiffening of arteries, development of atherosclerotic plaques
Urinary	↓ in peak bladder capacity, ↑ in residual urine, ↓ in renal blood flow, ↓ in glomerular filtration rate, ↑ in urinary frequency including nocturia, prostatic hypertrophy, ↓ in pelvic muscle tone
Gastrointestinal	Dental changes, ↓ in number of taste buds, ↓ in peristalsis, ↓ in gastric acid secretion, ↓ in absorption
Endocrine	↓ in utilization of insulin, ↓ in estrogen and testosterone
Special senses	Impaired night vision and color discrimination, ↓ in peripheral vision, ↑ in sensitivity to glare, lens opacity, ↓ in high-frequency hearing ability, difficulty in speech discrimination of such high-pitched sounds as *s, z, sb,* and *ch*
Sexual	↓ in penile sensitivity, slower and weaker erection, ↓ in ejaculatory volume, ↑ in refractory period in men, ↓ in vascularity and fat content of vaginal walls, ↓ in size of vagina, atrophic vaginitis

Adapted from Sloane PD: Normal aging. In Ham RJ, Sloane PD, editors: *Primary care geriatrics,* ed 2, St Louis, 1992, Mosby. Also adapted from Lincoln R: Promotion of health in the elderly. In Long BC, Phipps WJ, Cassemeyer VL, editors: *Medical-surgical nursing: a nursing process approach,* ed 3, St Louis, 1993, Mosby.

⟳ Nutritional Assessment

Nutrition is one of the most essential aspects in life for all. Diet, whether therapeutic or regular, has a major impact on a person's health, maintenance, and recovery from an illness. Nutritional behavior is a lifestyle that is influenced by culture; it must be considered as the nurse provides advice and guidance to individuals and families.

Anthropometric Measurements

Muscle mass measurements are obtained by measuring the arm circumference of the nondominant upper arm. The arm hangs freely at the side, and a measuring tape is place around the midpoint of the upper arm, between the acromion of the scapula and the olecranon of the ulna. The centimeter circumference is recorded and compared with standard values (Table 2).

The combined midarm circumference and triceps skinfold calculations provide an estimate of midarm muscle areas that can be a useful indicator for determining protein-energy malnutrition. These measurements can also be used to monitor interventions and changes in the nutritional status of elders regardless of race.

Table 2

Percentage of standard	Male	Female
Mid–upper arm circumference (in centimeters)		
90	26.33	25.7
80	23.4	22.8
70	20.5	20.0
60	17.6	17.1
STANDARD	29.3	28.5
Tricep skinfold (in millimeters)		
90	11.3	11.9
80	10.0	13.2
70	8.8	11.6
60	7.5	9.9
STANDARD	12.5	16.5

Modified from Keithley JK: Proper nutritional assessment can prevent hospital malnutrition. *Nurs '79* 92:70, 1979. In Ebersole P, Hess P: *Toward healthy aging: human needs and nursing response,* ed 4, St Louis, 1994, Mosby.

Body fat is assessed by measuring specific skinfolds with Lange or Harpenden calipers. Two areas are accessible for measurement. One area is the midpoint of the upper arm, the triceps area, which is also used to obtain arm circumference. The nondominant arm is again used. The nurse lifts the skin with the thumb and forefinger so that it parallels the humerus. The calipers are placed around the skinfold, 1 cm below where the fingers are grasping the skin. Two readings are averaged to the nearest half centimeter. Results should be compared with standard values. If there is a neuropathologic condition or hemiplegia after a stroke, the unaffected arm should be used for obtaining measurements.

The second and more accurate site is immediately below the tip of the scapula. This area provides uniformity of the fat layer. The skin immediately below the tip of the scapula is grasped with the thumb and forefinger, the calipers applied, and two consecutive readings obtained and averaged in the same manner as the triceps measurement.

Nutritional Self-Assessment

Complete the following self-assessment to help you look at the role of nutrition in your life now. Circle the numbers that best indicate you and your life during the last year:

	Almost never	Seldom	Often	Almost always
1. I read the labels for ingredients on foods I consume	1	2	3	4
2. I have two meatless days a week	1	2	3	4
3. I eat food without salting it	1	2	3	4
4. My meals include nonfat or lowfat milk and dairy products	1	2	3	4
5. I limit my meals at fast food restaurants to twice a week	1	2	3	4
6. I limit myself to three alcoholic drinks per week (including wine or beer)	1	2	3	4
7. I limit my caffeine use to three times per week (coffee, tea, cola drinks, etc.)	1	2	3	4
8. I limit sweet desserts to three times per week	1	2	3	4
9. My typical meals include fresh fruits and raw vegetables	1	2	3	4
10. Mealtimes are pleasant to me	1	2	3	4

Some suggestions for how you might learn from this self-assessment:

1. Connect all the circles down the length of the page. Look at the pattern that your connected line makes. You might also turn your page sideways to get an even more clear visual picture of nutrition in your life right now. What does it seem to be saying to you?

2. Now add up your total score: _____
   Circle which range it was in:

              10-19   20-29   30-40

   If your score was in the 10-19 range you might want to make some changes in your nutritional life. Which aspects do you think need the most work? How many "1's" did you mark on this assessment? These might serve as a clue to help you think about making changes in this area of your life.

3. How would you like this self-assessment to look 6 months from now? Are you interested in planning toward those improvements?

4. Remember to congratulate yourself for the ways in which you are providing good nutrition for yourself. Give yourself a pat on the back; go out and eat something "good" as a way to congratulate yourself.

Modified from Baldi S, Costell S, Hill L, et al: *For your health: a model for self-care,* South Laguna, Calif, 1980, Nurses Model Health.

Family Nutritional Assessment Tool

Family members	Age	Educational level	Developmental level
1.			
2.			
3.			
4.			
5.			
6.			

Family's perception of health status (describe)

Nutritional practices

Who decides on the menu?
Who does the grocery shopping?
Who prepares the meals?
Number of meals consumed per day?
Describe mealtime (Who is present, when, where, and atmosphere)
Does mealtime serve a particular function? (For example, are the day's activities planned? Are problems discussed?)
Snacks consumed and frequency
Knows food sources from the food pyramid
24-hour food recall

Dietary fat

Use of red meat, fish, and poultry (once a week, three times, etc.)
How often do you eat cheese? What kinds do you purchase?
How often do you use cold cuts?
How often do you use fish/chicken? (Describe preparation)
How often do you use processed foods such as bakery products, frozen dinners?
How much milk or other dairy products do you consume? What types?

Cholesterol and saturated fat

How many eggs does the family eat per week?
What kind of fat do you use in cooking?
What kind of vegetable oil do you use?

Complex carbohydrates and fiber

How often do you eat fruit? How do you eat it (juices, fresh, canned)?
What kind of vegetables do you eat (canned, frozen, fresh)?
What kind of bread do you eat (whole grain, white)?

Sugar consumption

Do you use sugar in cooking? Do you buy candy, pastries, sweetened cereals?

From Bomar P: *Nurses and family health promotion: concepts, assessment and interventions,* ed 2, Philadelphia, 1996, Saunders.

Family nutritional assessment tool—cont'd

Family members	Age	Educational level	Developmental level

Sodium

How often do you use processed foods (canned or packaged such as macaroni and cheese)?

Do you add salt to food?

Alcohol consumption

How often do you use alcohol?

Caffeine

How much coffee and tea do you drink per day?

Supplements

Do you take vitamins or mineral supplements? What and how much? Reason.

Cultural influences

"Special" foods

Eating habits unique to culture

Family food preferences or restrictions

Economics

Do you receive any supplementary income to purchase food items?

Eating problems

Do you have problems with indigestion, vomiting, nausea, sore mouth?

Do you have any difficulty swallowing liquids or solids or chewing and feeding yourselves?

Medications

Are you on any medications? Do they affect your appetite or weight?

Weight

Has weight changed in the last 6 months? How much? Describe events associated with the change.

Elimination pattern

Describe bowel and urinary patterns

Activity and exercise patterns

Usual daily/weekly activities of family members

Source of nutrition information

Magazines, family member, schools, health food store

Family work patterns

Do family members work outside of the home? Type of work and hours

Family nutritional assessment tool—cont'd

Family members	Age	Educational level	Developmental level

Physical assessment

Describe appearance of the family

Height

Weight

Blood pressure

Pulse/respirations

Percent body fat (or body mass index)

Relative weight $\frac{\text{actual weight} \times 100}{\text{ideal weight}}$

Example: 160 (actual weight) $\times 100 = 16,000$

(16,000 divided by ideal weight of $140 = 114\%$)

The closer relative weight is to 100%, the better.

120–139 mild obesity

140–159 moderate obesity

160+ severe obesity

Family strengths/weaknesses

(Identify nutritional concerns of the family)

Barriers to change? Are there reasons why the family cannot change the
problem area?

Assessment summary

Check problem area or potential problems

1. Dietary fat
2. Cholesterol and saturated fat
3. Complex carbohydrates and fiber
4. Sugar
5. Sodium
6. Alcohol
7. Caffeine
8. Supplements
9. Cultural influences
10. Economics
11. Eating problems
12. Medications
13. Weight changes
14. Elimination pattern
15. Activity and exercise
16. Nutrition resources
17. Work patterns
18. Notes of concern

Nursing diagnosis

Family nutritional assessment tool—cont'd

Family members	Age	Educational level	Developmental level

Plan and intervention

Evaluation

Supplementary assessment for obesity problems

Physical assessment (height, weight, body fat composition, blood pressure, pulse, respirations)

Highest and lowest weight

Why do you want to lose?

What are the contributing factors to weight gain?

Family weight history
    Maternal
    Paternal

Eating patterns

Diets attempted

Medical problems associated with obesity

Activity level

Developmental stage, stresses, significant life events

Nursing diagnosis

Goal

Plan

Evaluation

Nutritional Screening Guide

Level I Screen

		Measurement abnormal	
	Value	Yes	No
Height (in.) **Weight (lb.)**			
Percent desirable body weight			
Weight loss or gain in 6 mo			
Dietary data			
Does not have enough food each day			
Number of days per month without any food			
Poor appetite			
Usually eats alone			
Difficulty chewing or swallowing			
Problems with mouth, teeth, or gums			
Housebound			
Eats milk or milk products daily			
Eats fruits and vegetables daily			
On a special diet			
Usual daily food intake (optional)			
Less than 2 servings of milk or dairy products			
Less than 2 servings of meat/ poultry/fish/eggs			
Less than 2 servings of fruit/juice			
Less than 3 servings of vegetables			
Less than 6 servings of bread/ cereals/grains			

From Ebersole P, Hess P: *Toward healthy aging: human needs and nursing response,* ed 4, St Louis, 1994, Mosby.

Level I Screen—cont'd

| | | Measurement abnormal | |
	Value	Yes	No
More than 2 ounces of alcohol for men			
More than 1 ounce of alcohol for women			
Living environment			
Income less than $6000/year/ person			
Lives alone			
Concerned about home security			
Inadequate heating or cooling			
No stove or refrigerator			
Unable or prefers not to spend money on food			
Functional status—needs assistance with			
Bathing			
Dressing			
Continence			
Toileting			
Eating			
Ambulation			
Transportation			
Food preparation			

Identified problems should be referred to the appropriate health care professional such as physician, nurse, social worker, dietitian, dentist, or case manager.

Refer to a Physician If There Is
An involuntary increase or decrease in weight of greater than 10 lb in the past 6 mo
A body weight that is 20% above or below desirable body weight

Refer to a Dietitian for Food-related Problems.

Repeat This Screen Yearly or If a Major Change in Status Occurs.

Level II Screen
In-depth assessment (performed in medical settings)
Additional information to be obtained after referral to a physician or other qualified health care professional

		Measurement abnormal	
	Value	Yes	No
Height (in.) **Weight (lb.)**			
Percent desirable body weight			
Body mass index			
Weight loss or gain in 6 mo			
Dietary data			
Does not have enough food each day			
Number of days per month without any food			
Poor appetite			
Usually eats alone			
Special dietary needs			
Self-defined			
Prescribed			
Problems with compliance/ meeting special needs			
Multiple diet prescriptions			
Other unusual dietary practices			
Usual daily food intake (optional)			
Less than 2 servings of milk or dairy products			
Less than 2 servings of meat/ poultry/fish/eggs			
Less than 2 servings of fruit/juice			
Less than 3 servings of vegetables			
Less than 6 servings of bread/ cereals/grains			
More than 2 ounces of alcohol for men			
More than 1 ounce of alcohol for women			

Level II Screen—cont'd

	Value	Measurement abnormal	
		Yes	No
Laboratory and anthropometric data			
Serum albumin less than 3.5 g/dl			
Serum cholesterol less than 160 mg/dl			
Serum cholesterol greater than 240 mg/dl			
Triceps skinfold thickness below 10% of desirable			
Midarm muscle circumference below 10% of desirable			
Clinical features			
Difficulty chewing or swallowing			
Problems with mouth, teeth, or gums			
Skin changes that suggest malnutrition			
Angular stomatitis			
Glossitis			
History of bone pain			
Bone fractures			
Living environment			
Income less than $6000/year/person			
Lives alone			
Concerned about home security			
Inadequate heating or cooling			
No stove or refrigerator			
Unable or prefers not to spend money on food			

Level II Screen—cont'd

	Value	Measurement abnormal	
		Yes	No
Functional status—needs assistance with			
Bathing			
Dressing			
Continence			
Toileting			
Eating			
Ambulation			
Transportation			
Food preparation			
Shopping			
Mental/cognitive status			
Mini–mental examination indicates impairment (score <26)			
Depression scale suggests depression (Beck <15, GDS >5)			
Drug use			
More than 3 prescription drugs			
More than 3 nonprescription drugs			
Vitamin and mineral supplements			

Criteria for the Recognition of Common Problems from Completion of the Screen

Is there weight loss or is the client underweight?
Weight loss greater than 10% in last 6 months
Body weight less than 80% of desirable weight
Triceps skinfold thickness below the 10th percentile
Midarm muscle circumference below 10th percentile

Level II Screen—cont'd

Is there evidence of protein energy (hypoalbuminemic) malnutrition?
Serum albumin less than 3.5 g/dl

Is there evidence suggesting osteoporosis or mineral deficiency?
History of bone pain or bone fractures
Patient housebound

Is there evidence of hypovitaminosis or mineral deficiency?
Angular stomatitis, glossitis, or bleeding gums
Inadequate intakes of fruit and vegetables
Pressure ulcers

Is there evidence of obesity or hypercholesterolemia?
Weight greater than 120% of desirable weight
Serum cholesterol greater than 240 mg/dl

Should the client be referred to a dietitian or community nutrition program?
Food intake inappropriate, inadequate, or excessive
Problems complying with specialized diet
Need for nutrition-specific counseling or education, related to specific diseases
Functionally dependent for eating or food-related activities of daily living

Identified Problems Should Be Referred to the Appropriate Health Care Professional Such as a Physician, Nurse, Social Worker, Dietitian, Dentist, or Case Manager.

Nutritional Self-Care Activities Throughout the Life Span

Developmental stage	Nutritional considerations	Self-care activities
Infancy	Feeding experiences promote bonding with significant others.	Hold baby close during feeding. Feed promptly when hunger noticed.
	Iron stores are depleted by 4-5 mo.	Add iron supplement 4-5 mo.
	Primary teeth begin erupting at about 6 mo	Introduce solid foods 4-6 mo. Begin with strained, mushy foods. Progress to bite-size food by 10-12 mo.
		Introduce new foods one at a time at weekly intervals to screen for allergy.
		Offer foods from six exchanges by end of first year.
	Overweight infants have increased incidence of lower respiratory infection and an increased number of fat cells.	Allow child to determine quantity of foods.
	Underweight infants have slow bone growth, delayed calcification, slow fat deposition, retarded growth of lean body mass, smaller reserve, and higher susceptibility to illness.	Allow, encourage child to self-feed when able. Encourage physical activity.
	Infants who drink cows' milk are subject to dehydration during hot weather or during illness with vomiting, fever, or diarrhea.	Give fluid supplements: water or electrolyte solution.
	Skim milk lacks calories and linoleic acid and results in an increased renal solute load for infants.	Limit use of skim milk before 1 yr of age.

Continued.

From Jelliffe DB: Protein in Cow's Milk, *Nutrition and the MD*, 3(4):2, 1977; Kandzari J, Howard J: *The well family: a developmental approach to assessment*, Boston, 1981, Little, Brown, pp 167-222; Knittle JL: Obesity in childhood: a problem in adipose tissue cellular development, 81:1048, 1972; Neumann CG: Obesity in infancy—prevention and management, *Nutrition and the MD*, 1(9):1, 1975; Wenck DA, Baren M, Dewan SP: *Nutrition*, Winick M: Nutrition and aging, *Contemp Nut* 2(6), 1977. From Hill L, Smith N: *Self care nursing*, 1988, Prentice Hall.

Nutritional self-care activities throughout the life span—cont'd

Developmental stage	Nutritional considerations	Self-care activities
Toddler	Toddlers eat less than infants because of change in rate of growth.	Use serving size rule: one teaspoon or bite of each food for each year of age.
	Coordination can be poor and eating messy.	Offer finger foods.
		Offer praise for self-feeding.
	Molars may not have erupted.	Avoid inappropriate foods: tough, stringy foods, nuts, popcorn, peanut butter, raw carrots, hot dogs.
	Iron is often deficient in diet.	Offer iron supplements, foods high in iron.
	Toddler begins to identify and model food habits.	Provide good modeling of nutritional self-care.
Preschool	Activity level strongly influences amount of foods consumed. May "play too hard to eat."	Make nutritious snacks.
		Offer foods cut in finger-sized pieces.
	Likes to make choices and help prepare foods.	Have child help prepare meal, set table.
		Begin nutrition education.
	Suspicious of new foods.	Arouse interest in foods. Talk about it when buying, storing, preparing.
		Model good nutritional self-care.
	May dislike "strong-tasting" foods.	Introduce small amounts of spicy foods, broccoli, cabbage, and so forth.
School-age		*Child*
	Appetite may be low or fluctuate.	Gain new skills in balancing own energy input and output.
	Sedentary children become overweight.	
	Beginning to eat away from nuclear family.	Learn to avoid foods with caffeine and stimulants.
	Stable mealtimes may be difficult to maintain as activities increase.	Choose healthy snacks.

	Nutrition may affect school performance. Some nutritious snacks such as peanut butter or dried fruit may also promote tooth decay.	*Parent* Provide for dental self-care. Provide nutritious snacks. Model nutrition self-care. Praise wise choices. Encourage physical activity.
Adolescence	Most common nutritional problems are tooth decay, anemia, and obesity. Key period in acquiring adult habits. American obsession with thinness may precipitate fad diets, bulimia, or anorexia nervosa. Strenuous physical activity requires additional calories, fluids. Growth spurts and periods of heavy appetite vary widely. Many adolescents have sound nutritional knowledge.	*Adolescent* Provide for own iron intake. Balance own energy input/output. Model nutrition self-care for peers/family. Provide for adequate fluid/caloric intake. *Parent* Provide for dental self-care. Support self-care activities. Continue nutrition education. Praise wise choices. Allow to budget, plan, shop, and prepare family foods.
Young adulthood	Leaving home for college, job, marriage New responsibility for budgeting, planning, preparing foods. Metabolic rate leveling off. Caloric intake tied to activity level.	Model nutrition self-care for peers/family. Plan eating out carefully. Increase skills in budgeting and shopping. Alter intake in response to changes in exercise and stress levels.
Pregnancy/lactation	Mother's nutritional status affects the health of fetus, infant. Adequate calories, fluid, nutrient intake to meet demands of developing fetus and nursing infant.	Increase water intake to 6-8 glasses per day, more in hot weather. Eat regularly 5-6 times per day to develop regular supply of nutrients, fluids, calories. Balance energy input and output.

Continued.

Nutritional self-care activities throughout the life span—cont'd

Developmental stage	Nutritional considerations	Self-care activities
Pregnancy/lactation—cont'd		Avoid alcohol, caffeine, over-the-counter drugs. Use LaLeche League for additional information, support.
Middle age	Nutrition-related conditions may surface during this time: cardiovascular disease, diabetes mellitus, gallbladder disease,-liver disease. Changing lifestyle: decreased child-care responsibilities, career involvement, slower physical pace. Metabolic rate decreasing. Body image changing.	Maintain exercise program to offset decreasing metabolic rate. Keep alcohol, caffeine intake at a minimum. Provide for regular mealtimes and break times. Balance energy input and output. Maintain calcium intake to prevent osteoporosis.
Later adulthood	Aging process affects nutritional planning: decrease in taste sensitivity, decrease in gastric secretion, decrease in metabolic rate, declining body mass. Food selection may be attached to memories: e.g., may like dill pickles because of the memory of growing and canning cucumbers. Food purchases are influenced by changing financial status, ability to get to and from marketplace, physical stamina to prepare foods, interest in food preparation (particularly if living alone), ability to chew and digest foods, and beliefs of nutritional models. Aging adults generally need more protein, iron, calcium, vitamins A and C, folic acid, and fiber. They usually need less fat, sugar, sodium, and fewer calories.	Balance energy input and output. Limit fatty, spicy foods as needed. Limit sugar intake. Eat small, more frequent meals. Use available services such as meals-on-wheels, senior centers, food stamp programs to provide supplementary assistance. Consider strengths and limitations when planning diet. Use selected convenience foods when necessary. Encourage eating with another, sharing of food preparation.

Nutritional Assessment of the Elderly

Dietary history	Medical and socioeconomic history	Clinical evaluation	Laboratory evaluation
1. Number of daily meals; regularity 2. Usual daily diet 3. Supplemental vitamins or minerals; protein concentrate 4. General nutritional knowledge; sources of information	1. Chronic disease or disability; occupational hazard exposure; use of tobacco, alcohol, or drugs 2. Symptoms such as bleeding, fainting, loss of memory, shortness of breath, headache, pain, changed bowel habits; altered sight or hearing and condition of teeth or dentures 3. Self-administered or prescribed therapy such as a vitamins, alcohol, drugs, food fads, prescription items, eyeglasses, or hearing aids 4. Names, addresses, and phone numbers of persons providing medical or health care 5. Living situation: lives alone or with spouse or companion; house, apartment or senior citizen housing 6. Sources of income	1. Height and weight; obesity or physical wasting 2. Blood pressure, pulse rate, and rhythm 3. Skin color and texture 4. Anthropometric measurement of mid–upper arm circumference and tricep or subscapular skinfold 5. Condition of teeth or dentures and oral hygiene 6. Mental state during interview and examination 7. Vision and hearing assessments 8. Any gross evidence of neglect	1. Hemoglobin level or hematocrit ratio 2. Blood or urine sugar analysis 3. Urinalysis (color, odor, bile, and sediment by gross inspection), pH, glucose, albumin blood, and acetone by stick test 4. Feces (color, texture, gross blood; occult blood by guaiac test)

From Nutritional assessment in health programs, *Am J Public Health* 63(suppl):74, Nov 1973; Miller CA: *Nursing care of older adults*, Glenview, Ill, 1990, Scott Foresman/Little Brown Higher Education; Cape ROT: In *The Merck manual of geriatrics*, Rahway, NJ, 1990, Merck Sharpe & Dohme Research Laboratories. In Ebersole P, Hess P: *Toward healthy aging: human needs and nursing response*, ed 4, St Louis, 1994, Mosby.

Age-Related Gastrointestinal Changes, Outcomes, and Illness Prevention, Health Promotion, and Maintenance Approaches

Age-related changes	Outcomes	Illness prevention, health promotion, and maintenance
Decreased acuity of taste	Dry mouth	Take in adequate fiber in diet
Decreased salivary production with increased alkalinity	Diminished taste	Adequate exercise
Brittle teeth/retracted gingiva	Pale gums	Bowel training
Less effective chewing	Vermilion border of mouth missing	No or little use of laxative
Decreased esophageal and intestinal motility	Atrophy of gums with loss of teeth or decay	Good oral care
Decrease in gastric secretions	Difficulty chewing	Suck on ice chips or hard candy
Loss of elasticity in intestinal wall	Decreased appetite	Hold cold water in mouth before swallowing
Decreased blood flow to intestines	Thirst	Use sodium-free flavorings
Reduced blood flow to liver	Coughing or choking	Consult dentist once or twice a year
Loss or diminished anal sphincter control	Dysphagia	Use soft-bristled toothbrush and dental floss
	Nausea/vomiting	For dentures, brush to clean between teeth

Weaker neural impulses to lower bowel

Heartburn/indigestion
Diarrhea
Constipation
Fecal impaction
Malnutrition
Drug toxicity

Cut food into small pieces, chew thoroughly
Have abdominal pain evaluated
Increase dietary fiber, fluids, and exercise
Have a regular meal pattern
Respond promptly to the urge to defecate
Report any change in bowel routine
Manage diet within budget
Use meals on wheels if needed
Use dietary supplements
Recognize signs of drug toxicity for drugs taken

Fewer taste buds

Food tastes bland
Overseasons food

Encourage social dining
Nutritional supplementation
Use herbs for seasoning, lemons, spices (nonsalty)

From Ebersole P, Hess P: *Toward healthy aging: human needs and nursing response*, ed 4, St Louis, 1994, Mosby.

Disorders Associated with Dietary Excesses

Disease	Nutritional factor
Heart disease	Fats, cholesterol, calories
Cerebrovascular disease	Fats, cholesterol, sodium
Cancer (varies by site)	Calories, alcohol, fats, vitamin A, beta carotene, vitamin C, fiber
Diabetes mellitus	Carbohydrates, fats, calories
Liver disease and cirrhosis	Alcohol
Atherosclerosis	Fats, cholesterol, calories
Dental caries	Refined and simple sugars

From Simons-Morton B, O'Hara N, Simons-Morton D: Promoting healthful diet and exercise behaviors in communities, schools, and families, *Fam Comm Health* 9(3):4, 1986.

Recommended Dietary Allowances for Normal Infants during the First Year

	0-6 mo	6-12 mo
Weight		
kg	6	9
pounds	13	20
Height		
cm	60	71
inches	24	28

Nutrient	RDA	RDA
Protein, g	13	14
Vitamin A, μg RE*	375	375
Vitamin D, μg†	7.5	10
Vitamin E, mg TE‡	3	4
Vitamin K, mg	5	10
Ascorbic acid, mg	30	35
Thiamine, mg	0.3	0.4
Riboflavin, mg	0.4	0.5
Niacin, mg NE§	5	6
Vitamin B_6, mg	0.3	0.6
Vitamin B_{12}, μg	0.3	0.5
Folacin, μg	25	35
Calcium, mg	400	600
Phosphorus, mg	300	500
Magnesium, mg	40	60
Iodine, μg	40	50
Iron, mg	6	10
Zinc, mg	5	5
Selenium, μg	10	15

*Retinol equivalents. 1 retinol equivalent = 1 μg retinol or 6 μg betacarotene.
†As cholecalciferol, 10 μg cholecalciferol = 400 IU of vitamin D.
‡Alpha-tocopherol equivalents. 1 mg D-alpha-tocopherol = 1 alpha-TE.
§1 NC (niacin equivalent) is equal to 1 mg of niacin or 60 mg of dietary tryptophan.

Reproduced, with permission, from Food and Nutrition Board: *Recommended Dietary Allowances,* ed 10, rev 1989, Washington, DC, 1990, National Research Council, National Academy of Sciences. From Ingalls JA, Salerno MC: *Ingalls and Salerno's maternal and child health nursing,* ed 8, St Louis, 1995, Mosby.

Recommended Dietary Allowances for Growth (National Research Council, 1989 Version)

	Age (yr)	Weight (kg)	Weight (lb)	Height (cm)	Height (in.)	Energy (kcal)	Protein (g)	Vit. A (µg RE)	Vit. D (µg)	Vit. E (mg α-TE)
Infants	0-0.5	6	13	60	24	650	13	375	7.5	3
	0.5-1	9	20	71	28	850	14	375	10	4
Children	1-3	13	29	90	35	1300	16	400	10	6
	4-6	20	44	112	44	1800	24	500	10	7
	7-10	28	62	132	52	2000	28	700	10	7
Males	11-14	45	99	157	62	2500	45	1000	10	10
	15-18	66	145	176	69	3000	59	1000	10	10
Females	11-14	46	101	157	62	2200	46	800	10	8
	15-18	55	120	163	64	2200	44	800	10	8

		Water-soluble vitamins								Minerals				
	Age (yr)	Vit. C (mg)	Thiamin (mg)	Riboflavin (mg)	Niacin (mg NE)	Vit. B₆ (mg)	Folate (µg)	Vit. B₁₂ (µg)	Calcium (mg)	Phosphorus (mg)	Magnesium (mg)	Iron (mg)	Zinc (mg)	Iodine (µg)	Selenium (µg)

	Age (yr)	Vit. C (mg)	Thiamin (mg)	Riboflavin (mg)	Niacin (mg NE)	Vit. B_6 (mg)	Folate (µg)	Vit. B_{12} (µg)	Calcium (mg)	Phosphorus (mg)	Magnesium (mg)	Iron (mg)	Zinc (mg)	Iodine (µg)	Selenium (µg)
Infants	0-0.5	30	0.3	0.4	5	0.3	25	0.3	400	300	40	6	5	40	10
	0.5-1	35	0.4	0.5	6	0.6	35	0.5	600	500	60	10	5	50	15
Children	1-3	40	0.7	0.8	9	1.0	50	0.7	800	800	80	10	10	70	20
	4-6	45	0.9	1.1	12	1.1	75	1.0	800	800	120	10	10	90	20
	7-10	45	1.0	1.2	13	1.4	100	1.4	800	800	170	10	10	120	30
Males	11-14	50	1.3	1.5	17	1.7	150	2.0	1200	1200	270	12	15	150	40
	15-18	60	1.5	1.8	20	2.0	200	2.0	1200	1200	400	12	15	150	50
Females	11-14	50	1.1	1.3	15	1.4	150	2.0	1200	1200	280	15	12	150	45
	15-18	60	1.1	1.3	15	1.5	180	2.0	1200	1200	300	15	12	150	50

From Williams SR: *Essentials of nutrition and diet therapy*, ed 6, St Louis, 1994, Mosby.

Recommended Dietary Allowances for Adults (National Research Council, 1989 Version)

	Age (yr)	Weight (kg)	Weight (lb)	Height (cm)	Height (in.)	Protein (g)	Energy (kcal)	Vit A (µg RE)	Vit D (µg)	Vit E (mg α-TE)	Vit K (µg)
Males	19-24	72	160	177	70	58	2900	1000	10	10	70
	25-50	79	174	176	70	63	2900	1000	5	10	80
	51+	77	170	173	68	63	2300	1000	5	10	80
Females	19-24	58	128	164	65	46	2200	800	10	8	60
	25-50	63	138	163	64	50	2200	800	5	8	65
	51+	65	143	160	63	50	1900	800	5	8	65

	Age (yr)	Vit C (mg)	Thiamin (mg)	Riboflavin (mg)	Niacin (mg NE)	Vit B6 (mg)	Folate (µg)	Vit B12 (µg)	Calcium (mg)	Phosphorus (mg)	Magnesium (mg)	Iron (mg)	Zinc (mg)	Iodine (µg)	Selenium (µg)
Males	19-24	40	1.5	1.7	19	2.0	200	2.0	1200	1200	350	10	15	150	70
	25-50	40	1.5	1.7	19	2.0	200	2.0	800	800	350	10	15	150	70
	51+	40	1.2	1.4	15	2.0	200	2.0	800	800	350	10	15	150	70
Females	19-24	30	1.1	1.3	15	1.6	180	2.0	1200	1200	280	15	12	150	55
	25-50	30	1.1	1.3	15	1.6	180	2.0	800	800	280	15	12	150	55
	51+	30	1.0	1.2	13	1.6	180	2.0	800	800	280	10	12	150	55

From Williams SR: *Essentials of nutrition and diet therapy*, ed 6, St Louis, 1994, Mosby.

Recommended Nutrient Intakes for Canadians

Summary examples of recommended nutrient intake based on age and body weight expressed as daily rates

Age	Sex	Energy (kcal)	Thiamin (mg)	Riboflavin (mg)	Niacin NE	n-3 PUFA (g)	n-6 PUFA (g)	Weight (kg)	Protein (g)	Vit. A RE
0-4 mo	Both	600	0.3	0.3	4	0.5	3	6.0	12*	400
5-12 mo	Both	900	0.4	0.5	7	0.5	3	9.0	12	400
1 yr	Both	1100	0.5	0.6	8	0.6	4	11	13	400
2-3 yr	Both	1300	0.6	0.7	9	0.7	4	14	16	400
4-6 yr	Both	1800	0.7	0.9	13	1.0	6	18	19	500
7-9 yr	M	2200	0.9	1.1	16	1.2	7	25	26	700
	F	1900	0.8	1.0	14	1.0	6	25	26	700
10-12 yr	M	2500	1.0	1.3	18	1.4	8	34	34	800
	F	2200	0.9	1.1	16	1.2	7	36	36	800
13-15 yr	M	2800	1.1	1.4	20	1.5	9	50	49	900
	F	2200	0.9	1.1	16	1.2	7	48	46	800
16-18 yr	M	3200	1.3	1.6	23	1.8	11	62	58	1000
	F	2100	0.8	1.1	15	1.2	7	53	47	800
19-24 yr	M	3000	1.2	1.5	22	1.6	10	71	61	1000
	F	2100	0.8	1.1	15	1.2	7	58	50	800
25-49 yr	M	2700	1.1	1.4	19	1.5	9	74	64	1000
	F	1900	0.8	1.0	14	1.1	7	59	51	800
50-74 yr	M	2300	0.9	1.2	16	1.3	8	73	63	1000
	F	1800	0.8§	1.0§	14§	1.1§	7§	63	54	800

75+ yr M	2000	0.8	1.0	14	1.1	7	69	59	1000
F‖	1700	0.8§	1.0§	14§	1.1§	7§	64	55	800
Pregnancy (additional)									
First trimester	100	0.1	0.1	0.11	0.05	0.3		5	0
Second trimester	300	0.1	0.3	0.22	0.16	0.9		20	0
Third trimester	300	0.1	0.3	0.22	0.16	0.9		24	0
Lactation (additional)	450	0.2	0.4	0.33	0.25	1.5		20	400

NE, Niacin equivalents; PUFA, polyunsaturated fatty acids; RE, retinol equivalents.
*Protein is assumed to be from breast milk and must be adjusted for infant formula.
†Infant formula with high phosphorus should contain 375 mg of calcium.
‡Breast milk is assumed to be the source of the mineral.
¶Smokers should increase vitamin C by 50%.
§Level below which intake should not fall.
‖Assumes moderate physical activity.

From Scientific Review Committee: Nutrition recommendations, *Health and Welfare*, Ottawa, 1990. In Williams SR: *Nutrition and diet therapy*, ed 7, St Louis, 1993, Mosby.

Recommended nutrient intakes for Canadians—cont'd

Age	Sex	Vit. D (µg)	Vit. E (mg)	Vit. C (mg)	Folate (µg)	Vit. B$_{12}$ (µg)	Calcium (mg)	Phosphorus (mg)	Magnesium (mg)	Iron (mg)	Iodine (µg)	Zinc (mg)
0-4 mo	Both	10	3	20	25	0.3	250†	150	20	0.3‡	30	2‡
5-12 mo	Both	10	3	20	40	0.4	400	200	32	7	40	3
1 yr	Both	10	3	20	40	0.5	500	300	40	6	55	4
2-3 yr	Both	5	4	20	50	0.6	550	350	50	6	65	4
4-6 yr	Both	5	5	25	70	0.8	600	400	65	8	85	5
7-9 yr	M	2.5	7	25	90	1.0	700	500	100	8	110	7
	F	2.5	6	25	90	1.0	700	500	100	8	95	7
10-12 yr	M	2.5	8	25	120	1.0	900	700	130	8	125	9
	F	2.5	7	25	130	1.0	1100	800	135	8	110	9
13-15 yr	M	2.5	9	30	175	1.0	1100	900	185	10	160	12
	F	2.5	7	30	170	1.0	1000	850	180	13	160	9
16-18 yr	M	2.5	10	40¶	220	1.0	900	1000	230	10	160	12
	F	2.5	7	30¶	190	1.0	700	850	200	12	160	9

19-24 yr	M	2.5	10	40¶	220	1.0	800	1000	240	9	160	12
	F	2.5	7	30¶	180	1.0	700	850	200	13	160	9
25-49 yr	M	2.5	9	40¶	230	1.0	800	1000	250	9	160	12
	F	2.5	6	30¶	185	1.0	700	850	200	13	160	9
50-74 yr	M	5	7	40¶	230	1.0	800	1000	250	9	160	12
	F	5	6	30¶	195	1.0	800	850	210	8	160	9
75+ yr	M	5	6	40¶	215	1.0	800	1000	230	9	160	12
	F	5	5	30¶	200	1.0	800	850	210	8	160	9
Pregnancy (additional)												
First trimester		2.5	2	0	200	1.2	500	200	15	0	25	6
Second trimester		2.5	2	10	200	1.2	500	200	45	5	25	6
Third trimester		2.5	2	10	200	1.2	500	200	45	10	25	6
Lactation (additional)		2.5	3	25	100	0.2	500	200	65	0	50	6

Summary of Nutrients for Health

Nutrient	Important sources of nutrient	Provide energy	Build and maintain body cell	Regulate body processes	Deficiency symptoms	Toxicity symptoms
Protein Essential amino acids	Meat, poultry, fish Beans and peas Eggs Cheese Milk	Supplies 4 cal/g	Constitutes part of the structure of every cell, such as muscle, blood, and bone; supports growth and maintains healthy body cells	Constitutes part of enzymes, some hormones and body fluids, and antibodies that increase resistance to infection	Protein calorie malnutrition	Elevated uric acid and urea in serum
Carbohydrate Fiber Starch Sugar	Cereal Potatoes Beans Corn Bread Sugar	Supplies 4 cal/g Major source of energy for central nervous system	Supplies energy so protein can be used for growth and maintenance of body cells	Unrefined products supply fiber—complex carbohydrates in fruits, vegetables, and whole grains—for regular elimination	Poor GI function	Flatulence, trace mineral deficiencies
Fat	Shortening, oil Butter, margarine Salad dressing	Supplies 9 cal/g	Constitutes part of the structure of every cell	Assists in fat utilization Provides and car-	Essential fatty acid deficiency	Obesity

	Sources	Functions	Deficiency	Notes
	Sausages	ries fat-soluble vitamins (A, D, E, and K)		
Fat-soluble vitamins Vitamin A (Retinol)	Liver Carrots, pumpkin Sweet potatoes Greens Butter, margarine	Assists formation and maintenance of skin and mucous membranes that line body cavities and tracts, such as nasal passages and intestinal tract, thus increasing resistance to infection	Eye, skin, bone and blood disorders	Toxic at 25-100 times recommended dosage
		Functions in visual processes and forms visual purple, thus promoting healthy eye tissues and eye adaptation in dim light		
Vitamin D	Exposure to sunlight; fortified milk, fish	Activates calcium and phosphorous	Neuromuscular—Cramps, muscle twitching	
Vitamins E, K	Food fats, vegetable oils, nuts, fish	Antioxidants—affect cell aging nd immune system; wound healing, modified blood fats		
Water-soluble vitamins Vitamin C	Broccoli Orange Grapefruit	Aids in utilization of iron	Skin, blood, digestive, neurologic disorders	Usually nontoxic
		Forms cementing substances, such as collagen, that hold		

Continued.

Adapted from Poleman CN, Capra CI: *Shakelton's nutrition essentials and diet therapy*, ed 5, Philadelphia, 1984, Saunders; and Nestle M: *Nutrition in clinical practice*, Greenbrae, Calif, 1985, Jones Medical Publications.

Summary of nutrients for health—cont'd

Nutrient	Important sources of nutrient	Provide energy	Build and maintain body cell	Regulate body processes	Deficiency symptoms	Toxicity symptoms
Water-soluble vitamins—cont'd						
(ascorbic acid)	Papaya Mango Strawberries		body cells together, thus strengthening blood vessels, hastening healing of wounds and bones, and increasing resistance to infection			
Thiamin (B$_1$)	Lean pork Nuts Fortified cereal products	Aids in use of energy		Functions as part of a coenzyme to promote the utilization of carbohydrate Promotes normal appetite Contributes to normal functioning of nervous system	Skin, blood, digestive, neurologic disorders	
Riboflavin (B$_2$)	Liver Milk Yogurt Cottage cheese	Aids in use of energy		Functions as part of a coenzyme in the production of energy within body cells	Skin, blood, digestive, neurologic disorders	

Nutrient	Sources	Function		Deficiency/Other
Niacin (B₆)	Liver Meat, poultry, fish Peanuts Fortified cereal products	Aids in use of energy	Promotes healthy skin, eyes, and clear vision Functions as part of coenzyme in fat synthesis, tissue respiration, and utilization of carbohydrate Promotes healthy skin, nerves, and digestive tract Aids digestion and fosters normal appetite	Skin, blood, digestive, neurologic disorders
Minerals Calcium	Milk, yogurt Cheese Sardines and salmon with bones Collard, kale, mustard, and turnip greens		Combines with other minerals within a protein framework to give structure and strength to bones and teeth Assists in blood clotting Functions in normal muscle contraction and relaxation, and normal nerve transmission	Bone loss Osteoporosis Periodontal disease Muscle spasms Toxic at high dosage

Continued.

Summary of nutrients for health—cont'd

Nutrient	Important sources of nutrient	Provide energy	Build and maintain body cell	Regulate body processes	Deficiency symptoms	Toxicity symptoms
Iron	Enriched farina Prune juice Liver Dried beans and peas Red meats	Aids in use of energy	Combines with protein to form hemoglobin, the red substance in blood that carries oxygen to and carbon dioxide from the cells Prevents nutritional anemia and its accompanying fatigue Increases resistance to infection	Functions as part of enzymes involved in tissue respiration	Anemia, weakness, fatigue	Bronze coloration, liver damage, severe diabetes

Dietary Guidelines for All Americans

What should Americans eat to stay healthy? These guidelines, published by the U.S. departments of Agriculture and Health and Human Services, reflect recommendations of nutrition authorities who agree that enough is known about the effect of diet on health to encourage certain dietary practices. The guidelines are as follows:

- Eat a variety of foods.
- Maintain a healthy weight.
- Choose a diet low in fat, saturated fat, and cholesterol.
- Choose a diet with plenty of vegetables, fruits, and grain products.
- Use sugars only in moderation.
- Use salt and sodium only in moderation.
- Children and adolescents should not drink alcoholic beverages.

The *Dietary Guidelines* suggest at least the following number of servings from each of these food groups:

Vegetables	3-5 servings
Fruits	2-4 servings
Breads, cereals, rice, and pasta	6-11 servings
Milk, yogurt, and cheese	2-3 servings*
Meats, poultry, fish, dried beans and peas, eggs, and nuts	2-3 servings

---

*People aged 12 through 24 years should have three or more servings daily of foods rich in calcium.

From *FDA Consumer,* Sept. 1993, Pub. No. (FDA) 92-2257.

The Food Guide Pyramid

What Is the Food Guide Pyramid?

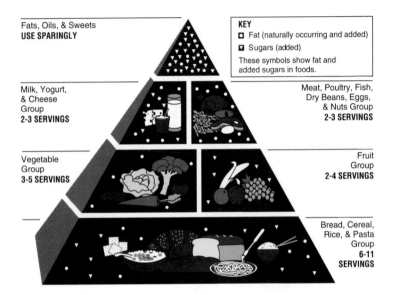

Fats, Oils, & Sweets
USE SPARINGLY

KEY
☐ Fat (naturally occurring and added)
◪ Sugars (added)

These symbols show fat and added sugars in foods.

Milk, Yogurt, & Cheese Group
2-3 SERVINGS

Meat, Poultry, Fish, Dry Beans, Eggs, & Nuts Group
2-3 SERVINGS

Vegetable Group
3-5 SERVINGS

Fruit Group
2-4 SERVINGS

Bread, Cereal, Rice, & Pasta Group
6-11 SERVINGS

The Pyramid is an outline of what to eat each day. It's not a rigid prescription, but a general guide that lets you choose a healthful diet that's right for you.

The Pyramid calls for eating a variety of foods to get the nutrients you need and at the same time the right amount of calories to maintain a healthy weight.

The Pyramid also focuses on fat because most American diets are too high in fat, especially saturated fat.

From USDA, No. 252, 1992, Rockville, Md.

How To Make the Pyramid Work for You

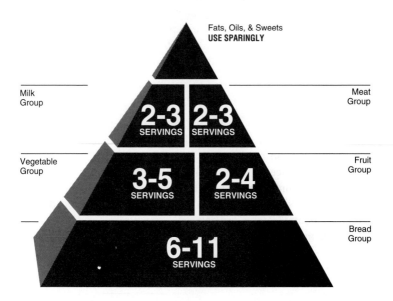

How Many Servings Are Right For Me?

The Pyramid shows a range of servings for each major food group. The number of servings that are right for you depends on how many calories you need, which in turn depends on your age, sex, size, and how active you are. Almost everyone should have at least the lowest number of servings in the ranges.

The following calorie level suggestions are based on recommendations of the National Academy of Sciences and on calorie intakes reported by people in national food consumption surveys.

For adults and teens

- 1600 calories is about right for many sedentary women and some older adults.
- 2200 calories is about right for most children, teenage girls, active women, and many sedentary men. Women who are pregnant or breast-feeding may need somewhat more.
- 2800 calories is about right for teenage boys, many active men, and some very active women.

From USDA, No. 252, 1992, Rockville, Md.

For young children

It is hard to know how much food children need to grow normally. If you're unsure, check with your doctor. Preschool children need the same variety of foods as older family members do but may need less than 1600 calories. For fewer calories they can eat smaller servings. However, it is important that they have the equivalent of 2 cups of milk a day.

For you

Now, take a look at the following table. It tells you how many servings you need for your calorie level. For example, if you are an active woman who needs about 2200 calories a day, 9 servings of breads, cereals, rice, or pasta would be right for you. You'd also want to eat about 6 ounces of meat or alternates per day. Keep total fat (fat in the foods you choose as well as fat used in cooking or added at the table) to about 73 grams per day.

If you are between calorie categories, estimate servings. For example, some less active women may need only 2000 calories to maintain a healthy weight. At that calorie level, 8 servings of breads would be about right.

Sample Diets for a Day at Three Calorie Levels

	Lower (about 1600)	Moderate (about 2200)	Higher (about 2800)
Bread group servings	6	9	11
Vegetable group servings	3	4	5
Fruit group servings	2	3	4
Milk group servings	2-3*	2-3*	2-3*
Meat group† (ounces)	5	6	7
Total fat (grams)	53	73	93
Total added sugars (teaspoons)	6	12	18

*Women who are pregnant or breast-feeding, teenagers, and young adults to age 24 need 3 servings.
†Meat group amounts are in total ounces.

From USDA, No. 252, 1992, Rockville, Md.

What Counts As a Serving?

Food groups

Bread, cereal, rice, and pasta

| 1 slice of bread | 1 ounce of ready-to-eat cereal | ½ cup of cooked cereal, rice, or pasta |

Vegetable

| 1 cup of raw leafy vegetables | ½ cup of other vegetables, cooked or chopped raw | ¾ cup of vegetable juice |

Fruit

| 1 medium apple, banana, orange | ½ cup of chopped, cooked, or canned fruit | ¾ cup of fruit juice |

Milk, yogurt, and cheese

| 1 cup of milk or yogurt | 1½ ounces of natural cheese | 2 ounces of process cheese |

Meat, poultry, fish, dry beans, eggs, and nuts

| 2-3 ounces of cooked lean meat, poultry, or fish | ½ cup of cooked dry beans, 1 egg, or 2 tablespoons of peanut butter count as 1 ounce of lean meat |

From USDA, No. 252, 1992, Rockville, Md.

Four Major Dietary Guidelines

Guideline category	US Dept. of Agriculture/US Dept. of Health and Human Services	American Heart Association	American Cancer Society	National Research Council
Weight/calories	Maintain desirable weight.	Adjust caloric intake to achieve and maintain ideal body weight.	Avoid obesity.	—
Fat and cholesterol	Avoid too much fat, saturated fat, and cholesterol.	Reduce total fat calories by a substantial reduction in dietary saturated fatty acids. Substantially reduce dietary cholesterol.	Cut down on total fat intake.	The consumption of both saturated and unsaturated fat should be reduced from its present level (approximately 40%) to 30% of total calories in the diet.
Alcohol	If you drink alcoholic beverages, do so in moderation.		Be moderate in consumption of alcoholic beverages.	If alcoholic beverages are consumed, should be done in moderation.
Starch, carbohydrate, fiber	Eat foods with adequate starch and fiber. Avoid too much sugar.	Increase dietary carbohydrate.	Eat more high-fiber foods such as whole grain cereals, fruits, and vegetables.	Include fruits, vegetables, and whole grain cereal products in the daily diet.

Variety	Eat a variety of foods.	—	Include foods rich in vitamins A and C in the daily diet. Include cruciferous vegetables such as cabbage, broccoli, brussels sprouts, kohlrabi, and cauliflower in the diet.	Include fruits, vegetables, and whole grain cereal products in the daily diet.
Sodium	Avoid too much sodium.	Reduce dietary sodium.	—	—
Salt-cured, smoked, pickled, or nitrate-cured	—	—	Be moderate in consumption of salt-cured, smoked, and nitrate-cured foods.	The consumption of food preserved by salt-curing, pickling, or smoking should be minimized.

From Simons-Morton B, O'Hara N, Simons-Morton D: Promoting healthful diet and exercise behaviors in communities, schools, and families, *Fam Comm Health* 9(3):4, 1986.

PART THREE

INDICATORS OF RISK

Indicators of risk are valuable as predictors of potential health problems. The nurse is always aware of changes in behavior, state of usual (normal) lifestyle, and resulting health status of clients. Risk indicators can cue the nurse toward appropriate anticipatory guidance and interactions.

 Abuse

Substance Abuse

Characteristics of Substances of Abuse

Substance	Route (most common first)	Common street name	Dependence: physical/ psychologic	Use: signs and symptoms	Overdose: signs and symptoms	Withdrawal: signs and symptoms	Special considerations/ consequences of use
Depressants							
Alcohol	Ingestion	Booze, brew, juice, spirits	Yes/Yes	Depression of major brain functions such as mood, cognition, attention, concentration, insight, judgment, memory, affect, and emotional rapport in interpersonal relationships. Extent of depression is dose dependent and ranges from slight lethargy through the various levels of anesthesia and death. Tranquilization, sedation, and sleep. Psychomotor impairment, increased reaction time, interruption of hand-eye coordination, motor ataxia, nystagmus.	Unconsciousness, coma, respiratory depression, death	General depressant withdrawal syndrome: tremors, agitation, anxiety, diaphoresis, increased pulse and blood pressure, sleep disturbance, hallucinosis, seizures, delusions, DTs (severe tremors, delirium, disorientation, visual hallucinations, extremely elevated temperature, vomiting, and diarrhea). Postacute withdrawal: mood swings, difficulty sleeping, impaired cognitive functioning, increased emotionality, overreaction to stress.	Chronic alcohol use leads to serious disruptions in most organ systems: malnutrition and dehydration; vitamin deficiency leading to Wernicke's encephalopathy and alcoholic amnestic syndrome; impaired liver function, including hepatitis and cirrhosis, esophagitis, gastritis, pancreatitis; osteoporosis; anemia; peripheral neuropathy; impaired pulmonary function; cardiomyopathy; myopathy; disrupted immune system; and brain damage.
Barbiturates	Ingestion Injection	Barbs, beans, black beauties, blue angels, candy, downers, goof balls, G.B., nebbies, reds, sleepers, yellow jackets, yellows	Yes/Yes				

	Route	Common names	Dependence (Physical/Psychological)	Effects	Overdose	Withdrawal	Long-term effects
Benzodiazepines	Ingestion Injection	Downers	Yes/Yes	Decreased REM sleep leading to more dreams and sometimes nightmares. Benzodiazepines have minimal cardiovascular and respiratory effects.		Low-dose benzodiazepine withdrawal: therapeutic dose for no more than 6 months; subtle symptoms, peak in about 12 days; wax and wane for 6-12 months; several symptom-free days, followed by acute anxiety, dilated pupils, elevated pulse, and blood pressure. High-dose benzodiazepine withdrawal: peaks in 2 to 3 days for short-acting drugs and 5 to 8 days for longer-acting; symptoms usually gone in 2 weeks	High susceptibility to other dependencies. Dependence on barbiturates and benzodiazepines may develop insidiously; users may underreport the actual amount taken because of guilt about multiple prescriptions and abuse.
Marijuana	Smoking Ingestion	Acapulco gold, aunt mary, broccoli, dope, grass, grunt, hay, hemp, herb, J, joint, joy stick, killer weed, maryjane, pot, ragweed, reefer, smoke, weed	No/Yes	Altered state of awareness, relaxation, mild euphoria, reduced inhibition, red eyes, dry mouth, increased appetite, increased pulse, decreased reflexes, panic reaction.	Toxic/psychosis	None	Pulmonary problems. Interference with reproductive hormones. May cause fetal abnormalities.

Continued.

From Stuart GW, Sundeen SJU: *Principles and practice of psychiatric nursing*, ed 5, St Louis, 1995, Mosby.

Characteristics of substances of abuse—cont'd

Substance	Route (most common first)	Common street name	Dependence: physical/ psychologic	Use: signs and symptoms	Overdose: signs and symptoms	Withdrawal: signs and symptoms	Special considerations; consequences of use
Stimulants							
Amphet-amines	Ingestion Injection	A, AMT, bam, bennies, crystal, diet pills, dolls, eye-openers, lid poppers, pep pills, purple hearts, speed, uppers, wake-up	Yes/Yes	Sudden rush of euphoria, abrupt awakening, increased energy, talkativeness, elation. Agitation, hyperactivity, irritability, grandiosity, pressured speech. Diaphoresis, anorexia, weight loss, insomnia. Increased temperature, blood pressure, and pulse.	Seizures. Cardiac arrhythmias, coronary artery spasms, myocardial infarctions, sharp increase in blood pressure and temperature that can lead to cardiovascular shock and death	Crash: depression, agitation, anxiety, and intense drug craving followed by fatigue, depression, loss of drug desire, insomnia, desire for sleep followed by prolonged sleep then extreme hunger, renewed drug cravings, anergia, and anhedonia, which may increase for 1 to 4 days.	Certain amphetamines prescribed for attention deficit hyperactivity disorder in children because of a paradoxic depressant action. May be used alternately with depressants. Psychosis that does not clear may indicate preexisting vulnerability.
Cocaine	Inhalation Smoking Injection Topical	Bernice, bernies, big C, blow, C, charlie, coke, dust, girl, heavy, jay, lady, nose candy, nose powder, snow, sugar, white lady Crack = conan, freebase, rock,	Yes/Yes	Tachycardia, ectopic heartbeats, chest pain. Urinary retention, constipation, dry mouth. High dose: slurred, rapid, incoherent speech. Stereotypic movements, ataxic gait, teeth grinding,		Pattern varies widely among patients; anxiety, depression, irritability; fatigue may last several weeks; craving may return; relapse is a risk	Cocaine use may lead to multiple physical problems: destruction of the nasal septum related to snorting; coronary artery vasoconstriction; seizures; cerebrovascular accidents; tran-

Substance	Street names	Methods of use	Effects	Overdose	Dependence	Withdrawal	Complications
	toke, white cloud, white tornado		illogical thought processes, headache, nausea, vomiting. Toxic psychosis: paranoid delusions in clear sensorium; auditory, visual, or tactile hallucinations (may scratch at nonexistent bugs). Very labile mood. Unprovoked violence.			Sometimes a user stops stimulants purposely to decrease tolerance, decreasing the amount needed to get high.	sient ischemic episodes; sudden death related to respiratory arrest, myocardial infarction, or status epilepticus. Intravenous use of stimulants may lead to the serious physical consequences described under Opiates.
Opiates							
Heroin	H, horse, harry, boy, scag, shit, smack, stuff, white junk, white stuff	Injection, Ingestion, Inhalation			Yes/Yes	Initially drug craving, lacrimation, rhinorrhea, yawning, diaphoresis. In 12–72 hr: sleep disturbance, mydriasis, anorexia, piloerection, irritability, tremor, weakness, nausea, vomiting, diarrhea, chills, fever, muscle spasms (especially in legs), flushing, spontaneous ejaculation, abdominal pain, hypertension, increased rate and depth of respirations.	Intravenous use leads to high risk for infection with bloodborne pathogens, such as HIV or hepatitis B. Other infections (e.g., skin abscesses, phlebitis, cellulitis, and septic emboli causing pneumonia, pulmonary abscess, or subacute bacterial endocarditis) may occur as a result of lack of asepsis or contaminated substances. Adulterants (e.g., talc, starch, strychnine) are deposited in the lungs, causing impaired function.
Morphine		Injection	Euphoria, relaxation, relief from pain, "nodding out" (apathy, detachment from reality, impaired judgment, and drowsiness); constricted pupils, nausea, constipation, slurred speech, respiratory depression	Unconsciousness, coma, respiratory depression, circulatory depression, respiratory arrest, cardiac arrest, death. Anoxia can lead to brain abscess			
Meperidine		Injection, Ingestion					
Codeine		Ingestion, Injection					
Opium		Smoking, Ingestion					
Methadone		Ingestion					

Continued.

Characteristics of substances of abuse—cont'd

Substance	Route (most common first)	Common street name	Dependence: physical/ psychologic	Use: signs and symptoms	Overdose: signs and symptoms	Withdrawal: signs and symptoms	Special considerations; consequences of use
Opiates—cont'd							
						Protracted withdrawal: changes in respirations and temperature, decreased self-esteem, anxiety, depression, and abnormal responses to stressful situations. Lasts up to 6 months.	Chronic use leads to lack of concern about physical well-being, resulting in malnutrition and dehydration. Criminal behavior may occur to acquire money for drugs. Multiple drug use is common.
Hallucinogens	Ingestion Smoking	Acid, big D, blotter, blue heaven, cap, D, deeda, flash, L, mellow yellows, microdots, paper acid, sugar, ticket, yellow	No/No	Distorted perceptions and hallucinations in the presence of a clear sensorium. Distortions of time and space, illusions, depersonalization, mystical experiences, heightened sense of awareness. Extreme mood labil-	Rare with LSD: convulsions, hyperthermia, death	None	Flashbacks may last for several months. Permanent psychosis may occur.

				ity. Tremor, dizziness, piloerection, paresthesias, synesthesia, nausea and vomiting. Increased temperature, pulse, blood pressure, and salivation. Panic reaction, "bad trip."		
Phencyclidine (PCP)	Smoking Ingestion	Angel dust, DOA, dust, elephant, hog, peace pill, supergrass, tic tac	No/No	Intensively psychotic experience characterized by bizarre perceptions, confusion, disorientation, euphoria, hallucinations (in clouded sensorium), paranoia, grandiosity, agitation. Anesthesia. Apparent enhancement of strength and endurance. Rage reactions. May be agitated and hyperactive with tendency toward violence and antisocial behavior or catatonic and withdrawn or vacillate between the two conditions. Red, dry skin; dilated pupils, nystagmus, ataxia, hypertension, rigidity, and seizures.	Seizures, coma, and death	None If flashbacks occur, they are mild and usually not disturbing.

The Five Stages of Substance Abuse

Stage	Drugs	Sources	Frequency	Feelings	Behavior	Treatment
0: Curiosity	None	Available—but not used	—	Curiosity	Risk taking, desire for acceptance	Optimal time; anticipatory guidance to develop good coping skills and strong self-esteem; clear family guidelines on drug and alcohol use; drug education
1: Experimentation	Tobacco, alcohol, marijuana	House supply, friends, siblings	Weekend use for recreational purposes	Excitement, pleasure, few consequences; learning how easy it is to feel good	Lying, little change	Drug education; attention to societal messages; reduction of supply; strict, loving rules at home; establishment of drug-free alternative activities

2: Regular use	As above, plus hashish or oil, tranquilizers, sedatives, amphetamines	Buying	Progresses to midweek use; purpose is to get high	Excitement followed by guilt	Mood swings, faltering school performance, truancy, changing peer groups, changing style of dress	Drug-free self-help groups (Alcoholics or Narcotics Anonymous); family involvement; psychiatric counseling unhelpful unless family therapy and aftercare provided
3: Psychologic or chemical dependency	As above, plus stimulants, hallucinogens	Selling to support habit; possibly stealing or prostitution in exchange for drugs	Daily	Euphoric highs followed by depression, shame, guilt, and perhaps suicidal thoughts	Pathologic lying; school failure; family fights; involvement with the law over curfew, truancy, vandalism, shoplifting, driving under the influence, breaking and entering, violence	Inpatient or foster care programs that require family involvement and provide aftercare

Continued.

Adapted from MacDonald DI: *Pediatric Rev* 10:89, 1988. In Stuart GW, Sundeen SJ: *Principles and practice of psychiatric nursing*, ed 5, St Louis, 1995, Mosby.

The five stages of substance abuse—cont'd

Stage	Drugs	Sources	Frequency	Feelings	Behavior	Treatment
4: Using drugs to feel "normal"	As above; any available drug, including opiates	Any way possible	All day	Euphoria rare and harder to achieve; chronic depression	Drifting, with repeated failures and psychologic symptoms of paranoia and aggression; frequent overdosing, blackouts, amnesia; chronic cough, fatigue, malnutrition	Inpatient or foster care programs that require family involvement and provide aftercare

Brief Drug Abuse Screening Test (B-DAST)

Instructions: The following questions concern information about your involvement with and abuse of drugs. Drug abuse refers to (1) the use of prescribed or over-the-counter drugs in excess of the directions and (2) any nonmedical use of drugs Carefully read each statement and decide whether your answer is yes or no. Then circle the appropriate response.

YES   NO   1. Have you used drugs other than those required for medical reasons?

YES   NO   2. Have you abused prescription drugs?

YES   NO   3. Do you abuse more than one drug at a time?

YES   NO   4. Can you get through the week without using drugs (other than those required for medical reasons)?

YES   NO   5. Are you always able to stop using drugs when you want to?

YES   NO   6. Have you had "blackouts" or "flashbacks" as a result of drug use?

YES   NO   7. Do you ever feel bad about your drug abuse?

YES   NO   8. Does your spouse (or parents) ever complain about your involvement with drugs?

YES   NO   9. Has drug abuse ever created problems between you and your spouse?

YES   NO   10. Have you ever lost friends because of your use of drugs?

YES   NO   11. Have you ever neglected your family or missed work because of your use of drugs?

YES   NO   12. Have you ever been in trouble at work because of drug abuse?

YES   NO   13. Have you ever lost a job because of drug abuse?

YES   NO   14. Have you gotten into fights when under the influence of drugs?

YES   NO   15. Have you engaged in illegal activities in order to obtain drugs?

YES   NO   16. Have you ever been arrested for possession of illegal drugs?

YES   NO   17. Have you ever experienced withdrawal symptoms as a result of heavy drug intake?

From Skinner HA: *Addict Behav* 7:363, 1982. In Stuart GW, and Sundeen SJ: *Principles and practice of psychiatric nursing,* ed 5, St Louis, 1995, Mosby.

YES NO 18. Have you had medical problems as a result of your drug use (e.g., memory loss, hepatitis, convulsions, bleeding)?

YES NO 19. Have you ever gone to anyone for help for a drug problem?

YES NO 20. Have you ever been involved in a treatment program specifically related to drug use?

The CAGE Questionnaire

- Have you ever felt you ought to **C**ut down on your drinking?
- Have people **A**nnoyed you by criticizing your drinking?
- Have you ever felt bad or **G**uilty about your drinking?
- Have you ever had a drink first thing in the morning to steady your nerves or get rid of a hangover (**E**ye-opener)?

Scoring: One "yes" answer calls for further inquiry. Two "yes" answers suggest an alcohol abuse problem.

From Ewing JA: *JAMA* 252(14):1905–1907, 1984. Copyright 1984 by the American Medical Association. Reprinted by permission In Stuart GW, Sundeen SJ: *Principles and practice of psychiatric nursing,* ed 5, St Louis, 1995, Mosby.

Selected Drugs Commonly Abused and Symptoms of Abuse

Drug category	Street names	Methods of use	Symptoms of use	Hazards of use
Marijuana/hashish	Pot, grass, reefer, weed, Columbian, hash, hash oil, sinsemilla, joint	Most often smoked; can also be swallowed in solid form	Sweet, burnt odor Neglect of appearance Loss of interest, motivation Possible weight loss	Impaired memory, perception Interference with psychologic maturation Possible damage to lungs, heart, and reproduction and immune systems Psychologic dependence
Alcohol	Booze, hooch, juice, brew	Swallowed in liquid form	Impaired muscle coordination, judgment	Heart and liver damage Death from overdose Death from car accidents Addiction
Amphetamines* Amphetamine Dextroamphetamine Methamphetamine	Speed, uppers, pep pills Bennies Dexies Moth, crystal Black beauties	Swallowed in pill or capsule form, or injected into veins	Excess activity Irritability; nervousness Mood swings Needle marks	Loss of appetite Hallucinations; paranoia Convulsions; coma Brain damage Death from overdose

Continued.

*Includes look-alike drugs resembling amphetamines that contain caffeine, phenylpropanolamine (PPA), and ephedrine.

From Blue Cross & Blue Shield Association, Chicago, Ill. In McKenry LM, Salerno E: *Mosby's pharmacology in nursing,* ed 19, St Louis, 1995, Mosby.

Selected drugs commonly abused and symptoms of abuse—cont'd

Drug category	Street names	Methods of use	Symptoms of use	Hazards of use
Cocaine	Coke, snow, toot, white lady, crack	Most often inhaled (snorted); also injected or swallowed in powder form, smoked	Restlessness, anxiety Intense, short-term high followed by dysphoria	Intensive psychologic dependence Sleeplessness; anxiety Nasal passage damage Lung damage Death from overdose
Nicotine	Coffin nail Butt, smoke	Smoked in cigarettes, cigars, and pipes, snuff, chewing tobacco	Smell of tobacco High carbon monoxide blood levels Stained teeth	Cancers of the lung, throat, mouth, esophagus Heart disease; emphysema
Barbiturates Pentobarbital Secobarbital Amobarbital	Barbs, downers Yellow jackets Red devils Blue devils	Swallowed in pill form or injected into veins	Drowsiness Confusion Impaired judgment Slurred speech Needle marks Constricted pupils	Infection Addiction with severe life-threatening withdrawal symptoms Loss of appetite Death from overdose Nausea
Narcotics Dilaudid, Percodan Demerol, Methadone		Swallowed in pill or liquid form, injected	Drowsiness Lethargy	Addiction with severe withdrawal symptoms Loss of appetite Death from overdose

Drug	Slang names	How administered	Symptoms	Effects
Morphine Heroin Codeine	Dreamer, junk, smack, horse School boy	Injected into veins, smoked Swallowed in pill or liquid form	Needle marks	Anxiety; depression Impaired memory, perception Death from accidents Death from overdose
Hallucinogens PCP (Phencyclidine)	Angel dust, killer weed, supergrass, hog, peace pill	Most often smoked; can also be inhaled (snorted), injected, or swallowed in tablets	Slurred speech; blurred vision, uncoordination Confusion, agitation Aggression	
LSD	Acid, cubes, purple haze	Injected or swallowed in tablets		
Mescaline Psilocybin	Mesc, cactus Magic mushrooms	Usually ingested in their natural form	Dilated pupils Delusions; hallucinations Mood swings	Breaks from reality Emotional breakdown Flashback
Inhalants Gasoline Airplane glue Paint thinner Nitrites Amyl Butyl	Poppers, locker room, rush, snappers	Inhaled or sniffed, often with use of paper or plastic bag or rag	Poor motor coordination Impaired vision, memory, and thought processes Abusive, violent behavior Slowed thought Headache	High risk of sudden death Drastic weight loss Brain, liver, and bone marrow damage Anemia, death by anoxia

Leading 10 Drugs Abused in the United States*

Emergency room†

Males
1. alcohol in combination
2. cocaine
3. heroin/morphine
4. marijuana/hashish
5. acetaminophen
6. diazepam (Valium)
7. aspirin
8. alprazolam (Xanax)
9. methamphetamine/speed
10. OTC sleep acids

Females
1. alcohol in combination
2. cocaine
3. acetaminophen
4. aspirin
5. alprazolam (Xanax)
6. heroin/morphine
7. diazepam (Valium)
8. codeine combinations
9. amitriptyline (Elavil)
10. fluoxetine (Prozac)

Medical examiners‡

Males
1. PCP/PCP combinations
2. marijuana/hashish
3. heroin/morphine/opiates
4. methamphetamine/speed
5. inhalants/solvents/aerosols
6. amphetamines
7. glutethimide (Doriden)
8. alcohol in combination
9. cocaine
10. oxycodone

Females
1. fluoxetine (Prozac)
2. pentobarbital (Nembutal)
3. flurazepam (Dalmane)
4. meperidine (Demerol)
5. thioridazine (Mellaril)
6. lorazepam (Ativan)
7. desipramine (Norpramin)
8. alprazolam (Xanax)
9. imipramine (Tofranil)
10. meprobamate (Miltown)

*Tradenames are in parentheses; many of these products are also available under their generic names.
†1990 data collected from 533 emergency rooms in 21 U.S. metropolitan areas. A total of 110,448 emergency room drug abuse episodes (occurrences resulting in a medical crisis) were reported.
‡1990 data from 135 medical examiners located in 27 U.S. metropolitan areas. A total of 5830 drug abuse related deaths were reported.

From McKenry LM, Salerno E: *Mosby's pharmacology in nursing,* ed 19, St Louis, 1995, Mosby.

Physical Abuse

Types of Child Abuse

	Definition	Characteristics
Physical abuse	Nonaccidental injury of a child	Physical injury at variance with history or explanation given; repeated pattern of physical punishment with short- or long-term effects
Emotional abuse	Nonphysical, often verbal, assault on a child—usually critical, demeaning, and emotionally devastating	Attack inflicted by parent or other adult, often as part of a continuing pattern
Sexual abuse	Use of a child for sexual purposes, including incest, rape, molestation, prostitution, or pornography	Nonabusing parent or other family members often aware of the abuse (and might be criminally liable if they do nothing to stop it)
Adolescent abuse	Physical, emotional, or sexual abuse inflicted on an adolescent	Adolescent who runs away from home; abusing parent often considers abuse justified

Adapted from Mott SR, James SR, Sperhac AM: *Nursing Care of Children and Families*, ed 2, Menlo Park, Calif, 1990, Addison-Wesley.

Components of Report of Child Maltreatment

Aspect of report	Example
Reason for suspicion or assessment of incident	Child's comments; nature or extent of injury
Behaviors observed and by whom	Teacher's report; circumstances of discovery (e.g., "child found alone by police in car")
Quality of parent-child relationship (if observed)	Any comforting measure noted or lacking (e.g., "father speaks in loud tones and uses threatening language")
What family has been told (to assist in follow-up for all team members)	Purpose of Child Protective Services (if family is unaware of report, explain rationale)
What protection team should do first	Possible interventions (e.g., assess home and risks to siblings; investigate and enlist possible community supports)

Adapted from Mott SR, James SR, Sperhac AM: *Nursing Care of Children and Families,* ed 2, Menlo Park, Calif, 1990, Addison-Wesley.

Parental Risk Factors for Child Maltreatment

Risk factor	Assessment finding
Lack of nurturing experience	Inadequate experience with parenting (e.g., multiple foster homes)
	Parent neglected or abused as a child
	Parent expected to meet high demands of own parents as a child
Lack of knowledge or normal growth and development	Inability to read "cues" of child
	Impatience when child does not respond as expected; unreasonable discipline
	Unrealistically high expectations for the child
Isolation	Inadequate use of supports
	Inability to identify resources
	Unknown to others in community
Low self-esteem	Lack of trust, particularly of authority figures
	Expect rejection
High vulnerability to criticism	History of family violence in family of origin or in current family system (e.g., spouse abuse)
	Impulsive
Many unmet needs	Feelings of being unloved or having unresponsive spouse, unstable marriage, or no marriage at all
	Youthful marriage, forced marriage, unwanted pregnancy
Multiple stressors	Poverty, unemployment, substandard housing, lack of job opportunities
	Inadequate clothing and insufficient food
Substance abuse	Abuse of alcohol or drugs
Role reversal	Emotional immaturity, lack of patience, inability to make judgments
	Preoccupied with self
	Depression
	Dependent on others

Adapted from Mott SR, James SR, Sperhac AM: *Nursing Care of Children and Families,* ed 2, Menlo Park, Calif, 1990, Addison-Wesley. In Olds S, London M, Ladewig P: *Maternal-newborn nursing,* ed 4, Reading, 1992, Addison-Wesley.

Pedophile Victimizers

Clinical profile

May be authority figures to child victims.

Are often but not always related to child victims.

Often have a history of having been physically abused as children.

Tend to have had a distant father-son relationship.

Tend to have had few friends while growing up.

Are characteristically described as shy, unassertive, passive, fearful about their competence in an adult sexual relationship.

Seek sexual gratification in ways that are least threatening to their fragile self-concept.

Some are sadistic or psychotic and brutalize or murder their victims.

From Haber J et al: *Comprehensive psychiatric nursing,* ed 4, St Louis, 1992, Mosby.

Methods Used to Pressure Children into Sexual Activity

The child is offered gifts or privileges.

The adult misrepresents moral standards by telling the child that it is "okay to do."

Isolated and emotionally and socially impoverished children are enticed by adults who meet their needs for warmth and human contact.

The successful sex offender pressures the victim into secrecy regarding the activity by describing it as a "secret between us" that other people may take away if they find out.

The offender plays on the child's fears, including fear of punishment by the offender, fear of repercussions if the child tells, and fear of abandonment or rejection by the family.

From Wong DL: *Whaley and Wong's nursing care of infants and children,* ed 5, St Louis, 1995, Mosby.

Talking with Children Who Reveal Abuse

Provide a private time and place to talk.

Do not promise not to tell; tell them that you are required by law to report the abuse.

From Wong DL: *Whaley and Wong's nursing care of infants and children,* ed 5, St Louis, 1995, Mosby.

Do not express shock or criticize their family.

Use their vocabulary to discuss body parts.

Avoid using any leading statements that can distort their report.

Reassure them that they have done the right thing by telling.

Tell them that the abuse is not their fault, that they are not bad or to blame.

Determine their immediate need for safety.

Let the child know what will happen when you report.

Warning Signs of Abuse

Physical evidence of abuse or neglect, including previous injuries

Conflicting stories about the "accident" or injury from the parents or others

Cause of injury blamed on sibling or other party

An injury inconsistent with the history, such as a concussion and broken arm from falling off a bed

History inconsistent with child's developmental level, such as a 6-month-old turning on the hot water

A complaint other than the one associated with signs of abuse (e.g., a chief complaint of a cold when there is evidence of first- and second-degree burns)

Inappropriate response of caregiver, such as an exaggerated or absent emotional response; refusal to sign for additional tests or agree to necessary treatment; excessive delay in seeking treatment; absence of the parents for questioning

Inappropriate response of child, such as little or no response to pain; fear of being touched; excessive or lack of separation anxiety; indiscriminate friendliness to strangers

Child's report of physical or sexual abuse

Previous reports of abuse in the family

Repeated visits to emergency facilities with injuries

From Wong DL: *Whaley and Wong's nursing care of infants and children,* ed 5, St Louis, 1995, Mosby.

Signs and Symptoms of Physical Abuse

Indication of abuse	Assessment findings
Bruises or welts on ears, eyes, mouth, lips, torso, buttocks, genital areas, calves	Injuries may be in shape of object used to produce them (e.g., sticks, belts, hairbrushes, buckles)
	Injuries located on parts of body not usually injured, such as bruising behind the ear, bleeding into the conjunctiva or retina, pinch marks on genitals (normal bruises commonly appear on forehead, shins, knees, elbows)
	Injuries often in various stages of healing
Burns	Shape suggests type of burn
Immersion burns	Immersion burns on feet have "socklike," on hands "glovelike," on buttocks or genitalia "donutlike" appearance
Pattern burns	Pattern suggests object used (e.g., iron, stove grate, electric burner, heater); small, circular burns on feet, face, hands, chest, or buttocks suggest cigar or cigarette
Friction burns	Friction burns on legs, arms, neck, or torso may be caused by child having been tied up with rope
Scald burns	Caused by hot liquid poured over trunk or extremities; multiple splash marks may appear on body; depth of burn varies with temperature of liquid, length of contact, and presence of clothing
Fractures of skull, face, nose, orbit, long bones, ribs	Multiple or spiral fractures caused by twisting motion
	Evidence of epiphyseal separations and periosteal shearing
	Shaft fractures from direct blows
	Fractures may be in various stages of healing if earlier fractures went untreated
Lacerations or abrasions on mouth, lips, gums, eyes, genitals	Human bitemarks, especially those of adult size, may be evident
	Torn frenulum in infant from forcing object into mouth
	Puncture wounds or deep scratch marks from fingernails around face or genital area

Adapted from Mott SR, James SR, Sperhac AM: *Nursing Care of Children and Families,* ed 2, Menlo Park, Calif, 1990, Addison-Wesley.

Signs and symptoms of physical abuse—cont'd

Indication of abuse	Assessment findings
Head trauma	Evidence of increased intracranial pressure in infant (e.g., bulging fontanelle) Subdural hematomas from being dropped on the head or from receiving blows to the head; if abuse is repetitive, separation of cranial sutures may be evidence because of chronic subdural hematoma Areas of baldness and swelling from hair being pulled out when dragging the child by the hair
Neck trauma	Limited range of motion from whiplash injury from being shaken Dislocation of subluxation of neck
Somatic	Persistent vomiting or abdominal pain Rigid abdomen caused by internal bleeding Shock
Child's behaviors	Extreme aggressiveness or withdrawal; wariness of adults; fear of going home; apprehension when other children cry Appears disinterested or frightened of parents, shows no emotion when parents leave or return Indiscriminate friendliness and immediate affection shown toward anyone providing attention Vacant stare, no eye contact Surveys environment but remains motionless Stiffens when approached as if expecting punishment of a physical nature Inappropriate response to painful procedures

Abuse Assessment Screen

1. Have you ever been emotionally or physically abused by your partner or someone important to you?   Yes   No
2. Within the last year, have you been hit, slapped, kicked, or otherwise physically hurt by someone?   Yes   No
   If yes, by whom _____
   Number of times _____
3. Since you have been pregnant, have you been hit, slapped, kicked or otherwise physically hurt by someone?   Yes   No
   If yes, by whom _____
   Number of times _____
   Mark the area of injury on body map.

4. Within the last year, has anyone forced you to have sexual activities?   Yes   No
   If yes, by whom _____
   Number of times _____
5. Are you afraid of your partner or anyone you listed above?   Yes   No

From Creasia JL, Parker B: *Conceptual foundations of professional nursing practice*, St Louis, 1991, Mosby.

Definitions of Elder Abuse

Source	Definition
O'Malley, Segal, and Perez (1979), adapted from Connecticut Department of Aging	Abuse: the willful infliction of physical pain, injury, or debilitating mental anguish; unreasonable confinement; or deprivation by a caretaker of services that are necessary to maintain mental and physical health.
Block and Sinnott (1979)	1. Physical abuse: malnutrition; injuries, e.g., bruises, welts, sprains, dislocations, abrasions, or lacerations.
	2. Psychologic abuse: verbal assault, threat, fear, isolation.
	3. Material abuse: theft, misuse of money or property.
	4. Medical abuse: withholding of medications or aids required.
Douglass, Hickey, and Noele (1980)	1. Passive neglect: being ignored, left alone, isolated, forgotten.
	2. Active neglect: withholding of companionship, medicine, food, exercise, assistance to bathroom.
	3. Verbal or emotional abuse: name calling, insults, treating as a child, frightening, humiliation, intimidation, threats.
	4. Physical abuse: being hit, slapped, bruised, sexually molested, cut, burned, physically restrained.
Lau and Kosberg (1979)	1. Physical abuse: direct beatings; withholding personal care, food, medical care; lack of supervision.
	2. Psychologic abuse: verbal assaults, threats, provoking fear, isolation.
	3. Material abuse: monetary or material theft or misuse.
	4. Violation of rights: being forced out of one's dwelling or forced into another setting.
Wolf and Pillemer (1984)	1. Physical abuse: infliction of physical pain or injury, physical coercion (confinement against one's will), e.g., slapped, bruised, sexually molested, cut, burned, physically restrained.
	2. Psychologic abuse: the infliction of mental anguish, e.g., called names, treated as child, frightened, humiliated, intimidated, threatened, isolated.

Continued.

Definitions of elder abuse—cont'd

Source	Definition
	3. Material abuse: the illegal or improper exploitation or use of funds or other resources.
	4. Active neglect: refusal or failure to fulfill a caretaking obligation, including a conscious and intentional attempt to inflict physical or emotional stress on the elder, e.g., deliberate abandonment, or deliberate denial of food or health-related services.
	5. Passive neglect: refusal or failure to fulfill a caretaking obligation, excluding a conscious and intentional attempt to inflict physical or emotional distress on the elder, e.g., abandonment, nonprovision of services.

From Fulmer T, O'Malley FA: *Inadequate care of the elderly: a health care perspective on abuse and neglect*, New York, 1987, Springer. In Edelman CL, Mandle CL: *Health promotion throughout the lifespan*, ed 3, St Louis, 1994, Mosby.

Signs of Elder Mistreatment

Contusions

Lacerations

Abrasions

Fractures

Sprains

Dislocations

Burns

Oversedation

Anxiety

Overmedication or
undermedication

Decubiti

Untreated but previously
treated conditions

Dehydration

Misuse of medications

Malnutrition

Freezing

Poor hygiene

Depression

Adapted from O'Malley TA, et al: *Ann Intern Med* 98:998, 1983; Fulmer T, O'Malley TA: *Inadequate care of the elderly: a health care perspective on abuse and neglect,* New York, 1987, Springer. In Edelman CL, Mandle CL: *Health promotion throughout the lifespan,* ed 3, St Louis, 1994, Mosby.

Danger Assessment

Several risk factors have been associated with homicides (murder) of both batterers and battered women in research that has been conducted after the killings have taken place. We cannot predict what will happen in your case, but we would like for you to be aware of the danger of homicide in situations of severe battering and for you to see how many of the risk factors apply to your situation. (The "he" in the questions refers to your husband, partner, ex-husband, ex-partner, or whoever is currently physically hurting you).

___ **1.** Has the physical violence increased in frequency over the past year?

___ **2.** Has the physical violence increased in severity over the past year or has a weapon or threat with weapon been used?

___ **3.** Does he ever try to choke you?

___ **4.** Is there a gun in the house?

___ **5.** Has he ever forced you into sex when you did not wish to do so?

___ **6.** Does he use drugs? By drugs I mean "uppers" or amphetamines, speed, angel dust, cocaine, "crack," street drugs, heroin, or mixtures.

From Campbell J, Humphreys J: *Nursing care of survivors of family violence,* St Louis, 1993, Mosby.

__ **7.** Does he threaten to kill you or do you believe he is capable of killing you?

__ **8.** Is he drunk every day or almost every day? (In terms of quantity of alcohol.)

__ **9.** Does he control most or all of your daily activities? For instance, does he tell you who you can be friends with, how much money you can take with you shopping, or when you can take the car? (If he tries, but you do not let him, check here__)

__ **10.** Have you ever been beaten by him while you were pregnant? (If never pregnant by him, check here__)

__ **11.** Is he violently and constantly jealous of you? (For instance, does he say, "If I can't have you, no one can.")

__ **12.** Have you ever threatened or tried to commit suicide?

__ **13.** Has he ever threatened or tried to commit suicide?

__ **14.** Is he violent toward the children?

__ **15.** Is he violent outside of the home?

__   **Total yes answers**

Thank you. Please talk to your nurse, advocate, or counselor about what the danger assessment means in terms of your situation.

History of Elder—Possible Indicators of Potential or Actual Elder Abuse

Area of assessment	At-risk responses or indicators of possible abuse/neglect
Primary concern/reason for visit	Historical data that conflict with physical findings
	Acute or chronic psychologic or physical disability
	Inability to participate independently in activities of daily living
	Inappropriate delay in bringing elder to health care facility
	Reluctance on the part of caregiver to give information on elder's condition
	Inappropriate caregiver reaction to nurse's concern (overreacts, underreacts)
Family health	
Elder	Substance abuse
	Grew up in a violent home (abused as child, spouse; abused children)
	Excessive dependence of elder on child(ren)
Child(ren) of elder	Were abused by parents as children
	Antagonistic relationship with elder
	Excessive dependence on elder
	Substance abuse
	History of violent relationship with other siblings or spouse
Siblings	Antagonistic relationship between siblings
	Excessive dependence of one or more siblings on another or each other
Other family members and family relations	Other history of abuse or neglect or violent death

Continued.

From Campbell J, Humphreys J: *Nursing care of survivors of family violence,* St Louis, 1993, Mosby.

History of elder—possible indicators of potential or actual elder abuse

Area of assessment	At-risk responses or indicators of possible abuse/neglect
Household	Violence and aggression used to resolve conflicts and solve problems
	Past history of abuse or neglect among family members
	Poverty
	Few or no friends or neighbors or other support systems available
	Excessive number of stressful situations encountered during a short period of time (unemployment, death of a relative or significant other, etc.)
Health history of elder	
Child	History of chronic physical or psychologic disability
Midlife	History of chronic physical or psychologic disability
Nutrition	History of feeding problems (gastrointestinal disease, food preference idiosyncracies)
	Inappropriate food or drink
	Dietary intake that does not fit with findings
	Inadequate food or fluid intake
Drugs/medications	Drugs/medications not indicated by physical condition
	Overdose of drugs or medications (prescribed or over-the-counter)
	Medications not taken as prescribed
Personal/social	Caregiver has unrealistic expectations of elder
	Social isolation (little or no contact with friends, neighbors, or relatives; lack of outside activity)
	Substance abuse
	History of spouse abuse (as victim or abuser)
	History of antagonistic relationships mong family members (between family members in general, including elder)

Large age difference between elder and spouse
Large number of family problems
Excessive dependence on spouse, children, or significant others

Discipline
  Physical
    Belief that the use of physical punishment is appropriate
    Threats with an instrument as a means to punish
    Use of an instrument to administer physical punishment
    Excessive, inappropriate inconsistent physical punishment
    History of caregiver or others "losing control" or "hitting too hard"

Emotional/violation of rights
    Fear-provoking threats
    Infantilization
    Berating
    Screaming
    Forced move out of home
    Forced institutionalization
    Prohibiting marriage
    Prevention of free use of money
    Isolation

Sleep
Elimination
Illness
    Chronic illness or handicap
    Disability requiring special treatment from caregiver and others

Operations/hospitalization
    Operations or illness that required extended or repeated hospitalizations
    Caregiver's refusal to have elderly hospitalized
    Caregiver overanxious to have elder hospitalized

Continued.

History of elder—possible indicators of potential or actual elder abuse—cont'd

Area of assessment	At-risk responses or indicators of possible abuse/neglect
Diagnostic tests	Caregiver's refusal for further diagnostic tests
	Caregiver's overreaction or underreaction to diagnostic findings
Accidents	Repeated
	History of preceding events that do not support actual injuries
Safety	Appropriate safety precautions not taken, especially in elders known to be confused, disoriented, or with physical disabilities restricting mobility
Health care utilization	Infrequent
	Caregiver overanxious to have elder hospitalized
	Health care "shopping"
Review of body systems	

Child History—Indicators of Potential or Actual Child Abuse and Neglect

Area of assessment	At-risk responses
Primary concern/reason for visit	Historical data that do not fit with physical findings
	Vague complaints about child
	Inappropriate delay in bringing child to health facility
	Reluctance on the part of the parent to give information
	Inappropriate parental reaction to nurse's concern (overreacts or underreacts)
	Hyperactivity
Family health history	
Parents	Grew up in a violent home (abused as child, observed mother or siblings abused)
	Low self-esteem
	Violence between adults
	Little knowledge of child development and care
	Substance abuse
	Adolescent birth of child
Siblings	History of abuse or neglect of siblings
	Large family
	History of sudden infant death
	Several young, dependent children in family
Other family members	Other history of violence or violent death

Continued.

From Campbell J, Humphreys J: *Nursing care of survivors of family violence*, St. Louis, 1993, Mosby.

Child history—indicators of potential or actual child abuse and neglect—cont'd

Area of assessment	At-risk responses
Household	Violence and aggression used to resolve conflicts and solve problems
	Poverty
	Single parent
	Very young parent (early teens)
	No friends, neighbors, or other support systems available
	Problems between parents, especially over childrenOther stressors
	Unemployment
	Illness in the family
	History of child foster home or other institutional placement for abuse/neglect
Child health history	
Prenatal	Unwanted pregnancy
	Difficult or complicated pregnancy
	Early adolescent parent
	Wanted a baby so that "I would have someone to love"
	Little or no prenatal care
Birth	Cesarean section
	Prematurity
	Low birth weight
	Birth defect
	Immediate separation of parents and child
	Child not of preferred sex or appearance
Neonatal	Separation of parents and child
	Complications or identification of health problem

Category	Indicators
Nutrition (if necessary include 24-hour dietary recall)	History of feeding problems (frequent change of formula, colic, difficult to feed)
	Inappropriate food, drink, or drugs
	Dietary intake that does not fit with physical findings
	Inadequate or excessive food or fluid intake
	Obesity, anorexia, or bulimia
Personal/social	Negative description of child (different, troublesome, difficult)
	Parent has unrealistic expectations of child
	Multiple school absences
	Difficulty in school
	Depression
	History of phobias, running away from home, or delinquent acts
	Poor peer relationships or no peer relations
	Sexual problems in child (excessive or public masturbation, age-inappropriate sexual play, promiscuity)
	History of pregnancy
	Substance abuse
Discipline	Use of physical punishment, especially in an infant or adolescent
	Use of an object to administer physical punishment
	Excessive, inappropriate, inconsistent physical punishment
	History of parent "losing control" or "hitting too hard"
Sleep	"Doesn't sleep," "Awake all night"
	Consistent history of inadequate sleep for age
Elimination	Inappropriate, excessive home treatment of constipation
	Enuresis
	Violent or excessively severe toilet training
Growth and development	History of excessive autostimulation
	"Hyperactivity"

Continued.

Child History—Indicators of potential or actual child abuse and neglect—cont'd

Area of assessment	At-risk responses
Child health history—cont'd	
Growth and development—cont'd	Learning Disability
	Developmental delays
	Excessive aggression or passivity
Illness	Disability requiring special treatment from parents
	History of multiple, unexplained illnesses
	History of menstrual disorders
Operations/hospitalization	Operations or illness that required extended hospitalization
	Operations for rupture of internal organs (spleen, liver)
	Parent refusal to have child hospitalized
	Significant delay in seeking hospitalization
	History of suicide attempt
	History of overdose, even in young children
	History of multiple, unexplained operations or hospitalizations
Diagnostic tests	Evaluation for failure to thrive or other problem that would explain injuries or lack of weight gain
	History of multiple evaluations or diagnostic tests for unexplained illnesses
	Severe anemia
	Elevated lead level
Diagnostic tests	Parent refusal for further diagnostic studies
	Parent insistence on further, unwarranted diagnostic studies
Accidents	Repeated
	History of preceding events does not support actual injuries

Area of assessment	At-risk responses
Safety	No age-appropriate safety precautions
	History of poisoning
Immunizations	None or only a few
Health care utilization	Parent "shops" for hospital care
	No consistent provider
	Significant delay in seeking health care for serious problems
Review of body systems	Changes in previously reported data
	Pertinent data not previously reported

Indicators of Potential or Actual Wife Abuse from History

Area of assessment	At-risk responses*
Primary concern/reason for visit	Unwarranted delay between time of injury and seeking treatment
	Inappropriate spouse reactions (lack of concern, overconcern, threatening demeanor, reluctance to leave wife, etc.)
	Vague information about cause of injury or problem; discrepancy between physical findings and verbal description of cause; obviously incongruous cause of injury given
	Minimizing serious injury
	Seeking emergency room treatment for vague stress-related symptoms and minor injuries
	Suicide attempt; history of previous attempts
Family health history	
Family of origin	Traditional values about women's role taught
	Spouse abuse or child abuse (may not be significant for wife but should be noted)
Children	Children abused
	Physical punishment used routinely and severely with children
	Children are hostile toward or fearful of father
	Father perceives children as an additional burden
	Father demands unquestioning obedience from children
Partner	Alcohol or drug abuse
	Holds machismo values
	Experience with violence outside of home, including violence against women in previous relationships
	Low self-esteem; lack of power in workplace or other arenas outside of home
	Uses force or coercion in sexual activities
	Unemployment or underemployment
	Extreme jealousy of female friendships, work, and children, as well as other men; jealousy frequently unfounded

	Stressors such as death in family, moving, change of jobs, trouble at work
	Abused as a child or witnessed father abusing mother
Household	Poverty
	Conflicts solved by aggression or violence
	Isolated from neighbors, relatives; few friends; lack of support systems
Past health history	Fractures and trauma injuries
	Depression, anxiety symptoms, substance abuse
	Injuries while pregnant
	Spontaneous abortions
	Psychophysiological complaints
	Previous suicide attempts
Nutrition	Evidence of overeating or anorexia as reactions to stress
	Sudden changes in weight
Personal/social	Low self-esteem; evaluates self poorly in relation to others and ideal self, has trouble listing strengths, makes negative comments about self frequently, doubts own abilities
	Expresses feelings of being trapped, powerlessness, that the situation is hopeless, that it is futile to make future plans
	Chronic fatigue, apathy
	Feels responsible for spouse's behavior
	Holds traditional values about the home, a wife's prescribed role, the husband's prerogatives, strong commitment to marriage
	External locus of control orientation, feels no control over situation, believes fate or other forces determine events

Continued.

---

*At-risk responses are derived from clinical experiences and review of the literature.

From Campbell J, Humphreys J: *Nursing care of survivors of family violence,* St Louis, 1993, Mosby.

Indicators of potential or actual wife abuse from history—cont'd

Area of assessment	At-risk responses*
Personal/social—cont'd	Major decisions in household made by spouse, indicates far less power than he has in relationship, activities controlled by spouse, money controlled by spouse
	Few support systems, few supportive friends, little outside home activity, outside relationships have been discouraged by spouse or curtailed by self to deal with violent situation
	Physical aggression in courtship
Sleep	Sleep disturbances, insomnia, sleeping more than 10 to 12 hours per day
Elimination	Chronic constipation, diarrhea, or elimination disturbances related to stress
Illness	Frequent psychophysiologic illnesses
	Treatment for mental illness
	Use of tranquilizers, mood elevators, or antidepressants
Operations/hospitalization	Hospitalizations for trauma injuries
	Suicide attempts
	Hospitalization for depression
	Refusals of hospitalization when suggested by physician
Personal safety	Handgun(s) in home
	History of frequent accidents
	Does not take safety precautions
Health care utilization	No regular provider
	Indicates mistrust of health care system

Review of systems	Headache, undiagnosed gastrointestinal symptoms palpitations, other possible psychophysiologic complaints
	Sexual difficulties, feels husband is "rough" in sexual activities, lack of sexual desire, pain with intercourse
	Joint pain or other areas of tenderness, especially at the extremities
	Chronic pain
	Pelvic inflammatory disease

Indicators of Potential or Actual Violence in a Family from Nursing History

Area of assessment	At-risk responses
Information from genogram	Severe physical punishment or husband-wife violence in parental families of origin
	Violent death or serious injury from violence in genogram
	Family members in parental families of origin using violence outside the home
	Wife abuse in husband's previous marital relationship
Family structure	Single-parent home
	Dependent grandparent in home
	Blended family (involving stepparents or step-children)
Family resources	Unemployment; poverty
	Inadequate housing
	Elderly member with controlled resources
	Financial problems
	Total control of monetary resources by male head of household
	Perception of inadequate "fit" of family resources to family demands
Family role	Rigid traditional sex roles
	Individual or family dissatisfaction with roles family expects individuals to fulfill
	Roles incompatible
	Roles rigid, unchangeable
Family boundaries	Boundaries rigid; mistrust of all outsiders
Family communication patterns	Family communications nonnurturing; destructive to some members
	Communications ambiguous
	Lack of communication among family members

Family conflict resolution patterns	Extensive use of verbal aggression; many threats of violence
	Evidence of physical aggression used in husband-wife, parent-child, sibling-sibling, or parent-grandparent conflict resolution
Family power distribution	Autocratic decision making by father
	Children have no power
	Grandparent in home who is powerless
	Frequent power struggles
Family values	Violence considered acceptable or valued
	Great incongruence of values among family members or between family and society
	Differing values among family members considered intolerable
Emotional climate	High tension in home
	Lack of visible affection
	Scapegoating
	High anxiety in family member(s)
	Lack of support between family members
	Frequent disparagement between family members
Division of labor	Rigid division of labor according to sex
	Members highly dissatisfied with division of labor
Support systems	Family isolation
	Family inhibitions to helpseeking
	Children not forming close, supportive peer relationships (especially same-sex peer relationships)
	Lack of support systems considered useful for direct aid, emotional support, or affirmation

Continued.

From Campbell J, Humphreys J: *Nursing care of survivors of family violence*, St Louis, 1993, Mosby.

Indicators of potential or actual violence in a family from nursing history—cont'd

Area of assessment	At-risk responses
Support systems—cont'd	Relatives are highly critical; tension among extended family
	Sudden withdrawal by adolescent from social activity and peers
	Violence in extended family
Developmental stages	More than one family member facing difficult developmental crisis
	Lack of knowledge in parents of what to expect at various developmental stages in children, selves, and grandparents
Stressors	At-risk scores on stress scale
	Lack of successful coping mechanisms to deal with stress in the past
	Situational crises
	Stress-related physical symptoms in family members
Socialization of children	Physical punishment used
	Only one parent disciplines children
	Lack of nurturance of children
	Children displaying aggressive behavior, at home or outside of home
	Juvenile delinquency or sexual promiscuity in children
Health history	Frequent trauma injuries to family members
	Adolescent suicide attempts
	Serious illness in a family member
	History of treatment for mental illness or vaginal trauma
	History of venereal disease or genital trauma in children
	Drug or alcohol abuse
	Substance abuse in adolescents

Indicators of Potential or Actual Violence in a Family from Nursing Observation

Area of assessment	At-risk observations
General considerations	Observations differ significantly from information gathered on history
Family resources	Family members inadequately clothed and groomed
	One family member inadequately clothed or groomed, but the rest are not
	Household totally disorganized and family members indicate displeasure with the lack of organization
Family roles	One parent looks at the other to hold major interaction with children
	One parent answers all questions
	One parent looks to other for approval before answering questions
Family communication patterns	Members continually interrupt each other
	Members answer questions for each other; one member never talks for himself or herself
	Negative nonverbal behavior in other members when one family member is speaking
	Members frequently misunderstand each other
	Members do not listen to each other
Family conflict resolution	Verbal aggression used in front of nurse
Family power distribution	Members act afraid of another member
	One person makes all decisions
	Power struggles

Continued.

Indicators of potential or actual violence in a family from nursing history—cont'd

Area of assessment	At-risk responses
Emotional climate	Nonverbals unhappy, anxious, fearful
	Excessive physical distance maintained between members
	Members never touch each other
	Tense atmosphere
	Secretive atmosphere
	Voice tones sharp, nonaffectionate, disparaging

From Campbell J, Humphreys J: *Nursing care of survivors of family violence*, St Louis, 1993, Mosby.

Parenting Profile Assessment

	YES	NO	UNSURE
ASSESSMENT MADE OF CLIENT (VIA MOTHER)			
MODERATE TO SEVERE DISCIPLINE AS A CHILD (5)			
PAST OR PRESENT SPOUSAL ABUSE (3)			
PERCEPTION OF STRESS (4, 5)			
MODERATE TO SEVERE LIFE CHANGE UNIT SCORE (4, 5)**			
HIGH SCHOOL EDUCATION OR LESS (3)			
RARE INVOLVEMENT OUT OF HOME (1.25)			
LITTLE OR NO PRENATAL CARE (2.5)			
DOES NOT FEEL GOOD ABOUT HERSELF (3.5)			
FEELS LIKE RUNNING AWAY (3)			
AGE AT FIRST BIRTH UNDER 20 (2)			
ASSESSMENT MADE OF FAMILY (VIA MOTHER)			
UNLISTED OR NO PHONE (1)			
DIFFICULTY COMMUNICATING WITH FAMILY MEMBERS (3.5)			
HISTORY OF UNEMPLOYMENT OVER A TWO-MONTH PERIOD (OF USUAL PROVIDER) (2)			
CURRENTLY UNDER OR UNEMPLOYED (USUAL PROVIDER) (2)			
FAMILY INVOLVEMENTS WITH POLICE (2)			
LESS THAN $20,000 A YEAR INCOME (2.5)			
ASSESSMENT MADE OF DISCIPLINE METHODS (VIA MOTHER)***			
CURSES AT CHILD(REN) WHEN DISCIPLINING (3.5)			
CHILD(REN) SHOWS EVIDENCE OF PUNISHMENT POST DISCIPLINING (3) (CUTS, BRUISES, MISSED SCHOOL)			
PERCEIVES DISCIPLINE OF CHILDREN AS HARSH (3)			
CALLS CHILD(REN) NAMES WHEN DISCIPLINING (3.5)			

SCORING OF RISK ASSESSMENT:

SCORES FOR EACH VARIABLE ARE LOCATED IN PARENTHESIS BESIDE THE VARIABLE. THE SCORES MATCH THE SCORING VALUE ON THE ORIGINAL DATA COLLECTION INSTRUMENT.

FOR EACH YES ANSWER ADD IN THE APPROPRIATE SCORE. UNSURE STATEMENTS ARE NOT SCORED. OVER 3 UNSURES QUESTION THE VALIDITY OF THE RISK ASSESSMENT SCORE

AFTER TOTALING THE SCORE FOR EACH INDIVIDUAL VARIABLE REVIEW THE ASSESSMENT FOR THE <u>PRESENCE OF ALL THE FOLLOWING FIVE VARIABLES:</u>

> INCOME UNDER $20,000 A YEAR
> HIGH SCHOOL EDUCATION OR LESS
> FAMILY INVOLVEMENTS WITH POLICE
> PERCEIVES DISCIPLINE OF CHILD(REN) AS HARSH
> MODERATE OR SEVERE LIFE CHANGE UNIT SCORE**

ALERT FOR ABUSE:

POSSIBLE PARENTING PROBLEMS AND RISK FOR CHILD ABUSE: OVER 21 POINTS OR THE PRESENCE OF ALL THE ABOVE FIVE VARIABLES (THESE FAMILIES REQUIRE A FOLLOW-UP HOME VISIT).

MINIMAL PARENTING PROBLEMS AND LOW RISK FOR CHILD ABUSE: UNDER 21 POINTS AND A LACK OF ONE TO FIVE OF THE ABOVE VARIABLES. (FOLLOW-UP FOR FAMILIES IS OPTIONAL).

UNCERTAIN RISK: NO ADDITIONAL CHILDREN AT HOME FOR IMMEDIATE ASSESSMENT OF DISCIPLINE METHODS BY MOTHER OR THREE OR MORE UNSURES CHECKED. (FOLLOW-UP REQUIRED FOR ADDITIONAL INFORMATION.)

> *TIMING OF A REPEAT HOME ASSESSMENT IS INDICATED BY THE AT-RISK STATUS OF THE MOTHER. A REASSESSMENT OF VARIABLES MAY BE REQUIRED TO DETERMINE ADDITIONAL AREAS OF RISK AND NECESSARY INTERVENTIONS.
>
> **TOOL TO ASSESS LIFE CHANGE UNIT SCORE MUST ACCOMPANY THIS TOOL.
>
> *** IF ASSESSMENT MADE IN HOSPITAL BETWEEN MOTHER AND FIRST NEWBORN, OBSERVATIONS OF THIS AREA WILL NEED TO BE DEFERRED UNTIL HOME FOLLOW-UP.

CHECK APPROPRIATE BOX:

☐ POSSIBLE PARENTING PROBLEMS
☐ RISK FOR CHILD ABUSE

☐ MINIMAL PARENTING PROBLEMS
☐ LOW RISK FOR CHILD ABUSE

☐ UNCERTAIN RISK

☐ FOLLOW-UP SCHEDULE FOR

From Anderson CL: *Appl Nurs Res* 6(1):31-38, 1993.

Administering the Parenting Profile Assessment

The majority of questions can be answered yes/no by the mother (or father) through a simple interview (either in the hospital or in the home). Observations of disciplining techniques with children at home or in other settings may be necessary along with observations of children for documentable signs of abuse, such as bruises. To determine moderate to severe Life Change Unit (LCU) scores, the Social Readjustment Rating Scale (SRRS) is used.

The SRRS, developed by Holmes and Rahe (1967), is useful in determining stressful life events. The 43 life events listed indicate or require some change and consequent coping behavior in the life of the individual. Each event has been assigned an LCU value depending on the amount of social readjustment one needs in the face of the event. Events listed include such items as death of a spouse (100 LCU), marriage (50 LCU), trouble with in-laws (29 LCU), or change in social activities (18 LCU). Holmes and Rahe found that LCU scores of 150 to 199 indicate mild stress; LCU scores of 200 to 299 indicate moderate stress; and LCU scores of 300+ indicate high stress and major life crises.

As a frequently used tool to assess stress levels, the SRRS was selected as a companion tool with the parenting profile assessment (PPA) to assess potential parenting problems. When assessing families, both tools can be presented with content in a yes/no format providing easily administered tools in a short period of time.

LCU scores for each individual are totaled and determined as mild, moderate, or severe. A check in the appropriate place of the PPA under the yes column indicates moderate or severe stress. A check in the no column indicates mild stress (or a score of under 200). After all items of the PPA are assessed, a risk assessment is made. Unsure answers are not scored, and three or more unsure answers will question the validity of the tool and the accuracy of the information. All items on the PPA have scores. Total the scores for the items according to the yes answers checked. Follow-up for families is indicated if a score of over 21 or if a yes answer applies to the following five items: (a) income under $20,000.00/year, (b) high school education or less, (c) family involvements with police, (d) disciplining of children perceived as harsh, and (e) moderate or severe LCU score.

First-time parents will need assessments made when the child is older. Clinicians must be cautioned that the PPA is a guideline for potential services and not a diagnostic tool. It is possible that parents who are not or never will be abusive will have high scores, and parents who abuse their children may score low. Tools may be obtained from the author.

Criteria for Possible Aggression

Criteria	Behavior	Comment
Increase in motor agitation	Pacing Inability to sit still Sudden cessation of motor activity	These are attempts to discharge aggressive impulses via large muscle activity. The stillness is uncomfortable, like the "calm before a storm." Stillness is an attempt to contain the energy and prevent an outburst.
Threatening verbalization or gestures toward real or imagined objects	Verbal abuse toward actual persons who are seen as threats; paranoid statements and self-protective actions	Verbal aggression is less destructive than physical aggression and discharges some aggressive impulses
	Aggressiveness in response to threatening visual or auditory hallucinations	Such hallucinations are bizarre, threatening, unfamiliar, or confusing. Many persons with psychoses live comfortably with an entourage of familiar "voices" that do not precipitate aggressive reactions.
	Aggressiveness in response to delusional thinking	The degree of aggression is related to how desperately the client perceives the need to protect the self.
Intensification of affect	Tense expression Jumpiness Elated expression Rapid, intense mood swings	Such intensification indicates loss of control, especially if accompanied by laughing.

Continued.

From Haber J et al: *Comprehensive psychiatric nursing*, ed 4, St Louis, 1992, Mosby.

Criteria for possible aggression—cont'd

Criteria	Behavior	Comment
History of assaultive behavior	Has acted aggressively in the past	One who has been aggressive is likely to be so again.
	Has never been assaultive in the past	One who has never been aggressive and suddenly becomes so may be suffering from organic illness.
Use of alcohol or addictive drugs	Intoxication with drugs or alcohol	Client can act out rage when inhibitions are dissolved.
	Withdrawal from drugs or alcohol	Aggression is due to irritability of the central nervous system.
Presence of acute organic brain syndrome	Sudden rise or fall in level of consciousness	
	Disorientation as to time, place, person	Sense of time is lost first.
	Impairment of recent memory	Especially significant where no memory impairment existed before.
	Auditory hallucinations	Such are heard coming from under the bed or outside the door. "Voices," out of earshot, as the
	Talking to self or objects of hallucination	voice of God or sounds from another planet, indicate functional mental disorder.
	Kinesthetic hallucinations, such as feeling as if bugs are crawling on skin or worms are moving around in brain or abdomen	Staying with the client and providing a supportive, nurturing environment helps the client tolerate the sensations. Medication may be prescribed.
	Visual hallucinations	Aggression in the presence of visual hallucinations is in self-defense.
	Abnormal muscle movements such as tics, jerks, tremors, akinesia	These are significant only where none existed before and may indicate an impending seizure

Criteria	Behavior	Comment
Expanding personal space	Sudden backing away from others, as if there is not enough space, or experience of suffocation Moving away from others and maintaining the distance with hostile verbalization	The person's need for much more personal space should be respected. Moving into the expanded personal space will precipitate aggression.

🔵 Mental Health

Major Depressive Disorder Subgroups

Subgroup	Essential features	Diagnostic implications	Treatment implications	Prognostic implications
Psychotic	Hallucinations Delusions	More likely to become bipolar than nonpsychotic types May be misdiagnosed as schizophrenia	Antidepressant medication plus a neuroleptic is more effective than are antidepressants alone. ECT is very effective	Usually a recurrent illness Subsequent episodes are usually psychotic Psychotic subtypes run in families Mood-incongruent features have a poorer prognosis
Melancholic	Anhedonia Unreactive mood Severe vegetative symptoms	May be misdiagnosed as dementia More likely in older patients	Antidepressant medication is essential ECT is 90% effective	If recurrent, consider maintenance medications
Atypical	Reactive mood Overeating/weight gain Oversleeping Rejection sensitivity Heavy limb sensation Fewer episodes	Common in younger patients May be misdiagnosed as personality disorder	TCAs may be less effective; MAOIs are preferred ?SSRIs preferred	Unclear

Seasonal	Onset, fall Offset, spring Recurrent	More frequent in non-equatorial latitudes Pattern occurs in major depressive and bipolar disorders	Medications have questionable efficacy Psychotherapy has questionable efficacy Phototherapy is an option	Recurs
Postpartum psychosis/depression	Acute onset (<30 days) in postpartum period Severe labile mood symptoms 1/1000 is psychotic form	Often heralds a bipolar disorder	Hospitalize Treat medically	50% chance of recurring in next postpartum period

ECT, Electroconvulsive therapy; TCA, tricyclic antidepressant; MAOIs, monoamine oxidase inhibitors; SSRIs, selective serotonin reuptake inhibition.

From Depression Guideline Panel: *Depression in primary care*, vol 1, *Detection and diagnosis. Clinical practice guideline*. no 5, Rockville, Md. 1993, US Department of Health and Human Services. Public Health Service Agency for Health Care Policy and Research, pub no 93-0550. In Stuart GW, Sundeen SJ: *Principles and practice of psychiatric nursing*, ed 5, St Louis, 1995, Mosby.

Behaviors Associated with Depression

Affective	Physiologic	Cognitive	Behavioral
Anger	Abdominal pain	Ambivalence	Aggressiveness
Anxiety	Anorexia	Confusion	Agitation
Apathy	Backache	Inability to concentrate	Alcoholism
Bitterness	Chest pain	Indecisiveness	Altered activity level
Dejection	Constipation	Loss of interest and motivation	Drug addiction
Denial of feelings	Dizziness	Self-blame	Intolerance
Despondency	Fatigue	Self-depreciation	Irritability
Guilt	Headache	Self-destructive thoughts	Lack of spontaneity
Helplessness	Impotence	Pessimism	Overdependency
Hopelessness	Indigestion	Uncertainty	Poor personal hygiene
Loneliness	Insomnia		Psychomotor retardation
Low self-esteem	Lassitude		Social isolation
Sadness	Menstrual changes		Tearfulness
Sense of personal worthlessness	Nausea		Underachievement
	Overeating		Withdrawal
	Sexual nonresponsiveness		
	Sleep disturbances		
	Vomiting		
	Weight change		

From Stuart GW, Sundeen SJ: *Principles and practice of psychiatric nursing,* ed 5, St Louis, 1995, Mosby.

Disorders that Cause Depression

Disorder	Examples
Neoplasm	Carcinomatosis, cancer of the pancreas, primary cerebral tumor, cerebral metastasis
Infection	Tuberculosis, subacute bacterial endocarditis, neurosyphilis, hepatitis, encephalitis, postencephalitic states
Cardiovascular disease	Post–myocardial infarction, congestive heart failure
Metabolic disorders	Hyperthyroidism, hypothyroidism, hyperparathyroidism, Cushing's disease, Addison's disease, hyponatremia, hypokalemia, pernicious anemia, severe anemia (any cause), protein deficiency, avitaminosis (especially vitamin B deficiencies), diabetes, uremia, hepatic disease, Wilson's disease
Degenerative disease	Parkinson's disease, Huntington's disease, primary degenerative dementia
Miscellaneous conditions	Pancreatitis, collagen vascular disorders, chronic subdural hematoma
Drug effects	Neuroleptics, barbiturates, meprobamate, benzodiazepines, alcohol, steroids, L-dopa, digitalis, methyldopa, reserpine, propranolol, hydralazine, guanethidine, clonidine

From Lehmann HE: *Psych Clin North Am* 5:33, 1982.

Differences between Anxiety and Depression

Anxiety	Depression
Predominantly fearful or apprehensive with feelings of dread	Predominantly sad or hopeless with feelings of despair
Difficulty falling asleep (initial insomnia)	Early morning awakening (late insomnia) or hypersomnia
Phobic avoidance behavior	Diurnal variation (feels worse in the morning)
Rapid pulse and psychomotor and autonomic hyperactivity	Slowed speech and thought processes
Breathing disturbances	Delayed response time
Tremors and palpitations	Psychomotor retardation (agitation may also occur)
Sweating and hot or cold spells	Loss of interest in usual activities
Faintness, light-headedness, dizziness	Inability to experience pleasure
Depersonalization (feelings of detachment from one's body)	Thoughts of death or suicide
Derealization (feeling that one's environment is strange, unreal, or unfamiliar)	Negative appraisals are pervasive, global, and exclusive
Negative appraisals are selective and specific and do not include all areas of life	Sees the future as blank and has given up all hope
Sees some prospects for the future	Regards mistakes as beyond redemption
Does not regard defects or mistakes as irrevocable	Absolute in negative evaluations
Uncertain in negative evaluations	Global view that nothing will turn out right
Predicts that only certain events may go badly	

From Stuart GW, Sundeen SJ: *Principles and practice of psychiatric nursing,* ed 5, St Louis, 1995, Mosby.

Dealing with Depression: The Nursing Process and Maslow's Hierarchy of Need

Needs	Assessment	Identifying problems	Establishing goals	Intervention	Evaluation
Physiologic needs Food/fluid Shelter/warmth Air Rest/sleep Avoidance of pain Sex	Usual and present nutritional, elimination, sleep, and sexuality patterns Physical activity— exercise pattern Emotional pain and discomfort Suicide potential Physical health Medications	Nutritional deficit Dehydration Constipation Sleep pattern disturbance Sexual dysfunction Self-destructive behavior Medications or physical illnesses that may cause depression	Establishing and maintaining adequate biologic functioning in areas of sleep, nutrition, and elimination Relief from emotional pain and discomfort Elimination of drug- or disease-induced depression	Assist with ADLs Support of self-care abilities Encouragement to start a physical activity regimen Teach side effects of antidepressants Treat medical problems under poor control Change medications that may cause depression	Feelings of physical satiation Homeostasis Optimal physical health
Safety and security needs Feel free from danger Need for a predictable, lawful, orderly world Need to feel in control	Home environment assessment Mental status examination Assessment of visual acuity and hearing Knowledge of disease process Physical mobility	Perceived inability to control feelings or behavior Perceived powerlessness Translocation syndrome Cognitive impairment Alteration in sensory perceptions Impaired physical mobility	Establish predictability and structure in environment Maintenance of a safe environment Realistic understanding of disease course and expected outcome Reversal of treatable confusion	ECT, hospitalization, antidepressive medications for the severely depressed Avoid relocations when possible Correct environmental hazards Encourage a structured daily routine Instruct about disease course and prognosis	Feeling in control of one's disease and optimistic about the future Confidence in the future Feelings of safety, peace, security, protection, lack of danger and threat

Continued.

Dealing with depression: the nursing process and Maslow's hierarchy of need—cont'd

Needs	Assessment	Identifying problems	Establishing goals	Intervention	Evaluation
Need for love, belonging, and affection Need for contact and intimacy Need for friends Need for a feeling of having a place, "belonging" Need for interactions with others	Family relationships and members Friends that are supportive Recent losses Present and past social interaction	Disruption in significant relationships Social isolation Lack of contact with or absence of significant others Alterations in socialization with reduced social interactions	Maintenance of significant relationships with family and friends Establish community support system Resumption of previous level of social activity	Encourage social interactions that have been enjoyed in the past Encourage interactions with family members, friends, and health care providers Provide reassuring, supportive atmosphere	Feelings of loving and being loved, of being one of a group, of acceptance
Need for esteem and self-respect Need for achievement, mastery, and competence Need for reputation or prestige, appreciation, and dignity Need for love of self	Amount of pleasurable pursuits Emotional or mood assessment Role patterns Coping—stress tolerance pattern Attitude about self, the world, the future	Negative feelings or conception of self Loss of significant roles Unrealistic self-expectations Anxiety Lifestyle change Dependency on others	Acceptance of realistic limitations Establish appropriate roles Achieve self-acceptance Accept ownership of consequences of one's own behavior	Teach problem-solving skills Cognitive therapy Promote self-care Counseling Behavior therapy Relaxation techniques	Feelings of self-confidence, worth, strength, capability, and adequacy, of being useful and necessary in the world
Need for self-actualization Need for beauty Need for self-expression Need for new situations and stimulation	Occupation, job history Value-belief patterns	Distress of human spirit Loss of zest for life	Expression of self through meaningful recreational activities Exploring new interests	Encourage a nonrestrictive environment Provide beauty in environment Read to the sick or hard of hearing Music	Autonomy Freshness of appreciation Creativeness Spontaneity Feelings of self-fulfillment

From Ronsman K: *J Gerontol Nurs* 13(12):21, 1987. In Ebersole P, Hess P: *Toward healthy aging: human needs and nursing response*, ed 4, St Louis, 1994, Mosby.

Changes Symptomatic of Moderate Depression

Affective Changes

Mood is despondent, dejected, gloomy.

Self-esteem is low.

Feelings of helplessness, powerlessness, and ineffectiveness are common.

Activities ordinarily enjoyed bring no pleasure.

The joy of life has left.

Anger and anxiety may be experienced.

Diurnal variation in depression or anxiety occur—certain times of day (morning or evening) are either better or worse.

Cognitive Changes

Thoughts are slowed.

Concentration becomes difficult.

Indecisiveness and self-doubt are common.

Thoughts tend to be ruminative; the same issues and content are repeated with absence of goal-directed thinking or recognition of alternatives.

Interests narrow.

Thoughts reflect an obsessional quality.

A pessimistic outlook that includes self-blame creates an attitude of hopelessness about the possibility of change or motivation to change.

Suicidal thoughts may intrude as an aspect of hopelessness.

Behavioral Changes

Social withdrawal ranges from a reluctance to socialize or interact with others to a withdrawal from school, work, and community involvement.

Tears and irritability may be present for no apparent reason.

Changes in personal hygiene, including bathing and cleanliness and coordination of clothes.

Psychomotor retardation (slowing of movement and speech) or agitated aimless activity such as pacing may occur.

Use of drugs or alcohol may increase.

Suicidal gestures and attempts such as repeated car accidents and self-inflicted lacerations and abrasions may occur, as well as overeating, smoking, and drug and alcohol abuse.

From Haber J et al: *Comprehensive psychiatric nursing,* ed 4, St Louis, 1992, Mosby.

Physiologic Changes

Headaches

Chest or back pain

Indigestion, nausea, vomiting, constipation

Anorexia and weight loss or overeating and weight gain

Amenorrhea

Decreased sexual desire and responsiveness

Sleep disturbances that include

    Difficulty falling asleep (initial insomnia)

    Waking up during the night (middle insomnia)

    Early morning awakening (terminal insomnia)

    Hypersomnia (excessive sleeping)

    Feelings of fatigue and weakness regardless of the amount of rest (parasomnia)

Changes Symptomatic of Severe Depression

Affective Changes

Despair and hopelessness are predominant, with no light at the end of the tunnel.

Flat affect, an emotional expression that is unchanging regardless of what occurs.

Feelings of worthlessness; the person has no value to self or others

Feelings of guilt; assumes responsibility for real or imagined wrongdoings.

Sense of isolation, loneliness, and being cut off from human connectedness.

Feels overwhelmed by any task.

An overwhelming feeling of bottomless emptiness.

Dysphoric mood, intense and pervasive unhappiness and sadness.

Cognitive Changes

Confusion, inability to concentrate or make decisions.

No motivation to mobilize oneself.

Self-blame and self-deprecation.

Suicidal thoughts occur as a solution to the hopelessness of one's situation; the wish to die is common. However, because of the depth of the depression, severely depressed people rarely have the energy or clarity of thought to organize and act on such thoughts. If the energy and clarity of thought are present, the risk of suicide is high.

From Haber J et al: *Comprehensive psychiatric nursing,* ed 4, St Louis, 1992, Mosby.

Delusions usually condemn these people's feelings of worthlessness, guilt (e.g., being punished for an imagined sin), and powerlessness. Somatic delusions may be related to parts of the body being diseased or eaten away.

Hallucinations are usually auditory and consist of harsh, unpleasant background noise rather than voices with specific messages.

Behavioral Changes

Psychomotor retardation can progress to the degree that motor activity comes to a near halt; such people can sit immobile for hours or walk slowly and with great effort, showing a robotlike appearance.

Frantic, aimless, agitated movements can also occur, including pacing and gestures such as hair pulling and rubbing of skin, hair, or clothing.

Poverty of speech includes a sharp decrease in amount of speech, with increased pauses and low, monotonous vocal pitch.

Inattention to hygiene and grooming results in an unkempt, disheveled, or dirty appearance.

Social withdrawal from family, friends, and colleagues.

Physiologic Changes

Elimination is sluggish; constipation and urinary retention are common.

Amenorrhea; lack of sexual interest and impotence.

Anorexia and lack of energy and motivation to prepare food and eat result in severe weight loss.

Insomnia—initial, middle, or terminal; terminal insomnia is most common, with person feeling worse in the morning and better as the day progresses.

Assessing Risk of Suicide

Behavior or symptom	Intensity of risk		
	Low	Moderate	High
Anxiety	Mild	Moderate	High, or panic state
Depression	Mild	Moderate	Severe
Isolation, withdrawal	Vague feelings of depression, no withdrawal	Some feelings of helplessness, hopelessness, and withdrawal	Hopeless, helpless, withdrawn, and self-depreciating
Daily functioning	Fairly good in most activities	Moderately good in some activities	Not good in any activities
Resources	Several	Some	Few or none
Coping strategies, devices being utilized	Generally constructive	Some that are constructive	Predominantly destructive
Significant others	Several who are available	Few or only one available	Only one or none available
Psychiatric help in past	None, or positive attitude toward	Yes, and moderately satisfied with outcome	Negative view of help received
Lifestyle	Stable	Moderately stable or unstable	Unstable
Alcohol, drug use	Infrequently to excess	Frequently to excess	Continual abuse
Previous suicide attempts	None, or of low lethality	None to one or more of moderate lethality	None to multiple attempts of high lethality
Disorientation, disorganization	None	Some	Severe
Hostility	Little or none	Some	Severe
Suicidal plan	Vague, fleeting, thoughts but no plan	Frequent thoughts, occasional ideas about a plan	Frequent or constant thought with a specific plan

From Hatton CL, Valente SM: *Suicide: assessment and intervention*, ed 2, Norwalk, Conn, 1984, Appleton-Century-Crofts. In Haber J et al: *Comprehensive psychiatric nursing*, ed 4, St Louis, 1992, Mosby.

Risk Factors Related to Suicide

Depression
Other mood disorders
Schizophrenia
Other psychoses
Delusions, hallucinations
Delirium
Neurologic disorders
Organic brain disorders
Personality disorders
Impulse control disorders
Use of or withdrawal from alcohol or drugs
Anxiety
Stress, acute or chronic
Isolation
Loss of physical health
   Acute loss of function
   Chronic loss of function
Loss of a significant other
Loss of self-esteem
Loss of social and economic resources
Internal conflicts
   Guilt
   Ambivalence
Isolation
   Physical
   Social
Family dysfunction
   Acute—crisis
   Chronic

From Haber J et al: *Comprehensive psychiatric nursing,* ed 4, St Louis, 1992, Mosby.

Clues of Suicidal Risk in Adolescents

Depressive equivalents are symptoms associated with depression: delinquency, aggressiveness, sexual promiscuity, running away, drug or alcohol use, headaches, abdominal pain, accident proneness, fatigue, slow speech, anorexia, sloppiness, and preoccupation with death.

From Edelman CL, Mandle CL: *Health promotion throughout the lifespan,* ed 3, St Louis, 1994, Mosby.

Verbal clues are statements that indicate the adolescent is thinking of suicide: "This world would be better off without me"; "I won't be around anymore."

Behavioral clues are actions that indicate the adolescent might be contemplating suicide; resigning from organizations, giving away cherished belongings, writing suicide notes, or exhibiting sudden changes in usual patterns of behavior (the good student who begins to fail, the quiet student who becomes aggressive).

Risk Factors for Suicidal Behavior*

Factor	High risk	Low risk
Age	Over 45 years or adolescent	25 to 45 years or under 12 years
Sex	Male	Female
Marital status	Divorced, separated, or widowed	Married
Socialization	Isolated	Socially active
Occupation	Professional workers (medicine, dentistry, law) or student	Blue collar workers
Employment	Unemployed	Employed
Physical illness	Chronically or terminally ill	No serious medical problems
Mental illness	Depression, delusions, or hallucinations	Personality disorder
Drug and alcohol use	Intoxicated or addicted	Neither intoxicated nor addicted
Previous attempts	At least one	None
Plan	Definite plan specified	Vague plan
Method	Violent means: shooting, hanging, or jumping	Nonviolent means: drugs, poison, or carbon monoxide
Availability of means	Readily available	Not yet obtained

*Risk factors are relative and intended as a guide to assessment. **Low** risk never means **no** risk.

From Stuart GW, Sundeen SJ: *Principles and practice of psychiatric nursing,* ed 5, St Louis, 1995, Mosby.

Suicide/Self-Harm Assessment

Directions:

1. Assess each key factor and current admission precipitated by attempt.
2. Circle one (of three) descriptor for each factor that BEST describes the client.
3. Add the points for each circled item plus current admission precipitated by suicide attempt to obtain the total score.
4. Add RN's subjective appraisal of risk score to total score.

Key factors	High risk (1:1)	Moderate risk (q15min observation)	No precautions
Contract for safety	Unwilling to contract OR Unable to contract because of impaired reality testing (e.g., hallucinations, delusions, dementia, delirium, dissociation) 2	Contracts but is ambivalent or guarded 1	Reliably contracts for safety 0
Suicide plan	Has plan with actual OR potential access to planned method 2	Has plan without access to planned method 1	No plan 0
Plan lethality	Highly lethal plan (e.g., gun, hanging, jumping, carbon monoxide) 2	Low lethality of plan 1	Low lethality of plan (e.g., superficial scratching, head banging, pillow over face, biting, holding breath) 0
Elopement risk	High elopement risk 2	Low elopement risk 1	No elopment risk 0
Suicidal ideation	Constant suicidal thoughts 2	Intermittent or fleeting suicidal thoughts 1	No current suicidal thoughts 0

Continued.

Suicide/self-harm assessment—cont'd

Key factors	High risk (1:1)		Moderate risk (q15min observation)		No precautions	
Attempt history	Past attempts of high lethality	2	Past attempts of low lethality	1	No previous attempts	0
Symptoms (circle those that apply) Hopelessness Helplessness Anhedonia Guilt/shame Anger/rage Impulsivity	5-6 symptoms present	2	3-4 symptoms present	1	0-2 symptoms present	0
Current morbid thoughts (e.g., reunion fantasies, preoccupation with death)	Constantly	2	Frequently	1	Rarely	0

Current admission precipitated by suicide attempt: Yes 2   No 1

RN's subjective appraisal of risk:
Client replies not trustworthy, several nonverbal cues   4
Client replies questionably, trustworthy, at least 1 nonverbal cue   3
Client replies trustworthy   0
Scoring key: high risk precautions   = 10 or more
moderate risk precautions   = 4-9
no precautions   = 0-3

Total score _____

Assessed by (RN): _____

Date: _____

Time: _____

From Division of Psychiatric Nursing, Medical University of South Carolina. In Stuart GW, Sundeen SJ: *Principles and practice of psychiatric nursing*, ed 5, St Louis, 1995, Mosby.

Behavioral Characteristics of Borderline Personality Disorder

- Interpersonal relationships are both intense and unstable.
- Interpersonal behavior is characterized by devaluation, manipulation, dependency, and masochism.
- Manipulative suicide attempts are designed to ensure rescue by significant others.
- An unstable sense of self leads to failure to develop a sense of object constancy and a fear of abandonment. These contribute to fear of aloneness.
- Negative affects, including anger, sustained psychologic discomfort, and depression, reflect a basic sense of "badness."
- Occasional psychotic experiences are characterized by paranoia, regression, and dissociation.
- Impulsiveness occurs, with episodes of substance abuse and promiscuity.
- A history of low achievement is present.

From Stuart GW, Sundeen SJ: *Principles and practice of psychiatric nursing,* ed 5, St Louis, 1995, Mosby.

Behaviors Associated with Low Self-Esteem

Criticism of self or others
Decreased productivity
Destructiveness toward others
Disruptions in relatedness
Exaggerated sense of self-importance
Feelings of inadequacy
Guilt
Irritability or excessive anger
Negative feelings about one's body
Perceived role strain
Pessimistic view of life
Physical complaints
Polarizing view of life
Rejection of personal capabilities
Self-derision

From Stuart GW, Sundeen SJ: *Principles and practice of psychiatric nursing,* ed 5, St Louis, 1995, Mosby.

Self-destructiveness
Self-diminution
Social withdrawal
Substance abuse
Withdrawal from reality
Worrying

Dealing With Stress

Stress and Stressors

Quick! Can you identify which of the following are causes of stress: the fender bender during rush hour or getting a new car? Too much chocolate or a ringing telephone? Facing retirement or having a baby? Getting laid off or getting that incredible job you dreamed of? The correct answer: all of the above. In fact, the word "Quick!" at the beginning of this paragraph can cause stress in the tense, worried, or even enthusiastic reader. Stress is neither good nor bad. Stress is a general term used to describe change, and a stressor is anything that can cause a response in you, whether physically, mentally, or emotionally. Stressors, like stress, are neither good nor bad. They take on meaning only as you react to them. Stressors fall into three categories: environmental (that ringing telephone), physical (too much chocolate!), or psychologic (having a baby or a fender bender; both of these stressors tend to provoke an emotional response).

The Stress Response

So what happens when you're hit by a stressor? Physiologically, your body enters a state of arousal. For example, blood is diverted from the digestive functions to muscles to prepare the body for action. Nerve impulses signal the heart to beat harder and faster; blood pressure and pulse rate both rise. Changes occur in the movements of the stomach and intestines, and hormones secreted into the body mobilize sugar and blood, making more energy available to the brain and muscles. All of this is your body's effort to defend itself. Psychologically, you respond by trying to evaluate the emotional impact of the situation. This can calm you down or make you even more upset. This often depends, too, on the kind of stress you're experiencing: short-term or long-term. Short-term stress is a healthy kind of stress, because it represents a challenge or a threat, which causes an alarm reaction and elicits a response, which resolves the situation and eliminates the stress. Short-term stress is the kind of stress we were designed to deal with. Long-term stress is what causes the most trouble. All of us have a certain amount of long-term stress—experiences or situations that may never be resolved in our lifetime, such as coping with a chronic illness of a family member, financial problems, or conflict in the work site. But if this level of emotional arousal continues over a prolonged period, the body pays a price for the strain.

In a crisis, your doctor may prescribe therapy or medication. But for ongoing, daily stress situations, a variety of relaxation techniques or exercises can provide the individual in stress with nonmedical relief. These can range from passive or concentration responses (e.g., meditation, progressive relaxation, imagery, yoga, positive health promotion, vacations, and biofeedback) to active coping techniques (e.g., humor, reading, socializing with friends, exercising, and engaging in sports, music, art, or a craft). A few specific stress management techniques are outlined below. You can get more details on any of these from your physician or a stress management clinic or workshop.

Stress charting. A good first step is to "chart" or track down the stressors in your life, so that you are aware of where they come from. Sometimes the individual under stress discovers stressors that simply don't need to *be* stressors—causes that had simply not been noticed. The first step is to list all the stressors present and the area of life in which each stressor occurs (e.g., family members, friends, work, health, finances, social concerns, recreation, or church). Then each stressor is rated as to effect, using a scale of 1 to 5. Awareness gained from this exercise may motivate you to making decisions about lifestyle changes or in choosing relaxation techniques.

Progressive relaxation. A simple relaxation technique that can be done anywhere and at any time is progressive relaxation. Find a quiet, soothing, private place, and, with eyes closed, concentrate on relaxing each part of the body, beginning with the toes and concentrating on each muscle and joint, moving up the body and ending with the head. Some people like to imagine all the stress or pain leaving each muscle as it relaxes, finally visualizing the stress leaving the body through the top of the head. Others like to incorporate deep-breathing exercises into this practice. However you choose to do it, try to allow yourself time after this exercise to sit quietly for a few minutes before resuming your daily activities.

Acupuncture, acupressure, shiatsu, and reflexology. *Acupuncture* is based on the Chinese philosophy that all life is a microcosm of a vast, constantly changing, flowing circle of energy. The body can reach a balanced state only if both the "rising" energy (yang) and "descending" energy (yin) are flowing smoothly. *Acupressure,* the predecessor of acupuncture, is the term applied to a number of techniques of applying pressure to stimulate acupuncture points on the body. Both techniques release tension and relieve pain and are used to balance energy by applying needles or pressure to specific points. *Shiatsu* is an ancient form of manipulation administered by the thumbs, fingers, and palms, without any instruments, to correct internal malfunctioning, maintain health, and treat disease. *Reflexology* is a technique based on the premise that body organs have corresponding reflex points on other parts of the body.

Biofeedback. Biofeedback is a means of receiving feedback or a message from the body about internal physiologic processes, using specific techniques or equipment to read tension and to learn ways of releasing that tension when cues of stress response are identified.

Massage is a systematic manipulation of the body tissue that benefits the nervous and muscular systems, local and general circulation, skin, viscera, and metabolism. During massage the hands stimulate the sensory receptors of the skin and subcutaneous tissues, causing a series of reflex effects, including capillary vasodilation or constriction, relaxation or stimulation of voluntary muscle contraction, and possible sedation or stimulation of pain in an area far from the area touched.

Yoga is an Indian philosophic system that emphasizes the practice of special techniques to attain the highest degree of physical, emotional, and spiritual integration. Its practice can reduce blood pressure, lower pulse rate, reduce serum cholesterol, regulate menstrual flow and thyroid function, increase range of motion, reduce joint pain, and increase the feeling of well-being.

Self-hypnosis allows the individual to induce the feeling of warmth and heaviness associated with a trance state. The exercises can be used to increase resistance to stressors, reduce or eliminate sleep disorders, and modify pain reactions. The system has been found effective in treating disorders of the respiratory and gastrointestinal tracts and the circulatory and endocrine systems, and also in alleviating anxiety and fatigue.

Thought stopping is a behavioral modification technique useful when nagging, repetitive thoughts interfere with behavior and wellness. Such unwanted thoughts are interrupted with the command "Stop," and a positive thought is substituted.

Refuting irrational ideas. Everyone engages in almost continuous self-talk during waking hours. When this internal dialogue is accurate and realistic, wellness is enhanced; when it is irrational and untrue, stress occurs. Refuting these irrational ideas requires a series of steps: identifying what brought on the stress-inducing thought; writing down and identifying the negative thought and the emotion it brought on; writing down all evidence that the idea is false; predicting both the worst and best possible outcomes if the negative, irrational idea *were* true; and substituting alternative self-talk with positive, rational statements.

Centering refers to separating from outside influences to gain an inner reference or thought of stability, calm, and self-awareness; a sense of self-relatedness, a quiet place within self where the individual can feel integrated, unified, and focused. Centering reduces fatigue, stress, depression, or anger when working with others and increases self-control. It involves sitting quietly, relaxing tense spots in the body as you inhale and exhale, and concentrating on breathing until you feel calm.

Assertive communication/behavior. Assertiveness means expressing personal thoughts, feelings, and desires, defining and making known personal rights that are reasonable while respecting the other person. Workshops frequently help people learn this way of behaving. Assertive techniques are particularly helpful in the face of criticism and other negative reactions. These include admitting mistakes, without defensiveness but without agreeing to a specific change that you may not want; asking what specifically is bothersome about a behavior for which you are criticized; shifting the conversation back to the subject and away from an intense expression of negative emotions; postponing a conversation when it reaches an impasse; not responding to an inappropriate or irrational attack; and using humor or deflection.

Guided imagery can be defined as focused attention on an inner, mental picture or a statement of belief of what the individual wants to accomplish by being open to and responding to the language of the unconscious or the deeper body levels. It is similar to self-hypnosis in that it involves sitting in a quiet place, relaxing, and envisioning a peaceful, soothing scene that can maintain relaxation and a positive attitude. Guided imagery promotes emotional health by building self-awareness and increasing coping resources.

Symptoms of Stress

Physiologic/Behavioral

Increased heart rate
Rise in blood pressure
Dryness of mouth and throat
Sweating
Tightness of chest
Headache
Nausea/vomiting

Indigestion
Diarrhea
Trembling, twitching
Grinding of teeth
Insomnia
Anorexia
Fatigue
Slumped posture
Pain, tightness in neck and back muscles
Urinary frequency
Missed menstrual cycle
Reduced interest in sex
Accident proneness
Startle reaction
Hyperventilation

Affective

Irritability
Depression
Angry outbursts
Emotional instability
Poor concentration
Uninterest in activities
Withdrawal
Restlessness
Anxiety
Increased use of sarcasm
Tendency to cry easily
Nightmares
Suspiciousness
Jealousy
Decreased involvement with others
Bickering
Complaining, criticizing
Tendency to be easily startled
Increased smoking
Use of alcohol and drugs

Cognitive

Forgetfulness
Poor judgment
Poor concentration
Reduced creativity
Less fantasizing

Errors in arithmetic and grammar
Preoccupation
Inattention to details
Blocking
Reduced productivity

Strategies for Managing Stress

- Evaluate sources of stress at work and attempt to change them.
- Learn to manage time effectively.
- Limit overtime.
- Discuss and try to solve problems with co-workers.
- Try not to personalize criticisms. Remember, it is often the situation that is the problem, although you may be the target of their emotions.
- Rotate assignments of those who are difficult to care for.
- Recognize the symptoms of stress in yourself and seek the help of an objective party to assist you in discussing and managing your feelings.
- Learn techniques for controlling your response to stress (e.g., deep breathing, repeating a saying in your mind that helps you stay calm, counting to 25).
- Withdraw from the situation and seek help when you feel you may lose control.
- When you feel "burned out" or as though you cannot cope, talk to your supervisor about scheduling time off.
- Instead of coffee and cigarette breaks, enjoy breaks in which you do short relaxation exercises, recline in a quiet area, or listen to relaxation tapes.
- Eat a well-balanced diet; avoid junk foods.
- Exercise regularly.
- Do something for yourself to unwind between work and home.
- Take naps; allow ample time for sleep.
- Schedule leisure activities into your life; develop a hobby.
- Do not rely on cigarettes, alcohol, or drugs to assist in relaxation.
- Learn about meditation and relaxation exercises and attempt to build them into your life.

From Edelman CL, Mandle CL: *Health promotion throughout the lifespan,* ed 3, St Louis, 1994, Mosby.

Family Systems Stressor-Strength Inventory (FS³I)

Instructions for Administration

The Family Systems Stressor-Strength Inventory (FS³I) is an assessment/measurement instrument intended for use with families. It focuses on identifying stressful situations occurring in families and the strengths families use to maintain healthy family functioning. Each family member is asked to complete the instrument on an individual form prior to an interview with the clinician. Questions can be read to members unable to read.

Following completion of the instrument, the clinician evaluates the family on each of the stressful situations (general and specific) and the available strengths they possess. This evaluation is recorded on the family member form.

The clinician records the individual family member's score and the clinician perception score on the Quantitative Summary. A different color code is used for each family member. The clinician also completes the Qualitative Summary, synthesizing the information gleaned from all participants. Clinicians can use the Family Care Plan to prioritize diagnoses, set goals, develop prevention/intervention activities, and evaluate outcomes.

Family Name _____ Date _____

Family Member(s) Completing Assessment _____

Ethnic Background(s) _____

Religious Background(s) _____

Referral Source _____

Interviewer _____

Family Members	Relationship in Family	Age	Marital Status	Education (Highest degree)	Occupation
1. _____	_____	____	____	_____	_____
2. _____	_____	____	____	_____	_____
3. _____	_____	____	____	_____	_____
4. _____	_____	____	____	_____	_____
5. _____	_____	____	____	_____	_____
6. _____	_____	____	____	_____	_____

Family's current reasons for seeking assistance?

_____

_____

_____

From Berkey KM, Hanson SMH: *Pocket guide to family assessment and intervention*, St. Louis, 1991, Mosby. In Hanson SMH, Boyd ST: *Family health care nursing: theory, practice, and research*, Philadelphia, 1996, FA Davis.

Part I: Family Systems Stressors (General)

DIRECTIONS: Each of the 25 situations/stressors listed here deals with some aspect of normal family life. Each stressor has the potential for creating stress within families or between families and the world in which they live. We are interested in your overall impression of how these situations affect your family life. Please circle a number (0 through 5) that best describes the amount of stress or tension they create for you.

Stressors:	Not Apply	Little Stress	Medium Stress	High Stress		Clinician Perception Score
1. Family member(s) feel unappreciated	0	1	2	3	4	5
2. Guilt for not accomplishing more	0	1	2	3	4	5
3. Insufficient "me" time	0	1	2	3	4	5
4. Self-image/self-esteem/feelings of unattractiveness	0	1	2	3	4	5
5. Perfectionism	0	1	2	3	4	5
6. Dieting	0	1	2	3	4	5
7. Health/Illness	0	1	2	3	4	5
8. Communication with children	0	1	2	3	4	5
9. Housekeeping standards	0	1	2	3	4	5
10. Insufficient couple time	0	1	2	3	4	5
11. Insufficient family play-time	0	1	2	3	4	5
12. Children's behavior/discipline/sibling fighting	0	1	2	3	4	5
13. Television	0	1	2	3	4	5
14. Over scheduled family calendar	0	1	2	3	4	5
15. Lack of shared responsibility in the family	0	1	2	3	4	5
16. Moving	0	1	2	3	4	5
17. Spousal relationship (communication, friendship, sex)	0	1	2	3	4	5
18. Holidays	0	1	2	3	4	5
19. In-laws	0	1	2	3	4	5
20. Teen behaviors (communication, music, friends, school)	0	1	2	3	4	5
21. New baby	0	1	2	3	4	5
22. Economics/finances/budgets	0	1	2	3	4	5

Stressors:	Family Perception Score						Clinician Perception Score
	Not Apply	Little Stress	Medium Stress		High Stress		Score
23. Unhappiness with work situation	0	1	2	3	4	5	_____
24. Overvolunteerism	0	1	2	3	4	5	_____
25. Neighbors	0	1	2	3	4	5	_____

Additional Stressors: _____

Family Remarks: _____

Clinician: Clarification of stressful situations/concerns with family members. Prioritize in order of importance to family members:

_____

Part II: Family Systems Stressors (Specific)

DIRECTIONS: The following 12 questions are designed to provide information about your specific stress-producing situation/problem, or area of concern influencing your family's health. Please circle a number (1 through 5) that best describes the influence this situation has on your family's life and how well you perceive your family's overall functioning.

The specific stress-producing situation/problem or area of concern at this time is: _____

_____

Stressors:	Family Perception Score			Clinician Perception Score
	Little	Medium	High	Score
1. To what extent is your family bothered by this problem or stressful situations? (e.g., effects on family interactions, communication among members, emotional and social relationships)	1 2	3	4 5	_____

Family Remarks: _____

_____

	Family Perception Score			Clinician Perception
Stressors:	Little	Medium	High	Score

2. How much of an effect does this stressful situation have on your family's usual pattern of living ?   1   2   3   4   5   _____
(e.g., effects on lifestyle patterns and family developmental task)

     Family Remarks: _____

     _____

     Clinician Remarks: _____

     _____

3. How much has this situation affected your family's ability to work together as a family unit ?   1   2   3   4   5   _____
(e.g., alteration in family roles, completion of family tasks, following through with responsibilities)

     Family Remarks: _____

     _____

     Clinician Remarks: _____

     _____

Has your family ever experienced a similar concern in the past?
1. YES   If YES, complete question 4
2. NO   If NO, complete question 5

4. How successful was your family in dealing with this situation/problem/ concern in the past ?   1   2   3   4   5   _____
(e.g., workable coping strategies developed, adaptive measures useful, situation improved)

     Family Remarks: _____

     _____

     Clinician Remarks: _____

     _____

5. How strongly do you feel this current situation/problem/concern will affect your family's future ?   1   2   3   4   5   _____
(e.g., anticipated consequences)

Stressors:	Family Perception Score			Clinician Perception
	Little	Medium	High	Score

Family Remarks: _____

Clinician Remarks: _____

6. To what extent are family members able to help themselves in this present situation/problem/concern? (e.g., self-assistive efforts, family expectations, spiritual influence, & family resources)

   1   2   3   4   5 _____

   Family Remarks: _____

   Clinician Remarks: _____

7. To what extent do you expect others to help your family with this situation/problem/concern? .... (e.g., what roles would helpers play; how available are extra-family resources)

   1   2   3   4   5 _____

   Family Remarks: _____

   Clinician Remarks: _____

Stressors:	Family Perception Score			Clinician Perception
	Poor	Satisfactory	Excellent	Score

8. How would you rate the way your family functions overall? .... (e.g., how your family members, relate to each other and to larger family and community)

   1   2   3   4   5 _____

   Family Remarks: _____

   Clinician Remarks: _____

Stressors:	Family Perception Score			Clinician Perception
	Poor	**Satisfactory**	**Excellent**	**Score**

9. How would you rate the overall physical health status of each family member by name? (Include yourself as a family member; record additional names on back.)

a. _____ 1 2 3 4 5 _____
b. _____ 1 2 3 4 5 _____
c. _____ 1 2 3 4 5 _____
d. _____ 1 2 3 4 5 _____
e. _____ 1 2 3 4 5 _____

10. How would you rate the overall physical health status of your family as a whole? .... 1 2 3 4 5 _____

Family Remarks: _____

_____

Clinician Remarks: _____

_____

11. How would you rate the overall mental health status of each family member by name? (Include yourself as a family member; record additional names on back.)

a. _____ 1 2 3 4 5 _____
b. _____ 1 2 3 4 5 _____
c. _____ 1 2 3 4 5 _____
d. _____ 1 2 3 4 5 _____
e. _____ 1 2 3 4 5 _____

12. How would you rate the overall mental health status of your family as a whole? .... 1 2 3 4 5 _____

Family Remarks: _____

_____

Clinician Remarks: _____

_____

Part III: Family Systems Strengths

DIRECTIONS: Each of the 16 traits/attributes listed below deals with some aspect of family life and its overall functioning. Each one contributes to the health and well-being of family members as individuals and to the family as a whole. Please circle a number (0 through 5) that best describes the extent that the trait applies to your family.

My Family:	Not Apply	Seldom	Usually	Always	Clinician Perception Score
1. Communicates and listens to one another	0	1 2	3 4	5	_____

Family Remarks: _____

Clinician Remarks: _____

2. Affirms and supports one another	0	1 2	3 4	5	_____

Family Remarks: _____

Clinician Remarks: _____

3. Teaches respect for others	0	1 2	3 4	5	_____

Family Remarks: _____

Clinician Remarks: _____

4. Develops a sense of trust in members	0	1 2	3 4	5	_____

Family Remarks: _____

Clinician Remarks: _____

5. Displays a sense of play and humor	0	1 2	3 4	5	_____

Family Remarks: _____

Clinician Remarks: _____

| My Family: | Not Apply | | Family Perception Score | | | Clinician Perception |
		Seldom	Usually	Always		Score
6. Exhibits a sense of shared responsibility	0	1	2	3	4	5	_____

Family Remarks: _____

Clinician Remarks: _____

| 7. Teaches a sense of right and wrong .... | 0 | 1 | 2 | 3 | 4 | 5 | _____ |

Family Remarks: _____

Clinician Remarks: _____

| 8. Has a strong sense of family in which rituals and traditions abound ..... | 0 | 1 | 2 | 3 | 4 | 5 | _____ |

Family Remarks: _____

Clinician Remarks: _____

| 9. Has a balance of interaction among members .... | 0 | 1 | 2 | 3 | 4 | 5 | _____ |

Family Remarks: _____

Clinician Remarks: _____

| 10. Has a shared religious core .... | 0 | 1 | 2 | 3 | 4 | 5 | _____ |

Family Remarks: _____

Clinician Remarks: _____

| 11. Respects the privacy of one another .... | 0 | 1 | 2 | 3 | 4 | 5 | _____ |

Family Remarks: _____

Clinician Remarks: _____

My Family:	Not Apply	Seldom	Usually	Always			Clinician Perception Score
			Family Perception Score				
12. Values service to others ..	0	1	2	3	4	5	_____

Family Remarks: _____

_____

Clinician Remarks: _____

_____

13. Fosters family table time
and conversation 0   1   2   3   4   5   _____

Family Remarks: _____

_____

Clinician Remarks: _____

_____

14. Shares leisures time 0   1   2   3   4   5   _____

Family Remarks: _____

_____

Clinician Remarks: _____

_____

15. Admits to and seeks help
with problems 0   1   2   3   4   5   _____

Family Remarks: _____

_____

Clinician Remarks: _____

_____

16a. How would you rate the
overall strengths that ex-
ist in your family? 0   1   2   3   4   5   _____

Family Remarks: _____

_____

Clinician Remarks: _____

_____

16b. Additional Family Strengths: _____

_____

_____

_____

16c. Clinician: Clarification of family strengths with individual members:

_____

_____

_____

Scoring Summary
Section 1: family perception scores

INSTRUCTIONS FOR ADMINISTRATION: The Family Systems Stressor-Strength Inventory (FS³I) Scoring Summary is divided into two sections: Section 1, Family Perception Scores and Section 2, Clinician Perception Scores. These two sections are further divided into three parts: Part I, Family Systems Stressors: General; Part II, Family Systems Stressors: Specific; and, Part III, Family Systems Strengths. Each part contains a Quantitative Summary and a Qualitative Summary.

Quantifiable family and clinician perception scores are both graphed on the Quantitative Summary. Each family member has a designated color code. Family and clinician remarks are both recorded on the Qualitative Summary. Quantitative summary scores, when graphed, suggest a level for initiation of prevention/intervention modes: Primary, Secondary, and Tertiary. Qualitative summary information, when synthesized, contributes to the development and channeling of the Family Care Plan.

Part I family systems stressors (general). Add scores from questions 1 to 25 and calculate an overall numerical score for Family System Stressors (General). Ratings are from 1 (most positive) to 5 (most negative). The Not Apply (0) responses are omitted from the calculations. Total scores range from 25 to 125.

Family Systems Stressor Score: General

$$\frac{(\quad)}{25} \times 1 =$$

Graph score on Quantitative Summary, Family Systems Stressors: General, Family Member Perception. Color code to differentiate family members.

Record additional stressors and family remarks in Part I, Qualitative Summary: Family and Clinician Remarks.

Part II family systems stressors: specific.   Add scores from questions 1–8, 10 and 12 and calculate a numerical score for Family Systems through Stressors: Specific. Ratings are from 1 (most positive) to 5 (most negative). Questions 4, 6, 7, 8, 10, and 12 are reverse scored.* Total scores range from 10 to 50.

Family Systems Stressor Score: Specific

$$\frac{(\quad)}{10} \times 1 =$$

Graph score on Quantitative Summary: Family Systems Stressor: Specific (Family Member Perceptions). Color code to differentiate family members.

Summarize data from questions 9 and 11 (reverse scored) and record family remarks in Part II, Qualitative Summary: Family and Clinician Remarks

Part III family systems strengths.   Add scores from questions 1 to 16 and calculate a numerical score for Family Systems Strengths. Ratings are from 1 (seldom) to 5 (always). The Not Apply (0) responses are omitted from the calculations. Total scores range from 16 to 80.

$$\frac{(\quad)}{16} \times 1 =$$

Graph score on Quantitative Summary: Family Systems Strengths (Family Member Perception).

Record Additional Family Strengths and Family Remarks in Part III, Qualitative Summary: Family and Clinician Remarks.

Section 2: Clinician Perception Scores

Part I family systems stressors (general).   Add scores from questions 1 to 25 and calculate an overall numerical score for Family System Stressors (General). Ratings are from 1 (most positive) to 5 (most negative). The Not Apply (0) responses are omitted from the calculations. Total scores range from 25 to 125.

Family Systems Stressor Score: General

$$\frac{(\quad)}{25} \times 1 =$$

---

*Reverse Scoring:
   Question answered as (1) is scored 5 points
   Question answered as (2) is scored 4 points
   Question answered as (3) is scored 3 points
   Question answered as (4) is scored 2 points
   Question answered as (5) is scored 1 point

Graph score on Quantitative Summary, Family Systems Stressors: General (Clinician Perception).

Record Clinicians' clarification of general stressors in Part I, Qualitative Summary: Family and Clinician Remarks.

Part II family systems stressors: specific. Add scores from questions 1–8, 10, and 12 and calculate a numerical score for Family Systems Stressors: Specific. Ratings are from 1 (most positive) to 5 (most negative). Questions 4, 6, 7, 8, 10, and 12 are reverse scored.* Total scores range from 10 to 50.

Family Systems Stressor Score: Specific

$$\frac{(\quad)}{10} \times 1 =$$

Graph score on Quantitative Summary: Family Systems Stressor: Specific (Clinician Perceptions).

Summarize data from questions 9 and 11 (reverse order) and record Clinician Remarks in Part II, Qualitative Summary: Family and Clinician Remarks

Part III family systems strengths. Add scores from questions 1 to 16 and calculate a numerical score for Family Systems Strengths. Ratings are from 1 (seldom) to 5 (always).

The Not Apply (0) responses are omitted from the calculations. Total scores range from 16 to 80.

$$\frac{(\quad)}{16} \times 1 =$$

Graph score on Quantitative Summary: Family Systems Strengths (Clinician Perception).

Record Clinicians' clarification of family strengths in Part III, Qualitative Summary: Family and Clinician Remarks.

---

*Reverse Scoring:

Question answered as (1) is scored 5 points
Question answered as (2) is scored 4 points
Question answered as (3) is scored 3 points
Question answered as (4) is scored 2 points
Question answered as (5) is scored 1 point

Quantitative Summary Family Systems Stressors: General and Specific Family and Clinician Perception Scores

DIRECTIONS: Graph the scores from each family member inventory by placing an "X" at the appropriate location. (Use first name initial for each different entry and different color code for each family member.)

Scores for Wellness and Stability	Family Systems Stressors General	
	Family Member Perception Score	Clinician Perception Score
5.0		
4.8		
4.6		
4.4		
4.2		
4.0		
3.8		
3.6		
3.4		
3.2		
3.0		
2.8		
2.6		
2.4		
2.2		
2.0		
1.8		
1.6		
1.4		
1.2		
1.0		

*PRIMARY Prevention/Intervention Mode: Flexible Line 1.0–2.3
*SECONDARY Prevention/Intervention Mode: Normal Line 2.4–3.6
*TERTIARY Prevention/Intervention Mode: Resistance Lines 3.7–5.0
*Breakdowns of numerical scores for stressor pentration are suggested values

Scores for Wellness and Stability	Family Systems Stressors	
	Family Member Perception Score	**Clinician Perception Score**
5.0		
4.8		
4.6		
4.4		
4.2		
4.0		
3.8		
3.6		
3.4		
3.2		
3.0		
2.8		
2.6		
2.4		
2.2		
2.0		
1.8		
1.6		
1.4		
1.2		
1.0		

*PRIMARY Prevention/Intervention Mode: Flexible Line 1.0–2.3
*SECONDARY Prevention/Intervention Mode: Normal Line 2.4–3.6
*TERTIARY Prevention/Intervention Mode: Resistance Lines 3.7–5.0
*Breakdowns of numerical scores for stressor pentration are suggested values

Family Systems Strengths: Family and Clinician Perception Scores

DIRECTIONS: Graph the scores from the inventory by placing an "X" at the appropriate location and connect with a line. (Use first name initial for each different entry and different color code for each family member.)

Scores for Wellness and Stability	Family Systems Stressors	
	Family Member Perception Score	Clinician Perception Score
5.0		
4.8		
4.6		
4.4		
4.2		
4.0		
3.8		
3.6		
3.4		
3.2		
3.0		
2.8		
2.6		
2.4		
2.2		
2.0		
1.8		
1.6		
1.4		
1.2		
1.0		

*PRIMARY Prevention/Intervention Mode: Flexible Line 1.0–2.3
*SECONDARY Prevention/Intervention Mode: Normal Line 2.4–3.6
*TERTIARY Prevention/Intervention Mode: Resistance Lines 3.7–5.0
*Breakdowns of numerical scores for stressor pentration are suggested values

Qualitative Summary Family and Clinician Remarks
Part I: Family Systems Stressors: General

Summarize general stressors and remarks of family and clinician.
Prioritize stressors according to importance to family members.

_____
_____
_____
_____

Part II: Family Systems Stressors: Specific

A. Summarize specific stressor and remarks of family and clinician.

_____
_____
_____
_____

B. Summarize differences (if discrepancies exist) between how
    family members and clinician view effects of stressful situation on
    family.

_____
_____
_____
_____

C. Summarize overall family functioning.

_____
_____
_____
_____

D. Summarize overall significant physical health status for family
    members.

_____
_____
_____
_____

E. Summarize overall significant mental health status for family
    members.

_____
_____
_____
_____

Part III: Family Systems Strengths
Summarize family systems strengths and family and clinician remarks that facilitate family health and stability.

_____
_____
_____
_____

Family Care Plan*

Diagnosis General & Specific Family System Stressors	Family Systems Strengths Supporting Family Care Plan	Goals Family & Physician	Prevention/Intervention Mode		Outcomes Evaluation and Replanning
			Primary, Secondary, or Tertiary	Prevention/Intervention Activities	

*Prioritize the three most significant diagnoses

Indicators of Families at Risk for Dysfunction

Family Structure

Single-parent family with inadequate supports
Blended family with inadequate supports
Adoptive family with inadequate supports
Teenage family
Young family with several children close in age
Single parent with changing live-in partner
Family with peripheral spouse—viewed by spouse as unreliable, incompetent, tyrannical
Parental separation

Family Environment

Impoverished family
Multiproblem family
Immature parents
Member(s) with handicapping, chronic, or fatal disease
Migrant or highly mobile family
Employment instability of key family members
Violence-prone family
Chemically dependent family member(s)
Chronic marital discord

From Olds S, London M, Ladewig P: *Maternal-newborn nursing,* ed 4, Reading, 1992, Addison-Wesley.

Family Crisis-Oriented Personal Scales (F-COPES)

The Family Crisis Oriented Personal Evaluation Scales is designed to record effective problem-solving attitudes and behavior which families develop to respond to problems or difficulties.

DIRECTIONS

First, read the list of "Response Choices" one at a time.

Second, decide how well each statement describes your attitudes and behavior in response to problems or difficulties. If the statement describes your response *very well*, then circle the number 5 indicating that you STRONGLY AGREE; if the statement does not describe your response *at all*, then circle the number 1 indicating that you STRONGLY DISAGREE; if the statement describes your response to some degree, then select a number 2, 3, or 4 to indicate how much you agree or disagree with the statement about your response.

When we face problems or difficulties in our family, we respond by	Strongly disagree	Moderately disagree	Neither agree nor disagree	Moderately agree	Strongly agree
1. Sharing our difficulties with relatives	1	2	3	4	5
2. Seeking encouragement and support from friends	1	2	3	4	5
3. Knowing we have the power to solve major problems	1	2	3	4	5
4. Seeking information and advice from persons in other families who have faced the same or similar problems	1	2	3	4	5

Continued

From McCubbin HI, Olson DH, Larsen A: F-COPES: Family-crisis oriented personal Evaluation Scales. In McCubbin HI, Thompson AI, McCubbin MA: *Family assessment: resiliency, coping, and adaptation—inventories for research and practice*, Madison, Wis, 1996, University of Wisconsin.

Family crisis oriented personal scales (F-COPES)—cont'd

When we face problems or difficulties in our family, we respond by	Strongly disagree	Moderately disagree	Neither agree nor disagree	Moderately agree	Strongly agree
5. Seeking advice from relatives (grandparents, etc.)	1	2	3	4	5
6. Seeking assistance from community agencies and programs designed to help families in our situation	1	2	3	4	5
7. Knowing that we have the strength within our own family to solve our problems	1	2	3	4	5
8. Receiving gifts and favors from neighbors (food, taking in mail, etc.)	1	2	3	4	5
9. Seeking information and advice from the family doctor	1	2	3	4	5
10. Asking neighbors for favors and assistance	1	2	3	4	5
11. Facing the problems "head-on" and trying to get solution right away	1	2	3	4	5
12. Watching television	1	2	3	4	5
13. Showing that we are strong	1	2	3	4	5
14. Attending church services	1	2	3	4	5
15. Accepting stressful events as a factor of life	1	2	3	4	5
16. Sharing concerns with close friends	1	2	3	4	5
17. Knowing luck plays a big part in how well we are able to solve family problems	1	2	3	4	5
18. Exercising with friends to stay fit and reduce tension	1	2	3	4	5
19. Accepting that difficulties occur unexpectedly	1	2	3	4	5
20. Doing things with relatives (get-togethers, dinners, etc.)	1	2	3	4	5
21. Seeking professional counseling and help for family difficulties	1	2	3	4	5

	1	2	3	4	5
22. Believing we can handle our own problems	1	2	3	4	5
23. Participating in church activities	1	2	3	4	5
24. Defining the family problem in a more positive way so that we do not become too discouraged	1	2	3	4	5
25. Asking relatives how they feel about problems we face	1	2	3	4	5
26. Feeling that no matter what we do to prepare, we will have difficulty handling problems	1	2	3	4	5
27. Seeking advice from a clergyperson	1	2	3	4	5
28. Believing if we wait long enough, the problem will go away	1	2	3	4	5
29. Sharing problems with neighbors	1	2	3	4	5
30. Having faith in God	1	2	3	4	5

Scoring the instrument is done by summing the numbers circled for items in each subscale, except for items 17, 26, and 28, which are reversed. The subscales are acquiring social support (1, 2, 5, 8, 10, 16, 20, 25, 29); reframing (3, 7, 11, 13, 15, 19, 22, 24); seeking spiritual support (14, 23, 27, 30); mobilizing the family to acquire and accept help (4, 6, 9, 21); and passive appraisal (12, 17, 26, 28). A total coping score is the sum of the subscales and has a possible range from 29 to 145. The mean scores reported range from 91.24 to 95.64, and standard deviations are from 12.06 to 14.05.

The Worry Scale

Instructions: Below is a list of problems that often concern many Americans. Please read each one carefully. After you have done so, please fill in one of the spaces to the right with a check that describes how much that problem worries you. Make only one check mark for each item.

Things that worry me . . .

	Never	Rarely (1–2 times per month)	Sometimes (1–2 times per week)	Often (1–2 times a day)	Much of the time (more than 2 times a day)
Finances					
1. I'll lose my home					
2. I won't be able to pay for the necessities of life (such as food, clothing, or medicine)					
3. I won't be able to support myself independently					
4. I won't be able to enjoy the "good things" in life (such as travel, recreation, entertainment)					
5. I won't be able to help my children financially					
Health					
6. my eyesight or hearing will get worse					
7. I'll lose control of my bladder or kidneys					
8. I won't be able to remember important things					
9. I won't be able to get around by myself					
10. I won't be able to enjoy my food					
11. I'll have to be taken care of by my family					
12. I'll have to be taken care of by strangers					
13. I won't be able to take care of my spouse					
14. I'll have to go to a nursing home or hospital					
15. I won't be able to sleep at night					
16. I may have a serious illness or accident					
17. my spouse or a close family member may have a serious illness or accident					
18. I won't be able to enjoy sex					
19. my reflexes will slow down					
20. I won't be able to make decisions					
21. I won't be able to drive a car					
22. I'll have to use a mechanical aid (such as a hearing aid, bifocals, a cane)					
Social conditions					
23. I'll look "old"					
24. people will think of me as unattractive					
25. no one will want to be around me					
26. no one will love me anymore					
27. I'll be a burden to my loved ones					
28. I won't be able to visit my family and friends					
29. I may be attacked by muggers or robbers on the streets					
30. my home may be broken into and vandalized					
31. no one will come to my aid if I need it					
32. my friends and family won't visit me					
33. my friends and family will die					
34. I'll get depressed					
35. I'll have serious psychological problems					
Other worries					
36.					
37.					
38.					
39.					
40.					

From Powers CB, Wisocki PA, Whitbourne SK: *Gerontologist* 32(1):82, 1992. In Ebersole P, Hess P: *Toward healthy aging: human needs and nursing response,* ed 4, St Louis, 1994, Mosby.

Assessment Data for Crisis Intervention

The following instrument will assist the nurse and client in naming the problem that has resulted in a client crisis. It will help the nurse determine both the effect of the crisis on the client's normal level of functioning and potential dangers to the client's health. The data collected may indicate a need for referral.

Date _____

Name _____   Next of Kin _____

Age _____   Address _____

Address _____   Telephone no. _____

Telephone no. _____   Information obtained from:

Reliable historian   Client _____

    Yes _____   Next of kin _____

    No _____   Other _____

                                          Name _____

                                          Address _____

                                          Telephone no. _____

1. Identification of problem or crisis event
     Reason for seeking help:

     Time event occurred:
        Sudden onset _____
        Gradual onset _____

     Effects of crisis on client:

     Effects of crisis on client's significant others:

     Response to crisis event:

2. Perception of crisis event
     Meaning of crisis to client:

     Meaning of crisis to client's significant others:

     Changes in client's life because of the crisis:

From Detherage KS, Johnson SS: In Edelman CL, Mandle CL, editors: *Health promotion throughout the lifespan,* ed 3, St. Louis, 1994, Mosby.

Effects of crisis on client's goals:

Is client perceiving crisis in realistic manner?

3. Identification of external support resources available to client (Note supports that are most meaningful to client.)
Family:

Friends:

Clergy:

Community agencies:

Others:

4. Coping abilities
Usual methods of coping

Coping behaviors that can be used to relieve present crisis:

5. Is client homicidal? _____If yes, give details:

6. Is client suicidal? _____ If yes, give details:

7. Ego functioning
Memory:

Judgment:

Problem-solving ability:

Perceptions:

8. Mood (happy, sad, and so on)

9. Level anxiety
Mild _____
Moderate _____
Severe _____

Problems Exhibited by the Crisis-Prone Person

Difficulty in learning from experience

History of frequent crises, ineffectively resolved because of poor coping ability

History of mental disorder or other serious emotional disturbances

Low self-esteem, which may be masked by provocative behavior

Tendency toward impulsive "acting out" behavior (doing without thinking)

Marginal income

Lack of regular, fulfilling work

Unsatisfying marriage and family relations

Heavy drinking or other substance abuse

History of numerous accidents

Frequent encounters with law-enforcement agencies

Frequent changes in address

From Detherage KS, Johnson SS: In Edelman CL, Mandle CL, editors: *Health promotion throughout the lifespan,* ed 3, St. Louis, 1994, Mosby.

Early Warning Signs of Mental Health Problems in Infants and Young Children

Physical Symptoms

Delayed or disordered growth and development: poor weight gain; retarded skeletal growth; failure to thrive, which may occur even when food intake is adequate; obesity; weak rooting and grasping responses during feeding

Delayed acquisition, loss, or deviant nature of motor skills and activities (walking, self-feeding and dressing, right-left discrimination); control over sphincters; communication (use of speech; idioglossia, or barely comprehensible speech; stuttering or stammering; continued use of baby talk, socially inappropriate gestures, and other nonverbal modes); intellectual processes (illogical or impaired focal attention, that is, inability to attend to a task for an extended period of time; an inability to learn not attributable to physical or organic disabilities)

Specific organ-system symptoms: gastrointestinal disturbances (vomiting, poor absorption of food, diarrhea, colitis, constipation, anorexia, peptic ulcers), skin disturbances (rashes, hives, eczemas,

Norbeck J, Pothier P: In Haber J and others, editors: *Comprehensive psychiatric nursing,* ed 3, New York, 1987, McGraw-Hill.

warts, angioneurotic edema), respiratory disturbances (rhinorrhea, asthma, wheezing), endocrine disturbances (juvenile diabetes mellitus, thyroid disturbances), circulatory disturbances (headaches)

Behavioral Symptoms

Sleep disturbances: nightmares, night terrors, difficulty falling asleep, sleepwalking, excessive sleeping

Disturbances in activity-rest patterns

Eating disturbances: too much or too little food intake, disturbance in appetite, avoidance of foods, ingestion of inedible substances (pica), anorexia, bulimia

Elimination disturbances: enuresis, encopresis

Disturbed capacity to play: become upset with messy play; regressed selection and use of play materials; inability to stick to activities for age-appropriate time periods

Accident-proneness, excessive clumsiness

Excessive running and climbing; act as if "driven by a motor"

Habit patterns: nail biting, tics, hair pulling

Impulsive temper tantrums

Shy and withdrawn, apathetic

Restless, fidgety, easily distractible, low achievement in school

Aggressive and destructive: fail to respect the rights of others

Excessively ritualistic, perfectionistic tendencies

Asocial behavior: stealing, lying, setting fires

Sexually inappropriate behavior: exhibitionism; seductiveness; excessive or public masturbatory behavior; molesting other children; cross-gender dressing

Delayed or disturbed relationships with others: excessive isolation; inability to relate to peers and teachers; difficulty separating from mother or father; refusal to attend school (school phobia)

Does not seem to listen to others

Not affectionate; lack empathy toward others; not attached to others

Absence of age-appropriate guilt

Tendency to blame others

Excessive distress on separation or anticipated separation from attachment figure

Unrealistic worry about losing attachment figure

Unrealistic worry about anticipated situations

Mood disturbances: overreaction to minor stresses; sadness; prolonged anger; anxiousness; fears of familiar and new situations and persistent doubts about capacity to master these situations; pervasive mood of unhappiness; inappropriate feelings under normal conditions

Areas of Disordered Functioning in Anorexia Nervosa

1. **Disturbed body image and delusional body concept.** The young girl identifies with her emaciation, defending the skeleton-like appearance as normal, actively maintains it, and denies that it is abnormal. She indicates that it is rewarding to achieve and maintain this emaciated state. She is increasingly fearful of weight gain and interprets the concern of others as attempts to make her fat.

2. **Inaccurate and confused perception and interpretation of inner stimuli.** Inaccurate hunger awareness is pronounced. The adolescent does not recognize signs of nutritional need in herself and is unable to assess the amounts of food taken. She may feel "full" after only a few bites and derives pleasure from the refusal of food. A preoccupation and tremendous involvement with food and related activities are associated with this eating behavior; the girl frequently assumes all meal planning and preparation for others. Girls with anorexia nervosa often increase their activity to help counteract the possibility of weight gain. This hyperactivity may continue until emaciation is far advanced.

3. **Paralyzing sense of ineffectiveness that pervades all aspects of daily life.** Teenagers with anorexia nervosa are overwhelmed by a deep sense of ineffectiveness. They are convinced that they function only in response to demands and wishes of others rather than doing as they want or choose. They have always been compliant children, but careful analysis reveals this to be mechanical obedience and overconformity that is not recognized as a reflection of a serious problem—a self-doubt regarding their ability to stand up for themselves or even the right for self-assertion.

Modified from Bruch H: *Nutr Today* 13(5):14-18, 1978. In Wong DL: *Whaley and Wong's nursing care of infants and children,* ed 5, St Louis, 1995, Mosby.

Some Characteristics of Eating Disorders

Factors	Anorexia Nervosa	Bulimia
Food	Turns away from food to cope	Turns to food to cope
Personality	Introverted	Extroverted
	Avoids intimacy	Seeks intimacy
	Negates feminine role	Aspires to feminine role
Behavior	"Model" child	Often "acts out"
	Compulsive/obsessive	Impulsive
School	High achiever	Variable school performance
Control	Maintains rigid control	Loses control
Body image	Body distortion	Less frequent body distortion
Health	Denies illness	Recognizes illness
		Fluctuates
Weight	Body weight less than 85% of expected norm	Within 5 to 15 lb of normal body weight
Sexuality	Usually not sexually active	Often sexually active

From Wong DL: *Whaley and Wong's nursing care of infants and children,* ed 5, St Louis, 1995, Mosby.

Early Signs of Anorexia Nervosa

The adolescent

Consumes an inappropriate diet (excessively strict) or may refuse to eat altogether

Develops peculiar eating habits such as toying with food, food "rituals," preparing and forcing food on family members without eating any herself

Engages in excessive exercise, such as compulsive jogging, running up and down stairs, rigorous calisthenics to burn off calories—often to the point of exhaustion

Withdraws from social interaction—starts to spend all her time in her room studying, exercising, or otherwise occupied

Ceases to have menstrual periods after sudden or excessive weight loss—sometimes almost as soon as dieting begins

Takes laxatives, diuretics, or enemas to speed intestinal transit time to lose added weight and empty intestines to flatten abdomen

From Wong DL: *Whaley and Wong's nursing care of infants and children,* ed 5, St Louis, 1995, Mosby.

Vomits deliberately—may go to bathroom after a meal and turn on faucets to avoid being heard

Denies hunger even after eating practically nothing for days or even weeks

Develops a distorted body image—states she "feels fat" as she becomes increasingly thinner

Loses weight—growing girls fail to achieve the 25th percentile on normal growth curves

Diagnostic Criteria for Anorexia Nervosa

1. Refusal to maintain body weight at or above a minimally normal weight for age and height (e.g., weight loss leading to maintenance of body weight less than 85% of that expected; or failure to make expected weight gain during period of growth, leading to body weight less than 85% of that expected)

2. Intense fear of gaining weight or becoming fat, even though underweight

3. Disturbance in the way in which one's body weight or shape is experienced, undue influence of body weight or shape on self-evaluation, or denial of the seriousness of the current low body weight

4. In postmenarcheal females, amenorrhea (i.e., the absence of at least three consecutive menstrual cycles) (a woman is considered to have amenorrhea if her periods occur only after hormone, e.g., estrogen, administration)

Specify type:

Restricting: during the current episode of anorexia nervosa, the person has not regularly engaged in binge-eating or purging behavior (i.e., self-induced vomiting or the misuse of laxatives, diuretics, or enemas).

Binge eating/purging: during the current episode of anorexia nervosa, the person has regularly engaged in binge eating or purging behavior (i.e., self-induced vomiting or the misuse of laxatives, diuretics, or enemas).

From American Psychiatric Association: *Diagnostic and statistical manual of mental disorders,* ed 4 (DSM-IV), Washington, DC, 1994, The Association. In Wong DL: *Whaley and Wong's nursing care of infants and children,* ed 5, St Louis, 1995, Mosby.

Diagnostic Criteria for Bulimia Nervosa

1. Recurrent episodes of binge eating. An episode of binge eating is characterized by both of the following:
   a. Eating, in a discrete period of time (e.g., within any 2-hour period), an amount of food that is definitely larger than most people would eat during a similar period of time and under similar circumstances
   b. A sense of lack of control over eating during the episode (e.g., a feeling that one cannot stop eating or control what or how much one is eating)
2. Recurrent inappropriate compensatory behavior to prevent weight gain, such as self-induced vomiting; misuse of laxatives, diuretics, enemas, or other medications; fasting; or excessive exercise.
3. The binge eating and inappropriate compensatory behaviors both occur, on average, at least twice a week for 3 months.
4. Self-evaluation is unduly influenced by body shape and weight.
5. The disturbance does not occur exclusively during episodes of anorexia nervosa.

Specify type:

Purging: during the current episode of bulimia nervosa, the person has regularly engaged in self-induced vomiting or the misuse of laxatives, diuretics, or enemas.

Nonpurging: during the current episode of bulimia nervosa, the person has used other inappropriate compensatory behaviors, such as fasting or excessive exercise, but has not regularly engaged in self-induced vomiting or the misuse of laxatives, diuretics, or enemas.

From American Psychiatric Association: *Diagnostic and statistical manual of mental disorders,* ed 4 (DSM-IV), Washington, DC, 1994, The Association. In Wong DL: *Whaley and Wong's nursing care of infants and children,* ed 5, St Louis, 1995, Mosby.

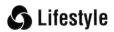 Lifestyle
Social Readjustment Rating Scale

Holmes and Rahe developed this scale to rate the amount of stress caused by many changes in life: major and minor, pleasant and unpleasant. To obtain your score, circle the ones that apply to you and then add up the total. Follow-up studies show that people who accumulate more than 200 points in a year are high risks for physical or psychologic stress-related illnesses.

Life event	Mean value
1. Death of spouse	100
2. Divorce	73
3. Marital separation from mate	65
4. Detention in jail or other institution	63
5. Death of a close family member	63
6. Major personal injury or illness	53
7. Marriage	50
8. Being fired at work	47
9. Marital reconciliation with mate	45
10. Retirement from work	45
11. Major change in the health or behavior of a family member	44
12. Pregnancy	40
13. Sexual difficulties	39
14. Gaining a new family member (e.g., through birth, adoption, oldster moving in)	39
15. Major business readjustment (e.g., merger, reorganization, bankruptcy)	39
16. Major change in financial state (e.g., a lot worse off or a lot better off than usual)	38
17. Death of a close friend	37
18. Changing to a different line of work	36
19. Major change in the number of arguments with spouse (e.g., either a lot more or a lot less than usual regarding child rearing, personal habits)	35
20. Taking out a mortgage or loan for a major purchase (e.g., for a home, business)	31
21. Foreclosure on a mortgage or loan	30
22. Major change in responsibilities at work (e.g., promotion, demotion, lateral transfer)	29
23. Son or daughter leaving home (e.g., marriage, attending college)	29
24. Trouble with in-laws	29

From Holmes TH, Rahe RH: *J Psychosom Res* 11, 1967.

Life event	Mean value
25. Outstanding personal achievement	28
26. Wife beginning or ceasing work outside the home	26
27. Beginning or ceasing formal schooling	26
28. Major change in living conditions (e.g., building a new home, remodeling, deterioration of home or neighborhood)	25
29. Revision of personal habits (dress, manners, associations, etc.)	24
30. Trouble with the boss	23
31. Major change in working hours or conditions	20
32. Change in residence	20
33. Changing to a new school	20
34. Major change in usual type or amount of recreation	19
35. Major change in church activities (e.g., a lot more or a lot less than usual)	19
36. Major change in social activities (e.g., clubs, dancing, movies, visiting)	18
37. Taking out a mortgage or loan for a lesser purchase (e.g., for a car, TV, freezer)	17
38. Major change in sleeping habits (a lot more or a lot less sleep, or a change in part of day when asleep)	16
39. Major change in number of family get-togethers (e.g., a lot more or a lot less than usual)	15
40. Major change in eating habits (a lot more or a lot less food intake, or very different meal hours or surroundings)	15
41. Vacation	13
42. Christmas	12
43. Minor violations of the law (e.g., traffic lights, jaywalking, disturbing the peace)	11

Family Inventory of Life Events and Changes (FILE)

Scoring for FILE is done[1] by totaling the numbers assigned for each item the client checks yes.

High score	= over 750	Inform family of high stress and offer
Moderate score	= 501-749	assistance in coping
Low score	= under 500	

From McCubbin HI, Thompson AI, McCubbin MA: *Family assessment: resiliency, coping, and adaptation—inventories for research and practice,* Madison, Wis., 1996, University of Wisconsin.

FILE—Family Inventory of Life Events and Changes
Hamilton I. McCubbin   Joan M. Patterson   Lance R. Wilson

Purpose

Over their life cycle, all families experience many changes as a result of normal growth and development of members and due to external circumstances. The following list of family life changes can happen in a family at any time. Because family members are connected to each other in some way, a life change for any one member affects all the other persons in the family to some degree.

> "Family" means a group of two or more persons living together who are related by blood, marriage, or adoption. This includes persons who live with you and to whom you have a long term commitment.

Directions

"Did the change happen in your family?"
Please read each family life change and decide whether it happened to any member of your family—including you.

- During the last year
First, decide if it happened any time during the last 12 months and check
Yes or no.

During last
12 months
Yes ☐ No ☐

Family Inventory of Life Events and Changes (FILE)   431

Family life changes		Did the change happen in your family?		Score
		During last 12 months Yes No		
I. Intrafamily strains				
1. Increase of husband/father's time away from family	46	☐	☐ 12	
2. Increase of wife/mother's time away from family	51	☐	☐	
3. A member appears to have emotional problems	58	☐	☐	
4. A member appears to depend on alcohol or drugs	66	☐	☐	
5. Increase in conflict between husband and wife	53	☐	☐	
6. Increase in arguments between parent(s) and child(ren)	45	☐	☐	
7. Increase in conflict among children in the family	48	☐	☐	
8. Increased difficulty in managing teenage child(ren)	55	☐	☐	
9. Increased difficulty in managing school age child(ren) (6-12 yr)	39	☐	☐	
10. Increased difficulty in managing preschool age child(ren) (2½-6 yr)	36	☐	☐	
11. Increased difficulty in managing toddler(s) (1-2½ yr)	36	☐	☐	
12. Increased difficulty in managing infant(s) (0-1 yr)	35	☐	☐	
13. Increase in the amount of "outside activities" that the child(ren) are involved in	25	☐	☐	
14. Increased disagreement about a member's friends or activities	35	☐	☐	
15. Increase in the number of problems or issues that do not get resolved	45	☐	☐	
16. Increase in the number of tasks or chores that do not get done	35	☐	☐	
17. Increased conflict with in-laws or relatives	40	☐	☐ 32	
II. Marital strains				
18. Spouse/parent was separated or divorced	79	☐	☐	
19. Spouse/parent has an "affair"	68	☐	☐	
20. Increased difficulty in resolving issues with a "former" or separated spouse	47	☐	☐	
21. Increased difficulty with sexual relationship between husband and wife	58	☐	☐ 36	

Subtotal 1 _____

Family life changes		Did the change happen in your family? During last 12 months		Score
		Yes	No	
III. Pregnancy and childbearing strains				
22. Spouse had unwanted or difficult pregnancy	45	☐	☐	
23. An unmarried member became pregnant	65	☐	☐	
24. A member had an abortion	50	☐	☐	
25. A member gave birth to or adopted a child	50	☐	☐ [45]	
IV. Finance and business strains				
26. Took out a loan or refinanced a loan to cover increased expenses	29	☐	☐	
27. Went on welfare	55	☐	☐	
28. Change in conditions (economic, political, weather) that hurts the family business	41	☐	☐	
29. Change in Agriculture Market, Stock Market, or Land Values that hurts family investments or income	43	☐	☐	
30. A member started a new business	50	☐	☐	
31. Purchased or built a home	41	☐	☐	
32. A member purchased a car or other major item	19	☐	☐	
33. Increasing financial debts caused by overuse of credit cards	31	☐	☐	
34. Increased strain on family "money" for medical/ dental expenses	23	☐	☐	
35. Increased strain on family "money" for food, clothing, energy, home care	21	☐	☐	
36. Increased strain on family "money" for child(ren) education	22	☐	☐	
37. Delay in receiving child support or alimony payments	41	☐	☐ [63]	
V. Work-family transitions and strains				
38. A member changed to a new job/career	40	☐	☐	
39. A member lost or quit a job	55	☐	☐	
40. A member retired from work	48	☐	☐	
41. A member started or returned to work	41	☐	☐	
42. A member stopped working for extended period (e.g., laid off, leave of absence, strike)	51	☐	☐	
43. Decrease in satisfaction with job/career	45	☐	☐	
44. A member had increased difficulty with people at work	32	☐	☐	
45. A member was promoted at work or given more responsibilities	40	☐	☐	
46. Family moved to a new home/apartment	43	☐	☐	
47. A child/adolescent member changed to a new school	24	☐	☐ [77] [78-01]	

Subtotal 2 _____

Family life changes		Did the change happen in your family?		Score
		During last 12 months		
		Yes	No	
VI. Illness and family "care" strains				
48. Parent/spouse became seriously ill or injured	44	☐	☐ [12]	
49. Child became seriously ill or injured	35	☐	☐	
50. Close relative or friend of the family became seriously ill	44	☐	☐	
51. A member became physically disabled or chronically ill	73	☐	☐	
52. Increased difficulty in managing a chronically ill or disabled member	58	☐	☐	
53. Member or close relative was committed to an institution or nursing home	44	☐	☐	
54. Increased responsibility to provide direct care or financial help to husband's or wife's parent(s)	47	☐	☐	
55. Experienced difficulty in arranging for satisfactory child care	40	☐	☐ [25]	
VII. Losses				
56. A parent/spouse died	98	☐	☐	
57. A child member died	99	☐	☐	
58. Death of husband's or wife's parent or close relative	48	☐	☐	
59. Close friend of the family died	47	☐	☐	
60. Married son or daughter was separated or divorced	58	☐	☐	
61. A member "broke up" a relationship with a close friend	35	☐	☐ [36]	
VIII. Transitions "in and out"				
62. A member was married	42	☐	☐	
63. Young adult member left home	43	☐	☐	
64. A young adult member began college (or post–high school training)	28	☐	☐	
65. A member moved back home or a new person moved into the household	42	☐	☐	
66. A parent/spouse started school (or training program) after being away from school for a long time	38	☐	☐ [41]	
IX. Family legal violations				
67. A member went to jail or juvenile detention	68	☐	☐	
68. A member was picked up by police or arrested	57	☐	☐	
69. Physical or sexual abuse or violence in the home	75	☐	☐	
70. A member ran away from home	61	☐	☐	
71. A member dropped out of school or was suspended from school	38	☐	☐ [50] [78-02]	

Subtotal 3 _____

Grand Total _____

Behavioral Health History

The Behavioral Health History assists the nurse in assessing the client's lifestyle risk factors, which may lead to illness or may complicate existing health factors.

Behavioral Health History
Social history

1. What organizations (community, church, lodge, social, professional, and so on) are you involved in? _____

   _____

2. List hobbies, skills, interests: _____
3. Do you live alone? ( ) Yes ( ) No
4. When did you last change residence? _____
5. (a) Marital status (circle one): single—married—divorced—widowed

   (b) Length of time _____
6. Were you ever in military service? ( ) Yes ( ) No

   (a) From ___ to ___ (b) Were you overseas during this time?

   ( ) Yes ( ) No
7. Has a close friend or immediate member of the family died within the past 2 years?

   ( ) Yes ( ) No
8. List names and addresses of relatives of close friends in this area, indicating if friend or relative _____

   _____

   _____

Patient profile

1. Number of years completed?   Elementary school ___

   High school ___ College ___
2. Customary occupation ___ Employer _____

   For how long? ___

   Is your work satisfying? ( ) No ( ) Yes

   Habits:

From Somers AR and others: *Patient Care,* June 15, 1979. Reproduced with permission, copyright Medical Economics Publishing, a division of Medical Economics Co., Montvale, N.J. All rights reserved. In Edelman CL, Mandle CL: *Health promotion throughout the lifespan,* ed 3, St Louis, 1994, Mosby.

3. Have you *ever* smoked cigarettes? ( ) No ( ) Yes
    a. How many? ( ) Less than ½ pack a day
    (check one)   ( ) About one pack a day
                     ( ) More than 1½ packs a day
    b. Do you smoke cigarettes now? ( ) No ( ) Yes
    c. For how long? ( ) Less than 5 years
    (check one)   ( ) 5-10 years
                     ( ) More than 10 years
4. Have you *ever* smoked cigars or a pipe? ( ) No ( ) Yes
    a. If Yes, how long? ( ) Less than 5 years
                           ( ) 5-10 years
                           ( ) More than 10 years
    b. Do you smoke cigars or a pipe now? ( ) No ( ) Yes
5. Do you drink alcohol (wine, beer, whiskey)? ( ) No ( ) Yes
    If Yes, how much per day on the average?
6. Have you sometimes in the past year gotten drunk on work days? ( ) No ( ) Yes
7. Have you sometimes in the past year had alcoholic drinks (wine, beer, whiskey) in the mornings? ( ) No ( ) Yes
8. How much coffee, tea, or cola do you drink?
    (check one)
    ( ) None
    ( ) Less than 6 glasses or cups per day?
    ( ) More than 6 glasses or cups per day?
9. Do you use seat belts? ( ) Never ( ) Sometimes ( ) Always
10. How many miles do you drive per year? _____
11. Exercise: Describe type and amount per week _____
_____
_____

12. How much sleep do you *usually* get per night?
    (check one) ( ) 7 hours per night or more
                  ( ) Less than 7 hours per night
13. Meals: Do you generally eat
    (check one) ( ) 3 regular meals per day?
                  ( ) 2 meals per day?
                  ( ) irregular meals?
FOR WOMEN: Do you examine your breasts each month for lumps?
        ( ) No ( ) Yes

Mortality Risk Appraisal

In each row, place a check in the box that best describes your current life situation or behavior.

Risk for cardiovascular disease

→ Increasing risk →

Risk factor:						
Sex and age	Female under 40	Female 40-50	Male 25-40	Female after menopause	Male 40-60	Male 61 or over
Family history (mother, father, brothers, sisters) — High blood pressure	No relatives with condition		One relative	Two relatives	Three relatives	
Heart attack	No relatives with condition		One relative with condition after 60	Two relatives with condition after 60	One relative with condition before 60	Two relatives with condition before 60
Diabetes	No relatives with condition			One or more relatives with maturity onset diabetes	One or more relatives with preadolescent or adolescent onset	
Blood pressure* — Systolic	120 or below	121-140	141-160	161-180	181-200	above 200
Diastolic	70 or below	71-80	81-90	91-100	101-110	above 110

Risk factor	No diagnosis	Maturity onset, controlled		Maturity onset, uncontrolled		Adolescent onset, controlled	Adolescent onset, uncontrolled
Diabetes*	No diagnosis	Maturity onset, controlled		Maturity onset, uncontrolled		Adolescent onset, controlled	Adolescent onset, uncontrolled
Weight*	At or slightly below recommended weight	10% overweight		20% overweight	30% overweight	40% overweight	50% overweight
Cholesterol*† level (mg/100 ml)	Below 180	181-200	201-220	221-240	241-260	261-280	Above 280
Serum triglycerides* (mg/100 ml) fasting	150 or below	151-400			401-1000	Above 1000	
Percent of fat in diet*	20%-30%	31%-40%			41%-50%	Above 50%	
Frequency of exercise* — Recreational	Intensive recreational exertion 35-45 min at least 4 times/wk	Moderate recreational exertion			Minimal recreational exertion	No recreational exertion	
Frequency of exercise* — Occupational	Intensive occupational exertion	Moderate occupational exertion			Minimal occupational exertion	Sedentary occupation	
Sleep patterns*	7 or 8 hr sleep/night			More than 8 hr sleep night		4-6 hr sleep/night	

*Indicates risk factors that can be fully or partially controlled.

†Serum lipid analysis is also recommended to determine low-density (beta) and high-density (alpha) lipoprotein levels.

Evidence suggests that high-density lipoprotein (HDL) carries cholesterol from tissues for metabolism and excretion. An inverse correlation appears to exist between HDL and coronary artery disease.

Mortality risk appraisal—cont'd

In each row, place a check in the box that best describes your current life situation or behavior.

Risk for cardiovascular disease → Increasing risk							
Risk factor:							
Cigarette smoking*	No./day	Nonsmoker	1-10/day	11-20/day	21-30/day	31-40/day	Over 40/day
	No. of yr smoked	Nonsmoker	Less than 10 yr	11-15/yr	16-20/yr	21-30/yr	31 yr or more
Stress*	Domestic	Minimal		Moderate	High		Very high
	Occupational	Minimal		Moderate	High		Very high
Behavior pattern* (particularly males)		**Type B** Relaxed, appropriately assertive, not time dependent, moderate to slow speech			**Type A** Excessively competitive, aggressive, striving, hyperalert, time dependent, loud, explosive speech		
Air pollution*		Low		Moderate	High		
Use of oral contraceptives* (females)		Do not use oral contraceptives		Under 40 and use oral contraceptives	Over 40 and use oral contraceptives		

Breast cancer (Women) — risk increases from left to right

Risk factor				
Age	20-29	30-39	40-49	50 or over
Race	Oriental	Black		Caucasion
Family history (grandmother, mother, sister)	None	Mother, sister, or grandmother	Mother and grandmother	Mother and sister
Onset of menstruation	Over 12 yr of age			Under 12 yr of age
Pregnancy* — Time	First pregnancy before 25	First pregnancy after 25		No pregnancies
Pregnancy* — No.	Three or more	One or two		None
Weight*	0%-40% overweight			Above 40% overweight
Personal history	No evidence of dysplasia or previous breast cancer	Breast dysplasia		Previous breast cancer

Lung cancer — risk increases from left to right

Risk factor						
Cigarette smoking* — No./day	Nonsmoker	1-10/day	11-20/day	21-30/day	21-40/day	Over 40/day
Cigarette smoking* — No. of yr smoked	Nonsmoker	Less than 10 yr	11-15 yr	16-20 yr	21-30 yr	31 or more yr
Occupational exposure to toxic chemicals*† — Length of exposure	Less than one yr	1-5 yr		6-10 yr	11-15 yr	Over 15 yr
Occupational exposure to toxic chemicals*† — Frequency and intesity of exposure	Low frequency and low intensity	Low frequency, moderate intensity		Moderate frequency, moderate intensity	Moderate frequency, high intensity (or vice versa)	High frequency, high intensity

*Indicates risk factors that can be fully or partially controlled.

†Chemicals such as asbestos, nickel, chromates, arsenic, chlormethly ethers, radioactive dust, petroleum or coal products, and iron oxide.

Mortality risk appraisal—cont'd

In each row, place a check in the box that best describes your current life situation or behavior.

Risk for malignant disease

→ Increasing risk →

Risk factor:				
Cervical cancer Onset of sexual activity*	After 28 yrs of age	22-27	16-21	Before 16 yrs of age
No. of sexual partners*	Two	Three		Four or more
Marital status*	Single		Married	
Sexual partner*	Circumcised		Uncircumcised	
Colorectal cancer Age	Below 45 yr of age		Above 45	
Personal history	No history of ulcerative colitis	Ulcerative colitis under 10 yr	Ulcerative colitis more than 10 yr	
Fiber content of diet*	High	Moderate	Low	
Weight* (men)	Less than 40% overweight		More than 40% overweight	
Rectal bleeding or black bowel movement	Never	Occasionally	Frequently	
Uterine and ovarian cancer Age	Below 45 yr of age		Over 45 yr of age	
Weight*	Less than 40% overweight		More than 40% overweight	

*Indicates risk factors that can be fully or partially controlled.

Risk factor					
Vaginal bleeding other than during menstrual period	Never		Occasionally		Frequently
Skin cancer — Complexion	Dark		Medium		Fair
Sun exposure (without protection)	Never or seldom		Occasionally		Frequently
Risk for auto accidents					
Alcohol consumption*	Nondrinker	Occasionally small to moderate consumption	Frequently small to moderate consumption	Occasionally heavy consumption	Frequently heavy consumption
Mileage driven/yr*	Under 5000 miles/yr	5001–10,000 miles/yr		10,001–20,000 miles/yr	Over 20,000 miles/yr
Use of seat belt*	Always	Usually		Occasionally	Never
Use of shoulder harness*	Always	Usually		Occasionally	Never
Use of drugs or medication that decrease alertness*	No use	Occasional use		Moderate use	Frequent use

*Indicates risk factors that can be fully or partially controlled.

Mortality risk appraisal—cont'd

In each row, place a check in the box that best describes your current life situation or behavior.

Risk factor: → Increasing risk →

Risk for malignant disease

Family history	No history		One family member		Two or more family members

Risk for suicide

Personal history*	Seldom experience depression	Periodically experience mild depression	Frequently experience mild depression	Periodically experience deep depression	Frequently experience deep depression
Access to hypnotic medication*	No access		Access to small or limited dosages		Unlimited access to large dosages

Risk for diabetes

Weight*	Desired weight	15% overweight	30% overweight	45% overweight	Above 45% overweight
Family history (parent or sibling)	None		Either parent or sibling		Both parent and sibling

*Indicates risk factors that can be fully or partially controlled.

Mortality risk appraisal—cont'd

Health Problem	(1) Total no. risk factors	(2) No. for which client is in highest risk level(s)*	(3) Percent for which client is in highest risk level(s) (col. 2 ÷ col. 1)
Cardiovascular disease	21†		
Breast cancer	8		
Lung cancer	4		
Cervical cancer	4		
Colorectal cancer	5		
Uterine or ovarian cancer	3		
Skin cancer	2		
Auto accidents	5		
Suicide	3		
Diabetes	2		

*High risk is risk within highest level of two to three levels within risk factor, or risk within highest two levels of four or more levels within risk factor.
†All subcategories under a given heading are counted individually. For example, Pregnancy—Time and Pregnancy—Number each count as a separate factor.

From Pender NJ: Health promotion in nursing practice, ed 3, Norwalk, Conn., 1966, Appleton & Lange.

Healthier People Health Risk Appraisal

Heath Risk Appraisal is an education tool. It shows you choices you can make to keep good health and avoid the most common causes of death for a person your age and sex. This Health Risk Appraisal is not a substitute for a checkup or physical exam that you get from a doctor or nurse. It only gives you some ideas for lowering your risk of getting sick or injured in the future. It is NOT designed for people who already have HEART DISEASE, CANCER, KIDNEY DISEASE, OR OTHER SERIOUS CONDITIONS. If you have any of these problems and you want a Health Risk Appraisal anyway, ask your doctor or nurse.

DIRECTIONS: To get the most accurate results answer as many questions as you can and as best you can. If you do not know the answer leave it blank. Questions with a * (star symbol) are important to your health but are not used to calculate your risks. However, your answers may be helpful in planning your health and fitness program.

1. SEX		❏ Male ❏ Female
2. AGE		[ ] Years
3. HEIGHT	(Without shoes)	[ ] Feet [ ] Inches
4. WEIGHT	(Without shoes)	[ ] Pounds
5. Body frame size		❏ Small ❏ Medium ❏ Large
6. Have you ever been told that you have diabetes (or sugar diabetes)		❏ Yes ❏ No
7. Are you now taking medicine for high blood pressure?		❏ Yes ❏ No
8. What is your blood pressure now?		[ ] / [ ] Systolic (High number)/Diastolic (Low number)
9. If you *do not* know the numbers, check the box that describes your blood pressure.		❏ High ❏ Normal or Low ❏ Don't Know
10. What is your TOTAL cholesterol level (based on a blood test)?		[ ] mg/dl
11. What is your HDL cholesterol (based on a blood test)?		[ ] mg/dl
12. How many cigars do you usually smoke per day?		[ ] cigars per day
13. How many pipes of tobacco do you usually smoke per day?		[ ] pipes per day
14. How many times per day do you usually use smokeless tobacco? (Chewing tobacco, snuff, pouches, etc.)		[ ] times per day
15. CIGARETTE SMOKING How would you describe your cigarette smoking habits?		❏ Never smoked ☞ Go to 18 ❏ Used to smoke ☞ Go to 17 ❏ Still smoke ☞ Go to 16

From The Carter Center of Emory University, Decatur, Georgia.

16. STILL SMOKE
    How many cigarettes a day do you smoke?
    GO TO QUESTION 18

    [   ] cigarettes per day ☞ Go to 18

17. USED TO SMOKE
    a. How many years has it been since you smoked cigarettes fairly regularly?

    [   ] years

    b. What was the average number of cigarettes per day that you smoked in the 2 years before you quit?

    [   ] cigarettes per day

18. In the next 12 months how many thousands of miles will you probably travel by each of the following: (NOTE: U.S. average = 10,000 miles)

    a. Car, truck, or van:

    [   ] ,000 miles

    b. Motorcycle:

    [   ] ,000 miles

19. On a typical day how do you USUALLY travel?
    (Check one only)

    ❑ Walk
    ❑ Bicycle
    ❑ Motorcycle
    ❑ Subcompact or compact car
    ❑ Midsize or full-size car
    ❑ Truck or van
    ❑ Bus, subway, or train
    ❑ Mostly stay home

20. What percent of the time do you usually buckle your safety belt when driving or riding?

    [   ] %

21. On the average, how close to the speed limit do you usually drive?

    ❑ Within 5 mph of limit
    ❑ 6-10 mph over limit
    ❑ 11-15 mph over limit
    ❑ More than 15 mph over limit

22. How many times in the last month did you drive or ride when the driver perhaps had too much alcohol to drink?

    [   ] times last month

23. How many drinks of alcoholic beverages do you have in a typical week?

    ☛ *(MEN GO TO QUESTION 33)*

    (Write the number of each type of drink)

    [   ] Bottles or cans of beer
    [   ] Glasses of wine
    [   ] Wine coolers
    [   ] Mixed drinks or shots of liquor

WOMEN

24. At what age did you have your first menstrual period?

    [   ] years old

25. How old were you when your first child was born?

    [   ] years old
    (If no children write 0)

26. How long has it been since your last breast x-ray (mammogram)?

    ❑ Less than 1 year ago
    ❑ 1 year ago
    ❑ 2 years ago
    ❑ 3 or more years ago
    ❑ Never

27. How many women in your natural family (mother and sisters only) have had breast cancer?	[ ] women
28. Have you had a hysterectomy operation?	❑ Yes ❑ No ❑ Not sure
29. How long has it been since you had a Pap smear test?	❑ Less than 1 year ago ❑ 1 year ago ❑ 2 years ago ❑ 3 or more years ago ❑ Never
★30. How often do you examine your breasts for lumps?	❑ Monthly ❑ Once every few months ❑ Rarely or never
★31. About how long has it been since you had your breasts examined by a physician or nurse?	❑ Less than 1 year ago ❑ 1 year ago ❑ 2 years ago ❑ 3 or more years ago ❑ Never
★32. About how long has it been since you had a rectal exam? ☛ (WOMEN GO TO QUESTION 34)	❑ Less than 1 year ago ❑ 1 year ago ❑ 2 years ago ❑ 3 or more years ago ❑ Never
MEN ★33. About how long has it been since you had a rectal or prostate exam?	❑ Less than 1 year ago ❑ 1 year ago ❑ 2 years ago ❑ 3 or more years ago ❑ Never
★34. How many times in the last year did you witness or become involved in a violent fight or attack where there was a good chance of a serious injury to someone?	❑ 4 or more times ❑ 2 or 3 times ❑ 1 time or never ❑ Not sure
★35. Considering your age, how would you describe your overall physical health?	❑ Excellent ❑ Good ❑ Fair ❑ Poor
★36. In an average week, how many times do you engage in physical activity (exercise or work which lasts at least 20 minutes without stopping and which is hard enough to make you breathe heavier and your heart beat faster)?	❑ Less than 1 time per week ❑ 1 or 2 times per week ❑ At least 3 times per week
★37. If you ride a motorcycle or all-terrain vehicle (ATV) what percent of the time do you wear a helmet?	❑ 75% to 100% ❑ 25% to 74% ❑ Less than 25% ❑ Does not apply to me
★38. Do you eat some food every day that is high in fiber, such as whole grain bread, cereal, fresh fruits or vegetables?	❑ Yes ❑ No
★39. Do you eat foods every day that are high in cholesterol or fat, such as fatty meat, cheese, fried foods, or eggs?	❑ Yes ❑ No

★40. In general, how satisfied are you with your life?	❑ Most satisfied ❑ Partly satisfied ❑ Not satisfied
★41. Have you suffered a personal loss or misfortune in the past year that had a serious impact on your life? (For example, a job loss, disability, separation, jail term, or the death of someone close to you.)	❑ Yes, 1 serious loss or misfortune ❑ Yes, 2 or more ❑ No
★42a. Race	❑ Aleutian, Alaska native, Eskimo or American Indian ❑ Asian ❑ Black ❑ Pacific Islander ❑ White ❑ Other ❑ Don't know
★42b. Are you of Hispanic origin such as Mexican-American, Puerto Rican, or Cuban?	❑ Yes ❑ No
★43. What is the highest grade you completed in school?	❑ Grade school or less ❑ Some high school ❑ High school graduate ❑ Some college ❑ College graduate ❑ Postgraduate or professional degree
★44. What is your job or occupation? (Check only one)	❑ Health professional ❑ Manager, educator, professional ❑ Technical, sales, or administrative support ❑ Operator, fabricator, laborer ❑ Student ❑ Retired ❑ Homemaker ❑ Service ❑ Skilled crafts ❑ Unemployed ❑ Other
★45. In what industry do you work (or did you last work)? (Check only one)	❑ Electric, gas, sanitation ❑ Transportation, communication ❑ Agriculture, forestry, fishing ❑ Wholesale or retail trade ❑ Financial and service industries ❑ Mining ❑ Government ❑ Manufacturing ❑ Construction ❑ Other

User's Guide to Interpreting the Health Risk Appraisal Report Form

Unhealthy habits lead to early death or chronic illness. Every year 1.3 million people die prematurely in the United States from conditions which could be prevented or delayed. This Health Risk Appraisal (HRA) may help you avoid becoming one of these statistics by giving you a prediction of your health risks related to your particular characteristics and habits.

Risk factors

Most chronic diseases develop slowly in the presence of certain risk factors. Risk factors are either controllable or uncontrollable. Uncontrollable risk factors include factors such as your age, sex, and the health history of your family. Controllable risk factors include lifestyle habits that you can change such as blood pressure, exercise, smoking, weight, cholesterol, and stress. You should focus on controllable risk factors.

Uncontrollable risk factors
1. Age
2. Sex
3. Heredity

Controllable risk factors
1. Blood pressure
2. Exercise
3. Smoking
4. Weight
5. Cholesterol
6. Stress

Choosing a habit to work on

Your Health Risk Appraisal is intended to encourage you to work on the habits you can change—to be the best that you can be. You don't have to change your entire lifestyle overnight—in fact, trying to change too many habits at once is probably the quickest way to discouragement and failure.

Health risk appraisal limits

Your Health Risk Appraisal does have limits. It is not a predictor, but rather an educational tool. It does not take into consideration whether or not you already have a medical condition and it does not consider more rare diseases and other health problems which are not fatal but can limit your enjoyment of life (such as arthritis).

What it does consider are the lifestyle factors over which you have a great degree of control and which account for a large number of premature deaths. Now that you are familiar with your particular health risks, it's time to do something about them!

Make a plan

Make a plan of how to change the habit you chose to work on. Write the plan down and keep it in sight. Be prepared for temptation! Observe the time, situation, or place that most often triggers your unhealthy habit and be ready to combat the urge when it appears. Let family and friends know of your goals, and ask for their encouragement.

Reward yourself

Rewards are an important part of changing behavior. Give yourself a reasonable reward when you accomplish your goal. Don't eat half a gallon of ice cream after losing 10 pounds! Choose a healthy and enjoyable reward. You've worked hard and are on the road to good health!

Lifestyle Questionnaire for School-Age Children

Activities that promote health	Yes	No	Sometimes
1. I sleep at least 8 hours every night.			
2. I brush my teeth twice a day.			
3. I visit the dentist every year.			
4. I watch less than 2 hours of TV every day.			
5. I exercise (running, biking, swimming, active sports) 1 hour every day.			
6. I eat fruits.			
7. I eat vegetables.			
8. I limit my intake of salty snacks and high-sugar snacks.			
9. I have a physical examination every 2 or 3 years.			
10. I stay away from cigarettes.			
11. I stay away from alcohol.			

Injury prevention	Yes	No	Sometimes
12. I wear a seat belt in an automobile.			
13. I look both ways when crossing streets.			
14. I follow bike safety rules.			
15. I stay away from lighters or matches.			
16. I never ride ATVs (all-terrain vehicles.)*			

*The American Academy of Pediatrics recommends that children do not ride on these vehicles.

In Potter PA, Perry AG: Fundamentals of nursing: concepts, process, and practice, ed 3, St Louis, 1993, Mosby.

Injury prevention—cont'd	Yes	No	Sometimes
17. I wear a helmet when I go on bike trips.			
18. I swim with a buddy.			
19. I wear a life jacket when I ride in a boat.			
20. I take medicine only with my parent's permission.			
21. I stay away from real guns.			
22. I tell my parents where I am going.			
23. I say "no" to drugs.			
24. Our home has a smoke detector that works.			
25. Our home has a fire extinguisher.			
26. If there is a fire, I know a safe way out of my house.			

Feelings	Yes	No	Sometimes
27. I think it is okay to cry.			
28. I enjoy my family.			
29. It is easy for me to fall asleep at night.			
30. My appetite is good.			
31. I like myself just the way I am.			

Lifestyle Assessment Questionnaire (National Wellness Institute)

Purpose

This assessment tool and the analysis it provides are designed to help you discover how the choices you make each day affect your overall health.

By participating in this assessment process, you will also learn how you can make positive changes in your lifestyle, enabling you to reach a higher level of wellness.

Some of the questions are personal. While you may leave them blank, the more information you provide about your current lifestyle, the more accurately the LAQ [Lifestyle Assessment Questionnaire] can assess your current level of wellness and risk areas.

Confidentiality

The National Wellness Institute, Inc. subscribes to the guidelines established by the Society of Prospective Medicine concerning confidentiality in the use of health risk appraisals and risk reduction systems. These guidelines specifically state that only the participant and health professionals authorized by the participant should receive copies of his/her own health risk appraisal results.

The National Wellness Institute, Inc. strongly encourages all users of the LAQ to strictly follow these guidelines and maintain the confidentiality of all answers.

What is Wellness?

Wellness is an active process of becoming aware of and making choices toward a higher level of well-being. **Remember,** leading a wellness lifestyle requires your **active involvement.** As you gain more knowledge about what enhances your well-being, you are encouraged to use this information to make informed choices which lead to a healthier life.

General Instructions

If you would like to have your test evaluated, **please write to the National Wellness Institute for the answer sheet.** Please make certain that you complete all of the information at the top of the answer sheet, including your zip code, group code, and social security number. If a group code has not been provided for you, leave this item blank.

Your questionnaire will be scored by an optical mark reading instrument; therefore, please use only a No. 2 (soft) pencil for marking your responses. To assure the most accurate results, follow the instructions shown on the answer sheet. If you do not wish to have your answers scored, please mark your answers on the following pages.

Section 1: Personal Data
Instructions

Please complete the following general information about yourself by marking your answers in the appropriate places on the LAQ answer sheet or circle the correct answer. Please take your time and read each question carefully.

1. Sex
   a) male
   b) female

2. Race
   a) White
   b) Black
   c) Hispanic
   d) Asian
   e) American Indian
   f) other
3. Age
4. Height (feet and inches)
5. Weight (pounds)
6. Body frame size
   a) small
   b) medium
   c) large
7. Marital status
   a) married
   b) widowed
   c) separated
   d) divorced
   e) single
   f) cohabiting
8. What was the total gross income of your household last year?
   a) under $12,000
   b) $12,000-$20,000
   c) $20,001-$30,000
   d) $30,001-$40,000
   e) $40,001-$50,000
   f) $50,001-$60,000
   g) over $60,000
9. What is the highest level of education you have completed?
   a) grade school or less
   b) some high school
   c) high school graduate
   d) some college or technical school
   e) college graduate
   f) postgraduate or professional degree
10. On the average day, how many hours do you watch television?
    a) 0 hours
    b) 1-3 hours
    c) 4-7 hours
    d) more than 8 hours
11. Where do you live?
    a) in the country
    b) in a city

    c) suburb

    d) small town

12. If you live in a city, suburb, or small town, what is the population?

    a) under 20,000

    b) 20,000-50,000

    c) 50,001-100,000

    d) 100,001-500,000

    e) over 500,000

Section 2: Lifestyle
Instructions

This section will help determine your level of wellness. It will also give you ideas for areas in which you might improve. Some questions touch on very personal subjects. Therefore, if you prefer to skip certain questions, you may. However, the more questions you answer, the more you will learn about your health and how to improve it.

Please respond to these statements using the following responses. If an item does not apply to you, do not mark it.

A *Almost always (90% or more of the time)*

B *Very often (approximately 75% of the time)*

C *Often (approximately 50% of the time)*

D *Occasionally (approximately 25% of the time)*

E *Almost never (less than 10% of the time)*

Physical exercise

Measures one's commitment to maintaining physical fitness.

1. I exercise vigorously for at least 20 minutes three or more times per week.

2. I determine my activity level by monitoring my heart rate.

3. I stop exercising before I feel exhausted.

4. I exercise in a relaxed, calm, and joyful manner.

5. I stretch before exercising.

6. I stretch after exercising.

7. I walk or bike whenever possible.

8. I participate in a strenuous activity (tennis, running, brisk walking, water exercise, swimming, handball, basketball, etc.).

9. If I am not in shape, I avoid sporadic (once a week or less often), strenuous exercise.

10. After vigorous exercise, I "cool down" (very light exercise such as walking) for at least five minutes before sitting or lying down.

Nutrition

Measures the degree to which one chooses foods that are consistent with the dietary goals of the United States as published by the Senate Select Committee on Nutrition and Human Needs.

11. When choosing nonvegetable protein, I select lean cuts of meat, poultry, fish, and low-fat dairy products.
12. I maintain an appropriate weight for my height and frame.
13. I minimize salt intake.
14. I eat fruits and vegetables, fresh and uncooked.
15. I eat breakfast.
16. I intentionally include fiber in my diet on a daily basis.
17. I drink enough fluid to keep my urine light yellow.
18. I plan my diet to insure an adequate amount of vitamins and minerals.
19. I minimize foods in my diet that contain large amounts of refined flour (bleached white flour, typical store bread, cakes, etc.).
20. I minimize my intake of fats and oils including margarine and animal fats.
21. I include items from all four basic food groups in my diet each day (fruits and vegetables; milk group; breads and cereals; meat, fowl, fish or vegetable proteins).
22. To avoid unnecessary calories, I choose water as one of the beverages I drink.
23. I avoid adding sugar to my foods. I minimize my intake of presweetened foods (sugarcoated cereals, syrups, chocolate milk, and most processed and fast foods).

Self-care

Measures the behaviors which help one prevent or detect early illnesses.

24. I use footgear of good quality designed for the activity or the job in which I participate.
25. I record immunizations to maintain up-to-date immunization records.
26. I examine my breasts or testes on a monthly basis.
27. I have my breasts or testes examined yearly by a physician.
28. I balance the type and amount of food I eat with exercise to maintain a healthy percent body fat.
29. I take action to minimize my exposure to tobacco smoke.
30. When I experience illness or injury, I take necessary steps to correct the problem.

31. I engage in activities which keep my blood pressure in a range which minimizes my chances of disease (e.g., stroke, heart attack, and kidney disease).
32. I brush my teeth after eating.
33. I floss my teeth after eating.
34. My resting pulse is 60 or less.
35. I get an adequate amount of sleep.
36. If I were to have sex, I would take action to prevent unplanned pregnancy.
37. If I were to have sex, I would take action to prevent giving and/or getting sexually transmitted disease.

Vehicle safety

Measures one's ability to minimize chances of injury or death in a vehicle accident.

38. I do not operate vehicles while I am under the influence of alcohol or other drugs.
39. I do not ride with drivers who are under the influence of alcohol or other drugs.
40. I stay within the speed limit.
41. I practice defensive driving techniques.
42. When traffic lights change from green to yellow, I prepare to stop.
43. I maintain a safe driving distance between cars based on speed and road conditions.
44. Vehicles which I drive are maintained to assure safety.
45. Because they are safer, I use radial tires on cars that I drive.
46. When I ride a bicycle or motorcycle, I wear a helmet and have adequate lights/reflectors.
47. Children riding in my car are secured in an approved car seat or seat belt.
48. I use my seat belt while driving or riding in a vehicle.

Drug usage and awareness

Measures the degree to which one functions without the unnecessary use of chemicals.

49. I use prescription drugs and over-the-counter medications only when necessary.
50. If I consume alcohol, I limit my consumption to not more than one drink per hour and no more than two drinks per day.
51. I avoid the use of tobacco.
52. Because of the potentially harmful effects of caffeine (e.g., coffee, tea, cola, etc.), I limit my consumption.

53. I avoid the use of marijuana.
54. I avoid the use of hallucinogens (LSD, PCP, MDA, etc.).
55. I avoid the use of stimulants ("uppers"—e.g., cocaine, amphetamines, "pep pills," etc.).
56. I avoid the use of nonmedically prescribed depressants ("downers"—e.g., barbituates, quaaludes, minor tranquilizers, etc.).
57. I avoid using a combination of drugs unless under medical supervision.
58. I follow the instructions provided with any drug I take.
59. I avoid using drugs obtained from illegal sources.
60. I understand the expected effect of drugs I take.
61. I consider alternatives to drugs.
62. If I experience discomfort from stress or tension, I use relaxation techniques, exercise, and meditation instead of taking drugs.
63. I get clear directions for taking my medicine from my doctor or pharmacist.

Social/environmental

Measures the degree to which one contributes to the common welfare of the community. This emphasizes interdependence with others and nature.

64. I conserve energy at home.
65. I consider energy conservation when choosing a mode of transportation.
66. My social ties with family are strong.
67. I contribute to the feeling of acceptance within my family.
68. I develop and maintain strong friendships.
69. I do my part to promote a clean environment (i.e., air, water, noise, etc.).
70. When I see a safety hazard, I take action (warn others or correct the problem).
71. I avoid unnecessary radiation.
72. I report criminal acts I observe.
73. I contribute time and/or money to community projects.
74. I actively seek to become acquainted with individuals in my community.
75. I use my creativity in constructive ways.
76. My behavior reflects fairness and justice.
77. When possible, I choose an environment which is free of **noise** pollution.
78. When possible, I choose an environment which is free of **air** pollution.

79. I participate in volunteer activities benefiting others.
80. I help others in need.
81. I beautify those parts of my environment under my control.
82. Because of limited resources, I do my part to conserve.
83. I recycle aluminum, glass, and paper products.
84. I involve myself with people who support a positive lifestyle.

Emotional awareness and acceptance

Measures the degree to which one has an awareness and acceptance of one's feelings. This includes the degree to which one feels positive and enthusiastic about oneself and life.

85. I have a good sense of humor.
86. I feel positive about myself.
87. I feel there is a satisfying amount of excitement in my life.
88. My emotional life is stable.
89. I am aware of my needs.
90. I trust and value my own judgment.
91. When I make mistakes, I learn from them.
92. I feel comfortable when complimented for jobs well done.
93. It is okay for me to cry.
94. I have feelings of sensitivity for others.
95. I feel enthusiastic about life.
96. I find it easy to laugh.
97. I am able to give love.
98. I am able to receive love.
99. I enjoy my life.
100. I have plenty of energy.
101. My sleep is restful.
102. I trust others.
103. I feel others trust me.
104. I accept my sexual desires.
105. I understand how I create my feelings.
106. At times, I can be both strong and sensitive.
107. I am aware when I feel angry.
108. I accept my anger.
109. I am aware when I feel sad.
110. I accept my sadness.
111. I am aware when I feel happy.
112. I accept my happiness.
113. I am aware when I feel frightened.
114. I accept my feelings of fear.
115. I am aware of my feelings about death.
116. I accept my feelings about death.

Emotional management

Measures the degree to which one controls and expresses feelings, and engages in effective, related behaviors.

117. I share my feelings with those with whom I am close.
118. I express my feelings of anger in appropriate ways.
119. I express my feelings of sadness in healthy ways.
120. I express my feelings of happiness in desirable ways.
121. I express my feelings of fear in appropriate ways.
122. I compliment myself for a job well done.
123. I accept constructive criticism without reacting defensively.
124. I set appropriate limits for myself.
125. I stay within the limits that I have set.
126. I recognize that I can have wide variations of feelings about the same person (such as loving someone even though you are angry with her/him at the moment).
127. I am able to develop close, intimate relationships.
128. I say "no" without feeling guilty.
129. I would feel comfortable seeking professional help to better understand and cope with my feelings.
130. I reduce feelings of failure by setting achievable goals.
131. I relax my body and mind without using drugs.
132. I can be alone without feeling lonely.
133. I am able to be spontaneous in expressing my feelings.
134. I accept responsibility for my actions.
135. I am willing to take the risks that come with making change.
136. I manage my feelings to avoid unnecessary suffering.
137. I make decisions with a minimum of stress and worry.
138. I accept the responsibility for creating my own feelings.
139. I can express my feelings about death.
140. I recognize grieving as a healthy response to loss.

Intellectual

Measures the degree to which one engages her/his mind in creative, stimulating mental activities, expanding knowledge, and improving skills.

141. I read a newspaper daily.
142. I read twelve or more books yearly.
143. On the average, I read one or more national magazines per week.
144. When I watch TV, I choose programs with informational/educational value.
145. I visit a museum or art show at least three times yearly.

146. I attend lectures, workshops, and demonstrations at least three times yearly.
147. I regularly use some of my time participating in hobbies such as photography, gardening, woodworking, sewing, painting, baking, art, music, writing, pottery, etc.
148. I read about local, state, national, and international political/public issues.
149. I learn the meaning of new words.
150. I engage in some type of writing activity such as a regular journal, letter writing, preparation of papers or manuscripts, etc.
151. I am interested in understanding the views of others.
152. I share ideas, concepts, thoughts, or procedures with others.
153. I gather information to enable me to make decisions.
154. I listen to radio and/or TV news.
155. I think about ideas different than my own.

Occupational

Measures the satisfaction gained from one's work and the degree to which one is enriched by that work. Please answer these items from your primary frame of reference, (e.g., your job, student, homemaker, etc.).

156. I enjoy my work.
157. My work contributes to my personal needs.
158. I feel that my job in some way contributes to my well-being.
159. I cooperate with others in my work.
160. I take advantage of opportunities to learn new work-related skills.
161. My work is challenging.
162. I feel my job responsibilities are consistent with my values.
163. I find satisfaction from the work I do.
164. I find healthy ways of reducing excessive job-related stress.
165. I use recommended health and safety precautions.
166. I make recommendations for improving worksite health and safety.
167. I am satisfied with the degree of freedom I have in my job to exercise independent judgments.
168. I am satisfied with the amount of variety in my work.
169. I believe I am competent in my job.
170. My co-workers and supervisors respect me as a competent individual.
171. My communication with others in my workplace is enriching for me.

Spiritual

Measures one's ongoing involvement in seeking meaning and purpose in human existence. It includes an appreciation for the depth and expanse of life and natural forces that exist in the universe.

172. I feel good about my spiritual life.

173. Prayer, meditation, and/or quiet personal reflection is/are important part(s) of my life.

174. I contemplate my purpose in life.

175. I reflect on the meaning of events in my life.

176. My values guide my daily life.

177. My values and beliefs help me to meet daily challenges.

178. I recognize that my spiritual growth is a lifelong process.

179. I am concerned about humanitarian issues.

180. I enjoy participating in discussions about spiritual values.

181. I feel a sense of compassion for others in need.

182. I seek spiritual knowledge.

183. My spiritual awareness occurs other than at times of crisis.

184. I believe in something greater or that I am part of something greater than myself.

185. I share my spiritual values.

Section 3: Health Risk Appraisal
Instructions

This section is intended to help you identify the problems most likely to interfere with the quality of your life. It will also show you choices you can make to stay healthy and avoid the most common causes of death for a person your age and sex.

This Health Risk Appraisal is not a substitute for a checkup or physical exam that you get from a doctor or nurse. It only gives you some ideas for lowering your risk of getting sick or injured in the future. It is NOT designed for people who already have HEART DISEASE, CANCER, KIDNEY DISEASE, OR OTHER SERIOUS CONDITIONS. If you have any of these problems and you want a Health Risk Appraisal anyway, ask your doctor or nurse to read this section (of the printout, if scored) with you.

If you don't know or are unsure of an answer, please leave that item blank.

1. Have you ever been told that you have diabetes (or sugar diabetes)?
   a. yes
   b. no

2. Does your natural mother, father, sister, or brother have diabetes?

    a. yes

    b. no

    c. not sure

3. Did either of your natural parents die of a heart attack before age 60? (If your parents are younger than 60, mark no).

    a. yes, one of them

    b. yes, both of them

    c. no

    d. not sure

4. Are you now taking medicine for high blood pressure?

    a. yes

    b. no

5. What is your blood pressure now?

    a. ____ systolic (high number)

    b. ____ diastolic (low number)

6. If you *do not* know the number, select the answer that describes your blood pressure.

    a. high

    b. normal or low

    c. don't know

7. What is your TOTAL cholesterol level (based on a blood test)? ____ (mg/dl)

8. What is your high-density lipoprotein (HDL) cholesterol level (based on a blood test)? ____ (mg/dl)

9. How many cigars do you usually smoke per day?

    ____

10. How many pipes of tobacco do you usually smoke per day?

    ____

11. How many times per day do you usually use smokeless tobacco (chewing tobacco, snuff, pouches, etc)?____

12. How would you describe your cigarette smoking habits?

    a. never smoked **Go to 15**

    b. used to smoke **Go to 14**

    c. still smoke **Go to 13**

13. How many cigarettes a day do you smoke?

    ____ cigarettes per day **Go to 15**

14. a. How many years has it been since you smoked cigarettes regularly?

       ____ years

    b. What was the average number of cigarettes per day that you smoked in the 2 years before you quit?

       ____ cigarettes per day

15. In the next 12 months, how many thousands of miles will you probably travel by each of the following?
    (NOTE: U.S. average = 10,000 miles)
    a. car, truck, or van: ____,000 miles
    b. motorcycle: ____,000 miles
16. On a typical day how do you USUALLY travel?
    (Check one only)
    a. walk
    b. bicycle
    c. motorcycle
    d. subcompact or compact car
    e. midsize or full-size car
    f. truck or van
    g. bus, subway, or train
    h. mostly stay home
17. What percent of the time do you usually buckle your safety belt when driving or riding?
    ____ %
18. On the average, how close to the speed limit do you usually drive?
    a. within 5 mph of limit
    b. 6-10 mph over limit
    c. 11-15 mph over limit
    d. more than 15 mph over limit
19. How many times in the last month did you drive or ride when the driver had perhaps too much alcohol to drink?
    ____ times last month
20. When you drink alcoholic beverages, how many drinks do you consume in an average day? (If you *never* drink alcoholic beverages, write 0.)
    ____ alcoholic beverages/average day
21. On the average, how many days per week do you consume alcohol?
    ____ days/week

(MEN GO TO QUESTION 31)
WOMEN ONLY (QUESTIONS 22-30)

22. At what age did you have your first menstrual period?
    ____ years old
23. How old were you when your first child was born (if no children, write 0)?
    ____ years old
24. How long has it been since your last breast x-ray (mammogram)?
    a. less than 1 year ago
    b. 1 year ago

    c. 2 years ago

    d. 3 or more years ago

    e. never

25. How many women in your natural family (mother and sisters only) have had breast cancer?

    _____ women

26. Have you had a hysterectomy?

    a. yes

    b. no

    c. not sure

27. How long has it been since you had a Pap smear test?

    a. less than 1 year ago

    b. 1 year ago

    c. 2 years ago

    d. 3 or more years ago

    e. never

28. How often do you examine your breasts for lumps?

    a. monthly

    b. once every few months

    c. rarely or never

29. About how long has it been since you had your breasts examined by a physician or nurse?

    a. less than 1 year ago

    b. 1 year ago

    c. 2 years ago

    d. 3 or more years ago

    e. never

30. About how long has it been since you had a rectal exam?

    a. less than 1 year ago

    b. 1 year ago

    c. 2 years ago

    d. 3 or more years ago

    e. never

WOMEN GO TO QUESTION 35
MEN ONLY (QUESTIONS 31-34)

31. About how long has it been since you had a rectal or prostate exam?

    a. less than 1 year ago

    b. 1 year ago

    c. 2 years ago

    d. 3 or more years ago

    e. never

32. Do you know how to properly examine your testes for lumps?

a. yes

b. no

c. not sure

33. How often do you examine your testes for lumps?
    a. monthly
    b. once every few months
    c. rarely or never

34. About how long has it been since you had your testes examined by a physician or nurse?
    a. less than 1 year ago
    b. 1 year ago
    c. 2 years ago
    d. 3 or more years ago
    e. never

35. How many times in the last year did you witness or become involved in a violent fight or attack where there was a good chance of a serious injury to someone?
    a. 4 or more times
    b. 2 or 3 times
    c. 1 time or never
    d. not sure

36. Considering your age, how would you describe your overall physical health?
    a. excellent
    b. good
    c. fair
    d. poor

37. In an average week, how many times do you engage in physical activity (exercise or work which lasts at least 20 minutes without stopping and which is hard enough to make you breathe heavier and your heart beat faster)?
    a. less than 1 time per week
    b. 1 or 2 times per week
    c. at least 3 times per week

38. If you ride a motorcycle or all-terrain vehicle (ATV), what percent of the time do you wear a helmet?
    a. 75% to 100%
    b. 25% to 74%
    c. less than 25%
    d. does not apply to me

39. Do you eat some food every day that is high in fiber, such as whole grain bread, cereal, fresh fruits, or vegetables?
    a. yes
    b. no

40. Do you eat foods every day that are high in cholesterol or fat, such as fatty meat, cheese, fried foods, or eggs?
    a. yes
    b. no

41. In general, how satisfied are you with your life?
    a. mostly satisfied
    b. partly satisfied
    c. not satisfied

42. Have you suffered a personal loss or misfortune in the past year that had a serious impact on your life? (For example, a job loss, disability, separation, jail term, or the death of someone close to you.)
    a. yes, 1 serious loss or misfortune
    b. yes, 2 or more
    c. no

Section 4: Topics for Personal Growth

This section will help you identify areas in which you would like more information. In response to your selection from the following topics, we will provide you with resources or services to meet your requests.

Select topics on which you would like information. (Maximum of 4 topics.)

1. Responsible alcohol use
2. Stop-smoking programs
3. Sexuality
4. Gay issues
5. Depression
6. Loneliness
7. Exercise programs
8. Weight reduction
9. Self-breast exam
10. Medical emergencies
11. Nutrition
12. Relaxation
13. Stress reduction
14. Parenting skills
15. Marital or couples problems
16. Assertiveness training (how to say "no" without feeling guilty)
17. Biofeedback for tension headache and pain
18. Overcoming fears (i.e., high places, crowded rooms, etc.)
19. Educational career goal setting/planning
20. Spiritual or philosophical values
21. Communication skills

22. Automobile safety
23. Suicide thoughts or attempts
24. Substance abuse
25. Anxiety associated with public speaking, tests, writing, etc.
26. Enhancing relationships
27. Time-management skills
28. Death and dying
29. Learning skills (i.e., speed-reading, comprehension, etc.)
30. Financial management
31. Divorce
32. Alcoholism
33. Men's issues
34. Women's issues
35. Medical self-care
36. Dental self-care
37. Self-testes exam
38. Aging
39. Self-esteem
40. Premenstrual syndrome (PMS)
41. Osteoporosis
42. Recreation and leisure
43. Environmental issues

IMPORTANT—If you have finished completing all sections of the LAQ, please make sure you have answered the questions in Section 1 requesting your sex, race, age, height, and weight. Results cannot be evaluated for the Health Risk Appraisal section without this information.

You and Your Lifestyle Are the Major Determinants for Joyful Living

The circle graph below indicates the factors which contribute to your enjoyment and quality of life. While medical professionals contribute

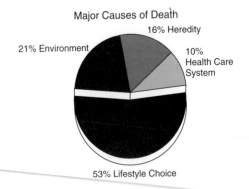

Major Causes of Death

to the quality of your life, this graph clearly shows that the majority of those factors which contribute to your well-being are controlled by you. As you make responsible, informed choices, your chances of improving your health and well-being increase.

The LAQ's Role . . .

We believe this instrument is useful in helping individuals identify the most likely causes of death and disability. More important, it identifies those areas of self-improvement which will lead to higher levels of health and well-being.

The areas assessed in the LAQ emphasize the importance of creating a balance among the many different aspects of your lifestyle. Each of these areas affects one another and determines your overall wellness status. Also, each provides an opportunity for learning, making responsible decisions, and personal growth.

We invite you to use the information provided by the LAQ to your best advantage to increase your level of wellness.

Words from the Past

Wellness is a term that has enjoyed growing popularity during the past several decades. Although the term was introduced relatively recently, the concept of prevention has been present for centuries. The following passages provide a brief glimpse of the wellness philosophy through the years. Wellness is a movement which has become a major part of modern culture and is the most important weapon available to combat lifestyle illnesses.

"For many years, while engaged in the practice of medicine, the author of this volume has been more and more impressed with the idea that the causes of suffering, diseases, and premature deaths, which we witness around us on every hand, lie near our own doors . . . and that the men and women of today, are, at least, equally as responsible for existing suffering, as those who have gone before them, and often much more so. In fact, he feels satisfied that by far the greatest portion of all the suffering, disease, deformity, and premature deaths which occur are the direct result of either the violation of, or the want of compliance with the laws of our being; calamities, which, were the requisite knowledge possessed by the community, can and should be avoided."

—JOHN ELLIS, M.D., 1859

"It is universally admitted at the present time that preventive medicine is of far greater importance than curative medication, and many of the most eminent members of the profession are devoting themselves exclusively to this branch."

—J. H. KELLOGG, M.D., 1902

"To ward off disease or recover health, men as a rule find it easier to depend on the healers than to attempt the more difficult task of living wisely."

—RENE DUBOS, Ph.D., 1959

"It's what you do hour by hour, day by day, that largely determines the state of your health; whether you get sick, what you get sick with, and perhaps when you die."

—LESTER BRESLOW, M.D., 1969

Therapeutic Exercise: Focus on Walking

What Exactly Is Meant by "Therapeutic Exercise"?

Therapeutic exercise is the motion of the body or its parts to achieve symptom-free movement and function. It is used to develop and retrain deficient muscles; to restore as much normal movement as possible to prevent deformity; to stimulate the functions of various organs and body systems; to build strength and endurance; and to promote relaxation.

Various theories and methods have been proposed to improve health through exercise and movement. Decreased physical activity, which may be the result of illness or treatment, can lead to anxiety, depression, weakness, fatigue, and nausea. Regular, moderate exercise can prevent these feelings and help a person feel energetic.

Aerobic exercise (the sustained rhythmic activity of large muscle groups, which entails using large amounts of oxygen) increases heart rate, stroke volume, respiratory rate, and relaxation of blood vessels. Cardiovascular fitness and increased stamina are the goals. Body fat is also reduced. Aerobic exercises include running, jogging, brisk walking, swimming, aquadynamics, and aerobic dance.

Always check with your doctor before beginning any exercise program and for help in choosing the type of exercise that is best for you. Whatever type you choose, the goal should be to maintain a regular, moderate exercise program to enhance physical and emotional health. The exercise should involve large muscle groups in dynamic movement for about 20 minutes 3 or more days a week. The exertion should be within limits appropriate to your physical status and needs. At the end of exercise you should feel replenished rather than bored, burned out, or excessively fatigued.

What Makes Walking a Good Form of Regular Exercise?

Walking allows for psychomotor expression without the hazards of contact sports and is adaptable to a wide range of weather or geographic conditions, schedules, personalities, and body types. It can be social or asocial, organized or unorganized as an activity. The long-term effects on joints and organs of regular, sustained, vigorous walking currently are unknown; physicians do report a lower incidence of the type of musculoskeletal damage resulting from the "pounding" effects of jogging.

Making Time for Exercising Regularly Is Hard. What Can I Do to Make It Easier?

There are two major obstacles to overcome in undertaking and maintaining an exercise program: making exercise part of a lifestyle and avoiding injury. Suggestions for making exercise a safe part of a lifestyle include the following:

1. Start in small increments, and keep it fun.
2. Avoid exercising for 2 hours after a large meal, and do not eat for 1 hour after exercising.
3. Include at least 10 minutes of warm-up and cool-down exercises.
4. Use proper equipment and clothing.
5. Post goals, pictures of the ideal self, and notes of encouragement in a readily seen place for self-encouragement.
6. Use visualization daily to picture successful attainment of exercise benefit (e.g., looking toned or graceful or achieving an ideal weight).
7. Keep records of weekly measures of weight, blood pressure, and pulse.
8. Focus on the rewards of exercise; keep a record of feelings, and compare differences in relaxation, energy, concentration, and sleep patterns.
9. Work with a peer or join a structured exercise class, running club, or fitness center. Spend more time with people dedicated to wellness.
10. Stop exercising or at least slow down and consult with a practitioner if any unusual, unexplainable symptoms occur.
11. Reward yourself for working toward exercise goals as well as attaining them. For example, after a month in an exercise program, buy a new pair of running shoes or treat yourself to a special wish.

What Does a Walking (or "Rhythmic Walking") Program Entail?

Rhythmic walking consists of walking briskly, arms swinging, so your whole body is involved in the rhythm of your movement and your heart rate is increased. It is a regular program to benefit every system of your body.

A good exercise plan starts slowly, allowing your body time to adjust. It is important that you do something to exercise the whole body on a regular basis. *Regular* means every day, or at least every other day; build up to about 20 minutes 3 or more days a week. The right kind of exercise never makes you feel sore, stiff, or exhausted.

We repeat: *first check with your physician.* Before starting a program, it is important to know if there are precautions you need to take. This is especially important if you have high blood pressure, diabetes, joint or bone problems, or heart disease. People with these conditions can exercise, but they must follow certain guidelines to do it safely.

Rhythmic walking is inexpensive. It requires no special equipment or uniforms. Wear comfortable clothes in which you can move freely. You must have the right kind of shoes. Running or jogging shoes or the shoes specially designed for walking are good. The wrong shoes can cause painful damage, such as tendonitis. Select shoes designed for walking, jogging, or running; look for a shock-absorbent cushioning midsole. A watch with a second hand to measure your heart rate is also important.

Everyone who exercises outside the home should carry identification and change for a telephone call and money for a taxi. Some people like to carry a small water bottle such as a plastic soda bottle. To carry these items, a small backpack or hip pack leaves your hands free to swing.

If it is wet, slippery, or hot, or if you feel unsafe walking in your neighborhood, enclosed shopping malls can be great places for walking. Some malls open early, before the shopping crowds arrive, especially for people who want to walk.

How Hard Should I Exercise?

Your heart rate is the best indicator of how hard your body is working. As you work harder, your heart rate increases; as you slow down, your heart rate decreases. You can take your pulse to measure your heart rate. To experience the benefits of exercise, you need to work hard enough to get your heart rate up to a certain point, calling the *training heart rate,* and keep it there. Your nurse or doctor can tell you what your training heart rate should be and how to take your own pulse. Find these two things out before beginning your exercise regimen.

How Long Should I Exercise?

It is important to start exercising slowly and build up gradually. If you have been very ill or have not been exercising on a regular basis, start with a 5- or 10-minute walk and add 2 minutes each week. If you are able to build up endurance without problems, work up to 45 minutes daily or every other day. More than 60 minutes of rhythmic walking daily is not necessary.

A good workout consists of three phases: warm-up, training period, and cool-down. The warm-up is necessary to prepare the body for exercise. Warm up by walking slowly. Next, begin rhythmic walking. This is your training period. Work up to your target heart rate, and walk steadily for your set period of time. Finally, walk slowly to cool off. The cool-down is necessary to help your body recover and to prevent soreness or stiffness.

If you are exercising correctly, you should never feel exhausted after the cool-down. If you do, slow down and take it easier next time. If you feel fatigued for hours after exercise or if you feel sore and stiff, you have done too much or exercised incorrectly.

Starting to Exercise for a Healthy Heart

If you are recovering from heart surgery or a heart attack, your doctor has probably prescribed a daily graduated walking program to help your recovery. This program is also good if you have not exercised in a long time and your doctor recommends walking to help control your blood pressure or reduce your chances of cardiovascular disease.

Daily exercise may be one of the best gifts you can give yourself. It improves circulation, lowers blood pressure, helps in a weight control program, and strengthens your muscles. It can also help you sleep better, feel more energetic, and increase your sense of well-being.

General Guidelines

1. If you are recovering from heart surgery or a heart attack, have someone with you for the first several weeks.
2. Wait at least 2 hours after eating.

3. Wear comfortable rubber-soled walking shoes and loose clothing.
4. Avoid extreme heat or cold. Don't exercise if the temperature is over 85° F (particularly if the humidity is over 75%) or under 20° F. During bad weather, walk in a covered shopping mall or gym.
5. Always begin with a 5-minute warm-up of stretching and slow walking.
6. Adopt a steady, rhythmic pace and keep it up. If you have attacks of leg cramps (claudication), you may need to alternate walking with rest periods.
7. Watch for signs of overexertion. Stop walking if any of these symptoms occurs: chest pain (angina), palpitations, irregular heartbeat, dizziness or light-headedness, shortness of breath for more than 10 minutes, nausea or vomiting, extreme fatigue, pale or splotchy skin, or "cold sweat." Call your doctor if these symptoms persist.
8. Cool down with light activity for 5 minutes; for example, if you are walking fast, slow down to a stroll.

Graduated Walking Program

Graduated walking programs are designed to slowly increase the time, distance, and walking pace. Because they begin very slowly, you may be tempted to skip ahead if you feel the schedule is "too easy." Don't. The graduated schedule allows your heart time to adjust to increasing amounts of work. Skipping ahead may overwork your heart. Carry out the program just as your doctor orders. If you develop symptoms of overexertion, return to the previous week's schedule until you are ready to progress.

You must know the exact distance to determine how fast you should walk. You can measure the distance on your car odometer. If you find you walk the distance in less time than the schedule specifies, slow your pace down next time. If it takes longer, you need to walk a little faster.

As soon as you stop walking, take your pulse. Your heart rate should not exceed the upper limit of the target heart rate set by your doctor. For many people, this is less than 115 beats per minute.

FIRST 9 WEEKS

Week	Walking Time	Distance
1	5 minutes	¼ mile
2	5 minutes	¼ mile
3	10 minutes	½ mile
4	10 minutes	½ mile
5	15 minutes	¾ mile
6	15 minutes	¾ mile

FIRST 9 WEEKS—cont'd

7	20 minutes	1 mile
8	20 minutes	1½ miles
9	30 minutes	2 miles

At this point, you are ready to extend your walking time. Because the exercise will be sustained for a longer time, your pace will need to be a little slower the first few weeks. By week 12, your walking speed will increase to a brisk walk.

WEEKS 10 to 12

Week	Walking Time	Distance
10	40 minutes	2 miles
11	40 minutes	2 miles
12	60 minutes	3 miles

You must continue with an exercise program after week 12. You should continue your walking program, join a medically supervised walk-jog program, or add another form of exercise to your program such as bicycling. Follow your doctor's advice about the best program for you.

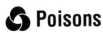 **Poisons**

Symptoms of Commonly Misused Drugs and Poisons

Amphetamine

Central nervous system (CNS) stimulation with restlessness, apprehension, irritability, delirium, hallucinations, tremors, and convulsions, followed by profound depression

Gastrointestinal (GI) distress

Dilated pupils, dry mouth

Antihistamines

CNS depression (children may be stimulated)

Atropine-like symptoms, dryness in mouth, fixed dilated pupils, flushing

GI distress

Aspirin

GI distress

Hyperventilation

Hyperpyrexia

Hypoprothrombinemia

Metabolic acidosis

Hypoglycemia

Barbiturates

Respiratory center depression with slow, shallow breathing; cyanosis often present

Circulatory depression and shock caused by depression of the vasomotor center, as well as direct action on smooth muscle in blood vessel wall

Water loss from skin and lungs; decrease in urine output; electrolytes variable

Chloral Hydrate

CNS depression

Cardiovascular depression

GI distress

Banana odor and blanching of lips

Modified from Chinn PL: *Child health maintenance: concepts in family-centered care,* ed 2, St Louis, 1979, Mosby. From Hancock LA, Fast GP, Murphy KE: Adolescence. In Edelman CL, Mandle CL, editors: *Health promotion throughout the lifespan,* ed 2, St Louis, 1990, Mosby.

"Knockout drops" are mixture of chloral and alcohol, producing potent depressant effect

Caustic effects with exophagitis (stricture) and gastritis

Codeine

CNS depression with muscular twitching and convulsions

Weakness, disturbed vision, miosis, dyspnea

Respiratory depression, collapse, coma

Ethyl Alcohol

CNS depression

Blood levels of 0.05%-0.15%—slight muscular incoordination and visual impairment and slowing of reaction time

Blood levels of 0.15%-0.3%—slurring of speech, definite visual impairment, muscular incoordination, sensory loss

Blood levels of 0.3%-0.5%—marked muscular incoordination, sensory loss, blurred or double vision, approaching stupor

At 5% concentration—coma, slowed and labored respiration, decreased reflexes, and sensory loss; death can occur

GI manifestations—one or more of the following:

Anorexia

Intermittent vomiting

Abdominal pain

Constipation

CNS manifestations—one or more of the following:

Irritability

Drowsiness

Persistent vomiting

Incoordination

Convulsions

Coma

Weakness or paralysis

Hypertension

Papilledema, optic atrophy, or both

Paralysis of one or more cranial nerves

Elevated cerebrospinal fluid (CSF) protein content

CSF plocytosis

Elevated CSF pressure

Hematologic manifestations—one or more of the following:

Hypochromic microcytic anemia

Significant degree of basophilic stippling of red blood cells

75%-100% red fluorescence in erythrocytes examined under ultraviolet light

Radiologic density at metaphyses of long bones

Marijuana

Exhilaration, euphoria, talkative, conjunctivitis, dryness of mouth
Later quiet, drowsy, sleepy
Chronic effects are tremors, anorexia, pallor, weakness, mental
  deterioration, with reduction of willpower and concentration
Users have odor of burnt rope on person or clothing

Meprobamate

CNS depression
Respiratory and cardiovascular collapse
Stupor, coma, hypotension, miosis, loss of reflexes

Morphine

Profound CNS depression from above downward and stimulation
  from below upward
Stupor, coma, miosis, slow and shallow respiration, cyanosis, tremors,
  convulsions
Severe retching and nausea

Nicotine

CNS stimulation followed by depression; clonic convulsions, fol-
  lowed by collapse and respiratory failure
GI distress, severe
Caustic effects on mouth, throat, esophagus, stomach

Parathion (Phosphate Ester Insecticides)

Nicotinic effects:
  Incoordination
  Fasciculation
  Paralysis
Muscarine effects:
  Miosis
  Sweating, salivation, tearing
  Pulmonary edema
  Bradycardia and hypertension
  Abdominal cramps, vomiting, diarrhea
General effects:
  Apathy
  Convulsions
  Coma

Poisoning

Poisoning from lead and poisonous plants is largely preventable. The nurse can use the following information to educate families and recommend precautionary measures.

Lead Poisoning

Effects of Lead Poisoning

Children: At low levels, the effects of lead poisoning may not be obvious. Nonetheless, low-level lead poisoning can slow a child's development, damage red blood cell production, and cause learning and behavioral difficulties, such as

- Excitability and hyperactivity
- Inability to pay attention
- Quick frustration

High levels may cause

- Central nervous system damage
- Kidney damage
- Reproductive system damage
- Anemia
- Deafness
- Blindness
- Coma
- Death

Adults (in addition to symptoms seen in children):

- Loss of hand-eye coordination
- Hypertension
- Stroke symptoms

There are usually no signs of lead poisoning, or they may be mistaken for flu or other illnesses. If present, symptoms may include

- Stomachache and cramps
- Irritability
- Fatigue
- Frequent vomiting
- Constipation
- Headache

Modified from State of Connecticut Department of Health Services, Lead Poisoning Prevention Program, Hartford, Connecticut, 1990.

- Sleep disorders
- Poor appetite

As more lead accumulates, clumsiness, weakness, and loss of recently acquired skills can occur.

Sources of Lead

Paint: Since 1977, household paints have contained far less than 1% lead. Previously, the lead content of paint was as high as 50%. Millions of American homes have some lead paint on the following surfaces:

- Windows and sills
- Doors, frames, and sills
- Walls and floors
- Stairs, railings, and banisters
- Woodwork, molding, and baseboards
- Porches and fences

Toys and furniture may also have lead paint.

Pipes and fixtures: Old water pipes may be made of lead, which can leach into drinking water. In buildings where lead soldering has been used on pipes and fixtures, water may be contaminated for up to 3 years (after plumbing installation or repair).

Other sources include:

- Dust from renovation, even a few houses away
- Antique pewter
- Drapery and window weights
- Battery casings
- Some folk medicines and folk cosmetics
- Some porcelain and pottery (especially imported)
- Dust or fumes from lead-stained glass, sandblasting
- Battery manufacturing

Steps for Prevention

- Be alert for chipping and flaking paint.
- Make sure child puts only safe, clean items in mouth.
- Feed well-balanced meals that are low in fat and high in iron, calcium, and zinc.
- Don't allow child to eat snow or icicles.
- Use safe interior paints on toys, walls, furniture, etc.
- Use pottery only for display if you're unsure about the glaze.
- Store food in glass, plastic, or stainless steel containers, not in open cans.

- Have your water tested, and draw drinking water only from the cold tap after allowing water to run for a few minutes (if you suspect lead danger).
- Have children wash hands before eating.
- Ask your local public health or housing/building official about an evaluation of lead hazards in your residence.
- *If you work with lead,* shower and change before coming home.
- Wash clothes separately from those of other family members.

Testing

Every child between the ages of 6 months and 6 years should be tested for lead at least once a year with a simple blood test. This may be done with a fingerstick or by venipuncture. If anyone in the household is diagnosed with lead poisoning, all other household members should be tested.

Screening for Lead Poisoning

Lead poisoning is one of the most common and preventable childhood environmental health problems in the United States. Although low-income, inner-city children have higher rates of lead poisoning, no socioeconomic group, geographic area, or racial or ethnic population is spared. In 1990, up to 3 million children under 6 years of age, 15% of all children in this age group, had blood lead levels greater than 10 µg/dl. Studies have shown associations between diminished intelligence, impaired neurobehavioral development, decreased hearing acuity, and growth inhibition and lead levels as low as 10 to 15 µg/dl.

Basics of Lead Screening

1. Risk assessment and counseling should begin during prenatal visits and continue after birth during regular office visits until at least the age of 6 years.
2. Each child's risk of lead toxicity should be evaluated. For this purpose, a structured set of questions such as that developed by the Centers for Disease Control (CDC) (Table 3) can be very helpful. If the answer to any of these questions is positive, the child is considered at high risk for exposure.

Clinician's Handbook of Preventive Services, Put Prevention into Practice Screening for Lead 1994.

Table 3 Recommended questions for assessing exposure risk

Does your child live in or regularly visit a house with peeling or chipping paint built before 1960? (This includes day care centers, preschools, homes of baby-sitters or relatives, etc.)

Does your child live in or regularly visit a house built before 1960 with recent, ongoing, or planned renovation or remodeling?

Does your child have a brother or sister, housemate, or playmate being followed or treated for lead poisoning (blood lead level ≥15 µg/dl)?

Does your child live with an adult whose job or hobby involves exposure to lead? (Such hobbies include ceramics, furniture refinishing, and stained glass work.)

Does your child live near an active lead smelter, battery recycling plant, or other industry likely to release lead?

Adapted from Centers for Disease Control: *Preventing lead poisoning in young children: a statement by the Centers for Disease Control,* Atlanta, 1991, Centers for Disease Control.

3. Screening by measurement of the blood lead level is more sensitive and specific than measurement of the erythrocyte protoporphyrin (EP) level. Blood lead levels <25 µg/dl cannot be reliably detected by EP testing. Elevated EP levels (≥35 µg/dl) require confirmation with blood lead testing.

4. Because of possible contamination of capillary specimens from environmental sources, venous blood samples are preferable to capillary sampling for blood lead levels. If capillary samples must be used, the precautions listed in Table 4 should be followed to minimize the chance of contamination. Elevated blood lead results (≥15 µg/dl) obtained on capillary specimens must be confirmed using venous blood. A child with a capillary lead level ≥70 µg/dl should be considered a medical emergency and retested with a venous sample immediately.

5. Blood lead test results can be interpreted and managed according to the CDC recommendations listed in Table 5.

6. Laboratories where blood is tested for lead levels should participate in a blood-lead proficiency testing program, such as the collaborative program between the Health Resources and Services Administration and CDC. Information on this program is available by calling (707) 488-7330.

7. Because iron deficiency can enhance lead absorption and toxicity, all children with blood lead levels ≥20 µg/dl should be tested for iron deficiency.

**Table 4 Recommendations for minimizing the contamination
of capillary blood samples obtained by finger stick**

Personnel who collect specimens should be well trained in and completely familiar with the collection procedure.

Puncturing the fingers of infants less than 1 year of age is not recommended. The heel is a more suitable site for these children.

If examination gloves are coated with powder, they should be rinsed with tap water.

The child's hand should be thoroughly washed with soap and water and then dried with a clean, low-lint towel.

Once washed, the finger or heel to be punctured should be cleansed with alcohol and not allowed to come into contact with any surface, including the child's other fingers.

Although its effectiveness in reducing contamination is under study, silicone spray can be used to form a protective layer between the skin and blood droplets.

The first droplet of blood, which contains tissue fluids, should be wiped off with sterile gauze or a cotton ball.

Do not collect blood that has run down the finger or onto the fingernail.

Contact between the skin and the collection container should be avoided.

Adapted from Centers for Disease Control: *Preventing lead poisoning in young children: a statement by the Centers for Disease Control,* Atlanta, 1991, Centers for Disease Control.

8. In addition to screening, it is important to provide guidance to parents about creating an environment safe from lead exposure for their children. Counseling should include advice on eliminating peeling or chipping paint, decreasing the lead content of water, preventing contact via hobbies or contaminated work clothing, remaining alert for pica behavior, and ensuring good hygiene. See Family Resources for publications to aid in counseling.

Family Resources

Getting the Lead Out. Food and Drug Administration. Superintendent of Documents, Consumer Information Center-3C, PO Box 100, Pueblo, CO 81002.

Home Buyer's Guide to Environmental Hazards. Environmental Protection Agency. Superintendent of Documents, Consumer Information Center-3C, PO Box 100, Pueblo, CO 81002.

Important Facts about Childhood Lead Poisoning Prevention. Centers for Disease Control and Prevention, Lead Poisoning Prevention Program, 1600 Clifton Rd., Atlanta, GA 30333; (707) 488-4880.

Table 5 CDC recommendations for follow-up of blood lead measurements

Class	Blood lead concentration (µg/dl)	Action	
I	≤9	Low risk:	6-35 months of age—Retest at 24 months of age (when blood levels peak), if resources allow. ≥36 and <72 months of age—Retesting not necessary unless history suggests exposure has increased.
		High risk:	6-35 months of age—Retest every 6 months. After two subsequent consecutive measurements are <10 µg/dl, or three are <15 µg/dl, retest once a year. ≥36 to 72 months of age—Retest once a year until sixth birthday.
IIA	10-14	Low risk:	6-35 months of age—Retest every 3-4 months. After two consecutive mesurements are <10 µg/dl or three are <15 µg/dl, retest once a year. ≥36 and <72 months of age—Retesting not necessary if all previous test results are <15 µg/dl, unless history suggests exposure has increased.
		High risk:	6-35 months of age—Retest every 3-4 months. After two consecutive measurements are <10 µg/dl or three are <15 µg/dl, retest once a year. ≥36 and <72 months of age—Retest once a year until sixth birthday.
IIB	15-19	Retest every 3-4 months. The family should be given education and nutritional counseling and a detailed environmental history should be taken to identify any obvious sources or pathways of lead exposure. If venous blood level is in this range in two consecutive tests 3-4 months apart, environmental investigation and abatement should be conducted, if resources permit.	

*Based on confirmatory blood lead level.

Adapted from Centers for Disease Control: *Preventing lead poisoning in young children: a statement by the Centers for Disease Control,* Atlanta, 1991, Centers for Disease Control.

Table 5   CDC recommendations for follow-up of blood lead measurements—cont'd

Class	Blood lead concentration (μg/dl)	Action
III	20-44*	Retest every 3-4 months. Conduct a complete medical evaluation, including iron deficiency testing. Environmental lead sources should be identified and eliminated. Pharmacologic treatment may be necessary.
IV	45-69*	Begin medical treatment and environmental assessment and remediation within 48 hours.
V	≥70*	Begin medical treatment and environmental assessment and remediation immediately.

What Everyone Should Know about Lead Poisoning. Alliance to End Childhood Lead Poisoning, 600 Pennsylvania Ave. SE, Suite 100, Washington, DC 20003 (individual copies); Channing L. Bete Co., Inc., 200 State Rd., South Deerfield, MA 01373; 1-800 628-7733 (bulk copies).

What You Should Know about Lead-Based Paint in Your Home. U.S. Consumer Product Safety Commission, Washington, DC 20207; 1-800 638-2666.

Provider Resources

Case Studies in Environmental Medicine: Lead Toxicity. Agency for Toxic Substances and Disease Registry, Division of Health Education, Mailstop E33, 1600 Clifton Rd., Atlanta, GA 30333; (707) 639-6205.

Preventing Lead Poisoning in Young Children: A Statement by the Centers for Disease Control. Centers for Disease Control and Prevention, Lead Poisoning Prevention Program, 1600 Clifton Rd., Atlanta, GA 30333; (707) 488-4880.

Blood-Lead Proficiency Testing Program. Centers for Disease Control and Prevention. (707) 488-4880.

Priority Groups for Screening Lead

- Children ages 6 to 72 months who live in or are frequent visitors to deteriorated housing built before 1960
- Children ages 6 to 72 months who live in housing built before 1960 with recent, ongoing, or planned renovation or remodeling
- Children ages 6 to 72 months who are siblings, housemates, or playmates of children with known lead poisoning
- Children ages 6 to 72 months whose parents or other household members participate in a lead-related occupation or hobby
- Children ages 6 to 72 months who live near active lead smelters, battery recycling plants, or other industries likely to result in atmospheric lead release

Poison Plants

A list of common house and garden plants is presented below. This is only a partial list, and some plants are known by more than one name. If you have questions about any plants not listed, call your local poison control center. There are many varieties of harmless plants that are possible to enjoy and still keep your children safe.

Nontoxic Plants

African violet	Dahlia	Lipstick plant
Air fern	Dandelion	Mountain ash
Aluminum plant	False aralia	Nasturtium
Aster	Fig leaf palm	Peperomia
Baby tears	Fuchsia	Petunia
Beauty bush	Gloxinia	Piggyback
Blood leaf	Hoya	Prayer plant
Boston fern	Hybiscus	Spider plant
Bridal veil	Impatiens	Spider aralia
Bromeliad	Inch plant	Swedish ivy
Christmas cactus	Jade	Yucca
Coleus	Kalanchoe	Zinnia
Coral bell	Lilac	

From USDHHS, PHS: *Preventing lead poisoning in young children,* 1991, CDC.

Modified from Connecticut Poison Center, Farmington, Connecticut, 1981, University of Connecticut Health Center.

Toxic Plants

The toxic parts of the plant are listed in parentheses using the key provided below. Where there is no code number, *all* parts are considered toxic.

1. Leaves, stems	**5.** Bulbs
2. Buds, berries	**6.** Seeds
3. Petals	**7.** Roots
4. Fruit, nuts	**8.** Bark

Acorns (1,2,4)
Amaryllis (5)
Angel trumpet
Azalea
Baneberry
Bird-of-paradise (1,2,5,6)
Bittersweet (1,4)
Black locust (1,5,8)
Bleeding heart
Bloodroot
Buckeye (3,4,6)
Buttercup
Caledium
Castor bean (1,6)
Christmas rose
Cowbane (7)
Crocus (1,3,5)
Crown of thorns
Daffodil
Daphne
Delphinium
Dogbane
Dumbcane
Elephant ear
Eucalyptus (1)
False parsley (7)

Four–o'clock (5,6,7)
Gladiolus (5)
Goldenrod (1,3)
Heather
Hellebore
Hemlock
Holly (1,2)
Hyacinth (5)
Indian corn
Indian poke
Ink berry
Iris
Jack-in-the-pulpit
Jasmine
Java bean
Jerusalem cherry (1,4)
Jequirity bean (6)
Jonquil
Juniper
Larkspur
Lily of the valley (1,3,4,7)
May apple
Mistletoe
Monk's hood
Morning glory
Mother-in-law

Mushrooms
Narcissus
Nightshade
Oleander (1,3)
Peony (7)
Philodendron
Poinsettia (1)
Poison ivy
Poison oak
Poison sumac
Pokeweed
Pothos
Privet (1,2)
Queen Ann's lace
Rhododendron
Rosary pea (2,4)
Skunk cabbage
Snow on the mountain
Spurge
Star-of-Bethlehem (3,5)
Sweet pea
Tobacco
Virginia creeper (2)
Wisteria (6)
Wolfsbane
Yew

What to Do If a Plant Poisoning Occurs

If you suspect that someone has ingested any amount of a plant that you believe is toxic or that you are unsure of, follow these guidelines:

1. Remove any plant parts from the person's mouth.
2. Give the person a small amount of water to drink.
3. Call the nearest Poison Control Center immediately. Don't wait for symptoms to develop.

Steps for Prevention

1. **Identify** all plants in your home and yard. This may be done by consulting a nursery, greenhouse, or florist. Show the plant to them.
2. **Label** the plants with proper names. You may want to write the name on tape and attach it to the pot. For the yard, you may want to make a map of the area indicating the name and location of each tree, plant, or bush. Keep this information handy in case of an emergency.
3. **Determine** which plants are safe and which are poisonous. Harmful plants should be kept well out of children's reach.
4. **Teach** children not to eat leaves, berries, buds, or flowers. Remind them to "look but don't lick—admire but don't pick."
5. **Store** all seeds and bulbs in a safe place.

Poisonous Parts of Common House and Garden Plants

Plant	Toxic part	Symptoms
Apple	Seeds	Releases cyanide when ingested in large quantities; may be fatal
Azalia	All parts	Nausea, vomiting, dyspnea, paralysis; may be fatal
Buttercup	All parts	Inflammation around mouth, stomach pains, vomiting, diarrhea, convulsions
Castor bean	Seeds	Burning of mouth and throat, excessive-thirst, convulsions; one or two seeds are near the lethal dose for adults
Croton	Plant juice	Gastroenteritis
Daffodil	Bulb	Nausea, vomiting, diarrhea; may be fatal
Dieffenbachia	All parts	Intensive burning and irritation of the mouth and tongue; death can occur if base of tongue swells enough to occlude air passages
English holly	Berries	Nausea, vomiting, diarrhea, central nervous system depression; may be fatal
English ivy	Leaves and berries	Dyspnea, vomiting, diarrhea, coma, and death
Hyacinth	Bulb	Nausea, vomiting, diarrhea; may be fatal
Iris	Underground stems	Digestive upset
Jasmine	All parts	Hallucinations, elevated temperature, tachycardia, paralysis
Lily of the valley	All parts	Arrhythmia, mental confusion, weakness, shock, and death
Mistletoe	Berries	Acute stomach and intestinal irritations with diarrhea; may be fatal
Oak tree	Acorns	Kidney failure, gastritis
Oleander	All parts	Digestive upset, bloody diarrhea, respiratory depression, cardiac arrhythmia, blurred vision, coma, and death

Continued.

From Edelman CL, Mandle CL: *Health promotion throughout the lifespan*, ed 3, St Louis, 1994, Mosby.

Poisonous parts of common house and garden plants—cont'd

Plant	Toxic part	Symptoms
Philodendron	All parts	Burning of lips, mouth, and tongue; swelling of tongue; dyspnea; kidney failure and death
Poinsettia	Leaves	Severe irritation to mouth, throat, and stomach; may be fatal
Potato	All green parts	Cardiac depression; may be fatal
Tomato	Green parts	Cardiac depression; may be fatal
Violet	Seeds	Taken in quantity, cathartic effects can be serious to infant
Yew	Foliage, seeds, bark	Nausea, vomiting, diarrhea, dyspnea, dilated pupils; death is sudden

Nursing Interventions to Prevent Plant Poisoning in Infants

- Keep plants out of reach of infants and young children.
- Never eat any part of a plant except those parts grown or sold as food.
- Keep jewelry made from unknown seeds or beans away from exploring infants.
- Learn to identify poisonous plants around your house and garden.
- Do not use unknown plants as medicines or teas.
- Pay close attention to infants at play inside and outside.
- Seek help whenever anyone chews or swallows a poisonous plant.
- Be aware that infants are more susceptible than adults to the effects of poisonous plants.

From Edelman CL, Mandle CL: *Health promotion throughout the lifespan,* ed 3, St Louis, 1994, Mosby.

Common Household Poisons

A checklist of poisonous products found in the home follows. Experience has shown that the products in *italic* type are the most dangerous poisons.

Kitchen

Aspirin
Drain cleaners (lye)
Furniture polish
Oven cleaner
Automatic dishwasher detergent
Ammonia
Powder and liquid detergents
Cleanser and scouring powders
Metal cleaners
Rust remover
Pills
Carpet and upholstery cleaners
Bleach
Vitamins

General

Plants
Flaking paint
Repainted toys
Broken plaster

Bedroom

Sleeping drugs
Tranquilizers
Other drugs
Jewelry cleaner
Cosmetics
Perfume
After-shave
Cologne

Reprinted, with permission, from *Poison primer,* Galveston, no date, Southeast Texas Poison Center.

Closets, Attic, Storage Places

*Rat poison, ant poison, and
    insecticides*
Mothballs

Laundry Room

Bleaches
Soap and detergents
Disinfectant
Bluing, dyes
Carbon tetrachloride

Bathroom, Garage, Basement

Aspirin
All drugs and pills
Drain cleaners (lye)
Iron pills
Toilet bowl cleaners
Shampoo, wave lotion, and sprays

Hand lotion
Creams
Nail polish and remover
Suntan lotions
Deodorants
Shaving lotions
Hair remover
Lye
Kerosene
Pesticides
Gasoline
Lighter fluid
Turpentine
Paint remover and thinner
Antifreeze
Lime
Paint
Weed killers
Fertilizers

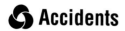 **Accidents**

Causes of Falls

Accidents
    True accidents (trips, slips, etc.)
    Interactions between environmental hazards and factors increasing
        susceptibility
Syncope (sudden loss of consciousness)
Drop attacks (sudden leg weaknesses, without loss of consciousness)
Dizziness or vertigo
    Vestibular disease
    CNS disease
Orthostatic hypotension
    Hypovolemia or low cardiac output
    Autonomic dysfunction
    Impaired venous return
    Prolonged bed rest
    Drug-induced hypotension
    Postprandial hypotension
Drug-related causes
    Diuretics
    Antihypertensives
    Tricyclic antidepressants
    Sedatives
    Antipsychotics
    Hypoglycemics
    Alcohol
Specific disease processes
    Acute illness of any kind ("premonitory fall")
    Cardiovascular
        Arrhythmias
        Valvular heart disease (aortic stenosis)
        Carotid sinus syncope
Neurologic causes
    Transient ischemic attack (TIA)
    Stroke (acute)
    Seizure disorder
    Parkinson's disease

From Kane R, Ouslander J, Abrass I: *Essentials of clinical geriatrics,* New York, 1994, McGraw-Hill.

Cervical or lumbar spondylosis (with spinal cord or nerve root compression)

Cerebellar disease

Normal-pressure hydrocephalus (gait disorder)

CNS lesions (e.g., tumor, subdural hematoma)

Idiopathic (no specific cause identifiable)

Risk Assessment for Falls Scale II (RAFS II)

Patient Name _____

Admission Date _____

Diagnoses _____

Sex _____ Age _____

Total Score _____
High Risk—14 or more

Categories	0	1	2	3	Score
(1) Assessment completed _____ days since admission		≥15 days	8-14 days	Admission to day 7	
(2) Years of age	<19	20-60	61-74	≥75	
(3) History of fall	No fall in last year	Fell in past 6 months	Fell in past 1-5 months	Fell in past 4 weeks	

Continued.

From Maas M, Buckwalter K, Hardy M: *Nursing diagnoses and intervention for the elderly*, Reading, 1991, Addison-Wesley.

Risk Assessment for Falls Scale II (RAFS II)—cont'd

Categories	0	1	2	3	Score
(4) Balance	Ambulates well alone	Ambulates alone with assistive device	Needs assist and assistive device OR help of 2 persons	Can stand and pivot only with help	
(5) Mental status	Oriented × 3	Oriented × 2 (person/place)	Oriented × 1 (person/self)	Disoriented	
(6) Agitation	No	Mild; uses abrasive language occasionally	Moderate; calls out and uses threatening language	Severe; combative; must be restrained	
(7) Depressed	No	Mild; feels blue, burned out; has poor appetite but no weight loss or sleep disturbances	Moderate; statements of low self-esteem; fatigue; sleep problems and poor appetite	Severe; poor concentration; preoccupied; poor appetite, with weight loss of ≥10 lb; apathy	
(8) Anxious	No	Mild; alert, motivated, restless, sleepless	Moderate; asks for reassurance; focuses on immediate concerns; has rapid speech; may repeat questions	Severe; very preoccupied; focuses on specific details; exhibits psychomotor behavior; complains of feelings of choking or paranoia	

	Normal	Corrected by glasses or monocular vision (blind in 1 eye/ lazy eye)	Blurred/cataract/ glaucoma	Visual field cut (hemi- anopsia, scotoma, tunnel vision)	
(9) Vision					
(10) Communication	Normal	Hearing loss	Speech disorder: dysphasia/ language barrier	Both hearing and speech disorder or language barrier	
(11) Medications (check category of medi- cine)	No effectors	CV effector	CNS effector	Both CV and CNS ef- fectors prescribed	
CV meds Diuretic Beta blocker Digitalis prep Vasodilator Other (name)	CNS meds Tranquilizers Hypnotic/analgesic sedative Psychotropic (e.g., Haldol) Other (name)				
(12) Chronic diseases (check) Cardiovascular CNS Pulmonary Cancer Other (Name)	None	1	2	3 or more	

Continued.

Risk Assessment for Falls Scale II (RAFS II)—cont'd

Categories	0	1	2	3	Score
(13) Urinary Nocturia ≥2 per night Urgency—sudden strong urge Frequency ≥6 times per day	None	1	2	All 3	

Total: _____

Scoring the Risk Assessment for Falls Scale

In the risk assessment for falls scale (RAFS), the degree of risk is directly proportional to the RAFS score; that is, the risk increases as the score increases. The critical score for the samples that have been tested has been 14 and above. However, this score should be determined for specific elderly groups by scoring the patients and then prospectively following them to determine if those with a score of less than 14 fall. If elderly persons with the lower scores fall, a decision must be made. Is the incidence frequent enough to reduce the critical score?

Based on the admission nursing assessment, the RAFS should be completed during the first 24 hours after admission and preferably during the first 8 hours. Early assessment is crucial because, for most individuals, the risk for falling is greatest during the first days of hospitalization or admission to an extended care facility. Review each category and, using the operational definitions, score each category 0–3 or 0–2 in the category of days since admission. If the score is 14 or more, the elderly patient is at high risk. If there is an area that needs to be assessed over a longer period of time—such as depression—this segment can be delayed, but the rest of the instrument should be completed in the event the elderly patient is at increased risk from the other categories and therefore should be on precautions.

Reassessment should occur at predetermined intervals, for example, if the elder's condition has deteriorated overall or in certain categories such as mental status. This elderly individual's score may have increased to a point of being at risk. Also, special precautions may be discontinued if the elderly patient's condition has improved and the risk is changed.

Once scoring has been completed, the elder also should be evaluated for risk of trauma if a fall should occur. Elderly persons who are at great risk of sustaining significant trauma should be carefully evaluated and basic measures should be taken despite a marginal RAFS score. For example, if the elderly person has some type of bleeding disorder, a fall may cause significant bleeding. Thus this individual should receive education about falls and should be instructed to request assistance when walking if the individual has any problems with ambulation.

Assessment for Clients Who Fall

1. Current medical problems_____
_____
_____

2. Medications_____
_____
_____

3. Is there a previous history of falls?
   ____ Yes ____ No
   If yes:
   Number of previous falls ____
   Is there a pattern?
   ____ Yes ____ No
   Frequency
   _____

   Time of day
   _____

   Position
   _____

   Activity
   _____

   Circumstances
   _____
   _____

4. Circumstances surrounding current fall
   Time of day
   _____

   Location
   _____

   Relationship to specific activities (e.g., toileting, climbing or descending stairs, exercise, turning head)
   _____
   _____
   _____

   Witness(es)
   _____
   _____
   _____

From Kane R, Ouslander J, Abrass I: *Essentials of clinical geriatrics,* New York, 1994, McGraw-Hill.

Environmental hazards (e.g., poor lighting, loose rug, uneven floor, other obstacles)

_____

_____

_____

5. Client's description of and reasons for the fall (in client's words)

_____

_____

_____

_____

6. Questions to the client (or witness)
   a. Did you know you were going to fall?
      ____ Yes ____ No
   b. After you fell, did you know what happened?
      ____ Yes ____ No
   c. Did you lose consciousness (pass out)?
      ____ Yes ____ No
      If yes, how long were you unconscious? ____ minutes.
      Were you aware of what happened after you awoke?
      ____ Yes ____ No
      Had you lost control of your bowel or bladder?
      ____ Yes ____ No
   d. Were you able to get up right away?
      ____ Yes ____ No
   e. Did you have any pain or injury after the fall?
      ____ Yes ____ No
   f. Did you do any of the following just before the fall?
      ____ Trip
      ____ Slip
      ____ Stand up quickly
      ____ Turn your head suddenly
      ____ Cough
      ____ Urinate
      ____ Have a bowel movement
      ____ Eat a large meal
   g. Did you have any of the following symptoms just before you fell?
      ____ Light-headedness
      ____ Vertigo (spinning around the room or vice versa)
      ____ Palpitations
      ____ Shortness of breath
      ____ Weakness or numbness on one side of the body

_____ Sudden weakness of both legs
_____ Slurred speech
_____ Difficulty saying what you wanted to say
_____ Strange smells
_____ Flashing lights (scotomata)

7. Physical assessment
   a. Postural vital signs

	Supine	Sitting	Standing
Blood pressure	___ / ___	___ / ___	___ / ___
Pulse	_____	_____	_____
Blood pressure other arm		___ / ___	

   b. Skin
      _____ Bruises
      _____ Diminished turgor
   c. Vision
      _____ Adequate for independent ambulation
      _____ Limits mobility, but still independent
      _____ Inadequate for independent ambulation
   d. Neck
      _____ Supple
      _____ Full range of motion
      _____ Symptoms with rotation
   e. Cardiovascular
      _____ Arrhythmia
      _____ Murmur suggestive of aortic stenosis
      _____ Signs of heart failure (Describe: _____
      _____)
      _____ Carotid bruit(s)
   f. Musculoskeletal
      _____ Trauma or suspected fracture
      _____ Deformity
      _____ Limited range of motion
      _____ Joint inflammation
   g. Podiatric
      Are any of the following impairing ambulation?
      _____ Callouses
      _____ Bunions
      _____ Nail deformity
      _____ Ulceration
      _____ Poorly fitted or otherwise inadequate shoes

h. Neurologic
____ Abnormal mental status
____ Focal neurologic sign(s)
____ Muscular weakness
____ Muscular rigidity/spasticity
____ Bradykinesia
____ Resting tremor
____ Peripheral neuropathy
____ Ataxia, finger to nose
____ Ataxia, heel to shin
Describe positive findings: _____

_____

i. Mobility
____ Ambulates independently
____ Uses aid
     ____ Cane
     ____ Quad-cane
     ____ Walker
____ Wheelchair, able to transfer independently
____ Wheelchair, needs help to transfer

j. Stability and gait

	Normal	Abnormal
Sitting balance	____	____
Rising from sitting to standing	____	____
Standing balance with eyes open	____	____
Standing balance with eyes closed (Romberg test)	____	____
Initiation of walking	____	____
Length of stride	____	____
Distance feet apart	____	____
Turning	____	____
Sitting down	____	____

Describe positive findings:

_____

_____

_____

8. Diagnostic studies

Test/procedure	Result
_____	_____
_____	_____
_____	_____

Test/procedure	Result

Fall Risk Factors for Elders

In the community	In an institution
Environmental hazards	Acute and severe chronic illness, debilitation
Female or single (incidence increases with age)	Functional limitations in self-care activities
Sedative and alcohol use, psychoactive medications	Women (75 years and older)
Previous falls, unsteadiness, dizziness	Multiple disorders and medications
Acute and recent illness	Recent relocation, unfamiliar with facility
Pathologic conditions, drop attacks	Wheelchair bound
Cognitive impairment, disorientation	Sensory deficits
Disability of lower extremities	Impaired locomotion
Abnormalities of balance and gait	Predisposing physiologic and psychologic conditions
Foot problems	Preoccupation with stressors
Depression, anxiety	Anxiety related to previous falls
Decreased vision or hearing	Confusion, dementia
Fear of falling	Urinary urgency, particularly nocturia
Terminal drop (dies in following year to 2 years)	
Recent relocation	
Assistive devices needed for walking	
Skeletal and neuromuscular changes that predispose to weakness and postural imbalance	

Community: from Tinetti et al (1988); Craven and Bruno (1986). Institution: from Craven and Bruno (1986); Kaufmann (1985) and Barbieri, 1983; and Fife et al, 1984. In Ebersole P and Hess P: Toward healthy aging: Human needs and nursing response, ed. 4, St Louis, 1994, Mosby.

Types of Falls

1. Slips and trips: the patient may falsely attribute the fall to these causes when in reality it is due to a physical deficit.
2. Falls while attempting a difficult maneuver (such as climbing over a bed rail).
3. Syncope: the loss of consciousness immediately precedes the fall and may itself be preceded by a brief interval of giddiness or unsteadiness.
4. Seizure: the loss of consciousness accompanies the fall. It may be preceded by an aura. It may or may not be accompanied by clonic movements and incontinence.
5. Drop attack: sudden loss of muscular tone without loss of consciousness.
6. Vertigo: the patient experiences true dizziness (the room seems to spin) and falls to one side or the other.
7. Sliding off furniture: caused by weakness or somnolence.

From Wieman H, Calkins E: Falls. In Calkins E, Davis P, Ford M, editors: *The practice of geriatrics,* Philadelphia, 1986, Saunders. In Ebersole P, Hess P: *Toward healthy aging: human needs and nursing response,* ed 4, St Louis, 1994, Mosby.

Measures to Prevent Falls

Stairs

Install treads with a uniform effective depth of 9 inches and 9-inch risers (vertical face of a step).

Install uniform-textured or plain-color surfaces on each tread.

Mark edge of tread with a built-in or painted strip that contrasts noticeably with remainder of tread.

Ensure proper lighting of each tread. Block sun or light bulb glare with translucent shades or screen, or use lower-wattage bulbs.

Ensure adequate headroom so user need not duck to negotiate stairway.

Design door at stairway entrance or exit so that door swings away from stairs.

Remove protruding objects (coat hooks, shelves, light fixtures, etc.) from stairway walls.

Maintain outdoor steps and walkways in firm condition, free of splinters, cracks, and holes.

From Archea et al: *Guidelines for stair safety,* NBS Building Ser. 120, 1979, Washington, DC, US Government Printing Office.

Handrails

Install smooth but slip-resistant handrail at least 2 inches from wall so user can grasp it.

Secure handrail firmly to support user's weight, especially at top and bottom of stairway.

Install grab bars in bathroom near toilet and tub. Place nonskid mat or strips in tub.

Floor Coverings

Secure all carpeting, mats, and tile. Place nonskid backing under small rugs.

Measures to Prevent Fire and Burns

Do not smoke in bed or when sleepy.

When cooking, do not wear loose-fitting clothing (bathrobes, nightgowns, pajamas).

Set thermostats for water heater or faucets so that the water does not become too hot.

Install a portable hand fire extinguisher in the kitchen.

Keep access to outside door(s) unobstructed.

Identify emergency exits in public buildings.

If you consider entering a boarding or foster home, check to see that it has smoke detectors, a sprinkler system, and fire extinguishers.

Wear clothing that is nonflammable or treated with a permanent flame-retardant finish.

Fabrics of animal hair, wool, or silk are less flammable.

Use several electrical outlets to avoid overloading.

From Age Page, 1980, Bulletin of National Institute on Aging.

General Safety Precautions

More deaths in the United States are caused by accidents than most people realize. In fact, accidents are the leading cause of death for children in this country. Yet about 90% of all accidents are preventable. Most households would reduce their annual need for emergency medical treatment if they would simply observe general safety precautions in a few key lifestyle areas.

Take time to check your own surroundings for potential hazards, and reduce or eliminate them. Below are some general guidelines for preventing common accidents. These guidelines encompass motor vehicles, sports and recreation, electrical and mechanical equipment, preventing falls, poisonings and ingestions, fire, and swimming pools. Use this as a checklist to evaluate your safety standards.

Motor Vehicles

Naturally all automobiles should be maintained in good mechanical condition. Seat belts should be worn at all times; never start the car until everyone has buckled up. You'll be surprised at how little time it takes for your friends and family to start buckling up automatically whenever they ride with you! Look carefully in front and in back of the car before accelerating, and make sure all car doors are locked when a child travels in your car. Young children should never be left alone in a car, and heavy or sharp objects should not be placed on the same seat with a child. Small children should ride in a car seat appropriate for their age.

Sports and Recreation

Many accidents in sports and recreation could be prevented by keeping equipment in good condition and proper working order.

We live in a rushed age. We often go directly from work to recreation or sports programs. Still, train yourself always to stop by the locker room first: always wear appropriate clothing and shoes (if needed) for the activity. You'll prevent a lot of injuries over the years by simply taking a few minutes before you play. Once involved in the sport or activity of your choice, do not attempt activities beyond your physical endurance. Injuring yourself will simply put you further back on the fitness scale.

Finally, keep all firearms and ammunition locked up.

Electrical and Mechanical Equipment

Only devices approved by Underwriters' Laboratories should be installed, and they should be inspected periodically. Dry your hands before touching appliances, and keep radios, fans, portable heaters, and hair dryers out of the bathroom. Discourage children from playing with or being in an area where appliances or power tools (e.g., washing machine, clothes dryer, saw, or lawn mower) are being used. Disconnect appliances after using them and before attempting minor repairs. Avoid overloading electrical circuits.

Keep garden equipment and machinery in a restricted area. As soon as each child in your household is old enough, teach him or her how to use the equipment properly.

Preventing Falls

You might be surprised at the number of broken bones that are a result of falls in or around the house each year. These are not only painful, time consuming, and expensive to fix—they can also be pretty embarrassing! Here are a few quick tips for saving bones, medical bills, and face: Keep stairs well lighted and free of clutter; provide sturdy railings. Anchor small rugs securely, and use rubber mats in the bathtub and shower. Use only sturdy ladders for climbing.

Poisonings and Ingestions

Poisonings and ingestions are the most common type of household accident among children and the elderly, but they can happen to anyone. Here are a few general guidelines: When cleaning, never mix bleaches with ammonia, vinegar, and other household cleaners. Label all medications clearly, and childproof your home by placing medications out of reach of children. But, just in case, keep emergency medical numbers clear, up-to-date, and easy to find.

Fire

Figure out an adequate fire escape plan, and routinely conduct home fire drills. Teach each child the escape routes as soon as he or she is old enough.

Keep a pressure-type hand fire extinguisher on each floor of your household. Instruct all family members who are old enough in its use. In addition, teach children about the danger of smoke inhalation. Use such slogans as "Stop, drop, and roll."

Communicable and Infectious Diseases

Recommended Childhood Immunization Schedule—United States, January–June, 1996

Vaccines are listed under the routinely recommended ages. Bars indicate range of acceptable ages for vaccination. Shaded bars indicate *catch-up vaccination:* at 11–12 years of age, hepatitis B vaccine should be administered to children not previously vaccinated, and varicella zoster virus vaccine should be administered to children not previously vaccinated who lack a reliable history of chickenpox.

Vaccine	Birth	1 mo	2 mos	4 mos	6 mos	12 mos	15 mos	18 mos	4-6 yrs	11-12 yrs	14-16 yrs
Hepatitis B	Hep B-1	Hep B-2			Hep B-3					Hep B[2]	
Diphtheria, tetanus, pertussis[3]			DTP	DTP	DTP	DTP[3] (DTaP at 15+ m)			DTP or DTaP	Td	
Haemophilus influenzae type b[4]			Hib	Hib	Hib[4]	Hib[4]					
Polio[5]			OPV[5]	OPV	OPV	OPV			OPV		
Measles, mumps, rubella[6]						MMR			MMR[6] or MMR[6]		
Varicella zoster virus vaccine[7]							Var			Var[7]	

1. *Infants born to HBsAg-negative mothers* should receive 2.5 μg of Merck vaccine (Recombivax HB) or 10 μg of SmithKline Beecham (SB) vaccine (Engerix-B). The 2nd dose should be administered ≥1 mo after the 1st dose.

   Infants born to HBsAG-positive mothers should receive 0.5 mL Hepatitis B Immune Globulin (HBIG) within 12 hr of birth, and either 5 μg of Merck vaccine (Recombivax HB) or 10 μg of SB vaccine (Engerix-B) at a separate site. The 2nd dose is recommended at 1-2 mo and the 3rd dose at 6 mo.

   Infants born to mothers whose HBsAg status is unknown should receive either 5 μg of Merck vaccine (Recombivax HB) or 10 μg of SB vaccine (Engerix-B) within 12 hr of birth. The 2nd dose of vaccine is recommended at age 1 mo and the 3rd dose at 6 mo.

2. Adolescents who have not previously received 3 doses of hepatitis B vaccine should initiate or complete the series at the 11-12 year-old visit. The 2nd dose should be administered at least 1 mo after the 1st dose, and the 3rd dose shold be administered at least 4 mo after the 1st dose and at least 2 mo after the 2nd dose.

3. DTP4 may be administered at 12 mo of age, if at least 6 mo have elapsed since DTP3. DTaP (diphtheria and tetanus toxoids and acellular pertussis vaccine) is licensed for the 4th and/or 5th vaccine dose(s) for children age ≥15 mo and may be preferred for these doses in this age group. Td (tetanus and diphtheria, toxoids, adsorbed, for adult use) is recommended at age 11-12 if at least 5 yr have elapsed since the last dose of DTP, DTaP, or DT.

4. Three *H. influenzae* type b (Hib) conjugate vaccines are licensed for infant use. If PRP-OMP (pedvaxHIB [Merck]) is administered at 2 and 4 mo of age, a dose at 6 mo is not required. After completing the primary series, any Hib conjugate vaccine may be used as a booster.

5. Oral poliovirus vaccine (OPV) is recommended for routine infant vaccination. Inactivated poliovirus vaccine (IPV) is recommmded for persons with a congenital or acquired immune deficiency disease or an altered immune status as a result of disease or immunosupressive therapy, as well as their household contacts, and is an acceptable alternative for other persons. The primary 3-dose series for IPV should be given with a minimum interval of 4 wk between the 1st and 2nd doses and 6 mo between the 2nd and 3rd doses.

6. The 2nd dose of MMR is routinely recommended at age 4-6 yr or at age 11-12 yr, but may be administered at any visit, provided at least 1 mo has elapsed since receipt of the 1st dose.

7. Varicella zoster virus vaccine (Var) can be administered to susceptible children any time after age 12 mo. Unvaccinated children who lack a reliable history of chickenpox should be vaccinated at the 11-12 year-old visit.

Approved by the Advisory Committee on Immunization Practices (ACIP), the American Academy of Pediatrics (AAP), and the American Academy of Family Physicians (AAFP).

Approved by the Advisory Committee on Immunization Practices (ACIP), the American Academy of Pediatrics (AAP), and the American Academy of Family Physicians (AAFP).

Summary of Sexually Transmitted Diseases

I. *Candida albicans*
   A. Etiologic agent: Gram-positive fungus—*Candida Albicans.*
   B. Mode of spread: Sexual contact; nonsexual: drugs-diabetes, pregnancy, oral contraceptives.
   C. Incubation period: Unknown.
   D. Clinical picture:
      Male: itching, irritating discharge, plaque of cheesy material under foreskin.
      Female: vaginal discharge: thick, white, cheesy, or curdlike material; vulval skin red and excoriated.
   E. Laboratory test: Wet prep.
   F. Treatment: Nystatin (Mycostatin) vaginal tablets, miconazole (Monostat Vaginal Creme).
   G. Complications and sequelae. Relapse of problem, especially when pregnant, infection of newborn if mother not treated; superficial infection of skin and mucus membranes.
   H. Nursing education message to emphasize:
      1. Client should arrange to return for other tests, arrange of test-of-cure in 14 days.
      2. Client should use good genital hygiene. For women, pantyhose serves as occlusive dressing, creating heat and moisture.

II. Genital warts (*Condyloma acuminata*)
   A. Etiologic agent: Infectious papovavirus (DNA virus).
   B. Mode of spread: Autoinoculations; sexual contact.
   C. Incubation period: Prolonged, month or more.
   D. Clinical picture: Digitating, papular, pedunculated lesions growing beneath or on prepuce, at external meatus or on glans and coronal sulcus. Lesions may be red or dirty gray and may remain singular and discrete; however, more often are in clusters.
   E. Laboratory test: Microscopically.
   F. Treatment: 20%-25% podophyllin in tincture of benzoin, desiccaction, surgery.
   G. Contacts: Examination of fingers, mouth, genitals of contact.

Modified from U.S. Department of Health and Human Services, Public Health Service, Centers for Disease Control: *Sexually transmitted disease summary,* Washington, D.C., 1982, U.S. Government Printing Office. Modified from Edelman CL, Mandle CL: *Health promotion throughout the lifespan,* ed 3, St Louis, 1994, Mosby.

H. Complications and sequelae:
1. Lesions may enlarge and produce tissue destruction.
2. Giant condyloma, although histologically benign, may simulate carcinoma.
3. In pregnancy, warts enlarge, are extremely vascular, and may obstruct the birth canal, necessitating cesarean section.

I. Nursing education message to emphasize:
1. Client should return for weekly or biweekly treatment and follow-up until lesions have resolved.
2. Partners should be examined for warts.
3. Client should abstain from sex or use condoms at time of therapy.

III. *Herpes genitalis*
A. Etiologic agent: Herpesvirus type 2.
B. Mode of spread: Autoinoculations; sexual contact.
C. Incubation period: 2-10 days maximum.
D. Clinical picture:
1. Primary: large, discrete vesicles on erythematous base; painless inguinal adenopathy; vesicles rupture; stage lasts 4-6 weeks.
2. Recurrent: clusters of small vesicles, more itchy than painful; lasts couple of hours to 10 days; no adenopathy.

E. Laboratory test: Tzanck test.
F. Treatment: No specific treatment; treat symptomatically.
G. Contacts: No specific follow-up.
H. Complications and sequelae:
1. Males and females: neuralgia, meningitis, ascending myelitis, urethral strictures, and lymphatic suppuration may occur.
2. Females: possibly an increased risk for cervical cancer and fetal wastage.
3. Neonates: Virus from an active genital infection may be transmitted during vaginal delivery, causing congenital herpes. Congenital herpes ranges from clinically inapparent infections, to local infections of eyes, skin, or mucous membranes, to severe, disseminated infection that may involve the central nervous system. Infection has high infant fatality rate, and many survivors have ocular or neurologic sequelae.

I. Nursing education message to emphasize:
1. Client should keep involved area clean and dry.
2. Because both initial and recurrent lesions shed high

concentrations of virus, clients should abstain from sex while symptomatic.

3. Undetermined but presumably small risk of transmission also exists during asymptomatic intervals. Condoms may offer some protection.

4. Annual Pap smears are recommended. Pregnant women should make their obstetricians aware of any history of herpes.

IV. *Molluscum contagiosum*

A. Etiologic agent: Pox virus group—DNA virus.

B. Mode of spread: Direct contact.

C. Incubation period: 14-50 days, average 30 days.

D. Clinical picture: Waxy, globular papule, pinhead to pea-size or larger; lesions elevated, shiny, translucent, and firm with no increase; pigmentation in center of lesions is small, dark colored with umbilication, from which curdlike substance may be expressed.

E. Laboratory test: Examination of crushed smear, wafer bodies.

F. Treatment: Desiccation or curetage of lesion.

G. Contacts: Examine contacts.

H. Complications and sequelae:

1. Secondary infection, usually with staphylococci, may occur.

2. Lesions rarely greater than 10 mm in diameter.

I. Nursing education message to emphasize:

1. Client should return for reexamination 1 month after treatment so that any new lesions can be removed.

2. Partners should be examined.

V. Nongonococcal urethritis (NGU)

A. Etiologic agent: *Chlamydia* group in half of cases.

B. Mode of spread: Sexual contact.

C. Incubation period: 1-3 weeks.

D. Clinical picture:

1. Male: frequency of micturition, watery mucoid urethral discharge, symptoms more mild than gonococcal urethritis.

2. Female: commonly a symptomatic carrier, vaginal discharge, dysuria, frequency of micturition.

E. Laboratory test: Smears and cultures.

F. Treatment: Broad-spectrum antibiotics.

G. Contacts: Treat steady partner.

H. Complications and sequelae:

1. Urethral strictures.

2. Prostatitis.

    3. Epididymitis.

    4. Chlamydial NGU may be transmitted to female sexual partners, resulting in mucopurulent endocervicitis and pelvic inflammatory disease.

    5. If pregnancy, risk of spontaneous abortion, stillbirth, and postpartum fever.

    6. Neonatal chlamydial infections such as ophthalmia or pneumonia may be acquired during delivery from infected endocervix.

  I. Nursing education message to emphasize:

    1. Client should understand how to take any prescribed oral medication. If tetracycline is prescribed, take 1 hour before or 2 hours after meals, and avoid dairy products, antacids, iron, other mineral-containing preparations, and sunlight.

    2. Client should return for test-of-cure or evaluation 4-7 days after completion of therapy, or earlier if symptoms persist or recur.

    3. Refer sexual partners for examination and treatment.

    4. Client and partners avoid sex until cured.

    5. Client should use condoms to prevent future infections.

VI. *Pediculus pubis*

  A. Etiologic agent: *Pthirus pubis:* grayish ectoparasite 1-4 mm long with claws for clinging to hair.

  B. Mode of spread: Sexual contact, occasionally from towels, clothing, toilet seats.

  C. Incubation period: Approximately 4 weeks.

  D. Clinical picture: Intense itching, irritation of skin, pinhead-size blood spots on underwear, nits attached to hair.

  E. Laboratory test: Identification of organism on body.

  F. Treatment: Kwell shampoo, lotion, creme.

  G. Contacts: To be examined and treated.

  H. Complications and sequelae:

    1. Secondary excoriations.

    2. Lymphadenitis.

    3. Pyoderma.

  I. Nursing education message to emphasize:

    1. Clothing and linen should be disinfected by washing them in hot water, by dry-cleaning them, or by removing them from human exposure for 1-2 weeks.

    2. Client should avoid sexual or close physical contact until after treatment.

    3. Client should ensure examination of sexual partners as soon as possible.

    4. Client should return if problem is not cured or if it recurs.

VII. Scabies
   A. Etiologic agent: *Sarcoptes scabiei:* female mite 0.3-0.4 mm, male somewhat smaller.
   B. Mode of spread: Prolonged, close contact with infected person.
   C. Incubation period: 4-6 weeks.
   D. Clinical picture: Severe itching that is worse at night, skin lesions papular and vesicular, burrows appear as grayish or black, irregular lines.
   E. Laboratory test: Microscopic identification.
   F. Treatment: Kwell shampoo, creme, lotion.
   G. Contacts: Examine and treat all sexual contacts.
   H. Complications and sequelae:
      1. Secondary bacterial infection may occur, particularly with nephrogenic strains of streptococci.
      2. Norwegian or crusted scabies (with up to 2 million adult mites in crusts) pose risk for patients with neurologic defects and those who are immunologically incompetent.
   I. Nursing education message to emphasize:
      1. Clothing and linen should be disinfected by washing them with hot water, by dry-cleaning them, or by removing them from human exposure for 1-2 weeks.
      2. Client should avoid sexual or close physical contact until after treatment.
      3. Ensure examination of sexual partners as soon as possible.
      4. Client should return if problem is not cured or recurs.
VIII. *Trichomonas vaginalis*
   A. Etiologic agent: Protozoan with undulating membrane and four flagella.
   B. Mode of spread: Sexual contact.
   C. Incubation period: 4-28 days.
   D. Clinical picture:
      Male: slight itching, moisture on tip of penis, slight early-morning urethral discharge.
      Female: itching and redness of vulva and skin inside thighs, strawberry-like appearance of cervix, vaginal discharge watery, copious, frothy.
   E. Laboratory test: Wet prep.
   F. Treatment: Metronidazole (Flagyl).
   G. Contacts: Examine and treat steady partners.
   H. Complications and sequelae:
      1. Secondary excoriations.

    2. Recurrent infections common.

  I. Nursing education message to emphasize:

    1. Client should understand how to take or use any prescribed medications.

      a. With trichomoniasis or vaginitis: Client should avoid alcoholic beverages until 3 days after completion of metronidazole therapy.

      b. With vaginitis: If tetracycline is prescribed, client should take 1 hour before or 2 hours after meals and avoid dairy products, iron, other mineral-containing preparations, and sunlight.

      c. With candidiasis:

        (i) Client should wear sanitary pad to protect clothing.

        (ii) Client should store suppositories in a refrigerator.

        (iii) Client should continue taking medicine, even during menstrual period.

    2. Client should refer sexual partners for evaluation.

    3. Client should return if problem is not cured or recurs.

    4. Client should use condoms to prevent future infections.

IX. Gonorrhea

  A. Etiologic agent: *Neisseria gonorrhoeae:* gram-negative diplococcus.

  B. Mode of spread: Sexual contact.

  C. Incubation period: 1 day to 2 weeks, average 3-5 days.

  D. Clinical picture:

    Male: frequency of urination; usually dysuria; mucoid urethral discharges, purulent urethral discharge later.

    Female: red, swollen cervix in 75% of females; symptomatic purulent vaginal discharge; frequency of urination; dysuria.

    Anorectal and pharyngeal infections are common, may be symptomatic or asymptomatic.

  E. Laboratory test:

    Female: culture from cervix.

    Male: culture from urethra.

  F. Treatment: Intramuscular penicillin.

  G. Contacts: Examination and treatment of all contacts.

  H. Complications and sequelea:

    1. 10%-20% of women develop pelvic inflammatory disease and are at risk for its sequelae.

    2. Men are at risk for epididymitis, sterility, urethral stricture, and infertility.

3. Newborns are at risk for ophthalmia, scalp abscess at the site of fetal monitors, rhinitis, pneumonia, or anorectal infection.
4. All infected, untreated persons are at risk for disseminated gonococcal infections, which include septicemia, arthritis, dermatitis, meningitis, endocarditis.

I. Nursing education message to emphasize:
   1. Client should understand how to take any prescribed oral medication. If tetracycline is prescribed, take 1 hour before or 2 hours after meals and avoid dairy products, antacids, iron, other mineral-containing preparations, and sunlight.
   2. Client should return for test-of-cure 4-7 days after completing therapy.
   3. Client should refer sexual partners for examination and treatment.
   4. Client and partners avoid sex until cured.
   5. Client should return early if symptoms persist or recur.
   6. Client should use condoms to prevent future infections.

X. Syphilis
   A. Etiologic agent: *Treponema pallidum:* spirochete with 6-14 regular spirals and characteristic motility.
   B. Mode of spread: Sexual contact, prenatal syphilis, kissing, accidental inoculation.
   C. Incubation period: 10-90 days.
   D. Clinical picture:
      1. Primary: classic chancre is painless, indurated, and located at site of exposure. All genital lesions should be suspected to be syphilitic.
      2. Secondary: patients may have highly variable skin rash, mucus patches, condylomata lata, lymphadenopathy, or other signs.
      3. Latent: patients have no clinical signs.
   E. Laboratory test: Blood serology.
   F. Treatment: Penicillin.
   G. Contacts: Examine and treat all contacts.
   H. Complications and sequelae:
      1. Both late syphilis and congenital syphilis are complications because they are preventable with prompt diagnosis and treatment of early syphilis.
      2. Sequelae of late syphilis include neurosyphilis (general paresis, tabes dorsalis, focal neurologic signs), cardiovascular syphilis (thoracic aortic aneurysm, aortic insufficiency), and localized gumma formation.

I. Nursing education message to emphasize:
1. Client should understand how to take any prescribed oral medications. If tetracycline is prescribed, take 1 hour before or 2 hours after meals and avoid dairy products, antacids, iron, other mineral-containing preparations, and sunlight.
2. Client should return for follow-up serologies 3, 6, 12, and 24 months after therapy.
3. Client should refer sexual partners for evaluation and treatment.
4. Client and partners avoid sexual activity until cured.
5. Client should use condoms to prevent further infections.

Universal Precautions

Instruments

To prevent infection through cuts, punctures, and nonintact skin:

- Needles: Do not recap. Do not bend, break, or remove needle.
- Sharps/instruments: Take care when *using, cleaning,* and *disposing.*
- Disposal: Place disposable needle-syringe unit and sharps into puncture-resistant container *immediately after use.*

Barriers

To prevent infection through eyes, nose, mouth, and nonintact skin:

- Gloves: Use when likely to **touch** the body fluids. Gloves are available for phlebotomy. Change after *each* patient contact. Do not reuse exam/surgical gloves. Housekeeping gloves can be reused if intact and properly cleaned.
- Protective eyewear, mask: Use if body fluid **droplets in the air.**
- Gown: Use if body fluids are likely to **splash on clothing.**
- Resuscitation bag (or other ventilation device): Use to avoid mouth-to-mouth contact. The barriers you use will require some judgment for exposure risk in each clinical situation.
- Infectious waste-linen: Before transport—bag and label for disposal or decontamination per your local procedures.

Disinfecting

- Hand washing must be immediate and thorough: Before and after *each* contact. After removal of gloves and barriers. After exposure

Adapted from Connecticut Dept. of Public Health, Hartford, Connecticut.

to contamination. Wash other skin surfaces after contact or contamination.
- Spills: Clean and disinfect immediately—per policy.

Training will emphasize how *you* can work safely with hazards on your job to protect yourself, co-workers, and patients.

Universal Blood and Body Fluid Precautions

Because medical history and examination cannot reliably identify all clients infected with HIV or other blood-borne pathogens, blood and body-fluid precautions should be used consistently for *all* clients. This approach, previously recommended by CDC, referred to as *universal blood and body-fluid precautions* or *universal precautions,* should be used in the care of *all* clients, especially including those in emergency-care settings in which the risk of blood exposure is increased and the client's infection status usually is unknown.

1. All health care workers should routinely use appropriate barrier precautions to prevent skin and mucous-membrane exposure when contact with blood or other body fluids of any client is anticipated. Gloves should be worn for touching blood and body fluid, mucous membranes, or nonintact skin of all clients; for handling items or surfaces soiled with blood or body fluids; and for performing venipuncture and other vascular access procedures. Gloves should be changed after contact with each client. To prevent exposure of mucous membranes of the mouth, nose, and eyes, masks and protective eye wear or face shields should be worn during procedures that are likely to generate droplets of blood or other body fluids. Gowns or aprons should be worn during procedures that are likely to generate splashes of blood or other body fluids.

2. Hands and other skin surfaces should be washed immediately and thoroughly if contaminated with blood or other body fluids. Hands should be washed immediately after gloves are removed.

3. All health care workers should take precautions to prevent injuries caused by needles, scalpels, and other sharp instruments or devices during procedures; when cleaning used instruments; during disposal of used needles; and when handling sharp instruments after procedures. To prevent

---

Modified from Centers for Disease Control: Recommendations for prevention of HIV transmission in health-care settings, *MMWR Morb Mortal Wkly Rep* 36(suppl. 2S):35-185, 1987.

needle-stick injuries, needles should not be recapped, purposely bent, or broken by hand, removed from disposable syringes, or otherwise manipulated by hand. After they are used, disposable syringes and needles, scalpel blades, and other sharp items should be placed in puncture-resistant containers for disposal; the puncture-resistant containers should be located as close as practical to the use area. Large-bore reusable needles should be placed in a puncture-resistant container for transport to the reprocessing area.

4. Although saliva has not been implicated in HIV transmission, to minimize the need for emergency mouth-to-mouth resuscitation bags or other ventilation devices should be available for use in areas where the need for resuscitation is likely.

5. Health care workers who have exudative lesions or weeping dermatitis should refrain from all direct patient care and from handling equipment for patient care until the condition resolves.

6. Pregnant health care workers are not known to be at greater risk for contracting HIV infection than are health care workers who are not pregnant; however, if HIV infection develops during pregnancy, the infant is at risk of infection as a result of perinatal transmission. Because of this risk, pregnant health care workers should be especially familiar with and should strictly adhere to precautions to minimize the risk of HIV transmission.

Implementation of universal blood and body-fluid precautions for *all* clients eliminates the need for use of the isolation category of "blood and body fluid precautions" previously recommended by the CDC for clients known or suspected to be infected with blood-borne pathogens. Isolation precautions (e.g., for enteric and upper respiratory infections) should be used as necessary if associated conditions, such as infectious diarrhea or tuberculosis, are diagnosed or suspected.

These precautions should be used (1) in emergency departments and outpatient settings, including both physicians' and dentists' offices; (2) during cardiac catheterization and angiographic procedures; (3) during a vaginal or cesarean delivery or other invasive obstetric procedure in which bleeding may occur; and (4) during the manipulation, cutting, or removal of any oral or perioral tissues, including tooth structure, in which bleeding occurs or the potential for bleeding exists. The universal blood and body-fluid precautions listed here should be the minimum precautions for *all* invasive procedures.

Transmission of Infectious Agents

Transmission of infectious agents—Any mechanism by which an infectious agent is spread from a source or reservoir to a person. These mechanisms are as follows:

1) **Direct transmission:** Direct and essentially immediate transfer of infectious agents to a receptive portal of entry through which human or animal infection may take place. This may be by direct contact such as touching, biting, kissing, or sexual intercourse, or by the direct projection (droplet spread) of droplet spray onto the conjunctiva or onto the mucous membranes of the eye, nose, or mouth during sneezing, coughing, spitting, singing, or talking (usually limited to a distance of about 1 m or less).

2) **Indirect transmission:**
   a) Vehicle-borne—Contaminated inanimate materials or objects (fomites) such as toys, handkerchiefs, soiled clothes, bedding, cooking or eating utensils, surgical instruments or dressings; water, food, milk, and biological products including blood, serum, plasma, tissues, or organs; or any substance serving as an intermediate means by which an infectious agent is transported and introduced into a susceptible host through a suitable portal of entry. The agent may or may not have multiplied or developed in or on the vehicle before being transmitted.
   b) Vector-borne—(i) Mechanical: Includes simple mechanical carriage by a crawling or flying insect through soiling of its feet or proboscis or by passage of organisms through its gastrointestinal tract. This does not require multiplication or development . of the organism. (ii) Biological: Propagation (multiplication), cyclic development, or a combination of these (cyclopropagative) is required before the arthropod can transmit the infective form of the agent to humans. An incubation period (extrinsic) is required following infection before the arthropod becomes **infective.** The infectious agent may be passed vertically to succeeding generations **(transovarian transmission); transstadial transmission** indicates its passage from one stage of life cycle to another, as nymph to adult. Transmission may be by injection of salivary gland fluid during biting, or by regurgitation or deposition on the skin of feces or other material capable of penetrating through the bite wound or through an

From Benenson A, editor: *Control of communicable diseases manual,* ed 16, Washington, 1994, American Public Health Association.

area of trauma from scratching or rubbing. This transmission is by an infected nonvertebrate host and not a simple mechanical carriage by a vector as a vehicle. However, an arthropod in either role is termed a *vector.*

3) **Airborne:** The dissemination of microbial aerosols to a suitable portal of entry, usually the respiratory tract. Microbial aerosols are suspensions of particles in the air consisting partially or wholly of microorganisms. They may remain suspended in the air for long periods of time, some retaining and others losing infectivity or virulence. Particles in the 1 to 5 μm range are easily drawn into the alveoli of the lungs and may be retained there. Not considered as airborne are droplets and other large particles that promptly settle out (see Direct transmission, above).

a) Droplet nuclei—Usually the small residues that result from evaporation of fluid from droplets emitted by an infected host (see above). They may also be created purposely by a variety of atomizing devices, or accidentally as in microbiology laboratories or in abattoirs, rendering plants, or autopsy rooms. They usually remain suspended in the air for long periods of time.

b) Dust—The small particles of widely varying size that may arise from soil (as, e.g., fungus spores separated from dry soil by wind or mechanical agitation), clothes, bedding, or contaminated floors.

Insect Vectors of Disease

Mosquitos: malaria, yellow fever, dengue, filariasis, and equine and human encephalitis. Many mosquitos are also fierce biters, even if they do not carry diseases.

Biting flies: sandfly fever, leishmaniasis, bartonellosis, tularemia, African sleeping sickness, and onchocerciasis.

Lice: rickettsial diseases (epidemic typhus and trench fever) and relapsing fever.

Fleas: plague and rickettsial disease (endemic typhus) and some worm diseases.

Ticks: rickettsial diseases (Rocky Mountain spotted fever, Sao Paulo typhus, South African tick fever), tularemia, relapsing fever, tick typhus, and some forms of encephalitis.

Mites: tsutsugamushi disease and related forms of scrub typhus.

From Edelman CL, Mandle CL, editors: *Health promotion throughout the lifespan,* ed 2, St. Louis, 1990, Mosby.

Cone-headed bugs: Chagas' disease.

Miscellaneous nuisance biters: horseflies, stable flies, and bedbugs are fierce biters but are not associated with any diseases.

Houseflies and other non–blood-sucking flies: intestinal infections such as diarrheas, dysenteries, typhoid fever, cholera, yaws, and possibly poliomyelitis. These flies mechanically transmit diseases by contamination of the food supply with human and animal feces or other filth. Cockroaches also have a similar role in the transmission of enteric diseases.

Lyme Disease—Important Facts

Lyme disease is an infection caused by *Borrelia burgdorferi,* which can be transmitted by the bite of certain species of ticks. The disease often starts as a skin rash, and can progress to more serious stages involving joint, nerve, or heart tissue. Antibiotics are usually effective, especially if treatment starts early in the disease process. Lyme Disease has now been reported in at least 47 states in the United States and in many countries throughout the world.

The Tick

In the United States, two closely related tick species, *Ixodes scapularis* and *Ixodes pacificus,* have been identified as harboring and transmitting the disease-causing *Borrelia* to people and animals. *I. scapularis,* the black-legged tick, is found in the eastern United States and *I. pacificus,* the western black-legged tick, is on the west coast. Keep in mind that *Ixodes* species are smaller than the common American "dog" tick, which does not transmit the Lyme disease-causing spirochetes.

While spring and summer are the seasons when ticks are most active in the Northeast and Midwest, in certain climates, such as in parts of California, the tick is active all year long. A warm winter or a dry spring may increase the number of ticks in many regions.

The two *Ixodes* species are found in a variety of habitats, principally woodlands and bushy areas, where they feed on a variety of wild animals, such as birds, mice, and deer. Domestic animals, such as cats, dogs, horses, and cows, can also carry ticks.

The Bite and Transmission

Most people do not feel a tick biting nor the subsequent drawing of the blood it needs for nourishment. If left undisturbed, the tick will

From Pfizer, Inc, Lyme Disease, 1994, Groton, Conn.

remain attached to its host and become engorged with blood over the subsequent 2-4 days, eventually dropping off. If the *Ixodes* tick happens to be a carrier of the *Borrelia* spirochetes, it may transmit them to the host during this feeding process. Once in the body, the spirochetes can multiply. Not all ticks carry the spirochete, and a bite does not always result in the development of Lyme disease—even if the tick is a carrier.

Tick Removal

Remove the tick promptly; the sooner it is removed, the less the chance of infection. Use either a tick-removing device or fine-point tweezers. Do not squeeze the tick's body; grasp it where its mouth parts enter the skin and tug gently and repeatedly, until it releases its hold by withdrawing its barbed mouth part from the skin. Above all, be patient—proper tick removal takes time.

Save the tick in a covered jar of alcohol labeled with the date, the body location of the bite, and the place where the tick was acquired. Wipe the bite area with antiseptic or wash with soap and water. Call the local or state Board of Health to have the tick identified.

Symptoms

A typical early symptom of the disease is a slowly expanding red rash at the site of the tick bite. The rash usually appears within a week to a month after the bite, and it can slowly expand over several days. Sometimes there are multiple secondary skin rashes. This large rash should not be confused with the harmless red spot that usually is seen immediately after receiving the bite. Many people have a small spot of redness at the site of the bite, which is a normal sensitivity to the bite itself (if uncertain, contact a doctor).

Although a majority of infected persons develop the classic red rash, many do not. Other common symptoms of early Lyme disease (with or without the rash) are flu-like and include fatigue, headache, neck stiffness, jaw discomfort, pain or stiffness in muscles or joints, slight fever, swollen glands, or reddening of the eyes. A pregnant or nursing woman who is bitten by a tick or develops a rash or flu-like symptoms should contact her doctor.

If untreated, Lyme Disease can progress to more serious stages. In the later stages of the disease, the joints, the heart, and the central nervous system can be involved. One example is Lyme arthritis with attendant joint pain and swelling. These symptoms, which usually occur in a single joint, can go away after a few days and later recur in another joint. Heart symptoms can occur within one to three weeks after the rash and include dizziness, weakness, and an irregular heartbeat. Still other patients may develop weakness of facial muscles—drooping of an eyelid or a corner of the mouth, or inflammation of the eye.

Treatment

Lyme Disease is treatable. Naturally, it is easier to treat when it is detected early. However, even in its later stages the disease commonly responds to medication. Antibiotics are the treatment of choice, and the physician will choose the one that is best.

Keep in mind that the disease may be contracted repeatedly or a relapse may occur. Although research is underway on vaccines that could provide long-term protection, these are at least several years away from approval.

Prevention

Be aware of and avoid tick habitats, such as tall grass, bushes, brush, and woods. If in such habitats, wear shoes and appropriate clothing such as a hat, long-sleeved shirt, and long pants tucked into socks. The use of tick repellents on the outside of clothing may be helpful.

Before coming indoors, brush off clothing. Once inside, remove all clothing and check for ticks. Family members can help each other with such inspection. Remove and dispose of any unattached ticks. If a tick that is attached is found, follow the procedure outlined under the heading Tick Removal. Monitor the bite area and be alert for early symptoms, such as an expanding rash or flu-like signs, over the following month or so.

Since pets that are allowed outdoors can cause humans to come in contact with ticks, frequently inspect pets and remove any attached or unattached ticks; use tick-control products that veterinarians recommend. These preventive measures are important to help protect pets because they also can get Lyme disease.

Guidelines for Selected Common Communicable Diseases

Lyme Disease

Name:	Lyme borreliosis (Lyme disease). Tick-borne disease commonly occurs in the summer in forested areas.

Adapted from Benenson A, editor: *Control of communicable diseases manual,* ed 16, Washington, 1994, APHA.

Method of diagnosis:	Diagnosis is based on clinical findings and serologic tests. Typical initial lesion looks like a bull's eye (erythema migrans) that expands in an annular manner. Can lead to neurologic or cardiac symptoms and may be accompanied by fatigue, fever, and stiff neck.
Reservoir:	Wild rodents, deer, and other animals maintain the cycle, with larval and nymphal ticks feeding on small mammals and adult ticks on deer.
Mode of transmission:	Tick-borne. Transmission does not occur until the tick has fed for several hours.
Incubation:	From 3 to 32 days after tick exposure.
Preventive measures:	Educate the public in mode of transmission by ticks and the means of personal protection. Avoid tick-infested areas. Apply tick repellant (deet or autan) to pant legs and sleeves. Examine and remove any ticks promptly without crushing.
Control of patient:	Isolation—none. Remove all ticks carefully. Early stage can be treated with antibiotics.

Candidiasis (Thrush)

Name:	Candidiasis (thrush). Oral thrush is a common, usually benign condition. Clinical disease occurs when host defense is low.
Method of diagnosis:	Laboratory microscopic test shows yeast cells in infected tissue or fluid. Visual evidence of ulcers or patchlike lesions in mouth or vagina.
Reservoir:	Person/people.
Mode of transmission:	Contact with excretions of mouth, skin, vagina, and especially feces from clients or carriers.

Incubation: Varies; 2 to 5 days for thrush in infants.

Preventive measures: Detect and treat vaginal thrush during third trimester of pregnancy to prevent neonatal thrush. Early detection and local treatment of thrush in mouth, esophagus, or urinary bladder.

Control of patient: Isolation—none. Concurrent disinfection—of secretion and contaminated articles. Immunization—none. Specific treatment—topical nystation or oral clotrimazote (mycelex) troches. Occasionally intravenous therapy. Ketoconazole is effective if lesions involve skin or mucous membranes of esophagus, mouth, or vagina.

Chickenpox

Name: Chickenpox (varicella). This viral disease is rarely fatal; the most common cause of death in adults is primary viral pneumonia, and in children it is septic complications and encephalitis.

Method of diagnosis: Laboratory microscopic examination of virus by electron microscope when required.

Reservoir: People.

Mode of transmission: A high rate of transmission from person to person by direct contact, droplet, or airborne spread of respiratory secretions.

Incubation: From 2 to 3 weeks.

Preventive measures: Protect high-risk individuals from exposure.

Control of patient: Isolation—exclude from school for 1 week after eruption first appears. Concurrent disinfection—articles soiled by discharges from nose, throat, and lesions. Specific treatment—palliative treatment of vesicles with astringent bath may reduce

itching. Occasionally oral anti-
puritic medication given for severe
itching.

Acute Conjunctivitis

Name:	Conjunctivitis (pink eye). A common nonfatal bacterial infection of the eye.
Method of diagnosis:	Confirmation of clinical observation by microscopic examination of a stained smear of discharge or bacteriologic culture if required to differentiate from allergy or infection by adeno-virus echovirus.
Reservoir:	People.
Mode of transmission:	Contact with discharges from eye or upper respiratory tract of infected person. Contaminated fingers. Clothing or other articles including shared eye makeup applicators, multiple-dose eye medication droppers.
Incubation:	Usually 24 to 27 hours.
Preventive measures:	Personal hygiene and treatment of affected eyes
Control of patient:	Isolation—exclude children from school during acute stage. Drainage secretion precautions. Concurrent infection—of discharge and soiled articles. Immunization—none. Specific treatment—local application of antibiotic or sulfonamide ointment or drops depending on the infecting organism.

Tinea (Ringworm)

Name:	Dermatophytosis (tinea, ringworm). Common fungal infection that can occur on the scalp, under nails, on the body, groin or perianal area, and the feet.

Method of diagnosis:	Clinical observation of lesions. Scalp—mousy odor and yellowcrusts on scalp. Nails—nail thickens, discolors, and is brittle with buildup of caseous material under nail. Feet—scaling, cracking of skin between toes. Laboratory examination of scalp under ultraviolet lamp (Wood's lamp) for yellow-green fluorescence. For nails, body, and feet, scrapings in 10% potassium hydroxide and microscopic examination.
Reservoir:	Scalp—people, animals (especially dogs, cats, cattle). Nails—people. Body—people, animals, soil. Feet—people.
Mode of transmission:	Scalp—direct skin-to-skin contact or indirectly from contaminated barber's clippers, combs. Nails, body, feet—direct contact from infected person or indirectly from contaminated shower stalls or floors. Also body infection may be caused from lesions of animals.
Incubation:	Scalp—10 to 14 days. Nails—unknown. Body—4 to 10 days. Feet—unknown.
Preventive measures:	Educate people not to use combs or brushes of others, strict personal hygiene. Launder clothes and towels with hot water or fungicidal agent. Clean shower floors with cresol.
Control of patient:	Griseofulvin by mouth, topical antifungal powders or ointments.

Enterobiasis (Pinworm)

Name:	Enterobiasis (pinworm disease). Pinworms are a common intestinal infection, usually benign and highly contagious.
Method of diagnosis:	Diagnosis is made by applying transparent adhesive tape to the perianal

region and examining the tape microscopically for eggs.

Reservoir: People. Pinworms in animals are not
transmissible to a person.

Mode of transmission: Direct transfer of infective eggs by
hand from anus to mouth or indi-
rectly through clothing, bedding,
food, or other articles contaminated
with eggs.

Incubation: Life cycle is 4 to 6 weeks. Eggs become infective within a few hours
after being deposited at the anus and
survive less than 2 weeks outside
the host.

Preventive measures: Remove sources of infection by treatment. Daily morning showering pre-
ferred to tub baths. Frequent change
to clean underclothing, night clothes,
and bed sheets. Clean/vacuum house
daily for several days after treatment.
Education in personal hygiene, especially the need to wash hands before
eating or preparing food. Avoid
scratching bare anal area and nail biting. Reduce overcrowding in living
arrangements. Keep toilets clean.

Control of client: Isolation—none. Concurrent
disinfection—change bed linens and
underwear carefully to avoid dispers-
ing eggs into the air. Eggs killed at
temperatures of 131° F for a few
seconds; vacuum sleeping and living
area daily for several days.

Ascarias (Roundworm)

Name: Ascarias (roundworm infection). A
common infection of the small intestine with few symptoms.

Method of diagnosis:	Microscopic examination of eggs in feces or observation of adult if worms passed from anus, nose, or mouth.
Reservoir:	People or soil infected with roundworm eggs.
Mode of transmission:	Ingestion of infective eggs from soil contaminated with feces. Not from person to person. Contaminated soil may be carried on feet or footwear.
Incubation:	Lifecycle requires 4 to 8 weeks to complete. Feces contain eggs about 60 days after ingestion.
Preventive measures:	Educate the public to use toilet facilities. Provide proper disposal of feces, and prevent soil contamination in areas near homes or where children play. Good hand washing before eating or handling food.
Control of client:	Isolation—none. Specific antihelminthic medications.

Food Poisoning

Name:	Foodborne intoxication (salmonellosis, staphylococcal, botulism). Salmonellosis and staphylococcal illnesses are due to bacteria. Botulism is due to ingestion of toxin bacillus.
Method of diagnosis:	Salmonellosis—microscopic examination of fecal material. Staphylococcal—microscopic examination of vomitus, feces, or suspected food item. Botulism—laboratory examination of serum or feces showing the specific toxin.
Reservoir:	Salmonellosis—people and animals (poultry, cattle, rodents, turtles, dogs, cats). Staphylococcal—people. Botulism—agricultural products, marine sediment, and intestinal tract of animals and fish.

Mode of transmission:	Salmonellosis—ingestion of organism in food. Staphylococcal—ingestion of organism in food. Botulism—ingestion of food in which toxin has been formed (inadequate heating and canning of foods).
Incubation:	Salmonellosis—6 to 72 hours. Staphylococcal—30 minutes to 7 hours. Botulism—12 to 36 hours.
Preventive measures:	Strict hygiene of food handlers, kitchens. Hand washing before and after food preparation. Refrigeration of foods. Educate people on home canning technique (botulism).
Control of client:	Isolation—none. Vigorous hand washing after handling soiled diapers or linens. Report required to health authority. Exclude symptomatic individuals from food handling or at-risk patients. Rehydration and electrolyte replacement. Intravenous treatment often indicated for botulism. Specific antibiotic treatment may be appropriate for staphylococcal and salmonellosis infection.

Scabies

Name:	Scabies. An infectious disease of the skin caused by a mite or parasite.
Method of diagnosis:	Recover the mite from its burrows and examine with microscope.
Reservoir:	People.
Mode of transmission:	Transfer of parasite is direct skin-to-skin contact.
Incubation:	2 to 6 weeks before onset of itching in persons without previous exposure, 1 to 4 days after reexposure.
Preventive measures:	Isolation—exclude infested individuals from school or work until the day after treatment. Educate the public for good hygiene. Launder underwear,

clothing, and bed sheets used in the 48 hours before treatment.

Control of client: Application of topical solution (e.g., Kwell), cleanse, change to clean bedding and clothes.

Roseola

Name: Exanthema subitum (roseola—sixth disease). An acute viral infection usually in children under 4 years of age; nonthreatening.

Method of diagnosis: Clinical observation of a maculopapular rash and high fever.

Reservoir: People.

Mode of transmission: Not known.

Incubation: About 10 days.

Preventive measures: If exposed, immunocompromised people should be treated to avoid pneumonitis.

Control of client: Educate the public to use good hygiene and hand-washing techniques to reduce infections.

Rubella

Name: Rubella (German measles). A mild fertile viral infectious disease with a diffuse macular rash.

Method of diagnosis: Clinical observation and blood test.

Reservoir: People.

Mode of transmission: Airborne droplet spread of respiratory secretions.

Incubation: 16 to 18 days.

Preventive measures: Vaccinated with live attenuated vaccine. Educate public to encourage immunizations. Avoid contact with respiratory secretions of infected individual.

Control of client: Report to local health authority. Keep children out of school at least 4 days after appearance of rash.

Measles (Rubeola)

Name:	Measles. Hard measles or red measles.
Method of diagnosis:	Clinical observation, blood test for antibody level.
Reservoir:	People.
Mode of transmission:	Airborne by droplet spread, direct contact with nasal or throat secretion of infected persons.
Incubation:	About 10 days from exposure to onset of fever.
Preventive measures:	Vaccinate with live attenuated vaccine. Avoid respiratory secretions of infected individual. Educate the public to encourage immunization.
Control of client:	Report to health authority. Children should be kept out of school for at least 4 days after rash appears.

Giardiasis

Name:	Giardiasis. A protozoa infection of the upper small intestine often resulting in diarrhea and caused by contaminated water.
Method of diagnosis:	Diagnosed by identifying cysts or trophozoites in feces under a microscope.
Reservoir:	People and possibly beaver and other wild or domestic animals.
Mode of transmission:	Ingestion of cysts in fecally contaminated water. Person-to-person transmission occurs by hand-to-mouth transfer of cysts from feces of an infected person.
Incubation:	5 to 25 days, median 7 to 10 days.
Preventive measures:	Protect public water supplies at risk of human or animal fecal contamination. Sanitary disposal of feces. Boil water or treat with bleach or iodine

before drinking. Educate the public about good hand washing, especially child care personnel.

Control of client: Isolation—enteric precautions. Concurrent disinfection—sewage disposal system for feces. Treatment with flagyl or quinacrine.

Herpes Varicella

Name: Herpes varicella (shingles). Local evidence of inflammation and blistering along sensory nerve. Not life threatening, but lesions are painful. Occurs mostly in older adults. The same virus that causes chickenpox.

Method of diagnosis: Laboratory microscopic visualization of virus or isolation of virus in tissue culture.

Reservoir: People.

Mode of transmission: A low rate of transmission from vesicle fluid.

Incubation: From 2 to 3 weeks.

Preventive measures: Protect high-risk individuals from exposure.

Control of client: Isolation—none. Concurrent disinfection—articles soiled by discharges from lesions. Immunization—none. Specific treatment—vidarabine is effective if begun within 72 hours of onset in immunocompromised patient. Acyclovir is also effective.

Mumps

Name: Mumps. An acute viral infection of the salivary glands.

Method of diagnosis: Clinical observation. Occasionally blood test may be used.

Reservoir: People.

Mode of transmission:	By droplet spread and direct contact with saliva of an infected person.
Incubation:	About 2 to 3 weeks; often 18 days.
Preventive measures:	Administer live attenuated vaccine anytime after 1 year of age. Avoid contact with nose and throat secretions of infected individuals. Educate the public to encourage immunization.
Control of client:	Respiratory isolation for 9 days from onset of swelling. Dispose of articles soiled with nose and throat secretions.

Tuberculosis

Name:	Tuberculosis. A microbacterial disease usually affecting the lungs but will infect other organs.
Method of diagnosis:	Acid-fast bacilli from sputum observed under microscope.
Reservoir:	People, occasionally cattle.
Mode of transmission:	Expose to bacilli in airborne droplets from sputum of infected person.
Incubation:	From infection to a primary lesion in 4 to 12 weeks. Can remain latent for years.
Preventive measures:	Improve social conditions that increase risk of infection (overcrowding). Educate public about covering mouth when coughing. Dispose of sputum and secretion—tissues of infected person. Educate clients toward compliance in medication regime.
Control of client:	Report to health authority required. Most initial infections heal without treatment. Medication—isoniazid, rifampin, and other regimens used in active disease. Person with active disease should be isolated initially until treated with medication. Medication after for 1 year or more. Immunization (BCG) available in situa-

tions of continuous exposure to untreated or ineffectively treated patients with positive sputum pulmonary tuberculosis.

Pediculosis

Name:	Pediculosis (lice). A common infestation of the head, pubic area, or clothing seams.
Method of diagnosis:	Clinical observation. Nit egg can be seen and verified under a microscope.
Reservoir:	Infested people.
Mode of transmission:	Direct contact with an infested person.
Incubation:	Eggs of lice hatch in 7 days and reach maturity about 8 to 10 days after hatching.
Preventive measures:	Avoid physical contact with infested people, clothing, and bedding. Educate the public in laundering clothes or bedding in hot water (131° F) for 20 minutes or dry-cleaning. Regular inspection of children for head lice, especially for children in school and summer camp.
Control of client:	Isolation—physical contact isolation for 24 hours after application of effective insecticide. Examination of household and other close contacts. Laundering of infected clothes, bedding, cosmetic articles. Use Kwell, Pyrinate, RID, or similar agent, and repeat in 10 days.

Pertussis

Name:	Pertussis (whooping cough). An acute bacterial respiratory illness resulting in paroxysmal coughing.

Method of diagnosis:	Diagnosis based on microscopic examination of secretions swabbed from the nasopharynix.
Reservoir:	Infected people.
Mode of transmission:	Usually from direct contact with discharges from respiratory mucous membranes of infected person by airborne droplets.
Incubation:	Commonly 7 days and almost always within 10 days.
Preventive measures:	Active immunization series and education of public and especially parents for immunization of children.
Control of client:	Report to local health authority. Isolation for known cases. Terminal cleaning. Antibiotic therapy may shorten communicability.

Definition of Positive Mantoux Skin Test (5TU-PPD) in Children*

Reaction ≥5 mm

Children in close contact with persons who have known or suspected infectious cases of tuberculosis:

- Households with active or previously active cases if (1) treatment cannot be verified as adequate before exposure, (2) treatment was initiated after period of child's contact, or (3) reactivation is suspected

Children suspected to have tuberculous disease:

- Chest roentgenogram consistent with active or previously active tuberculosis
- Clinical evidence of tuberculosis

Children with immunosuppressive conditions† or HIV infection

Reaction ≥10 mm

Children at increased risk of dissemination from

- Young age: <4 yr of age

†Including immunosuppressive doses of corticosteroids.

---

*These recommendations should apply regardless of whether BCG has been previously administered.

From Report of the committee on infectious disease: Red Book, ed 23, Elk Grove, Ill, 1994, American Academy of Pediatrics.

- Other medical risk factors, including Hodgkin's disease, lymphoma, diabetes mellitus, chronic renal failure, and malnutrition

Children with increased environmental exposure:

- Born, or whose parents were born, in regions of the world where tuberculosis is highly prevalent
- Frequently exposed to adults who are HIV infected, homeless, users of intravenous and other street drugs, poor and medically indigent city dwellers, residents of nursing homes, incarcerated or institutionalized persons, and migrant farm workers

Reaction ≥15 mm

Children ≥4 yr of age without any risk factors

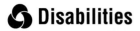 Disabilities

Case Management Process and Roles

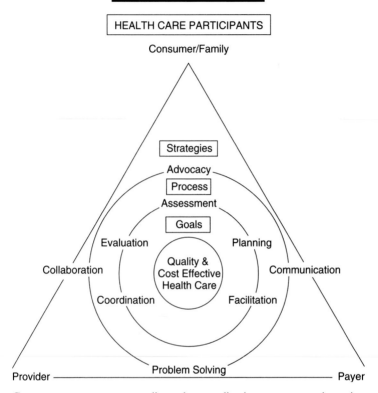

HEALTH CARE PARTICIPANTS

Consumer/Family

Strategies

Advocacy

Process

Assessment

Goals

Evaluation

Planning

Collaboration

Quality & Cost Effective Health Care

Communication

Coordination

Facilitation

Provider ——————— Problem Solving ——————— Payer

Case management: a process directed at coordinating resources and creating flexible, cost-effective health care options in collaboration with the treatment team for individuals and their families to facilitate optimum health care outcomes.

The specific activities of the case manager blend with the stages of the nursing process or clinical reasoning process to form a framework for nursing case management. Referring to the case management model developed by the National Task Force on Case Management, the process involves assessment, planning, facilitation, coordination, and evaluation.

From Hoeman S: *Rehabilitation nursing: process and application,* ed 2, St Louis, 1996, Mosby.

Nurse Case Management in Rehabilitation

Escalating health care costs have given rise to the development of new and more effective approaches to the delivery of health care services. One such approach, that of case management, has emerged as a significant trend in managed health care. Nurses, with their specialized knowledge and skills in caring for persons with disabilities, are in a unique position to serve as case managers for clients in acute, rehabilitation, and community settings.

Case management is the process of planning, organizing, coordinating, and monitoring the services and resources needed to respond to a client's health care needs. Case management does not usually involve hands-on nursing care of clients. By assessing, planning, implementing, coordinating, and evaluating, the rehabilitation nurse case manager ensures the delivery of cost-effective, quality health care services that helps the client move toward optimal health following a disabling illness or injury.

I. **Case management goals**
    A. The nurse case manager uses a goal-oriented approach emphasizing both quality and cost-effectiveness of services; goals include the following
       1. Outcomes of care
          a. Optimal functioning and independence in the least restrictive environment
          b. Prevention of complications
          c. Effective coping with the disability
          d. A successful return to work, school, and community
       2. System outcomes: Provision of timely, appropriate services by qualified service providers
       3. Minimization of health care costs
    B. The rehabilitation nurse case manager facilitates outcomes of case management
       1. As a *coordinator,* the case manager facilitates client access to health care services and coordinates and monitors all health care provided to the client; timely provision and continuity of services are essential to effective coordination
       2. As a *collaborator,* the nurse case manager collaborates with the facility-based and community-based rehabilitation teams through ongoing communication

From McCourt A, editor: *The rehabilitation nursing foundation of the association of rehabilitation nurses. The speciality practice of rehabilitation nursing: a core curriculum,* ed 3, 1993, Ill, 1993.

3. As an *educator,* the case manager promotes or provides the education of clients regarding their health status and prevention of complications or further disability; emphasis is placed on self-management and responsibility for health care needs

4. As an *advocate,* the nurse case manager strives to promote the client's optimal functioning and independence in the community

II. **Client characteristics and referral considerations**

 A. Early identification of clients is essential to successful case management and subsequent achievement of outcomes; ideally, this should occur at the onset of disability

   1. Internal, or facility-based, case managers typically serve all clients receiving care and initiate services on a client's admission

   2. External case managers receive referrals primarily from insurance carriers and other third-party payers

      a. These referrals are usually based on predetermined criteria used by the referral source and encompass clients with catastrophic illnesses or injuries, those at high risk for the long-term consequences of disability, and those with work-related illnesses or injuries

      b. External case managers often can facilitate early identification of clients needing case management through ongoing education of referral sources and reviews of claim files

 B. Clients of all ages are served by nurse case managers; those who provide services to children and older adult client populations need additional specialized knowledge

   1. Children served by case managers include those with disabilities at birth, those with developmental disabilities, and those with acquired catastrophic illness or injury

   2. Community reintegration of children with an emphasis on education is a major focus of the rehabilitation team and case manager

   3. Older adult clients include those who, through the case manager's coordination of appropriate services, can continue to function independently in their community

   4. The case manager facilitates placement when a client's remaining at home is no longer feasible

 C. Considerations in referring clients for case management

   1. The nature and severity of the illness or injury

      a. Catastrophic illness or injuries: Multiple trauma, burns, head injury, spinal cord injury, stroke, cancer, and AIDS

      b. Workers' compensation cases: Back injury, chronic pain, soft tissue or joint injury, or repetitive motion disorder

      c. Presence of secondary disability

  2. Type of treatment received or recommended

  3. Emotional and behavioral status

  4. Age

  5. Available social support systems

III. Role functions of the nurse case manager: Correspond to the phases of the nursing process

  A. Assessment

    1. A comprehensive assessment is completed on referral to the case manager; authorization, if necessary, is obtained before the assessment, which is performed in the client's home whenever possible

    2. Assessment data are collected from a variety of sources

      a. Interview with client and client's family

      b. Attending physician and other health care disciplines involved in client's care

      c. Review of medical records and school reports

      d. Employer contact in workers' compensation cases

    3. Areas of emphasis during assessment

      a. Present illness or injury as well as health status

        1) Diagnosis, prognosis, current treatment, and future treatment recommendations

        2) Functional abilities and activities of daily living

      b. Psychosocial status

        1) Emotional and behavioral response to illness or injury

        2) Roles, relationships, and family functioning

      c. Financial status

        1) Income sources

        2) Eligibility for additional funding sources

      d. Home environment

        1) Accessibility

        2) Safety

      e. Educational and vocational assessment

        1) Educational

          a) Current ability to read and write

          b) Level of education completed; degrees held

          c) Specialized training obtained in military service

          d) Eligibility for Department of Veterans Affairs training benefits

        2) Vocational

a) Past employment
  (1) Jobs held
  (2) Duration of employment
  (3) Reason(s) for leaving job(s)
  (4) Special skills attained
  (5) Union involvement
  (6) Client's verbalized or demonstrated attitude toward employer, co-workers, union
b) Transferable skills
  (1) Help determine client's vocational potential
  (2) Are determined by analyzing client's past work history
  (3) Can be determined by using various resources
    (a) Vocational Diagnosis and Assessment of Residual Employability (VDARE) worksheet
    (b) *Dictionary of Occupational Titles* (U.S. Department of Labor, Employment and Training Administration, 1991)
c) Job analysis
  (1) Formalized process for observing a job as it is performed and describing its characteristics, including its physical demands, working conditions, prerequisite general education, training time, and required aptitudes
  (2) A means to compare job characteristics with postinjury abilities
  (3) A method for observing or measuring a job's physical demands
    (a) Lifting
    (b) Carrying
    (c) Bending
    (d) Reaching
    (e) Grasping
    (f) Standing
    (g) Walking
    (h) Talking
    (i) Hearing
    (j) Seeing
  (4) Classifying physical demands as described in the *Dictionary of Occupational Titles* (U.S. Department of Labor, Employment and Training Administration, 1991)

(a) Sedentary (0 to 10 lb lifted frequently)
(b) Light (10 lb lifted frequently; 20 lb lifted occasionally)
(c) Medium (20 lb lifted frequently; 50 lb lifted occasionally)
(d) Heavy (50 lb lifted frequently; 100 lb lifted occasionally)
(e) Very heavy (more than 100 lb lifted frequently)

B. Planning
  1. Problems or nursing diagnoses are formulated from assessment data
  2. Rehabilitation plan is developed in partnership with the client, family, and facility-based or community-based rehabilitation team members
     a. Rehabilitation plan has several features
        1) Short- and long-term goals or expected outcomes that are patient centered
        2) Recommendations for care, treatment, and services
        3) Target dates for achievement of goals or outcomes
        4) Costs of services
        5) Treatment alternatives and associated costs
        6) Available community resources or alternate funding sources
        7) Discharge plans, when appropriate
     b. Community-based rehabilitation team members include
        1) Nurse case manager
        2) Rehabilitation counselor
        3) Claims representative for client's insurance carrier, third-party payer, or private funding source
        4) Employer or volunteer supervisor for noncompetitive placement
        5) School personnel
        6) Client's attorney
        7) Discharge planner
        8) Community health nurse
  3. Service providers are evaluated according to whether they offer quality services at reasonable cost
  4. Authorization for services usually is obtained through client's insurance carrier or third-party payer
  5. Long-term planning for catastrophic cases is done through development of life care plans
     a. Life care plans involve projection of comprehensive

needs and costs over the course of the lifetime of the person with a catastrophic illness or injury

    b. Life care plans are often used in litigation of catastrophic cases; however, most important, they serve to provide a framework for the long-term care needs of clients and families

    c. Life care plans include projections of future rehabilitation interventions and costs as the client ages, experiences a change in medical status, or requires periodic reinitiation of health care services

6. In workers' compensation cases, the primary goal is return to work

    a. A return-to-work hierarchy is used to determine an appropriate vocational goal

    b. Hierarchy includes return-to-work alternatives

      1) Same job and same employer

      2) Same job (modified) and same employer

      3) Different job and same employer

      4) Same job but different employer

      5) Same job (modified) but different employer

      6) Different job and different employer

      7) Different job involving retraining; employer could be either same or different

      8) Self-employment

C. Implementation

  1. Involves procurement and coordination of monitoring of the care, treatment, and services provided to the client

  2. Services can include various options

    a. Medical or surgical treatment

    b. Inpatient, outpatient, day treatment, or community reintegration rehabilitation programs

    c. Specialized rehabilitation programs for persons with head injuries, spinal cord injuries, burns, chronic pain

    d. Skilled, intermediate, or long-term nursing care

    e. Home health care

    f. Attendant care or assistance with behavioral management

    g. Home evaluation services and home modification

    h. Orthotic and prosthetic devices

    i. Durable medical equipment and supplies

    j. Psychologic services

    k. Outpatient or home-based physical, occupational, speech, or cognitive therapy; community skills or life skills training

  l. Independent or transitional living centers

  m. Hospice care

  n. Transportation services

  o. Meal programs

  p. Support groups

  q. Vocational services

   1) Work hardening

   2) Vocational evaluation

   3) Vocational counseling

   4) Job placement or supported employment

   5) Job modifications

   6) Work adjustment

   7) On-the-job training or job coaching

   8) Formal training

   9) Volunteer or noncompetitive placement

   10) Referral to vocational rehabilitation office

3. Community reintegration is addressed

  a. Access to community agencies is obtained

  b. Reentry to the home or an alternative living site is facilitated

4. Costs of services are negotiated, whenever possible, taking into account preferred provider organization (PPO) networks and mandated fee schedules

5. Services are coordinated through ongoing communication and collaboration among rehabilitation team members

  a. Case manager attends team staff meetings, whenever possible, in all settings

  b. Client progress is communicated by and to rehabilitation team members

D. Evaluation

1. Outcomes are evaluated and progress toward goal achievement is identified

2. Goals are modified when necessary

3. Successful goal achievement ideally determines the discontinuation of case management services or case closure; cases can be closed for various other reasons as well

  a. Client is unwilling to participate in services

  b. Attending physician is not receptive to case management

  c. Client's attorney is not receptive to case management

  d. Closure is requested by insurance carrier or third-party payer

  e. Funding has been exhausted

4. If goals are unable to be met or funding is exhausted, case manager must refer client to community agencies
5. Case closure in external case management includes a cost-benefit analysis
6. Case closure should also identify circumstances under which the case will be reopened
   a. Change in medical status
   b. Impact of aging
   c. Progression of illness
   d. Change in family structure
   e. Change in placement
   f. Reinitiation of rehabilitation services

IV. **Legislative and regulatory influences on case management**
   A. The nurse case manager must have knowledge of federal, state, and local governmental regulations and legislation and their impact on health care services
   B. The nurse case manager will encounter regulatory and service systems that require knowledge of the benefits provided
      1. Medicare
      2. Medicaid
      3. Private health care insurance
      4. Social Security disability
      5. Veterans Administration disability
      6. Workers' compensation
      7. State vocational rehabilitation programs
      8. Other federal, state, and local agencies
      9. Community groups
   C. Much legislation at the federal, state, and local levels affects case management practice
      1. Economic Opportunity Acts of 1964 and 1974: Initiated Head Start program; included children with disabilities in 1974
      2. Rehabilitation Act of 1973 and the amendments of 1978: Provided funding for variety of efforts
         a. Vocational rehabilitation
         b. Affirmative action efforts to employ qualified persons with disabilities
         c. Accessibility of federally funded building and transportation systems
         d. Funding for independent living
      3. Education for All Handicapped Children Act of 1975 and the amendments of 1986: Provided funding for educational assistance and early intervention programs for children with disabilities

    4. Americans with Disabilities Act of 1990: Mandated non-discrimination in the employment of persons with disabilities and barrier-free transportation systems and buildings

V. Current issues in case management

A. Quality assurance for case management practice
  1. Essential component of rehabilitation case management services
  2. Provides a mechanism for the case manager to evaluate the case management provided; aspects to be evaluated include the following
     a. Client outcomes
     b. System outcomes based on accepted standards of practice
     c. Client satisfaction
  3. Quality assurance data are used to strengthen ongoing provision of case management services

B. Governmental regulation of practice that includes scope of nurse case managers, state nurse practice acts, educational preparation, and referral or funding source guidelines

C. Legal and ethical issues influencing practice
  1. Many insurance claims involve litigation and thus attorneys are often actively involved in cases; attorneys are considered members of the rehabilitation team and should be kept informed of services provided to clients as well as the benefits of each service
  2. Complete and accurate documentation of all case management services provided is essential, because these records are admissible as evidence in a court of law
  3. When funding for case management services is terminated, referrals to community and government-supported agencies should be initiated

D. Accountability to clients
  1. In external case management (services are provided on a fee-for-service basis): Nurse case manager's services usually are retained by the insurance carrier or third-party payer, but may be retained by the family directly or by the attorney, trustee, or court-appointed guardian
     a. Case manager's primary responsibility is to the client
     b. Case manager's level of responsibility to the referral source should be defined before initiation of case management services; goals and outcomes of the case management services expected by the referral source and case manager should be identified in measurable terms

    2. In internal case management: Nurse case manager has a responsibility to all rehabilitation team members to ensure that all services provided are in the best interest of the client and directed toward discharge goals

E. Funding

    1. Claim dollars available for services to the client are often limited due to parameters of the policy

    2. The rehabilitation nurse case manager should be aware of a client's insurance policy limits because insurance carriers set aside reserves to pay claim costs

    3. Often the case manager is required to provide funding of services within the policy limits and thus must be proactive and creative in developing a rehabilitation plan for the client

    4. When funding is from a reinsurance source, the case manager must be familiar with monies available (e.g., trusts, annuities, estate funds) and recommend services accordingly throughout the client's life span

F. Regulation of case management practice

    1. Federal and state governments are beginning to determine some aspects of case management practice

    2. Credentialing of case managers: Professional bodies are also attempting to determine recommended education, experience, and certification

       a. A baccalaureate education

       b. A minimum of 2 years of clinical experience in rehabilitation or a related specialty

       c. Certification in rehabilitation nursing (Certified Rehabilitation Registered Nurse [CRRN] credential)

    3. Nurse case managers must take a strong leadership role in influencing future regulatory efforts

Access to Health Care Services

Access to health care historically has been a challenge to those with disabilities. Health care providers must be able to define strategies for obtaining health care services, identify the available financial resources, be knowledgeable regarding public laws governing access

From McCourt A, editor: *The rehabilitation nursing foundation of the association of rehabilitation nurses. The specialty of rehabilitation nursing: a core curriculum,* ed 3, Skokie, Ill, 1993.

to health care services, and assist those with disabilities in securing and using health care services.

I. **Access to health care for people with disabilities**
 A. Obstacles to health care services
  1. Geographic location
   a. Availability and transportation issues related to access to health care facilities and community resources
   b. Access to home-based care services
   c. Prohibitive cost of transportation services
   d. Limited public funds for assistance with obtaining vehicle modifications or purchasing a vehicle (e.g., a van with hand controls), which decreases access to health care services, especially in rural areas
  2. Architectural issues related to accessibility (including buildings and grounds)
   a. Parking lot accessibility and design
   b. Sidewalk accessibility
   c. Office building accessibility and design
   d. Health care facility accessibility and design
  3. Attitudes: Discrimination by health care providers toward older clients
   a. Age can impose additional limits on health care access secondary to payer source limits (e.g., Medicare coverage for home care services, equipment, and outpatient services)
   b. Elderly people often have additional and more complex health problems
   c. Discrimination can lead to poor self-esteem due to increased physical, social, and psychologic stressors
   d. Ageism may bring about job discrimination or loss of a job, with a subsequent loss of medical benefits
  4. Lack of information about care needs of those with disabilities
  5. Economic constraints
   a. Personal finances
    1) Loss of medical benefits, Supplemental Security Income (SSI), or Social Security Disability Insurance (SSDI) if a disabled person is employed and earns more than the allowable amount
    2) Possible reduction in Social Security benefits and medical benefits if a person with a disability marries
    3) Medical benefits that are now tied to income criteria and encourage disabled persons to be dependent on the system

   b. Unavailability of medical benefits for people with disabilities under Medicare until 2 years after the onset of the disability
      1) Discourages persons with disabilities from seeking health care services
      2) Raises possibility of disabled persons being without any medical benefits if they do not qualify for state assistance or Medicaid and thus contributes to increased numbers of indigent persons seeking health care services
      3) Raises possibility that people with disabilities will seek health care services only when health care needs are well advanced and require hospitalization
      4) Begins a cycle that increases the burden on health care providers to supply free care and contributes to an increase in the overall cost of health care services
   c. Limited eligibility for funding for attendant care
      1) Funding that is usually tied to eligibility for income assistance
      2) Long waiting periods that frequently last for 1 or 2 years
      3) Minimal reimbursement for attendants, which makes it difficult to recruit and retain qualified attendants
      4) Programs that require the clients to be able to manage their own workers independently and to handle training and payroll, which may not be possible for persons with severe disabilities or the elderly
      5) Strict definitions of what constitutes a disability that may disqualify many of those who need the services
   d. Ability to obtain needed equipment, supplies, and medications
      1) Dependence on insurance coverage
      2) Possible requirement of a down payment (in cash)
      3) Frequent limits on additional equipment covered by insurance
      4) Possible inability to obtain the necessary equipment (e.g., a padded commode chair with removable arms for a spinal cord injured person)
6. Limited funding for independent living arrangements (residential and nonresidential models)
   a. Continued limitation of funds for independent living centers (ILCs) despite their having been mandated by

the Rehabilitation, Comprehensive Services and Developmental Disabilities Amendments of 1978 (Public Law 95-602)

b. Some support through Medicaid Title XIX (state) funding for attendant assistance and community support services

c. The rarity of ILC programs in rural areas

7. Issues in attendant training

a. On-the-job training

b. Lack of regulations regarding worker qualifications

c. No supervision of work performance

d. Lack of public funding that would allow control over worker qualifications and performance

e. Lack of availability of attendants able to meet the specialized needs of the pediatric population

B. Limited health care services: Limits might arise due to attitudes, architectural designs, or reimbursement limits

1. Limited counseling services

a. Medical social worker services are usually available only through home care agencies

b. Few psychiatrists and psychologists make home visits

c. Reimbursement for counseling is limited

2. Special health care needs of people with disabilities

a. Obstetric and gynecologic services

1) Exam tables that are accessible to women with disabilities

2) Health care providers knowledgeable in obstetric and gynecologic areas

3) Specialized training for personnel (e.g., how to care for a spinal cord injured person who has had a baby)

b. Dental services

1) Offices that are architecturally accessible

2) Accessible, comfortable office chairs

3) Elimination of financial obstacles to preventive care (e.g., insurance such as Medicare or Medicaid that does not cover preventive care)

II. **Obtaining access to community resources and health care services (see Figure 1)**

A. Contact local governmental disability office, city commission, or city departments to determine public services available to persons with disabilities

1. Accessible housing

a. Established referral system in place

b. Technical assistance

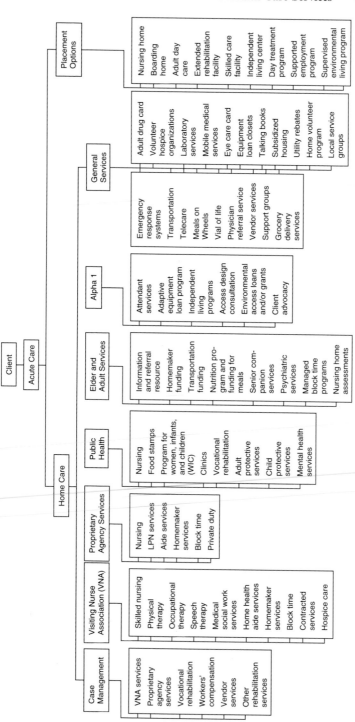

Figure 1
Gaining access to community resources.

    c. Development, design, and building assistance
    d. Home mortgage loans
    e. Availability of accessible public housing
    f. Funding for adaptations in private residences

2. Transportation
    a. Designated parking
    b. Private transportation services
    c. Public transportation (e.g., availability, accessibility)
    d. Reduced bus passes
    e. Paratransit
    f. Parking stickers

3. Advocacy
    a. Established advisory council
    b. Involvement of advocacy groups with community agencies
    c. Funding for programs
    d. Information exchange regarding disability issues (e.g., legislation)
    e. Appointment of persons with disabilities to governmental boards and commissions
    f. Legal assistance
    g. Public education regarding disability issues

4. Employment
    a. Affirmative action for hiring the disabled
    b. Training and placement assistance; supported employment services
    c. Funding for environmental modifications

5. Recreation
    a. Accessible community centers and leisure programs
    b. Special events focused on population with disabilities (e.g., wheelchair division of marathon races)

6. Supportive services
    a. Information and referral
    b. Counseling
    c. Personal care assistance programs
    d. Telecommunication devices for the deaf; sign language interpreters (e.g., at public hearings)
    e. Homemaker services
    f. Augmentative communication aids, adaptive toys, assistive technology
    g. Health screening services
    h. Funding for rehabilitation technology services and adaptive equipment

        i. Access to electronic bulletin-board systems

    7. Education

       a. Availability of educational opportunities

       b. Funding

       c. Building accessibility

       d. Programs for disadvantaged children

       e. Therapy services available in school systems (e.g., occupational therapy, speech and language therapy, physical therapy)

       f. Head Start program; early intervention programs

       g. Bilingual education

       h. Acquisition of equipment to supplement special education and related services; training in computer technology

       i. Self-help groups

       j. Playground accessibility; school environment modifications

       k. Specialized buses, cars, vans to meet the needs of school children

B. Contact other local agencies or health care professionals

    1. Social workers in hospitals, rehabilitation centers, extended-care facilities, government bureaus

    2. Department of health and human services

    3. Visiting nurse associations (VNAs)

    4. Case managers at private insurance companies

    5. Physicians' referral services

    6. Local bureau of elder and adult services

    7. Vendors

    8. Mental health department

    9. American Association of Retired Persons

    10. Department of Veterans Affairs

C. Contact public affairs departments of local media

III. Funding sources for gaining access to rehabilitation and supportive services in the community

A. Agencies and sectors receiving state funding through appropriation of monies or grants or through direct reimbursement

    1. VNAs and private not-for-profit home care agencies

    2. Alpha I (member of National Council on Independent Living)

       a. Is funded through state and federal monies

       b. Provides services to people with disabilities

         1) Peer support, attendant services, client advocacy

    2) Access to design consultation
       a) Education of design professionals and the public regarding legal requirements for creating accessible environments
       b) Building product information
       c) Design review
       d) Assessments of home after occupancy
    3) Environmental access grants and loans
    4) Loan program for adaptive equipment
       a) Low-interest loans
       b) Loans available to citizens and businesses to purchase technological aids that enhance independence in the home, workplace, or other environment
    5) Independent living programs: Provide instruction on and hands-on experience in transitional living skills
    6) Adapted vehicle driving evaluation and education
    7) Monitoring of access issues
       a) Watchdog project to correct building code violations and publicize standards for accessible design
       b) Statewide network of grassroots advocacy
       c) Group that informs the design and construction industries about legal requirements for building or remodeling public buildings and public housing
       d) Group that files complaints or litigation if corrective action is not taken

3. Proprietary (for-profit) agencies
4. Public health services
  a. Nursing services
    1) Home visits for health teaching and screening
    2) Clinics for blood pressure, screening, child immunizations, and flu vaccines
  b. Vocational rehabilitation
  c. Adult and child protective services
5. Elder and adult services
6. Transportation resources
  a. Public transportation
  b. Private organizations receiving state funds to purchase vans with lifts and to serve the elderly, those with disabilities, and those who have state benefits (e.g., Medicaid, paratransit)

7. Independent living programs
   a. Services vary according to locality and program
      1) Referral to housing and training in independent living skills
      2) Permanent residential, transitional residential, or temporary housing
      3) Attendant referral, training, or management training
      4) Client and system advocacy
      5) Disability awareness among community
      6) Equipment repair and referral
      7) Reduction of environmental barriers
      8) Promotion of consumer involvement in community activities and information and referral services
   b. Program components vary with each independent living program
8. Extended rehabilitation facilities, skilled nursing facilities, boarding homes
9. Vendor services
   a. Durable medical equipment
   b. Intravenous therapy: Hydration, total parenteral nutrition, antibiotics, blood and blood products, pain management
   c. Chemotherapy
   d. Medical supplies
   e. Oxygen or ventilator services
   f. Nutrition-related services
   g. Enteral feedings
10. Selective professional services
    a. Physicians' visits (office and home)
    b. Inpatient and outpatient hospital services
    c. Counseling services
    d. Outpatient phlebotomy services
    e. Mobile medical services (e.g., x-rays, electrocardiographs in the home)
    f. Eye care cards (e.g., funding for eye exams, eyeglasses)
11. Programs
    a. Adult day care
    b. Day treatment programs (e.g., for those with a head injury or with Alzheimer's disease)
    c. Supervised environmental living program
    d. Hospice
    e. Prosthetic and orthotic devices
B. Agencies and sectors receiving federal funding through

appropriation of monies, grants, or direct reimbursement to agencies for services that they provide

1. VNAs and private not-for-profit agencies providing home care services
2. Vendor services
3. Some independent living programs
4. Outpatient phlebotomy services
5. Physicians' visits (office and home)
6. Extended rehabilitation facilities
7. Hospice care
8. Prosthetic and orthotic devices
9. Mobile medical services
10. Inpatient and outpatient hospital services (acute and rehabilitation)
11. Outpatient rehabilitation services (e.g., hospital-based, VNA, private)

C. Department of Veterans Affairs services

1. Inpatient and outpatient hospital services
2. Pharmacy services
3. Vocational rehabilitation services
4. Nursing home care
5. Home health care
6. Orthotic and prosthetic devices
7. Durable medical and adaptive equipment
8. Services for the visually impaired
9. Home modifications for people with disabilities
10. Mortgage loans

D. Federal or state-subsidized assistance based on income, age, or disability

1. Adult drug cards
2. Subsidized housing
3. Utility and telephone rebates
4. Eye care cards
   a. Provide reimbursement for eye examinations and glasses
   b. Are unavailable for those holding state medical cards because they would duplicate some coverage
5. Health care services at public clinics (e.g., immunizations, flu vaccines)
6. Meals on Wheels program
7. Talking books

E. Elder and adult services

1. Services funded primarily for those over the age of 62 years

2. Age and income are the two main criteria for determining eligibility for programs
3. Services provided by typical senior companion program
   a. Respite care
   b. Running errands
   c. Taking clients out to do errands
   d. Light housekeeping

IV. **Nursing interventions to help clients gain access to health care resources**

A. Coordinating referrals to not-for-profit and private home care agencies
B. Identifying agencies that provide free care or sliding scale fees for services based on income and the duration of needed services
C. Arranging for social work services to assist with access to community systems for obtaining subsidized housing, Medicaid applications, SSI, SSDI, counseling services, advocacy assistance, equipment needs, and transportation and to find organizations that provide community services
D. Contacting the local department of human services regarding services available for rehabilitation care needs
E. Contacting legislators to support funding for transferring client to an ILC and for attendant training, as well as for supplemental funding that allows those with disabilities to work without a drastic reduction in or termination of medical benefits
F. Attending public hearings on issues affecting people with disabilities
G. Acting as a community advocate to promote increased environmental accessibility, decreased architectural barriers, increased access to public transportation, decreased cost of services to elderly clients on fixed incomes, and increased access to health care services
H. Making referrals to rehabilitation counselors, peer counselors, and those providing psychologic services
I. Contacting state disability office, commission(s), or department(s) for assistance
J. Promoting the education of health care providers and caregivers within facilities and the community
   1. Providing in-service education
   2. Consulting one-on-one with providers regarding health care issues, ways to manage individual clients' health care needs, and ways to promote access to health care services

3. Encouraging family involvement early in the rehabilitation process and teaching about equipment, procedures, medications, and ways to manage emergencies

4. Coordinating a home visit by the rehabilitation team to evaluate the need for home modifications, equipment, and ways to improve safety

5. Making referrals to appropriate community resources

6. Promoting interagency communication regarding rehabilitation needs, follow-up teaching needs, and previous nursing interventions in the event of a transfer to a different environment

7. Periodically reassessing and evaluating the client's ability to perform ADLs, changes in level of independence, health care needs, and barriers to gaining access to required services

8. Contacting health care providers in the community to determine access to buildings, cost of services, insurance coverage, ways to modify the office environment, and the availability of transportation

K. Speaking at service club meetings

L. Actively participating in professional organizations that support legislation and advocacy activities for people with disabilities (see Figure 2 for a list of laws governing access to rehabilitation services)

M. Promoting appointment of people with disabilities to public offices and commissions, and to private-sector industry and business boards

N. Helping clients with disabilities prepare testimony for legislative hearings

O. Participating in health planning endeavors and advocating for services that meet the needs of children and adults

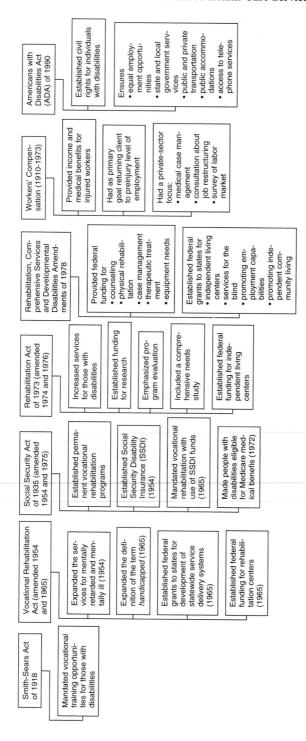

Figure 2
Laws governing access to rehabilitation services

Preserving Self: from Victim, to Client, to Disabled Person

The basic social psychologic process of "preserving self" explains the strategies used in each stage and requires deliberate action, focused energy, and tremendous effort and will. The strategies used to preserve self change in each stage of the model. At the beginning, when physical survival is in jeopardy, the strategies were primarily physical. Protecting self is a process of "taking time out" and of shutting down, in the stage of disruption. In the stage of enduring the self, it is passively learning to "take it" and to bear the treatments. Finally, in the stage of striving to regain the self, preserving the self is the work of regaining and redefining the self as a disabled person.

The stages of preserving self

Stage I Vigilance: becoming engulfed	Stage II Disruption: taking time out	Stage III Enduring the self: confronting and regrouping	Stage IV Striving to regain self: merging the old and the new reality
Being vigilant Experiencing clarity of thought Experiencing the expansion of time	Being in a shattered reality Experiencing memory gaps, "fog" Dreaming vividly, frequently bizarre, confused with reality	Learning to endure Living through pain and treatments Grasping the implications of the injury	Making sense Seeking information about the accident Recognizing it "could be worse"
Being directive, protecting the living, breathing self	Vacillating sleep/wake cycles Perceiving the world as changing and hostile	Trying to "bear it," learning to "take it" Learning to accept dependence	

Distancing subjective from objective body	Anchoring onto the significant other	Latching onto the significant other	Getting to know and trust the altered body
Observing dispassionately	Trying to "keep myself together"	Not tolerating being left alone	Learning limitations
Becoming two-personned		Seeking distraction	Viewing life beyond self
		Seeking encouragement	Revising/modifying life goals
		Seeking entertainment	
		Learning physical limitations	
Relinquishing to caregivers	Recognizing reality	Doing the work of healing	Accepting the consequences of the experience
Surrendering	Beginning the struggle	Living with setbacks and discouragement	Realizing they can "hack it"
Becoming calm		Keeping a score card	Evaluating meaning
		Refusing to accept the damage	Redefining self

From Morse JM, O'Brien B: *J Adv Nurs* 21:886-896, 1995.

Assessment of Equipment Needs for the Disabled Client

Activity	Problem	Equipment	Comments
Transfers	One-sided impairment	Sliding board	A smooth-surfaced wooden board with a center hole placed between client and transfer object. The board is placed under client's upper thigh.
	Lower extremity impairment	Sliding board, trapeze	
	All extremities impaired	Sliding board with one-person assist	
		Hoyer lift	The Hoyer lift is a hydraulic lift using a sling to hold client. It may also be useful with an overweight dependent client.
	Low endurance	Sliding board	
	Visual impairment	Not applicable*	Orientation to environment
	Auditory impairment	Not applicable	
Mobility	One-sided impairment	Manual wheelchair with one-hand drive, ambulatory with walker, cane (straight, narrow-base or wide-base quad), or crutches	
	Lower extremity impairment	Manual wheelchair (standard or sports model), ambulatory with braces and assistive devices	
	All extremities impaired	Manual wheelchair with lugs	Lugs allow client with limited grasp to propel a wheelchair. Lugs are protrusions from the rim of the wheelchair. Gloves are recommended to provide better traction.

		The various drive controls are specific to patient's functional ability. Breath and chin controls are used for client who have no function in upper extremities, but who have good head and neck control. The hand control can be adapted with differently shaped devices.
	Motorized wheelchair with specific drive control (hand, breath, chin)	
Low endurance	Manual wheelchair, motorized wheelchair, motorized scooter	Client must have good balance to operate motorized scooter.
Visual impairment	Seeing eye dog; cane	Orientation to environment. If a person leads the client, client must hold onto the person's upper arm and be given verbal cues.
Auditory impairment	Not applicable	
One-sided impairment	Toilet bars, raised toilet seat, bedpan, bedside commode, shower commode chair, toileting stick	The shower commode chair can be placed directly over toilet. The toileting stick is used by clients who have limited reach. It holds toilet paper and assists with cleaning.
Toileting Lower extremity impairment	Toilet bars, bedside commode, shower commode chair, suppository insertor, digital stimulator	These are used to assist client with limited mobility/grasp.

Continued.

*No specific equipment recommendations are required.

Bernstein L, et al: *Primary care in the home*, Philadelphia, 1987, JB Lippincott.

Assessment of equipment needs for the disabled client—cont'd

Activity	Problem	Equipment	Comments
Toileting—cont'd	All extremities impaired	Bedside commode, toileting stick, shower commode chair, suppository insertor, digital stimulator	
	Low endurance	Bedside commode	
	Visual impairment	Not applicable	Orientation to environment; consistency maintained with placement of objects
	Auditory impairment	Not applicable	
	Bedridden	Bedpan or urinal, absorbent pads	
Feeding	One-sided impairment	Dycem pad	Dycem pad is a nonskid rubber pad that prevents on object from skidding. It is placed beneath the object.
		Rocker knife	Rocker knife is a curved-blade kife that allows patient to cut food with one hand by using a rocking motion
		Scoop dish, plate guard	Both devices have high sides so patient can push food against the sides, preventing food from sliding off plate.
	Lower extremity impairment	Not applicable	
	All extremities impaired	Electric self-feeder	Electrically brings utensil to client's mouth.
		Utensils with built-up handles	Used for clients with decreased grasp.
		ADL/universal cuff, C-clip holder	Both devices wrap around palm of hand to hold utensils. They are used by clients who have limited or no grasp.

Low endurance	Long straw, mug	Pace activity level.
Visual impairment	Not applicable	Consistency in organization; verbal cuing exploration of dish; memory training. When cuing the individual, you must describe position of food, utensils, and beverage by associating the positions with the numbers on a clock.
Auditory impairment	Not applicable	
Hygiene		
Brushing hair/ combing hair		
One-sided impairment	Not applicable	
Lower extremity impairment	Not applicable	
All extremities impaired	Long-handled brush or comb, built-up handle, C-clip holder	
Low endurance	Not applicable	Pace activity level.
Visual impairment	Not applicable	
Auditory impairment	Not applicable	
Brushing teeth	One-sided impairment	Suction denture brush	Client needs to place toothbrush on counter to stabilize. Open toothpaste tube with one hand and squeeze onto toothbrush.
Lower extremity impairment	Not applicable	
All extremities impaired	Suction denture brush, built-up handle, C-clip holder, toothbrush	
Low endurance	Electric toothbrush	
Visual impairment	Use braille labels on items	
Auditory impairment	Not applicable	

Continued.

Assessment of equipment needs for the disabled client—cont'd

Activity	Problem	Equipment	Comments
Hygiene—cont'd			
Bathing	One-sided impairment	Long-handled sponge, suction nail brush, soap on a rope, wash mitt	
	Lower extremity impairment	Long-handled sponge	
	All extremities impaired	Long-handled sponge, suction nail brush, wash mitt, soap on a rope, digital read-out temperature faucets	Water temperature must be checked on *full* sensation areas. Nonskid surface is recommended in tub.
	Low endurance	Long-handled sponge	
	Visual impairment	Raised letters on faucets	Consistency in organization of supplies helpful.
	Auditory impairment	Not applicable	
	One-sided impairment	Electric shaver	
Shaving	Lower extremity impairment	Not applicable	
	All extremities impaired	Electric razor, C-clip holder for razor (manual or electric), shaving cream dispenser handle	The shaving cream dispenser handle is lever apparatus attached to spray nozzle to assist in pressing down. This is for clients with limited hand control.
		Built-up handle for manual razor	
	Low endurance	Electric razor	Decreases chance of cutting onseself
	Visual impairment	Electric razor	
	Auditory impairment	Not applicable	

Dressing		
Putting on lower extremity clothing	One-sided impairment	Dressing stick	Wooden stick with hook on the end to aid in reaching and hooking clothing
		Stocking aid	Oval-shaped plastic device with loops on top. Stocking is fitted over plastic, foot is placed into stocking, and loops are pulled upward.
	Lower extremity impairment	Dressing stick, reacher, trouser and sock pulls	The pulls are loops that are attached to clothing. Client places hand or wrist through loop. The wrist is used for pulling by clients who lack grasp.
		Leg lifter	The leg lifter may be either webbing or a strap to assist client in lifting leg for positioning to dress.
	All extremities impaired	Dressing stick, reacher, trouser pull, stocking aid, zipper pull	The zipper pull is a small loop or ring attached to the zipper for a client with limited hand control.
	Low endurance	Reacher	
	Visual impairment	Not applicable	Client sets up own system for identifying colors and styles, for example, by using a different knot on the label to distinguish clothing of different colors (e.g., red = 2 knots).
	Auditory impairment	Not applicable	
Putting on upper extremity clothing	One-sided impairment	Velcro closure for bras or shirts, front closing bra, button hook	
	Lower extremity impairment	Not applicable	

Continued.

Assessment of equipment needs for the disabled client—cont'd

Activity	Problem	Equipment	Comments
Putting on upper extremity clothing—cont'd	All extremities impaired	Velcro closure for bras, button hook, dressing stick	
	Low endurance	Not applicable	Pace activity level.
	Visual impairment	Not applicable	
	Auditory impairment	Not applicable	
Dressing			
Putting on shoes	One-sided impairment	Elastic laces, Velcro closure, long shoe horn, slip-on shoes	
	Lower extremity impairment	Not applicable	
	All extremities impaired	Elastic laces, Velcro closure, long shoe horn, slip-on shoes	
	Low endurance	Long shoe horn, Velcro closure, slip-on shoes	
	Visual impairment	Not applicable	
	Auditory impairment	Not applicable	
Communication	One-sided impairment	Low mounted telephone, portable telephones, shoulder rest for telephone, intercom systems, personal alarm systems	
	Lower extremity impairment	Low mounted telephone, portable telephone	

All extremities impaired	Dialing stick	Stick is placed in a hand splint or in the mouth to assist with dialing telephone.
	Push-button telephone, automatic dialer, speaker telephone, alternate telephone devices: MED Micro-dec, Prentke Romich, Du-it Mecca	The alternate telephone devices are used to gain access to telephone. The specific type of control depends on patient's upper extremity function.
Low endurance	Portable telephone	Place within easy access.
Visual impairment	Large number outlays for telephone with raised numbers or braille; automatic dialer	
Auditory impairment	Telecommunicator (teletype or telecommunication device)	This provides a visual display or printout of incoming messages when attached to the telephone. Telephone may also be installed with a light system to indicate incoming calls.
	Volume control on hand set	
Meal preparation		
One-sided impairment	Rocker knife; rehabilitation cutting board	The rehabilitation cutting board is a wooden board with two stainless steel nails projecting to secure food for cutting.
	Dycem pad	
	Cart	To transport food
	Cane holder	Holder clips onto cane to balance on the countertop.
All extremities impaired	Adapted utensils	Joint protection techniques for arthritics Utensils are adapted with built-up handles or clips to secure onto hand if client has poor control.

Continued.

Assessment of equipment needs for the disabled client—cont'd

Activity	Problem	Equipment	Comments
Meal preparation—cont'd			
		Dycem pad	
		Rehabilitation cutting board	
		Zim jar opener	
		Electric can opener	
		Lapboard	To transport items
		Reacher	
		Bag attached to wheelchair	
		Lower countertops	Modification for the wheelchair-bound patient
	Lower extremity impairment	Reacher, lapboard, bag attached to walker, lower countertops	
	Low endurance	High stool	Pace activity level. A high stool enables patient to sit while working, thereby decreasing energy expenditure.
	Visual impairment	Not applicable	Consistent organization, labeling, using touch, verbal cuing, marking dials, long oven mitts, memory training, orient to environment
	Auditory impairment	Not applicable	

PART FOUR

TEACHING TECHNIQUES AND ANTICIPATORY GUIDANCE

Anticipatory guidance and client teaching are central to public and community health nursing practice. The nurse draws from numerous sources for appropriate information to share with the client. The following items will assist in this endeavor.

Educational Techniques
Fundamentals of Teaching

Although no set rules can be laid down as absolute standards for effective teaching, the following suggestions are recommended:

1. Be trustworthy and consistent.
2. Have self-esteem and enthusiasm. Generate a sense that what you are teaching will benefit the learner.
3. Don't discuss your personal problems with a client.
4. Think through your teaching image. What do clients learn from your cleanliness (or lack of it), dress, posture, tone of voice, gestures, and yawns?
5. Know your teaching area. Organize and present your material so that clients feel you know what you are doing.
6. Review and evaluate your teaching methods for effectiveness.
7. Utilize available teaching methods, resources, various emotional climates, and referral systems when appropriate.
8. Record your teaching experience and share these notes with other

From Murray RB, Zentner JL: *Nursing assessment and health promotion,* Norwalk, Conn., 1993, Appleton & Lange.

staff members (or teachers from other disciplines) who may instruct the client.

9. Be realistic about teaching and learning. Accept good days and bad days. Sometimes you will be elated, sometimes depressed about results.

10. Respect the client as more important than a procedure, a potential disease process, or a research project.

11. If you ask the client to do something, explain why.

12. Distinguish between lack of intelligence and misunderstandings caused by cultural, ethnic, or religious differences, and do not equate intelligence level with educational level.

13. Strive for learning from inner motivation through recognition of need, not from outward pressure.

14. Practice sensing the moment of learning. A sense of appropriate timing is essential in teaching.

15. If you write instructions, write legibly.

16. Plan for interruption.

17. Don't overwhelm with technicalities.

18. Give reinforcement regarding progress.

19. Accept errors in the learning process without harsh judgment but with correct information.

20. Don't allow your racial bias to control your attitude about another's ability to learn.

21. Don't reinforce destructive thinking. When a client says, "My mother died of this disease," don't reply, "It's a real killer. My two aunts died from it too."

Tips on Teaching Clients

The following are four steps you can use in planning your teaching strategy:

1. Teach the **smallest amount** possible to do the job.
2. Make your point as **vivid** as you can.
3. Have the client **restate** and demonstrate the information.
4. **Review** repeatedly.

The following are important principles:

• Don't overstuff. Limit yourself to the essentials.

From Doak C, Doak L, Root J: *Teaching patients with low literacy skills,* Philadelpha, 1985, JB Lippincott.

- Give a little—get a little. Feedback and practice are the methods by which the learning takes place.
- Three or four items of instruction are enough at any one time for clients.
- Space the learning. Understanding takes time and practice.
- Anxiety is the enemy. Do everything you can to help your clients overcome it.
- Reward every possible step with encouraging words. Clients need all the help they can get!

Physiologic Changes from Aging and Alterations in Teaching Techniques

Aging changes	Teaching techniques
Reaction time	
Lengthens	• Slow pace of presentations; do not rush response; provide liberal practice time
	• Give smaller amounts of information at each session
	• Repeat information frequently
	• Use analogies relevant to individual
	• Give reinforcement to verbal instructions with handouts, videos, practice
Manual dexterity	
Decreases	• Use tape-recorded instructions
	• Select precut appliances
	• Use anatomic models
Vision	
Lens yellows and thickens	• Avoid blue and green paper or print for teaching materials
	• Use nonglossy paper
	• Use large print for instructions
	• Make sure eyeglasses are worn
	• Make handouts of most important points
Lens accommodation decreases	• Make sure eyeglasses are worn
	• Use magnifying mirror
	• Use large graphic representations and hand gestures

Pupils are smaller; decreased amount of light to retina	• Use soft white light to reduce glare • Focus light directly on objects • Have light source behind client
Decreased depth perception	• Mark pump sprayer with bright nail polish, toward direction of spray • Draw line with felt-tip pen to designate area of clamp placement and fill line of pouch • Use stoma guide strips • Allow for slightly larger pouch opening
Hearing Ability to discriminate sounds is reduced	• Speak more slowly • Use short sentences • Use *slightly* louder tone • Do not shout • Face client when speaking; do not cover mouth • Speak into client's ear
Ability to hear high frequencies and to distinguish consonant sounds (such as c, ch, f, s, sh, and z) is reduced	• Check whether hearing aid is worn • Determine whether client hears better with one ear • Maintain eye contact when speaking; make sure eyeglasses are being worn • Eliminate background noise • Allow time for client to repeat information

Adapted from Blaylock B: Enhancing self-care of the elderly client: practical tips for ostomy care. *J ET Nurs* 18:120, 1991. Used with permission. Added information from Welch-McCaffrey D: To teach or not to teach? Overcoming barriers to patient education in geriatric oncology. *Oncol Nurs Forum* 13:25-31, 1986. Also from Wilson CM et al: Educating the older cancer patient: obstacles and opportunities. *Health Educ Q* 10(suppl):76-87, 1984. From Boyle D: The elderly patient with cancer: teaching/learning considerations for ostomy, wound and continence management, *Progressions* 6(1):19, 1994.

Teaching Guidelines for the Elderly Client with Cancer

- Ask how much, who wants to know, and what is the priority learning need?
- Determine the amount of information useful in the past.
- Review the sociocultural mix of your client caseload; consider modifications needed in teaching materials.
- Consider environmental impediments before teaching.
- Teach in phases, not "all at once"; break topics down into manageable concepts.
- Anticipate possible adherence difficulties.
- Include the family in teaching sessions.
- Use peer educational approach when possible.
- Plan clear, concise, and repetitive instruction.
- Reinforce teaching, particularly if this diagnosis or current problem is a new one (within the last 6 months).

From Boyle D: The elderly patient with cancer: teaching/learning considerations for ostomy, wound and continence management, *Progressions* 6(1):19, 1994.

Health Learning Needs for Individuals of Different Health Status

Category of health content	Health status		
	Wellness	Acute illness	Chronic illness
Nutrition	Balancing nutrients Weight control Normal elimination Understanding nutrition labels	Adjustment for disease Changes in elimination Equipment to aid nutrition and elimination	Balancing nutrients Weight control Adjustment for disease Changes in elimination Equipment to aid nutrition and elimination
Exercise and rest	Regularity Amounts Methods to promote rest or exercise Incorporation into lifestyle	Hazards of immobility Adjustment for disease	Hazards of immobility Adjustment for disease Incorporation into lifestyle Energy conservation
Stress management	Self-responsibility Diversions Relaxation techniques Use of support systems	Self-responsibility Pain management Rest and sleep Personal space Use of support systems	Self-responsibility Pain management Diversions Relaxation techniques Use of support systems Financial management Handling social systems
Illness care	Identification and treatment of minor illness When to call a professional How to enter the health care system Over-the-counter medications	Illness related information: symptoms, treatment, tests, equipment, pain control, potential outcomes	Home care regimen Signs and symptoms of crisis When to call a professional How to enter the health care system

Continued.

From Whitman N et al: *Teaching in nursing practice*, Norwalk, Conn, 1986, Appleton-Century-Crofts.

Health learning needs for individuals of different health status—cont'd

Category of health content	Health status		
	Wellness	Acute illness	Chronic illness
Illness care—cont'd			Adaptation of treating minor illness due to chronic disease
			Over-the-counter medications/implications with chronic disease
			Prescription medications
Health monitoring	Seven signs of cancer	Symptom monitoring	Symptom monitoring
	Breast self-exam/testicular exam	Follow-up health care	Follow-up health care
	BP monitoring	When to call a professional	When to call a professional
	Eye exams		
	Dental exams		
	Physical exams		
Anticipatory guidance	Risk factors	Discharge needs: resumption of normal	Financial management
	Enviromental sensitivity	ADLs —diet, activity, work/school	Developmental crises
	Immunization	Prescription medications	Disease trajectories
	Parenting	Potential complications	Environmental sensitivity
	Developmental crises		
Safety	Home, work, auto	Ambulation	Locomotion
	Hygiene	Locomotion	Adaptive devices
	Avoiding carcinogens	Hygiene	Hygiene
	Environmental sensitivity	Environmental sensitivity	Home, work, auto
	Smoking	Dangers of equipment	Avoiding carcinogens
	Alcohol and other drug use/abuse	Smoking	Smoking
			Alcohol and other drug use/abuse

Client Teaching at Different Developmental Stages

The client's developmental stage will influence your teaching style and content. Keep this in mind when assessing learning needs and selecting appropriate teaching strategies.

Infant
Developmental tasks
- Develops attachment to primary caregiver
- Develops awareness of self as separate person
- Begins developing communication skills

What to ask
- Does the infant respond to the physical presence of his or her parents?
- How does infant communicate his or her needs and feelings?

What to look for
- Shows distress when family leaves
- Uses motor and verbal skills to communicate needs and feelings

Teaching approaches
- Teach the parents to participate in infant's care.
- Role-play caring, nurturing behavior for the parent to see.
- Use a security toy or pacifier to reduce the infant's anxiety and elicit cooperation.
- Help the parent view the world through the child's eyes.
- Praise the parents as appropriate.

Special concerns
- Immunizations
- Nutrition
- Elimination patterns
- Sleep patterns
- Skin integrity (diaper rash)

Toddler
Developmental tasks
- Develops sense of autonomy
- Further develops sense of self
- Begins developing socialization skills

From Lieberman AR: *Community and home health nursing,* 1990, Springhouse Corp.

What to ask

- Does the toddler prefer certain foods or activities?
- How does child acknowledge parental distress or approval?
- Does child play with other children or adults?

What to look for

- Willing to follow whims
- Plays alongside others or interacts with them
- Approaches others with show-and-tell items
- Enjoys interacting with parents through touching and hugging

Teaching approaches

- Involve the parent in helping the child make sense of the world. To illustrate your concepts, include simple, clear examples from child's everyday life (toys, cars, grocery stores).
- Teach the parents to participate in their child's care.
- Give the child simple, direct, and honest explanations.
- Use puppets or coloring books to explain procedures.
- Let the child play with equipment to reduce his anxiety.
- Let the child make appropriate choices about his treatment, such as choosing which side of his body for an injection.
- Freely praise the child as appropriate.

Special concerns

- Immunizations
- Nutrition
- Safety
- Exercise
- Dental hygiene

Preschooler
Developmental tasks

- Masters self-care skills
- Develops sense of purpose, self, sex, identity, and family relationship

What to ask

- Which self-care skills can the child perform?
- What's child's reaction to schedules and routines?
- What would the child like to be when he or she grows up?
- What's his or her favorite activity?
- Can child state his or her name and identify family members?

What to look for

- Occupies free time independently
- Participates in self-care activities
- Evaluates disapproval of others
- Initiates activities rather than just imitating others' actions

Teaching approaches

- Urge the parents to participate in child care.
- Use simple, neutral words to describe procedures and treatments.
- Encourage the child to fantasize to help plan his or her responses to possible situations.
- Use body outlines or dolls to show anatomic sites and procedures.
- Let the child handle the equipment before a procedure.
- Use play therapy as an emotional outlet and a way to test the child's sense of reality.
- Freely praise the child as appropriate.

Special concerns

- Immunizations
- Nutrition
- Sleep patterns
- Exercise
- Safety
- Dental hygiene
- Parental support

School-age child
Developmental tasks

- Further develops sense of self through achievement
- Develops sense of right and wrong
- Shows more interaction with peers

What to ask

- What does the child like to do most?
- What's child's favorite subject in school?
- Who's child's best friend? What kinds of things do they do together?
- What would child do if he or she found a lost item on the playground?

What to look for

- Talks about friends, family, and activities
- Interacts with others and initiates conversation

- Participates in self-care activities
- Attempts to improve his or her skills

Teaching approaches

- Use body outlines and models to explain body mechanisms and procedures.
- Explain logically why a procedure or treatment is necessary.
- Describe the sensations to anticipate during a procedure.
- Encourage the child's active participation in learning.
- Praise the child for cooperating.

Special concerns

- Nutrition
- Socialization within the school setting
- Hygiene practices
- Dental hygiene
- Safety

Adolescent
Developmental tasks

- Establishes self-identity
- Prepares for independent role in society
- Continues to develop relationships with peers of both sexes

What to ask

- Is the client in school? What are his or her plans after completing school?
- Who are the friends? Do they visit and participate in activities in the home?

What to look for

- Expresses individuality through appearance or activities
- Interacts with peers
- Communicates interest in school

Teaching approaches

- Ask the client if he or she wants parents present during teaching sessions and procedures.
- Give scientific explanations, using body diagrams, models, or videotapes.
- Encourage the client to verbalize his or her feelings or express them through artwork or writing.
- Offer praise appropriately.

Special concerns

- Nutrition
- Alcohol and drug abuse
- Sexuality and contraception
- Motor vehicle safety
- Sports and physical injury

Young Adult
Developmental tasks

- Establishes independence from parental figures
- Initiates a permanent lifestyle
- Maintains relationships with peers of both sexes
- Integrates values into career and socioeconomic constraints

What to ask

- Does the client live at home with parents or on his or her own? Does the client have his or her own family?
- Is the client employed or in school?

What to look for

- Forms role-appropriate relationships with family and peers
- Forms intimate relationship with another person
- Demonstrates concern for cost of care and treatment
- Freely asks questions regarding concerns
- Assists and directs health care plan

Teaching approaches

- Negotiate learning goals with the client.
- Include family members in teaching if acceptable to the client.
- Use the client's past experience as a learning resource.
- Use problem-centered teaching.
- Provide for immediate application of learning.
- Let the client test his or her own ideas, take risks, and be creative.
- Allow the client to evaluate his or her actions and change behavior.

Special concerns

- Economic stability
- Nutrition
- Exercise
- Time management

Middle-aged Adult
Developmental tasks

- Establishes socioeconomic status
- Helps younger and older persons
- Finds satisfaction through his or her work, as a citizen and family member, or as a care provider

What to ask

- What's the most satisfying thing in his or her life?
- Who are the important people in his or her life?
- Is client active in community affairs?

What to look for

- Participates in and directs health care plan
- Freely asks questions regarding concerns
- Demonstrates concern for family
- Expresses concern for the cost of care and treatment

Teaching approaches

- Essentially the same as for the young adult

Special concerns

- Nutrition
- Exercise or activity program
- Coping skills
- Knowledge of early signs of illness

Older Adult
Developmental tasks

- Forms mutually supportive relationships with grown children
- Adjusts to loss of friends or relatives
- Prepares for retirement
- Uses leisure time in satisfying way
- Adapts to aging

What to ask

- Does client have financial concerns?
- What are client's retirement plans?
- Does client have friends his or her own age?
- How does he or she feel about getting older?

What to look for

- Shows concern for children and grandchildren
- Keeps current on world events
- Participates in care and decision making

Teaching approaches

- Negotiate learning goals with the client.
- Include family members in teaching.
- Evaluate the client's memory deficit by asking for verbal feedback.
- Present one idea at a time, and have the client summarize information.
- Use simple sentences, concrete examples, and reminders, such as calendars or pillboxes. Speak slowly and distinctly.
- Position yourself to allow for direct eye contact.
- Use large-print materials and equipment with oversized numbers.

Special concerns

- Immobility
- Transportation
- Sensory losses
- Communicable infections
- Elimination patterns
- Dental hygiene
- Loneliness
- Home maintenance
- Nutrition

Implications for the Preschooler's Health Learning

Key developmental factors	Implications for health learning
Physical maturation	
Motor: Runs easily, beginning ability to balance	Able to be independent with basic self-care, still needs reminders
Expands environment	
Well-developed bowel and bladder control	
Hand–eye coordination	
Manipulation of large pencils and crayons still results in a degree of imprecision	
Able to build fairly complicated block structures	
Cognitive development	
Preoperational (Piaget)	Able to learn safety rules and rationale when explained simply and repeatedly
Communication:	
Vocabulary 1000-2000 words	Able to learn name, address, phone number
Still relies heavily on symbolism and mobility of play	
Vague understanding about bodily functions, interested in concepton and childbirth	Learns from actual situations, visual symbols (drawings, dolls, pictures), and sensory experiences
Curious	
Reality still not discriminated from fantasy	Use simple, concrete, nonthreatening terms
Egocentric	Elicit feedback through child's terms and play
Limited attention span	Answer questions honestly and in an accepting manner without embarrassment
Relates time to common events in daily life	
	Focus on the positive in relation to the child
	Brief—15 minutes maximum—learning sessions
	Relate events to known daily habits
Psychosocial development	
Initiative vs. guilt (Erikson)	Involve parents, remind of the role of parent modeling
Family remains of primary importance although other persons may be significant	Specify any body parts involved and sensory experiences
Imitation of same-sex parent role	
Fear of bodily injury	

From Whitman N et al: *Teaching in nursing practice,* Norwalk, Conn., 1986, Appleton-Century-Crofts.

Implications for the School-Age Child's Health Learning

Key developmental factors	Implications for health learning
Physical maturation	
Motor: Moves energetically but with increasing grace and balance. Able to participate in skilled sports	Can manage simple psychomotor tasks as young school-ager and manipulate more complex equipment such as insulin injections after age 8–9
Hand–eye coordination: Control and timing of motor movements well developed by age 8–9	
Cognitive development	
Concrete operations (Piaget)	Able to learn about healthful eating, injury control, sexuality, basic first aid, exercise regimens
Communication: Extensive vocabulary	
Understands cause and effect	Learns through language—verbal and some written—using known terms, diagrams, and models
Attention span expands to allow 2–3 hours work at a time	Often needs misconceptions clarified
Decision-making skills develop	
Develops orientation to past, present, and some future time	Should be given explanations of purpose and role in activity
	Lessons of 15–30 minutes work well
	Able to make simple decisions related to own health and illness
	Needs time to sort out new things
Psychosocial development	
Industry vs. inferiority (Erikson)	Praise is a good reinforcer
Expanding interaction with peers	May learn well in group setting
Competition, compromise, and co-operation develop	Privacy is important
Increased awareness of sexual self and own uniqueness	Allow control through some help in planning
Fears disability, loss of status, loss of control	

From Whitman N et al: *Teaching in nursing practice,* 1986, Appleton-Century-Crofts.

Implications for the Adolescent's Health Learning

Key developmental factors	Implications for health learning
Physical maturation	
Motor: near adult capacity Physical growth spurts may produce temporary clumsiness Hand–eye coordination: very discrete	Able to learn complex self-care skills Able to manipulate equipment for own medical treatments
Cognitive development	

Formal operations (Piaget)
Communication:
  Interprets language
  Understands satire and nuance
Understands complexities
Orientated to past, present, and future
	Able to learn about accident prevention, environmental safety, sexuality, and health problems such as acne, obesity, pregnancy, venereal disease, and substance abuse
	Learns through verbal and written language
	Able to understand complex models and diagrams
	Can understand implications of health state on future outcomes

Psychosocial development	
Identity vs. identity diffusion (Erikson) Struggles for independence and self-control Group acceptance very important Compares own appearance and function to an ideal image Exploring ideas for future life	Able to make own decisions related to health Allow control through help with planning as much as possible Adolescent and parents should be worked with separately Privacy extremely important

From Whitman N et al: *Teaching in nursing practice,* 1986, Appleton-Century-Crofts.

Implications for the Adult's Health Learning

Key developmental factors	Implications for health learning
Physical maturation	
Motor: During young adulthood systems function at peak	Able to be independent in all aspects of self-care and health decision making. Action may be influenced by economics, sociocultural practices, personal values
Some decrease in muscle tone during middle adulthood; outcome varies	
Hand–eye coordination: at best during young adulthood, declines not seen until late adulthood	
Energy: more quickly expended and more slowly recovered during middle adulthood	
Cognitive development	
Full cognitive capacity	Can handle a variety of levels of difficulty
Flexibility, past experience, and confidence help with learning	Experiential as well as written and verbal methods are useful
Learning motivated when it is meaningful and applicable	Identifies own readiness to learn
	Content should be relevant to existing life needs
Psychosocial development	
Intimacy vs. self-isolation (Erikson—young adult)	Needs to be involved with planning and directing learning
Generativity vs. self-absorption and stagnation (Erikson—mature adult)	Can use learning to cope with role changes, developmental changes in career, lifestyle alternatives; to prevent and manage illness
Lifestyle choices—career, family important	
Self-sufficiency of early adulthood expands to include social and civic responsibilities	

From Whitman N et al: *Teaching in nursing practice,* 1986, Appleton-Century-Crofts.

Implications for Health Learning in Late Adulthood

Key developmental factors	Implications for health learning
Physical maturation	
Sensory changes:	Distinct, large configurations in visual aids, glasses clean, accessible; good lighting
Decreased acuity and accommodation of vision	
Loss of perception of high tone sounds and some sound discrimination	Speak clearly, at a normal rate, close to learner; increase loudness as needed
Cognitive development	
Affected by motivation, interest, sensory alteration	Present content at a slow pace or foster self-pacing
Decreased speed of response	Allow adequate response time
Less efficient short-term memory	Provide repetition, opportunities for recall
Simultaneous activities disruptive	Short learning sessions
	Environment should eliminate distracting sights and sounds
Psychosocial development	
Ego integrity vs. despair (Erikson)	Establish reachable short-term goals
Well-developed lifestyle habits	
Changes in roles occur through retirement, loss of spouse (others) through death	Encourage participation in decision making and planning for learning
Changes in body image caused by effects of aging	Integrate new behaviors with previously established ones
	Family members should participate

From Whitman N et al: *Teaching in nursing practice,* 1986, Appleton-Century-Crofts.

Sign Language for Common Health Situations

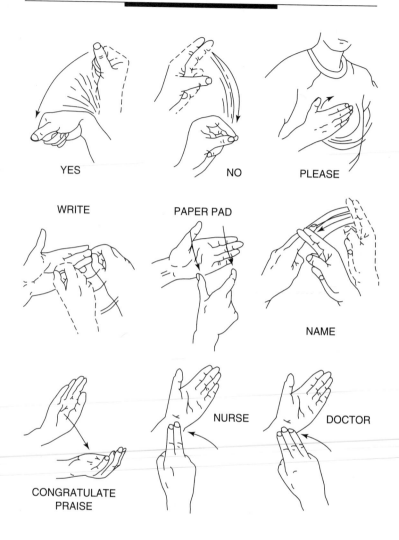

YES

NO

PLEASE

WRITE

PAPER PAD

NAME

CONGRATULATE
PRAISE

NURSE

DOCTOR

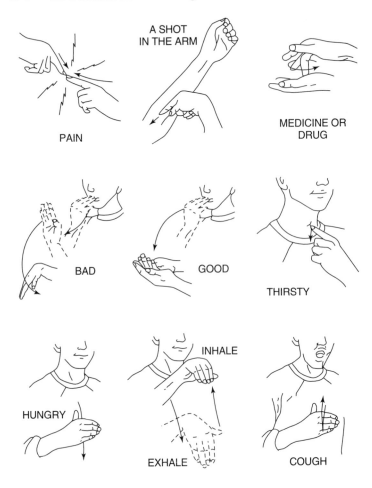

Tips for Communicating with a Hearing Impaired Person

The person who is hard of hearing must be made aware that someone is speaking to them. A hearing impaired person addressed from behind or at their side often cannot hear the speaker. Always get their attention first by touching the shoulder or arm gently and by approaching from the front. If the person has a "good" ear, move to that side before speaking.

Some practical hints for speaking to hearing-impaired person include the following:

- The speaker should position himself or herself directly in front of the person.
- The speaker should ensure good lighting so their face can be easily seen.
- Communication is visual; thus body language is essential.
- The speaker should use simple words and sentences.
- The speaker should not cover his or her mouth, chew gum, or eat when speaking.
- The speaker should have a paper to write out key words.
- When a hearing aid is used, the speaker should direct his or her speech to the battery unit of the listener's hearing aid (worn in the ear or as a body unit). The speaker should not shout, but should speak distinctly. A hearing aid is an amplifier, and it will distort sounds that are too loud.
- If a person uses sign language, the speaker should inquire which hand or arm is used for signing. This is especially important when planning for IV care.

Advantages and Disadvantages of Contraceptive Methods in the Adolescent

Method	Advantages	Disadvantages
Abstinence	100% effective in prevention of STDs and pregnancy	Peer pressure for sex
Withdrawal Withdrawal of penis before ejaculation	No medical visit needed	High failure rate Some seminal fluid often released before ejaculation Ejaculate at vaginal orifice may enter vagina No STD protection
Rhythm Refrain from intercourse during fertile period	Encourages couple participation	Requires a predictable menstrual cycle, unusual in early and middle adolescence No STD protection High failure rates
Barrier methods Condom *Male:* Penile covering to trap sperm *Female:* Inserted into vagina with base covering part of perineum	No prescription needed Easy to use STD protection No medical complications	Interrupts sex May have decreased sensations Requires consistent use
Diaphragm Cervical covering to prevent sperm from reaching eggs Used with spermicidal jelly	May be inserted 4 to 6 hours before sex Effective when used correctly Few medical complications May be reused	Little STD protection Requires fitting by medical personnel Requires body awareness and comfort with touching oneself for insertion

Method	Advantages	Disadvantages
Sponge Cervical covering Releases a spermicide	May be inserted up to 6 hours before sex Can be obtained without prescription	May increase incidence of urinary tract infection Minimal STD protection Requires body awareness and comfort with touching self May be difficult to remove Decreased effectiveness in parous woman
Spermicides Foam, jelly, cream, suppositories Inserted into vagina to kill sperm	Available without prescription Inexpensive Easy to use No major health concerns	High failure rate unless used with condom Interrupts sexual experience Messy
Oral contraceptives Estrogen and progesterone-like compounds that inhibit ovulation	Few medical complications in teens 99% effective if used correctly No interruption of sex Regulates menses, decreased dysmenorrhea and acne	Must use consistently Requires prescription Expensive No STD protection Small weight gain
Norplant Levonorgestrol slowly released into vascular system for 5 years Inhibits ovulation, thickens cervical mucosa; 6 small rods inserted into upper arm	No interruption of sex Long-term, highly effective protection against pregnancy Pregnancy prevention begins 24 hours after insertion Once removed, fertility returns immediately	No STD protection Significant weight gain Irregular menses Requires minor surgical procedure Expensive

From Wong DL: *Whaley and Wong's nursing care of infants and children*, ed 5, St Louis, 1995, Mosby.

Advantages and disadvantages of contraceptive methods in the adolescent—cont'd

Method	Advantages	Disadvantages
Depo Provera Progestin that suppresses hormonal cycle and prevents ovulation Injection given every 3 months	No interruption of sex Invisible method	No STD protection Significant weight gain Irregular menses or amenorrhea Decreased libido Fertility may be delayed Must return to care provider every 3 months for injection
Postcoital contraception Combined estrogen-progestin pill containing ethinyl estradiol; given within 72 hours of unprotected sex and repeated 12 hours later; prevents implantation	Useful in unplanned sexual intercourse	No STD protection May experience nausea Effectiveness dependent on phase of menstrual cycle Not intended for repeated use

Pelvic Muscle Exercises

The pelvic floor is made up of muscles responsible for holding the body's lower organs, including the bladder. Because we walk upright, quite a bit of pressure is put on these organs as we walk, exercise, cough, or pick up something. When these muscles are weakened by childbirth or hormonal changes (such as those caused by menopause) or as a result of surgery or lower back injury, small amounts of urine may leak with physical activity. This condition is called stress incontinence, and it affects many women and some men.

Stress incontinence may be controlled without surgery in many cases. Exercising the pelvic muscles is a good way to strengthen them. Pelvic exercises (sometimes called Kegel exercises, after Dr. Arnold Kegel) are an excellent way to improve the fitness of the pelvic floor muscles.

Pelvic Muscle Exercises for Women

First, it is important to locate and identify the correct muscles to exercise. The muscles you wish to exercise surround the urethra (the tube where urine leaves your body) and the vagina. You can find this muscle by practicing stopping your urine in midstream. Tighten (contract) the muscles to stop the urine; release the muscles to continue urination. Your nurse will help you locate the correct muscles. She may gently place a gloved finger in the vagina and ask you to contract the muscles around her finger, or she may use a special machine that helps you find and contract the correct muscles. The special machine uses sound or visual signals to help you understand how to contract and release the pelvic muscles. The nurse will also help you avoid tightening your abdominal or thigh muscles. Contracting these muscles will not help you strengthen the pelvic muscles.

It is helpful to practice Kegel exercises while urinating because correct muscle tightness will stop the flow of urine. During urination, tighten your muscles until the flow stops. The buttocks will be squeezed together. Hold back the flow for 3 to 5 seconds and then relax and start the flow of urine again. Repeat this stopping and starting of urinating flow 10 times, or until there is no more urine. Later you will be able to vary your muscle tightness from a rapid pace to a prolonged 10- to 30-second period.

As soon as you think you understand how to contract and release the pelvic muscles, here's how to proceed:

- Choose a time and place to exercise. You will need about 15 minutes to do your exercises.
- You will find the best position to do your exercises with practice. Some women prefer to sit or stand; others lie on the back with the head elevated on a pillow.
- Tighten the pelvic muscles as hard as you can.
- Hold the muscle tight for 10 seconds—you may find it helpful to count to 10—then relax the muscle for 10 seconds.
- Repeat this exercise 10 times.
- Ask your nurse or doctor how many times a day (repetitions) you need to perform the exercise (generally, it is best to begin with 10 repetitions and work up to 35 to 50 repetitions every other day). Remember that one repetition consists of 10 seconds of tightening and 10 seconds of relaxation.

You may wish to try a variation of this exercise.

- While sitting, standing, or lying with your head elevated, tighten and release the pelvic muscles in rapid succession. Repeat this 15 times.
- In the same position, tighten the pelvic muscles while you exhale. Hold the muscle for a count of 30. Repeat this exercise 10 times.

Nursing Counseling for Families about Enuresis

Enuresis is a common problem.

No serious physical problem is present, although the child may have a small or immature bladder.

It often is inherited; other family members may have had the same problem.

With time the child will be cured, usually by adolescence.

The child is not wetting the bed intentionally; it is not a conscious act.

The child wants to be dry.

The parents are not at fault.

If a treatment is tried, the child needs to be responsible for dealing with both the problem and the treatment.

Punishment when the child is wet should be replaced with praise when dry (positive reinforcement).

From Edelman CL, Mandle CL: *Health promotion throughout the lifespan,* ed 3, St Louis, 1994, Mosby.

A first simple treatment step that often is helpful is to not drink for 3 hours before bedtime and to urinate before bedtime. Some parents also wake the child to urinate before they go to bed.

A family plan for dealing with the wet bed and child can decrease family arguments. The plan may include who strips the bed, where sheets go, and so on. The child should play a major role in this process.

Keep It Simple—Reading Skills Rules

Clients with poor reading skills are more likely to understand written information presented at the fifth-grade reading level. Readability formulas may be useful as screening tools because they're easy to use and give quantitative ratings. The SMOG Readability Index is one such formula that's most often used by educators. It uses the average number of sentences and syllables in three 100-word passages to determine grade-level readability estimates. Following are some general tips:

- Use a conversational style and an active voice in writing. For example, say, "Use a measuring cup for vegetables" instead of "A measuring cup should be used for vegetables."
- Use short words and sentences whenever possible.
- State the topic of the paragraph in the first sentence so the client will know immediately what the paragraph is about.
- Limit the number of ideas on one page.
- Don't put words in all capital letters, handwriting, or a stylized typeface. Using 16- to 18-point type with uppercase and lowercase letters makes it easier to decode words.
- Break up long stretches of narrative with subtitles and captions.
- Write lists—don't bury sequential information or series of events or ideas in narrative form.
- Leave plenty of open white space on the printed page. This will help clients concentrate on the educational message by minimizing distracting elements.
- Use arrows, circles, and underlining to help focus attention on the message.
- Black print on white or yellow paper is the most easily read. In contrast, pale green, pink, and blue are difficult to read.
- Dull finishes are preferable to glossy paper.

From Fain J: When your patient can't read, *Am J Nurs* 94(6):160.

- Illustrations (with enough detail to emphasize the intended message) and photographs add appeal.
- Be sure pictures portray only intended messages.

SMOG Testing to Check Literacy Skills

The SMOG formula was originally developed by G. Harry McLaughlin in 1969. It will predict the grade-level difficulty of a passage within 1.5 grades in 68% of the passages tested. That may be close enough for your purposes. It is simple to use and faster than most other measures. The procedure is presented below.

Instructions

1. You will need 30 sentences. Count out 10 consecutive sentences near the beginning, 10 consecutive from the middle, and 10 from the end. For this purpose, a sentence is any string of words punctuated by a period (.), an exclamation point (!), or a question mark (?).
2. From the entire 30 sentences, count the words containing **three or more syllables,** including repetitions.
3. Obtain the grade level from Table 6, or you may calculate the grade level as follows: Determine the nearest perfect square root of the total number of words of three or more syllables and then add a constant of 3 to the square root to obtain the grade level.

Example:

Total number of multisyllabic (3 or more syllables) words	67	
Nearest perfect square	64	
Square root	8	
Add constant of 3	11	This is the grade level.

From Doak C, Doak L, Root J: *Teaching patients with low literacy skills,* Philadelphia, 1985, JB Lippincott.

Table 6 SMOG conversion table

Word count	Grade level
0-2	4
3-6	5
7-12	6
13-20	7
21-30	8
31-42	9
43-56	10
57-72	11
73-90	12
91-110	13
111-132	14
133-156	15
157-182	16
183-210	17
211-240	18

Developed by Harold C. McGraw, Office of Educational Research, Baltimore County Public Schools, Towson, Maryland.

Special Rules for SMOG Testing

- Hyphenated words are **one** word.
- For numerals, pronounce them aloud and count the syllables pronounced for each numeral (e.g., for the number 573, five = 1, hundred = 2, seventy = 3, and three = 1, or 7 syllables).
- Proper nouns should be counted.
- If a long sentence has a colon, consider each part of it as a separate sentence. However, if possible, avoid selecting that segment of the passage.
- The words for which the abbreviations stand should be read aloud to determine their syllable count (e.g., Oct. = October = 3 syllables).

SMOG on Shorter Passages

Sometimes it may be necessary to assess the readability of a passage of less than 30 sentences. You can still use the SMOG formula to obtain an approximate grade level by using a conversion number from Table 7 and then using Table 6 to find the grade level.

First count the number of sentences in your material and the number of words with three or more syllables. In Table 7, in the left-hand column, locate the number of sentences, and locate the conversion number in the column opposite. Multiply the word count found earlier by the conversion number. Use this number in Table 7 to obtain the corresponding grade level.

For example, suppose your material consisted of 15 sentences and you counted 12 words of three or more syllables in this material. Proceed as follows:

1. In Table 7, left-hand column, locate the number of sentences in your material. For your material, the number is 15.
2. Opposite 15 in the adjacent column, find the conversion number. The conversion number for 15 is 2.0.
3. Multiply your word count, 12, by 2 to get 24.
4. Now look at Table 6 to find the grade level. For a word count of 24, the grade level is 8.

Table 7 SMOG conversion for samples with fewer than 30 sentences

Number of sentences in sample material	Conversion number
29	1.03
28	1.07
27	1.1
26	1.15
25	1.2
24	1.25
23	1.3
22	1.36
21	1.43
20	1.5
19	1.58
18	1.67
17	1.76
16	1.87
15	2.0
14	2.14
13	2.3
12	2.5
11	2.7
10	3

From Doak C, Doak L, Root J: *Teaching patients with low literacy skills,* Philadelphia, 1985, JB Lippincott.

Guidelines for Using Interpreters

When clients speak a language different from that of the health care provider, an interpreter may be necessary to facilitate cross-cultural

From Randal DE: *Strategies for working with culturally diverse communities and clients,* Bethesda, Md, 1989, Association for the Care of Children's Health.

communication. Before or at the initial visit, it should be determined whether the adolescent or parents will require a translator. Persons for whom English is a second language may speak English with reasonable fluency but may not have sufficient linguistic skills to understand complicated information. Therefore it may still be beneficial to use an interpreter. The presence of an interpreter, however, does tend to complicate the interaction between the provider and the client. To facilitate this process, the following points should be considered.

How to Choose an Interpreter

1. Ideally, an interpreter should be trained in cross-cultural interpretation; trained in the health care field; proficient in the language of the client/parents and that of the provider; and able to understand and respect the cultures of the client/parents and of the provider. These interpreters are ideal because they not only translate the interaction but also bridge the culture gap.
2. In the absence of a trained interpreter, a volunteer should be used who has training in medical terminology, an understanding of the significance of the particular health matter he or she will be translating, and an understanding of the importance of confidentiality.
3. Bilingual hospital personnel should not be relied on if they have not had training as an interpreter.
4. Family members, especially those of a different age or sex from the client, should be used cautiously. Clients are often embarrassed to discuss intimate matters with members of the opposite sex or with younger or older members of their family. Family members may wish to censor what is said either to shield the client or to keep information within the family.
5. The health care provider should be sensitive to the client's right to privacy and his or her choice of who should act as an interpreter. Often there are problems when the interpreter is of a different social class, educational level, age, or sex or knows the client's parents.
6. If the interpreter is an influential leader of the client's community, the client and parents may be embarrassed to disclose certain information and concerned about confidentiality. In addition, the interpreter may act as a gatekeeper, believing it is appropriate to omit or add information around such key issues as premarital sex, birth control, use of medications, and the sharing of psychosocial problems.

How to Work with an Interpreter

1. The health care provider should meet regularly with the interpreter to keep communications open and facilitate an

understanding of the goals and purpose of the visit by the client. They should meet before meeting with the client and parents.

2. The interpreter should be encouraged to meet with the client and parents before the appointment to find out about the client's and parents' educational level and attitudes toward health and health care. This information can aid the interpreter in the depth and type of information and explanation that will be needed.

3. Short units of speech, not long involved sentences or paragraphs, should be used. Long, complex discussions of several topics in a single appointment are to be avoided.

4. Technical terminology, abbreviations, and professional jargon should be avoided.

5. Colloquialisms, abstractions, idiomatic expressions, slang, similes, and metaphors are also to be avoided.

6. The interpreter should be encouraged to translate the client's and parents' own words as much as possible, rather than paraphrasing or "polishing" it into professional jargon. This gives a better sense of the client's and parents' concept of what is going on, their emotional state, and other important information.

7. The interpreter should refrain from inserting his or her own ideas or interpretation or omitting information.

8. To check on the client's and parents' understanding and the accuracy of the translation, the client and parents should be asked to repeat instructions or whatever has been communicated in their own words, with the interpreter facilitating.

9. During the interaction, the health care provider should look at and speak directly to the client or parent, not the interpreter. The provider sits facing the client or parent, with the interpreter seated at an angle (as if equal points in a triangle). The provider should never talk through the interpreter, but ask questions directly to the client or parent, for example, "How can I help you today?" not "How can I help her today?" This allows the provider to express warmth and concern through nonverbal communication. Also, the provider should listen closely to the client and parents and observe their facial expressions, voice intonations, and body movements for cues that may aid in the health assessment.

10. Patience is necessary. An interpreted interview takes longer. Careful interpretation often requires that the interpreter use long explanatory phrases.

Even if an interpreter is used, there are ways that the health care provider can become more actively involved in the communication process.

1. Proper forms of address in the client and parents' language should

be used. This conveys respect for the client and parents and demonstrates willingness to learn about their culture.

2. The provider should learn basic words and sentences of the client and parents' language and become familiar with special terminology used by clients. Even though the provider can't speak well enough to communicate directly, the more he or she understands, the greater the chance that misinterpretations and misunderstandings in the interpreter-client-parent interchange will be detectable.

3. A positive tone of voice conveys interest in the client and parents. The provider must never be condescending, judgmental, or patronizing.

4. Important information should be repeated more than once. The reason or purpose for a treatment or prescription should always be given.

5. Verbal interaction should be reinforced with materials written in the client and parents' language and with visual aids.

6. Cross-cultural variations in nonverbal communication should be understood in order to avoid misunderstandings and unintentional offenses. This may include variations in silence, physical distance, eye contact, emotional expressiveness, and body movements.

Nursing Suggestions to Encourage Language Development in Preschoolers

Read to the child. Encourage the child to be an active listener by pausing at times during the story to ask such questions as, "What do you think will happen next?"; "Why do you think the boy said that?"; and "What would you do now?"

Praise the child's storytelling.

Always respond to the child's questions. At times a response must be delayed; for example, if the parent is driving in heavy traffic and the child asks a question that requires a complex answer, the parent might say, "That's a very good question, let's talk about that as soon as we get home." The parent should remind the child later of the question and respond if the child still is interested.

Never tease or criticize a child about his verbalizations. If the child is excited and talking so fast that he is fumbling over words, the parent might say, "I can't listen that fast. Slow down a little for me." This is much more encouraging than, "You talk too fast. No one can understand you."

From Edelman CL, Mandle CL: *Health promotion throughout the lifespan,* ed 3, St Louis, 1994, Mosby.

Play games that are language focused, such as naming the colors of houses or kinds of flowers as parent and child walk to the store.

Administration and Scoring of the Preschool Readiness Experimental Screening Scale (PRESS)

NAME	BIRTH DATE

SCHOOL	DATE

1. a. What color is grass?   _____
   b. What color is the sky if there are no clouds? _____
2. a. Repeat four numbers (one success in two _____
   tries): 4-1-7-3 or 3-8-6-4
   b. Recognize four tongue blades.   _____

3. a. Does Christmas come in the winter or the _____
   summer?
   b. Where is your heel?   _____

4. Draw a square (best success in two tries).   _____
5. a. Comprehension and performance   _____
   b. Personal-social maturity   _____
                          TOTAL _____

Comments:

PRESS General Outline and Record Form. The children were asked to reproduce a standard 1-inch square.

Introduction

As the child is placed on the examining table and the records and equipment are organized, the nurse says:

From Rogers WB Jr, Rogers RA: *Clin Pediatr* 11:10, 1972; and Rogers WB Jr, Rogers RA: *Clin Pediatr* 14:253, 1975. In Chinn PL: *Child health maintenance: concepts in family-centered care,* ed 2, St Louis, 1979, Mosby.

1. "Mrs. Smith, as I examine Johnny I will be asking him a few questions, so please don't talk to him for a few minutes." The nurse smiles and asks: "Ok?"
2. "Johnny, I hear you're going to start kindergarten soon. Do you think you'll like that?"

Knowledge of Colors

These questions are asked during the eye, ear, nose, throat (EENT) examination:

1. "I hear your teacher will want you to know colors. Do you know any colors yet?"
2. "If she asks you to color a house, what color should you make the grass?"
3. "And what color should you make the sky if there are no clouds?"

Knowledge of Numbers

These questions are asked during the heart and lung examination:

1. "If the teacher tells you some numbers, could you remember them and repeat them back to her?"
2. "I'm going to tell you some numbers. Now you remember them and say the same numbers right back to me." (4-1-7-3 and 3-8-6-4)
3. "If the teacher asks you to count, could you do that?"
4. "Tell me, how many tongue blades are there?" At this point place four tongue blades on the table beside the child.

Instructions for Use of PRESS*

Parents of preschoolers often ask how to tell if their child is ready for school or for a particular school program. School readiness can be thought of as the fit between the child's skill level, the child and family's psychosocial status, and the characteristics of the particular school program. Any questions about an individual child's readiness should only be answered after all of these components are addressed. The developmental testing used during the toddler years is less accurate as the child approaches school age. Some appropriate tools can help to identify the child's skill level.

A widely used tool is the *PRESS,* or *Preschool Readiness Experimental Screening Scale.* Determinations of its validity indicate that it is reliable in assessing school readiness. The nurse can administer it easily during a health assessment. The central concern is *not* measurement of intellectual level but rather screening for

---

*From Edelman CL, Mandle CL: *Health promotion throughout the lifespan,* ed 3, St Louis, 1994, Mosby.

developmental lags or abnormalities that would interfere with the child's ability to succeed in the academic and social world of school. The tool was constructed for the average capabilities of 5-year-old children but may be useful in estimating readiness in children slightly older or younger.

When obtaining more specific scores of developmental age is necessary, the nurse may use one of the screening tools specific to the preschool child. Such screening tools provide only a rough estimate of ability but may be useful in identifying those children who need more extensive evaluation of intellectual capacity.

Suggestions for Content of Education Program for Diabetes

a) General facts
   - Definition of diabetes mellitus
   - Basic anatomy and physiology
   - Basic metabolism of carbohydrates, protein and fats
   - Classification of diabetes (type I, type II, gestational, etc.)
b) Psychologic adjustment
   - Client self-assessment
   - What is "compliance?"
   - Successful adjustment and coping (living with a chronic disease, work, travel, and vacation)
   - Expressing feelings openly
   - Collaboration between client and health care team
c) Family involvement
   - Diabetes as a family challenge
   - Coping with feelings (client and family)
   - Learning to recognize and work with adverse family dynamics
   - Coping with the health care system
d) Nutrition
   - Learning to structure a daily diet
   - Learning a dietary system: exchange system, flexible diet, menu plans, others
   - Understanding dietary concepts: food content, food groups, glycemic indices, others
   - Defining, achieving, and maintaining weight goals
   - Special occasions—how to enjoy them
   - Nutritional resources

Bergenstal R: Complications of diabetes, *Caring* 3(11), 1988.

e) Exercise
- Benefits
- Methods
- Precautions
- Food and insulin adjustment
- Heart rate

f) Medications
- Goal of treatment
- Oral agents:
  Explanation of use
  Action
  Cautions
  Drug interactions
- Insulin:
  Explanation of use
  Action
  Cautions (especially Somogyi hypoglycemia)
  Strengths—purities
  Injection techniques
  Complications of treatment—hypoglycemia, antibodies, lipo-dystrophy
  Dose and timing

g) Relationship between nutrition/exercise/medication
- Putting it all together
- How each relates to the other

h) Monitoring
- Goals
- Kinds of monitoring available
- Strengths and limitations of each kind
- How to use monitoring to achieve and maintain good glucose control

i) Hyperglycemia and hypoglycemia
- Definition of hyperglycemia and hypoglycemia
- What to do for each
- When to call the health care team
- Prevention of each
- Record keeping

j) Illness
- Effect of illness on diabetes
- Monitoring glucose/ketones
- Sick day guidelines (including diet)
- When to call the health care team

k) Complications (prevent, treat, rehabilitate)
- Kinds of complications

- Possible causes of complications
- Self-care for prevention of complications
- Referral and treatment
- Rehabilitation

l) Hygiene (skin, teeth, feet, genitalia, etc.)
- Relationship to diabetes care
- Self-care measures to prevent complications

m) Benefits and responsibilities of care
- Maintaining short- and long-term life goals
- Client-professional care partnership
- Rights of the client
- Responsibilities of the client

n) Use of health care systems
- Ensuring prompt referral, coordinated care and continuing access to medical and educational services
- Identifying and using available resources

o) Community resources
- Agencies available
- Who, what, when, where to call
- Licensing and employment regulations
- Insurance considerations
- Use of local library

Sample Diabetes Client Education Record

Part I. Preprogram Assessment

This is to be completed by the diabetes client education staff member. It is *not* intended for client self-administration.

Client Demographics

NAME (LAST) _____ (FIRST) _____ (MIDDLE) _____ PHONE (___)

ADDRESS _____ (STREET) _____ (CITY) _____ (ZIP CODE)

SEX
___ 1 Male
___ 2 Female

YEAR BORN _____

ETHNIC GROUP
___ 1 Caucasian
___ 2 Black
___ 3 American Indian
___ 4 Asian or Pacific Islander
___ 5 Other

AGE WHEN DIAGNOSED _____

HEIGHT _____ (inches)

WEIGHT _____ (pounds)

TYPE OF DIABETES
___ 1 Type I
___ 2 Type II–Using insulin
___ 3 Type II–diet and/or oral agent
___ 4 Other _____

OCCUPATION _____

SPOUSE'S OCCUPATION _____

MEDICAL INSURANCE _____

DIABETES MANAGEMENT

___ Diet ___ Oral hypoglycemics ___ Exercise ___ Insulin

GENERAL HEALTH

___ 1 Excellent
___ 2 Good
___ 3 Fair
___ 4 Poor

Are you satisfied with your control?
___ No
___ Yes

MEDICATIONS FOR OTHER HEALTH PROBLEMS

No ___

If yes, please specify: _____

HEALTH PROBLEMS

___ Renal   ___ Infections
___ Hypertension ___ Neuropathy
___ Cardiac   ___ Contemplating pregnancy
___ Vascular   ___ Currently pregnant
___ Eyes

MONITORING/CONTROL HISTORY

	Method	Frequency
Blood glucose testing		
Urine glucose testing		
Urine ketone testing		

HEALTH CARE IN LAST 12 MONTHS

Hospital: Time(s) ___ Reason(s) ___
Emergency room visits: Time(s) ___ Reason(s) ___
Doctor office visits: Time(s) ___ Reason(s) ___
Date of last retinal exam _____

Nutritional History _____

Calories prescribed/day _____ Calories consumed/day _____

Continued.

Sample Diabetes Client Education Record—cont'd

HIGHEST LEVEL OF EDUCATION COMPLETED _____

YEAR OF PREVIOUS (DIABETES) EDUCATION _____ None _____ 19 _____

RELATIVES WITH DIABETES

_____ Parent(s)   _____ Grandparent(s)   _____ Brother(s) or sister(s)

_____ Identical twin   _____ Children

LIVING ARRANGEMENTS

_____ Alone   _____ With friends   _____ With family   _____ Other

PHYSICIAN (responsible for diabetes management) _____

DATE OF ENROLLMENT IN PROGRAM _____ / _____ 19 _____

PHYSICIAN'S SPECIALTY _____

_____ 1 General or family practice
_____ 2 Internist
_____ 3 Diabetologist/endocrinologist
_____ 4 Pediatrician
_____ 5 Obstetrician/gyneocologist
_____ 6 Other

REASONS FOR ENROLLMENT IN PROGRAM

_____ 1 Health professional referral
_____ 2 Health care agency referral
_____ 3 Self-referral/personal interest
_____ 4 Personal health reasons
_____ 5 Other

Medical History

Blood pressure _____   Blood glucose _____   HbA, _____

Exercise
_____ 1 Never
_____ 2 Every other week
_____ 3 1-2 days/week
_____ 4 3-5 days/week
_____ 5 6-7 days/week

Smoking
_____ 1 Never
_____ 2 Quit
_____ 3 Less than 1 pack/day
_____ 4 1 pack or more/day

Alcohol Use
_____ 1 Never
_____ 2 1-2 drinks/week
_____ 3 3-10 drinks/week
_____ 4 11 or more drinks/week

Meal Plan

Breakfast	Lunch	Dinner	Snacks	Exercise Snacks

% over ideal body weight _____

% under ideal body weight _____

Does own shopping
_____ No
_____ Yes

Does own cooking
_____ No
_____ Yes

Evaluation (Summary of evaluation data after completion of education program)

Skills _____   Attitudes _____

Knowledge _____

Planned Follow-up _____

At what interval: _____

Follow-up Method:
1. Phone
2. Letter
3. Home visit
4 Referral

Bergenstal R: Complications of diabetes, *Caring* 3(11), 1988.

The Relaxation Response

Content	Instructional activities	Evaluation
Describe the characteristics and benefits of relaxation	Discuss physiologic changes associated with relaxation and contrast these behaviors of anxiety	Client identifies own responses to anxiety Client describes elements of a relaxed state
Teach deep muscle relaxation through a sequence of tension-relaxation exercises	Engage the client in the progressive procedure of tensing and relaxing voluntary muscles until the body as a whole is relaxed	Client is able to tense and relax all muscle groups Client identifies those muscles that become particularly tense
Discuss the relaxation procedure of meditation and its components	Describe the elements of meditation and assist the client in using this technique	Client selects a word or scene with pleasant connotations and engages in relaxed meditation
Assist in overcoming anxiety-provoking situations through systematic desensitization	With client, construct a hierarchy of anxiety-provoking situations or scenes Through imagination or reality, work through these scenes using relaxation techniques	Client identifies and ranks anxiety-provoking situations Client exposes self to these situations while remaining in a relaxed state
Allow the rehearsing and practical use of relaxation in a safe environment	Role-play stressful situations with the nurse or other clients	Client becomes more comfortable with new behavior in a safe, supportive setting
Encourage client to use relaxation techniques in life	Assign homework of using the relaxation response in everday experiences Support success of client	Client uses relaxation response in life situations Client is able to regulate anxiety response through use of relaxation techniques

From Stuart GW, Sundeen SJ: *Principles and practice of psychiatric nursing*, ed 5, St Louis, 1995, Mosby.

Managing Pain without Drugs

There are several techniques you can use to relieve pain without taking drugs or to enhance the effect of your pain medication— **relaxation, imagery, distraction,** and **skin stimulation.**

Relaxation

Relaxation relieves pain by easing muscle tension. Easing muscle tension can also help you feel less tired and anxious and help other pain-relieving methods work better.

How to relax. Sit or lie down, preferably in a quiet place. Be sure you are comfortable. Do not cross your legs or arms.

Take a deep breath, and tense your muscles (you may tense up your whole body or concentrate on one set of muscles at a time, such as your facial muscles or those in your arms and hands).

Hold your breath, and keep your muscles tense.

Release your breath and your muscles at the same time. Let your body go limp (repeat for other muscle areas if you are concentrating on one set at a time).

You can add imagery (see below) or music to help you relax. Relaxation tapes are also available.

Don't be discouraged if relaxation doesn't help immediately. Practice the relaxation technique for 2 weeks before you give it up. If you find that it aggravates your pain, try another method.

Imagery

Imagery involves using your imagination to create mental scenes that use all your senses: sight, sound, touch, smell, and taste. You can imagine exotic locations or revisit one of your favorite places. You can create stories and characters to add to your scenes. Imagery can take your mind off your anxiety, boredom, and pain.

How to use imagery. Close your eyes. A few moments of the relaxation technique (see above) will help your body and mind prepare for imagery.

Let your mind begin forming its image. The following is an example of imagery:

Imagine that you are at the seashore. You are sitting in the wet sand; the afternoon sun is warm on your shoulders. The ocean rolls into the shore in gentle waves, and the water laps teasingly at your toes. A hungry pair of seagulls cry overhead and take swift, darting dives at a dog that is scavenging along the shore. Your tension lessens with each wave that touches your toes and retreats. You close your eyes and take a deep, slow breath of salt-filled air. You are completely relaxed. Stay on the beach as long as you like.

To end the image, count to three and open your eyes. Resume your regular activities slowly.

Distraction

A distraction is any activity that takes your mind off your pain and focuses your attention elsewhere. Doing crafts, reading a book, watching television, or listening to music through headphones can all help distract your mind. Distraction works well when you are waiting for drugs to take effect or if you have brief bouts of pain. Sometimes people can take their minds off their pain for long periods, especially if the pain is mild.

Skin Stimulation

Skin stimulation is used to block pain sensation in the nerves. Pressure, massage, hot and cold applications, rubbing, and mild electrical current are all ways to stimulate the skin. However, if you are undergoing radiation treatment, consult your doctor before applying any skin stimulation.

You can do skin stimulation at the site of the pain, near it, or on the opposite side of pain. For example, stimulating the left wrist when the right wrist is in pain can actually ease the pain in the right wrist.

Pressure. Using your entire hand, the heel of your hand, your thumb, your knuckles, or both hands, apply at least 15 seconds of pressure at the point where you feel pain. Keep trying spots around the painful area if you find no relief the first time. You may extend the time you apply pressure to 1 minute.

Massage. You or someone else can perform the slow, circular motions of massage. The feet, back, neck, and scalp can be massaged to relieve tension and pain anywhere in the body. Some people prefer to use oils or lotions during the massage. If deep massage is too uncomfortable, try light stroking. Do not massage red, raw, or broken skin.

Heat and cold. Some people prefer cold; others prefer heat. Use whichever works best for you. A convenient way to use cold is to freeze gel-filled packs and wrap them in towels. Ice cubes can also be used. Heat can be applied with a heating pad; hot, moist towels; or a hot water bottle or by taking a hot bath. Be careful not to burn your skin with water that is too hot or to go to sleep with a heating pad on. Don't expose your skin to intense cold for very long.

Transcutaneous electrical nerve stimulation. TENS can be used to eliminate or ease pain. A TENS unit is a pocket-sized, battery-operated device that provides a mild, continuous electrical current through the skin by the use of two to four electrodes, which are taped onto the skin. Lead wires connect the electrodes to the device. It is this mild electrical current that blocks or modifies the pain messages and replaces them with a buzzing, tingling sensation. It is also thought that TENS may stimulate the body's production of endorphin, a natural pain reliever.

Techniques for Preventing Aggression

1. Form and maintain a social norm against aggression. The entire unit must communicate a distinct disapproval of any form of verbal or physical aggression. Appropriate alternatives for expressing emotion and perceptions are taught and reinforced. Staff must be willing to openly explore valid criticisms of treatment and the milieu by clients and reinforce talking versus yelling, but aggression in any form is not tolerated. Staff must be available and accessible to clients who are struggling to maintain control and give clients time when they need it.

2. Be vigilant to recognize and manage transference and counter-transference issues on the part of staff and clients. *Transference* is a conscious or unconscious emotional response in which a client transfers onto another person feelings, wishes, and conflicts which originated in the client's own relationships with significant others. *Countertransference* is the other person's response to the transfer. For instance, Jan, a newly admitted client, interacted with the nurse, Jim, for about 2 minutes before she got angry. Jim asked whether he reminded her of somebody. "Yes, you do. You look and act just like my ex-husband. I really don't want to talk to you."

3. Ensure responsible involvement by psychiatrists during aggressive episodes. Psychiatrists are to be trained, along with the nursing staff, so that teamwork is ensured. The presence of psychiatrists for intervening in aggressive episodes is thought to contribute significantly to prevention of further episodes.

Staff need to be specifically trained to manage aggression to ensure the following: (1) increase teamwork and consistency of approach to clients, (2) decrease staff uncertainty about how to respond to aggression, (3) increase the management of risk and

From Haber J et al: *Comprehensive psychiatric nursing.* ed 4, St Louis, 1992, Mosby.

liability for clients and staff, (4) decrease the rate of injury of clients and staff, and (5) provide staff with response alternatives to aggression rather than relying on past modes of intervention.

The compassionate, intelligent care of aggressive clients requires clinicians to be skilled in the use of a variety of management techniques. Students and staff need courses in aggression management as much as they need courses in cardiopulmonary resuscitation.

4. Evaluate by means of thorough assessment each client's potential for aggression to help the staff plan specific care for those who are more likely to act out. Pay prompt attention to the significance of each aggressive episode, decreasing the likelihood of another aggression episode.

5. *Debriefing* is questioning of clients for the purpose of eliciting their thoughts and feelings about upsetting events after they occur. Staff continue to debrief with clients until the event is resolved and clients are free to turn their attention to their treatment issues. All the team members need to be cognizant of the initial event and the resolution of the issues over time.

Staff need to debrief with each other as well. Two processes occur for staff. Communicating feelings and perceptions needs to occur first; evaluation of how the staff managed the event evolves out of the debriefing. The purpose of evaluation is to become more proficient in managing aggressive episodes and working together as a team.

Alcohol Self-Care Activities

Sources
    Liquor, wine, beer, medications.
Positive effects
    Relaxation, vasodilation.
Problematic effects
    Danger of addiction; damage to liver, nervous system; congenital birth defects; precipitates hypertension in some people; continued overindulgence can destroy relationships, physical health.
Recommendations
    Do not use alcohol for insomnia or pain control.
    Limit to two servings per week.
    Measure intake by the ounce—not by glass.

From Hill I, Smith N: *Self-care nursing,* 1985, Prentice-Hall.

Self-care activities

Celebrate with sparkling fruit juices; they are festive for children also.

Drink dry white wine, mineral water, or exotic fruit drinks without alcohol.

Be aware of effect of ethyl alcohol on your body; validate with spouse, friends.

Know alcohol content of beverages.

Keep an ethyl alcohol diary for 6 months to determine drinking patterns.

Use a "stop drinking program" if needed.

Do not drink and drive.

Do not mix medications with alcohol.

Role model responsible behavior with ethyl alcohol to children; show them it is easy to have fun socially without drinking.

Learn and teach concepts of tolerance, dependence, intoxication.

Learn withdrawal symptoms, potential dangers.

Take turns being the driver for the evening when drinking with friends.

The Progression and Recovery of the Alcoholic in the Disease of Alcoholism

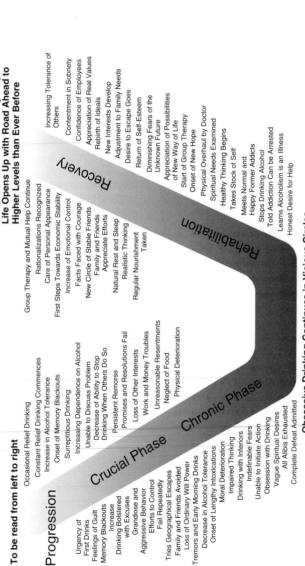

The Progression and Recovery of the Alcoholic in the Disease of Alcoholism. (From Jellinek EM: *QJ Stud Alcohol* 13:672, 1952. In Stuart GW, Sundeen SJ, *Principles and practice of psychiatric nursing*, ed 5, St. Louis, 1995, Mosby.)

Typical Characteristics of Codependence

- Overcommit self
- Feel compelled to help others solve their problems
- Feel overly responsible for other people's feelings, thoughts, actions, needs, and well-being
- Feel worthless when not productive
- Feel trapped in relationships
- Feel "crazy" and wonder what is "normal"
- Afraid of own anger
- Tired and lack energy
- Feel uncomfortable when a compliment is given
- Always try to please others, not self
- Try to control events and how other people should behave
- Find it difficult to express emotions and make decisions
- Wish there was more time for exercise, hobbies, and sports
- Constantly seeking approval and affirmation

Adapted from Zerwekh J, Michaels B: *Nurs Clin North Am* 24:109, 1989. In Stuart GW, Sundeen SJ: *Principles and practice of psychiatric nursing,* ed. 5, St Louis, 1995, Mosby.

Stages of Chemical Dependence

Characteristics	Early stage	Middle stage	Late stage
Pattern of use	Regular	Daily	Continuous
Motives for use	To relax, sleep, achieve euphoria	To feel "normal"	To avoid uncomfortable psychologic or physiologic states (to avoid withdrawal symptoms)
Tolerance	Tolerant	Tolerant	Lower threshold of tolerance
Dependence	Psychologic dependence	Psychologic dependence and possible physiologic dependence	Psychologic and physiologic dependence
Job performance	May be somewhat diminished	Decreased productivity	Impaired performance
Social and community relations	Arguments over use	Increasing isolation	Withdrawal from community activities and social relationships

Adapted from Jellinek EM: Phases of alcohol addiction, *Q J Stud Alcohol* 13:673–684, 1952. In Haber J et al: *Comprehensive psychiatric nursing,* ed 4, St Louis, 1992, Mosby.

Levels of Application of Preventive Measures

The chart below, developed by H.R. Leavell and E.G. Clark, shows the natural history of a disease as it relates to the three levels of prevention, then identifies specific activities that can be used for each level of prevention.

NATURAL HISTORY OF A DISEASE

Prepathogenesis period	Pathogenesis period
Interrelations among Agent, Host, and Environmental Factors →Stimulus	Early Pathogenesis →Early Lesions → Discernible Early Lesions → Advanced Disease →Convalescence

LEVELS OF PREVENTION

Primary prevention		Secondary prevention		Tertiary prevention
Health promotion	*Specific protection*	*Early diagnosis and prompt treatment*	*Disability limitation*	*Rehabilitation*
Health education Good standard of nutrition adjusted to developmental phase of life	Use of specific immunizations Attention to personal hygiene	Case-finding measures, individual and mass Screening surveys	Adequate treatment to arrest disease process and prevent further complications and sequelae	Provision of hospital and community facilities for retraining and education for maximum use of remaining capacities

Attention to personality development	Use of environmental sanitation	Selective examinations	Provision of facilities to limit disability and prevent death	Education of the public and industry to employ the rehabilitated
Provision of adequate housing, recreation, and agreeable working conditions	Protection against occupational hazards	Cure and prevention of disease processes		As full employment as possible
	Use of specific nutrients	Prevention of the spread of communicable diseases		Selective placement
Marriage counseling and sex education	Protection from carcinogens	Prevention of complications and sequelae		Work therapy in hospitals
Genetics	Avoidance of allergens	Shortened period of disability		Use of sheltered colony
Periodic selective examinations				

Adapted from Leavell HR, Clark EG: *Preventive medicine for the doctor in his community*, ed 3, New York, 1965, McGraw-Hill.

Criteria to Differentiate and Discriminate Among Preventive Approaches

| | Types of approaches | | |
| | **Primary** | **Secondary** | **Tertiary** |
Criteria	**Proactive pretherapeutic**	**Paraactive paratherapeutic**	**Reactive therapeutic**
1. Risk	Low to minimal	High: in need but not critical	Very high: critical
2. Reversibility	High: 100% to 66%	Medium 66% to 33%	Low to very low: 33% to 0%
3. Probability of breakdown	Low but potential	Medium but probable	High and real (actual)
4. Population	Nonclinical: labeled but not diagnosable	Preclinical and diagnosable	Clinical: critical and diagnosed
5. Ability to learn	High	Medium	Low
6. Goals	Increase competence and resistance to breakdown	Decrease stress and chance of crisis	Restore to minimum functioning
7. Type of involvement	Voluntary: many choices	Obligatory: decrease in choices	Mandatory: no other choices available
8. Recommendations	"Could benefit by it." "It would be nice."	"You need it before it's too late." "Recommend strongly that you do it."	"It is necessary." "Nothing else will work." "Other choices would be more expensive" (i.e., hospitalization, incarceration)
9. Cost	Low	Medium	High
10. Effectiveness	High(?)	Questionable yet to be found	Relatively low
11. Personnel	Lay volunteers and pre- and paraprofessionals	Middle-level professionals	Professionals
12. Types of intervention	General, learning, strengthening, enrichment	More specific to behavior, that is, programmed materials	Specialized therapy
13. Degree of structure	High	Medium	Low
14. Degree of specificity	General and topical	Individualized	Specific to the symptom

From L'Abate L: *Building family competence*, Newbury Park, Calif., 1990, Sage Publications.

Examples of Health Promotion Strategies to Dimensions of the Whole Person

Physical/physiologic	Emotional	Cognitive	Social	Spiritual/moral
Proper nutrition/fluid balance	Consistent warm, tender, nurturing of offspring	Promotion of curiosity and learning	Socialization processes	Values clarification
Balance of exercise-rest	Effective communication	Coping methods	Family, friend, peer relations	Acknowledgement of meaning and purpose of life
Immunizations	Effective guidance/discipline	Visualization	Group associations and processes	Establishment of belief system
Safety measures	Promotion of self-esteem, self-confidence, security	Imagery	Maintenance of cultural ties	Establishment of moral and ethical behaviors
Temperature control	Anxiety reduction measures	Health education		
Prevention of environmental hazards and pollution	Play, use of toys, leisure activities			
Cessation of habits destructive to health (smoking, alcohol or drug abuse, overeating)	Crisis resolution			
Health screening				

From Murray RB, Zentner JL: *Nursing assessment and health promotion,* 1993, Appleton and Lange.

Contraindications and Precautions to Vaccinations[a]

True contraindications and precautions	Not contraindications (vaccines may be administered)
General for all vaccines (DTP/DTAP, OPV, IPV, MMR, HIB, Hepatitis B)	*Not contraindications*
Contraindications	Mild to moderate local reaction (soreness, redness, swelling) following a dose of an injectable antigen
Anaphylactic reaction to a vaccine contraindicates further doses of the vaccine	Mild acute illness with or without low-grade fever
Anaphylactic reaction to a vaccine constituent contraindicates the use of vaccines containing that substance	Current antimicrobial therapy
Moderate or severe illnesses with or without a fever	Convalescent phase of illnesses
	Prematurity (same dosage and indications as for normal, full-term infants)
	Recent exposure to an infectious disease
	History of penicillin or other nonspecific allergies or family history of such allergies
Diphtheria, tetanus, pertussis or acellular pertussis (DTP/DTAP)	*Not contraindications*
Contraindications	Temperature of <40.5° C (105° F) following a previous dose of DTP
Endephalopathy within 7 days of administration of previous dose of DTP	Family history of convulsions[c]
Precautions[b]	Family history of sudden infant death syndrome
Fever of ≥40.5° C (105° F) within 48 hours after vaccination with a prior dose of DTP	Family history of an adverse event following DTP administration
Collapse or shocklike state (hypotonic-hyporesponsive episode) within 48 hours of receiving a prior dose of DTP	
Seizures within 3 days of receiving a prior dose of DTP[c]	

Persistent, inconsolable crying lasting ≥3 hours within 48 hours of receiving a prior dose of DTP

Oral polio (OPV)[d]

Contraindications	*Not contraindications*
Infection with HIV or a household contact with HIV	Breast-feeding
Known altered immunodeficiency (hematologic and solid tumors; congenital immunodeficiency; and long-term immunosuppressive therapy)	Current antimicrobial therapy
	Diarrhea

---

[a]This information is based on the recommendations of the Advisory Committee on Immunization Practices (ACIP) and those of the Committee on Infectious Diseases (Red Book Committee) of the American Academy of Pediatrics (AAP). Sometimes these recommendations vary from those contained in the manufacturer's package inserts. For more detailed information, providers should consult the published recommendations of the ACIP, AAP, and the manufacturer's package inserts.

[b]The events or conditions listed as precautions, although not contraindications, should be carefully reviewed. The benefits and risks of administering a specific vaccine to an individual under the circumstances should be considered. If the risks are believed to outweigh the benefits, the vaccination should be withheld; if the benefits are believed to outweigh the risks (e.g., during an outbreak or foreign travel), the vaccination should be administered. Whether and when to administer DTP to children with proven or suspected underlying neurologic disorders should be decided on an individual basis. It is prudent on theoretic grounds to avoid vaccinating pregnant women. However, if immediate protection against poliomyelitis is needed, OPV is preferred, although IPV may be considered if full vaccination can be completed before the anticipated imminent exposure.

[c]Acetaminophen given before administering DTP and thereafter every 4 hours for 24 hours should be considered for children with a personal or family history of convulsions in siblings or parents.

[d]No data exist to substantiate the theoretic risk of a suboptimal immune response from the administration of OPV and MMR within 30 days of each other.

[e]Persons with a history of anaphylactic reactions following egg ingestion should be vaccinated only with caution. Protocols have been developed for vaccinating such persons and should be consulted.

[f]Measles vaccination may temporarily suppress tuberculin reactivity. If testing cannot be done the day of MMR vaccination, the test should be postponed for 4 to 6 weeks.

From Centers for Disease Control and Prevention: General recommendations on immunization: recommendations of the Advisory Committee on Immunization Practices (ACIP) *MMWR* 43(RR-1):24–25, 1994. From Wong DL: *Whaley and Wong's nursing care of infants and children*, ed 5, St Louis, 1995, Mosby.

Contraindications and precautions to vaccinations—cont'd

True contraindications and precautions	Not contraindications (vaccines may be administered)
Immunodeficient household contact ***Precaution***[b] Pregnancy	
Inactivated polio (IPV) *Contraindication* Anaphylactic reaction to neomycin or streptomycin ***Precaution***[b] Pregnancy	
Measles, Mumps, Rubella (MMR)[d] *Contraindications* Anaphylactic reactions to egg ingestion and to neomycin[e] Pregnancy Known altered immunodeficiency (hematologic and solid tumors, congenital immunodeficiency, and long-term immunosuppressive therapy) ***Precautions***[b] Recent immune globulin administration Immune globulin products and MMR should not be given simultaneously; if unavoidable, give at different sites and revaccinate or test for seroconversion in 3 months; if IG is given first, MMR should not be given for at least 3–6 months, depending on the dose; if MMR is given first, IG should not be given for 2 weeks	*Not contraindications*[a] Tuberculosis or positive PPD skin test Simultaneous TB skin testing[f] Breast-feeding Pregnancy of mother of recipient Immunodeficient family member or household contact Infection with HIV Nonanaphylactic reactions to eggs or neomycin

Not contraindications[a]
Tuberculosis or positive PPD skin test
Simultaneous TB skin testing[f]
Breast-feeding
Pregnancy of mother of recipient
Immunodeficient family member or household contact
Infection with HIV
Nonanaphylactic reactions to eggs or neomycin

Haemophilus Influenzae type B (HIB)

Contraindications
Nonidentified

Not a contraindication
History of Hib disease

Hepatitis B virus (HBV)

Contraindication
Anaphylactic reaction to common baker's yeast

Not a contraindication
Pregnancy

[b] The events or conditions listed as precautions, although not contraindications, should be carefully reviewed. The benefits and risks of administering a specific vaccine to an individual under the circumstances should be considered. If the risks are believed to outweigh the benefits, the vaccination should be withheld; if the benefits are believed to outweigh the risks (e.g., during an outbreak or foreign travel), the vaccination should be administered. Whether and when to administer DTP to children with proven or suspected underlying neurologic disorders should be decided on an individual basis. It is prudent on theoretic grounds to avoid vaccinating pregnant women. However, if immediate protection against poliomyelitis is needed, OPV is preferred, although IPV may be considered if full vaccination can be completed before the anticipated imminent exposure.

[d] No data exist to substantiate the theoretic risk of a suboptimal immune response from the administration of OPV and MMR within 30 days of each other.

Body Mass Index

Body mass is the figure you get by dividing your weight in kilograms by the square of your height in meters.

1. To convert weight to kilograms, divide pounds without clothes by 2.2: _____ .
2. To convert to meters, divide your height in inches (without shoes) by 39.4 (   )_, then square it: _____ .
3. Divide (1) by (2). Body mass index = _____ .

For men, desirable body mass is 22–24. Above 28.5 is overweight; above 33 is seriously overweight.
For women, desirable body mass is 21–23. Overweight begins at 27.5, and seriously overweight is above 31.5.

From Phipps WJ et al: *Medical-surgical nursing: concepts and clinical practice,* ed 5. St Louis, 1995, Mosby.

Self-Help Devices

Grooming Devices

A long-handled comb: curved handle or built-up handle to enlarge it.*
Built-up handle hair brush.*
Extension mirror to be fit around client's neck. These can also be purchased with a magnifying mirror. They are available in department stores.
Fingernail brush. Mounts with two suction cups to adhere to cabinet or sink top. Allows the client to clean fingernails with the use of only one hand. This model can also be used in the kitchen for a vegetable brush.

Dressing Aids

Sock and stocking aids. These have long handles or straps, allowing the client to put on socks and stockings from a sitting position.
Long-handled shoe horn with built-up handle.* Put on shoes in a sitting position.
Elastic shoelaces. These permit shoes to be tied once. They come in various lengths and colors and allow lace shoes to be slipped on without tying.
Combination button aid and zipper pull. Built-up handle and wire loop

---

Walsh D: *Manual of home health care nursing,* Philadelphia, 1987, JB Lippincott.
*All built-up handles can be made by applying foam rubber curlers or pipe insulation or by applying bicycle handles.

on one end allow one-handed buttoning. Hook on the other end allows for zipper pull.

Dressing stick. This 24-inch stick with hooks on both ends assists in pulling up trousers, underclothing, and so on, for the client unable to bend.

Eating Aids

Dishes. Dishes are available with one side built up to allow food to be pushed up and trapped on cutlery. Entire sets of dishes are available in Melamine in attractive designs. A homemade plate guard can also be attached to the plates used by the client.

Cutlery. Handles can be built up by use of plastic foam curlers or narrow foam rubber pipe insulation, or they can be purchased with wood built-up handles.

Securing of straws: A bulldog clip can be secured to the edge of the glass and a straw inserted through the hole on the clip handle and into the liquid.

Cutting board. The corner of a cutting board can be built up with small pieces of wood or other material. It can be used to anchor bread for buttering or other items needing to be anchored.

A jar opener can be mounted in the kitchen for ease of opening jars with one hand.

Drinking cups. Large-handled mugs can be purchased. In addition, cups are available with nonspill tops and with large handles and holders that can be shaped to fit tumblers, soft-drink cans, and so forth.

A nonslip material (similar to that used in bathtubs) applied under dishes can be used at the table to prevent their slipping.

An adjustable cuff can be purchased that can be applied to the hand and various sizes of handles can be secured in the cuff. This is appropriate for persons having little or no grip.

Tablecloth clamps, purchased at the dime store and applied to the dining table, secure the table cloth and prevent it from slipping.

Nonslip placemats are available in various colors.

Large-handled vegetable peeler, large-handled food grater, and one-handed slicing knife and frame for slicing bread are available commercially.

A two-sided suction holder (for holding soap; available in the dime store) can also be used under plates and other dishes to hold them in place.

Communication and Security

Automatic night-lights are available.

Magnifiers of various magnitudes and sizes are commercially available.

Telephones can be amplified for adjustable volume control. Big-button telephones are available with hands-free speaker.

Wiring can be done in the home for hearing-impaired clients to allow a lamp to flash on and off when a doorbell or telephone rings.

Radio-controlled switches are available for remote control (up to 40 feet away) of lights, small appliances, and television.

Clothing

Regular gowns and pajama tops can be seamed down the back and attached with velcro or ties, for ease of application.

Large terrycloth and vinyl bibs with "gutters" to catch crumbs and spills are available or can be made.

Reachers

Simple long tongs (used for barbecue) often suffice to reach items beyond arm's length.

Other reachers have magnetic tips, easy gripping devices, and adjustable "jaws."

Wheelchair and Walker Accessories

A basket or bag can be applied to the front of a walker for carrying small items.

A small holder with a squeeze clamp to be applied to the front of the wheelchair, below the armrest, is available for carrying small items that fall easily.

A cup or soft-drink-can holder can be applied by putting a squeeze clamp on the front of the wheelchair below the armrest.

A lap board (available in dime stores) assists the wheelchair client to write and eat.

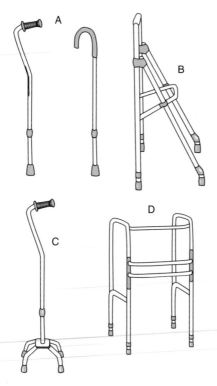

Assistive devices for ambulation. **A,** Straight canes. **B,** Pickup walker. **C,** Quad cane. **D,** Standard walker. (From Hoeman SP: *Rehabilitation nursing: process and application,* ed 2, St Louis, 1996, Mosby.)

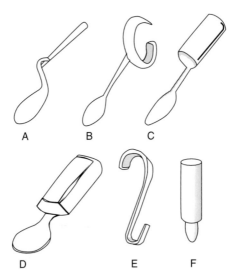

Hand manipulation aids. **A,** Swivel spoon. **B,** Vertical palm self-handle spoon. **C,** Built-up handle spoon. **D,** Universal cuff holds various utensils. **E,** Doorknob turner. **F,** Telephone dialing stick.

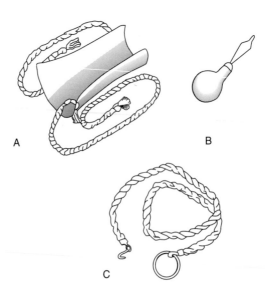

Dressing aids. **A,** Flexible sock and stocking aid. **B,** Button hook. **C,** Long reach zipper pull.

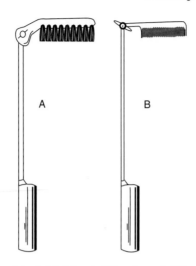

Adapted hairbrush (**A**) and comb (**B**).

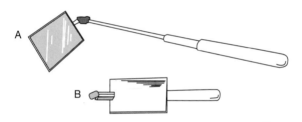

Long-handled skin inspection mirror (**A**) and reach zipper pull (**B**).

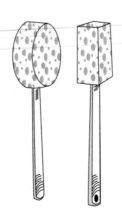

Long-handled bath sponge.

Quitting Smoking

Your doctor has told you to quit smoking. You want to, but you aren't sure of the best way. Perhaps you've tried before. Or you're afraid you'll gain weight.

What's the Best Way to Quit?

There are many ways to quit smoking, but you need only one thing—*the desire to quit.* Once you have that all-important ingredient, you will succeed.

You can quit "cold turkey," or you can set a quit date and taper off gradually over a 2-week period. Some people find it helpful to have support from others who are quitting at the same time. Your local chapter of the American Lung Association, the American Cancer Society, or the American Heart Association or a hospital in your community can help you locate a smoking cessation class. Or you can use the "buddy system"—make a pact with a friend who wants to quit and provide support for each other.

Many people find chewing nicotine gum or using a nicotine patch helpful for the first few weeks. Talk to your doctor about prescribing one of these for you.

Adopt as many techniques as you think will work for you, and use them all.

What about Withdrawal Symptoms?

Keep in mind that most smokers actually have a double addiction: physical and psychologic. You will need to deal with both aspects.

Physical withdrawal can be a problem for heavy smokers (more than one pack a day). The symptoms vary from one person to another, but common complaints are headaches, constipation, irritability, nervousness, trouble concentrating, and insomnia. You may even cough more for the first week after quitting as your cilia become active again. This is actually a sign that your body is healing itself.

You can do several things to ease the withdrawal symptoms. Although you may fear that you'll be craving a cigarette all the time, each urge actually lasts only 2 or 3 minutes. When it hits, do a minute or two of deep-breathing exercises to calm the urge; close your eyes, take a deep breath, and slowly let it out. If you still feel a craving, change your activity—walk around or do something that requires both hands, or do something that you especially enjoy.

Drink lots of water to help flush the toxins from your body. Eat a healthy, well-balanced diet. Many authorities say that eating less meat and more fresh vegetables and fruits helps reduce withdrawal symptoms. To combat aftermeal cravings, leave the table immediately and brush your teeth. Sugarless gum or hard candy, a toothpick, or unsalted, shelled sunflower seeds satisfy the oral craving without adding calories.

Daily exercise (unless your doctor advises you not to) will help relax you and hasten recovery from the effects of nicotine.

Try to avoid situations that you associate with smoking, such as a morning cup of coffee or a before-dinner drink. You may need to modify your habits for a while until the withdrawal period is over. This also means avoiding spending too much time around other smokers.

Write down all your reasons for quitting smoking to remind yourself whenever you're discouraged or tempted to smoke. Keep the list handy, and look at it often. And feel proud of yourself for quitting.

Won't I Gain Weight?

According to recent studies, only about one third of ex-smokers gain some weight; one third lose weight, and one third stay the same. The key to not gaining weight is not to eat every time you crave a smoke. As long as you maintain a well-balanced diet, don't snack between meals, and exercise, you shouldn't experience any weight problems.

What if I Fail?

Many people who have successfully quit smoking failed the first time they tried. Often they describe these "failures" as valuable learning experiences that helped them succeed the next time. Whatever you do, don't give up. More than 36 million Americans have already quit. You can, too.

Blood Pressure Recommendations
for Follow-Up and Classification—Adult

Classification of stages of high blood pressure for adults age 18 years or older*

Average DBP mm Hg	Average SBP mm Hg				
	<140	140-159	160-179	180-209	≥210
<90	No HBP	1	2	3	4
90-99	1	1	2	3	4
100-109	2	2	2	3	4
110-119	3	3	3	3	4
≥120	4	4	4	4	4

*Not taking antihypertensive durgs and not acutely ill. When systolic and diastolic pressure fall into different categories, the higher category should be selected to classify the individual's blood pressure status. For instance, 160/92 should be classified as stage 2, and 180/120 should be classified as stage 4. Isolated systolic hypertension (ISH) is defined as SBP ≥ 140 mm Hg and DBP < 90 mm Hg and staged appropriately (e.g., 170/85 mm Hg is defined as stage 2 ISH).

From the 5th Joint National Committee on detection, evaluation and treatment of high blood pressure, 1993, Heart, Lung and Blood Inst., NIH.

Recommendations for follow-up based on initial set of blood pressure measurements for adults age 18 and older

Initial screening blood pressure (mm Hg)*		Follow-up recommended†
Systolic	Diastolic	
<130	<85	Recheck in 2 years
130-139	85-89	Recheck in 1 year‡
140-159	90-99	Confirm within 2 months
160-179	100-109	Evaluate or refer to source of care within 1 month
180-209	110-119	Evaluate or refer to source of care within 1 week
≥210	≥120	Evaluate or refer to source of care immediately

*If the systolic and diastolic categories are different, follow recommendation for the shorter time follow-up (e.g., 160/85 mm Hg should be evaluated or referred to source of care within 1 month).

†The scheduling of follow-up should be modified by reliable information about past blood pressure measurements, other cardiovascular risk factors, or target-organ disease.

‡Consider providing advice about lifestyle modifications.

Classification of blood pressure for adults age 18 years and older after two or more reading*

Average DBP mm Hg	Average SBP mm Hg			
	<120	120-129	130-139	≥140
<80	Optimal†	Normal	High Normal	High
80-84	Normal	Normal	High Normal	High
85-89	High Normal	High Normal	High Normal	High
≥90	High	High	High	High

Category	Systolic mm Hg	Diastolic mm Hg
Normal	<130	<85
High normal	130-139	85-89
Hypertension‡		
Stage 1 (mild)	140-159	90-99
Stage 2 (moderate)	160-179	100-109
Stage 3 (severe)	180-209	110-119
Stage 4 (very severe)	≥210	≥120

*Not taking antihypertensive drugs and not acutely ill. When systolic and diastolic pressure fall into different categories, the higher category should be selected to classify the individual's blood pressure status. For instance, 160/92 should be classified as stage 2 and 180/120 should be classified as stage 4. Isolated systolic hypertension (ISH) is defined as SBP ≥ 140 mm Hg and DBP < 90 mm Hg and staged appropriately (e.g., 170/85 mm Hg is defined as stage 2 ISH). From the 5th Joint National Committee on detection, evaluation and of high blood pressure, 1993, Heart, Lung and Inst., NIH.
†Optimal blood pressure, with regard to cardiovascular risk, is SBP < 120 mm Hg and DBP < 80 mm Hg. However, unusually low readings should be evaluated for clinical significance.
‡Based on the average of two or more readings taken at each of two or more visits following an initial screening.

⑤ Screening Tools, Techniques, and Diagnostic Criteria

Vision, Hearing, and Language Screening Procedures

Method	Age	Procedure	Normal response
Vision			
Following	Infancy	Shine light or hold bright object directly in front of infant's line of vision; move slowly from side to side.	Follow light or bright object up to 180 degrees
Turn to light response	Infancy	Hold back of head to bright light source.	Eyes turn toward source of light
Optokinetic drum	Infancy	Twirl drum with stripes slowly in front of infant's eyes.	Nystagmus occurs.
Herschberg reflex (corneal light reflex)	Infancy through adolescence	Shine penlight into child's eyes; note where light reflex falls. For older children: have child focus and stare at point 14 inches and then 20 inches away before shining light into eyes.	Light reflex falls in same position in eye
Cover test	Toddler through adolescence	Have child focus on specified spot first 14 inches, then 20 inches away. While child is focusing, one eye is completely covered	No wandering or sharp jerky movement of eyes noted, indicating ability to focus

Continued.

Hogard NO: In Stanhope MJ, Lancaster J: *Community health nursing: process and practice for promoting health,* St Louis, 1992, Mosby.

Vision, hearing, and language screening procedures—cont'd

Method	Age	Procedure	Normal response
Cover test—cont'd		for 5 to 10 seconds. Cover is then removed and eye observed for movement. Procedure repeated for other eye.	
Snellen E	Preschool	Child is instructed to point finger in direction that the E or table legs are pointing from a distance of 20 feet. Test each eye separately, then together. Test as far down on chart as child can go.	Visual acuity of 20/30
Snellen alphabet	School age through adolescence	Child stands 20 feet from chart and reads letters. Each eye is tested separately and then together. Testing usually started at 20/30 or 20/40 line and child allowed to test as far down chart as possible. Passing score consists of reading majority of letters (or Es) on each line.	Visual acuity of 20/20
Hearing			
Startle reflex	Newborn	Loud noise or bang made near infant's ears.	Jumps at noise, blinks, cries or widens eyes

Tracks sound	3-6 months	Make noise, call name or sing.	Eyes shift toward sound; responds to mother's voice; coos to verbalization
Recognizes sound	6-8 months	As preceding, from out of line of vision.	Turns head toward sound; responds to name, babbles to verbalization
Localization of sound	8-12 months	Call name, or use tuning fork or say words.	Localizes source of sound; turns head (and body at times) toward sound, repeats words
Pure tone screening—play	Toddler to preschool	Demonstrate to child by putting headpones on and making believe you hear sound. As you say "I hear it," put a block in box or ring on holder. Put headphones on child and give block or ring to use. Sound a 50 dB tone at 1000 Hz and guide child's hand with block to box. When child can do this alone, beging screening. Set at 25 dB at 1000 Hz. If child responds, go to 2000, 4000, and 6000 Hz. Praise child and place new block in hand. Switch to other ear and test.	Should respond at 25 dB at any frequency
Pure tone audiometry	School age through adolescence	Explain procedure to child. Place headphones on ears. Test 1 ear at	Should respond at 25 dB at any frequency

Continued.

Vision, hearing, and language screening procedures—cont'd

Method	Age	Procedure	Normal response
Pure tone audiometry—cont'd		a time in sequence as preceding (i.e., 25 dB at 1000, 2000, 4000 and 6000 Hz). Have child raise hand to indicate sound is heard.	
Tuning fork test	Some preschoolers; school age through adolescence		
A. Weber test		Strike tuning fork to make it vibrate and place the stem in midline of scalp. Ask child if sound is same in both ears or louder in either ear.	Sound heard equally well in both ears
B. Rinne test		Strike tuning fork until it vibrates, place stem on child's mastoid until he no longer hears it. Then place vibrating fingers of fork 1 to 2 inches in front of concha. Ask child if he can still hear sound.	Sound from fingers of fork vibrating in air should be heard when child can no longer hear sound with stem against mastoid, i.e., air conduction is greater than bone conduction
Language			
Assessment of child's language comprehension	3 to 6 years	Child points to picture named by examiner Assesses single word vocabulary and two-word, three-word, and four-word phrases	Child able to name picture understandably

Peabody Picture Vocabulary Test	2½ to 18 years	Child looks at picture and points to one named by examiner	Child able to respond correctly by following directions
Preschool Language Scale	Birth to 3 years	Observation of child's performance	Depending on age level, child should be able to point to picture, follow direction, or manipulate objects
Expressive One Word Picture Vocabulary	2 to 12 years	Child looks at picture and names what is seen	Child able to follow directions and articulate response at age level

Landmarks of Speech, Language, and Hearing Ability During the Preschool Period

Age (months)	Receptive language	Expressive language	Related hearing ability
42	Up to 4200 words; knows words such as what, where, how, funny, we, surprise, secret, knows number concepts to 2, how to answer questions accurately, such as do you have a dog, which is the girl, what toys do you have.	Up to 1200 words in mostly complete sentences averaging four to five words per sentence; uses all 50 phonemes; 7% of sentences are compound or complex; averages 203 words per hour; rate of speech is faster; relates experiences and tells about activities in sequential order; uses words such as what, where, how, see, little, funny, they, we, he, she, several; can say a nursery rhyme; asks permission; 95% of speech is intelligible.	
48	Up to 5600 words; carries out three-item commands consistently; knows why we have houses, books, umbrella, key; knows nearly all colors, words such as somebody, anybody, even, almost, now, something, like, bigger, too, full name, one or two songs, number concepts to 4; understands most preschool stories; can complete opposite analogies, such as brother is a boy, sister is a	Up to 1500 words in sentences averaging five to six words per sentence; averages 400 words per hour; counts to 3, repeats four digits, names three objects, and repeats nine-word sentences from memory; names the primary colors, some coins; relates fanciful tales; enjoys rhyming nonsense words and using exaggerations; demands reasons why and how; questioning is at a	Begins to make the fine discriminations among similar speech sounds, such as the difference between *f* and *th* or *f* and *s*. Child has matured enough to be tested with an audiometer. At this age formal hearing testing usually can be carried out. Not only has hearing developed to its optimum level, but listening has also become considerably refined.

54

; in daytime it is light, at night it is _____.

Up to 6500 words; knows what a house, window, chair, and dress are made of and what we do with our eyes and ears; understands differences in texture and composition, such as hard, soft, rough, smooth; begins to name or point to penny, nickel, dime; understands if, because, why, when.

peak, up to 500 a day; passes judgment on own activity; can recite a poem from memory or sing a song; uses words such as even, almost, something, like, but; typical expressions might include I'm so tired, you almost hit me, now I'll make something else.

Up to 1800 words in sentences averaging five to six words; now averages only 230 words per hour—is satisfied with less verbalization; does little commanding or demanding; likes surprises; about 1 in 10 sentences is compound or complex, and only 8% of sentences are incomplete; can define 10 common words and count to 20; common expressions are I don't know, I said, tiny, funny, because; asks questions for information, and learns to manipulate and control persons and situations with language.

Continued.

Adapted from Chinn PL: *Child health maintenance: concepts in family-centered care*, ed 2, St Louis, 1979, Mosby. In Edelman CL, Mandle CL: *Health promotion through the lifespan*, ed 3, St Louis, 1994, Mosby.

Landmarks of speech, language, and hearing ability during the preschool period—cont'd

Age (months)	Receptive language	Expressive language	Related hearing ability
60	Up to 9600 words; knows number concepts to 5; knows and names colors; defines words in terms of use such as a horse is to ride; also defines wind, ball, hat, stove; understands words such as if, because, when; knows what the following are for: horse, fork, legs; begins to understand right and left.	Up to 2200 words in sentences averaging six words; can define ball, hat, stove, policeman, wind, horse, fork; can count five objects and repeat four or five digits; definitions are in terms of use; can single out a word and ask its meaning; makes serious inquiries—what is this for, how does this work, who made those, what does it mean; language is now essentially complete in structure and form; uses all types of sentences, clauses, and parts of speech; reads by way of pictures, and prints simple words.	

Nursing Suggestions to Encourage Language Development in Preschoolers

Read to the child. Encourage the child to be an active listener by pausing at times during the story to ask such questions as, "What do you think will happen next?"; "Why do you think the boy said that?"; and "What would you do now?"

Praise the child's storytelling.

Always respond to the child's questions. At times a response must be delayed; for example, if the parent is driving in heavy traffic and the child asks a question that requires a complex answer, the parent might say, "That's a very good question, let's talk about that as soon as we get home." The parent should remind the child later of the question and respond if the child still is interested.

Never tease or criticize a child about his verbalizations. If the child is excited and talking so fast that he is fumbling over words, the parent might say, "I can't listen that fast. Slow down a little for me." This is much more encouraging than, "You talk too fast. No one can understand you."

Play games that are language focused, such as naming the colors of houses or kinds of flowers as parent and child walk to the store.

From Edelman CL, Mandle CL: *Health promotion throughout the lifespan,* ed 3, St Louis, 1994, Mosby.

Nurse's Interventions for Screening Vision and Hearing of Preschoolers

Be skilled in the use of the equipment.

Avoid the term *test* because even some preschoolers have come to associate test with anxiety and possibly failure.

Allow the child to ask questions and examine the equipment.

Do vision and hearing screening early in the visit before anything intrusive or painful.

Do screening in a quiet, private area so the child is not distracted by people or noises.

Praise the child for cooperating.

From Edelman CL, Mandle CL: *Health promotion throughout the lifespan,* ed 3, St Louis, 1994, Mosby.

If the child becomes distracted or tired, take a brief break before
  beginning again.

Discuss the results of the screening with the child using simple,
  positive terms.

Clues for Detecting Visual Impairment

Cause	Behavior	Signs/symptoms
Congenital blindness	Does not follow a moving light; no orientation response to visual stimuli Does not initiate eye-to-eye contact with caregiver	Constant nystagmus Fixed pupils Marked strabismus Slow lateral movements
Refractive errors	Rubs eyes excessively Tilts head or thrusts head forward Has difficulty in reading or other close work Holds books close to eyes Writes or colors with head close to table Clumsy; walks into objects Blinks more than usual or is irritable when doing close work Is unable to see objects clearly Does poorly in school, especially in subjects that require demonstration, such as arithmetic	Dizziness Headache Nausea following close work
Strabismus	Squints eyelids together or frowns Has difficulty in focusing from one distance to another Inaccurate judgment in picking up objects	Diplopia Photophobia Dizziness

Continued.

From Wong DL, Whaley LF: *Clinical manual of pediatric nursing,* ed 4, St Louis, 1994, Mosby.

Clues for Detecting Visual Impairment—cont'd

Cause	Behavior	Signs/symptoms
Strabismus—cont'd	Unable to see print or moving objects clearly Closes one eye to see Tilts head to one side If combined with refractive errors, may see any of the above	Headache Cross-eye
Glaucoma	Mostly seen in acquired types—loses peripheral vision; may bump into objects that are not directly in front of him; sees halos around objects; may complain of mild pain or discomfort (severe pain, nausea, and vomiting if sudden rise in pressure)	Redness Excessive tearing (epiphora) Photophobia Spasmodic winking (blepharospasm) Corneal haziness Enlargement of the eyeball (buphthalmos)
Cataract	Gradually less able to see objects clearly May lose peripheral vision	Nystagmus (with complete blindness) Gray opacities of lens Strabismus

Denver Eye Screening Test

The Denver Eye Screening Test (DEST) tests visual acuity in children 3 years or older by using a single card for the letter E (20/30) from a distance of 15 feet. A complete instructional manual is available. General guidelines include the following:

1. Mark a distance of 15 feet for testing.
2. Use the large **E** (20/100) to explain and demonstrate the testing procedure to the child.
3. Use the small **E** for actual testing. Test each eye separately using the occluder.
4. Consider the results *abnormal* if the child fails to correctly identify the direction of the small **E** over three trials.
5. Test children from 2½ to 2¹¹/₁₂ years of age or those untestable with the letter **E** using the picture (Allen) cards. (Cooperative children as young as 2 years can also be tested.)
6. Show each card to the child at close range to make certain he can identify it.
7. Present the pictures at a distance of 15 feet for actual testing. Test each eye separately if possible.
8. Consider the results *abnormal* if the child fails to correctly name three of the seven cards in three to five trials.
9. Screen children from 6 to 30 months by testing for the following:
   a. Fixation (ability to follow a moving light source or spinning toy)
   b. Squinting (observation of the child's eyes or report by parent)
   c. Strabismus (report by parent and performance on cover and pupillary light reflex tests)
10. Consider the results *abnormal* if failure to fixate, presence of a squint, or failing two of the three procedures for strabismus.
11. Retest all children with abnormal findings. Refer those with a repeat failure.

From Wong DL, Whaley LF: *Clinical manual of pediatric nursing,* ed 4, St Louis, 1994, Mosby.

Tuning Fork Tests

Test and steps	Rationale

Weer's test (lateralization of sound)

Hold the fork at its base and tap it lightly against the heel of the palm.

Place the base of the vibrating fork on the top of the client's head or middle of forehead (see below).

Ask the client where sound is heard (on one or both sides).

A client with normal hearing hears sound equally in both ears or in midline of head. In conduction deafness, sound is heard in the impaired ear. In unilateral sensorineural hearing loss, sound is identified in the good ear.

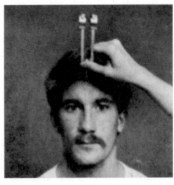

Rinne's test (comparison of air and bone conduction)

Strike the tuning fork against the knuckle (see below, left.)

Place the vibrating fork on the mastoid process (see below, left.)

Ask the client to inform you when sound is no longer heard.

Immediately place the vibrating fork close to the external ear meatus (see below, right.)

Ask the client to inform you if sound can be heard.

Normally, sound can be heard longer through air than through bone (positive Rinne). In conduction deafness, sounds through bone conduction can be heard after air conduction sounds become inaudible (negative Rinne). In sensorineural deafness, sound is heard longer through air.

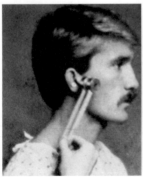 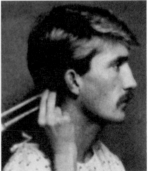

From Potter PA, Perry AG: *Fundamentals of nursing,* ed 3, St Louis, 1993, Mosby.

Normal Tooth Formation in the Child

Teeth	Lower (mandibular) appear at age	Upper (maxillary) appear at age
Primary		
Central incisors	5 to 7 months	6 to 8 months
Lateral incisors	12 to 15 months	8 to 11 months
Cuspids (canines)	16 to 20 months	16 to 20 months
First molars	10 to 16 months	10 to 16 months
Second molars	20 to 30 months	20 to 30 months
Total per jaw—10		
Total—20		
Permanent		
Central incisors	6 to 7 years	6 to 7 years
Lateral incisors	7 to 9 years	8 to 9 years
Cuspids (canines)	8 to 11 years	11 to 12 years
First bicuspids	10 to 12 years	10 to 11 years
Second bicuspids	11 to 13 years	10 to 12 years
First molars (6-year molars)	6 to 7 years	6 to 7 years
Second molars (12-year molars)	12 to 13 years	12 to 13 years
Third molars (wisdom teeth)	17 to 22 years	17 to 22 years
Total set—32		

From Ingalls AJ, Salerno MC: *Maternal and child health nursing,* St Louis, 1991, Mosby.

Median Age of Eruption	Median Age When Shed	THE PRIMARY TEETH
6-9 months	— 6-7 years —	Central Incisor
7-10 months	— 7-8 years —	Lateral Incisor
16-18 months	—10-12 years —	Cuspid
12-14 months	— 9-11 years —	First Molar
20-28 months	— 9-11 years —	Second Molar

Median Age of Eruption	THE PERMANENT TEETH
6-7 years —	Central Incisor
7-8 years —	Lateral Incisor
10-12 years —	Cuspid
10-11 years —	First Premolar (Bicuspid)
11-12 years —	Second Premolar (Bicuspid)
5½-6 years —	First Molar
12-13 years —	Second Molar
16-21 years —	Third Molar (Wisdom Tooth)

From Wong DL, Whaley LF: *Clinical manual of pediatric nursing,* ed 3, St Louis, 1990, Mosby.

Developmental Tools Used to Assess Children with Chronic Conditions

Type of screening tools	Test/source	Age level	Method	Comments
General development (social, emotional, cognitive, and co-ordination)	AAMD Adaptive Behavior Scale (school edition) Authors: K Nihiro, R Foster, M Shellhaas, H Leiland, N Lambert, and M Windmiller Source: CTB/McGraw-Hill Book Co	3-16 yr	Observation	• Used as a screening tool and for instruction planning • Can be an indicator in assessing children whose adaptive behavior indicates possible mental retardation, learning handicaps, or emotional disturbances
	Bayley Infant Scales Author: N Bayley Source: The Psychological Corp Harcourt, Brace, Jovanovich, Inc	2-30 mo	Observation/ demonstration	• Evaluates motor, mental, and behavior of the infant and toddler • Diagnoses normal vs retarded development • Requires a qualified practitioner to examine and evaluate the infant
	Bender Visual Motor Gestalt Test Author: L Bender Source: American Orthopsychiatric Association	≥3 yr	Demonstration	• Used as an evaluation tool for developmental problems in children, learning disabilities, retardation, psychosis, organic brain disorders

Carey Infant Temperament Questionnaire Author: WB Carey Source: WB Carey, MD 319 West Front St Media, PA 19063	4-8 mo	Interview	• Provides an objective measure of the infant's temperament profile • Fosters more effective interactions between parent and infant
Carey and McDevitt Revised Temperament Questionnaire (95 items, 6-pt frequency scale) 1. Toddler Temperament Scale Authors: W Fullard, SC McDevitt, and WB Carey Source: W Fullard, PhD Dept of Educational Psychology Temple University Philadelphia, PA 19122	1-3 yr	Interview	• Provides an objective measure of the child's temperament profile • Fosters more effective interactions between parent and child
2. Behavior Style Questionnaire Authors: SC McDevitt and WB Carey Source: SC McDevitt, PhD Devereux Center 6436 E Sweetwater Scottsdale, AZ 85254	3-7 yr	Interview	• Provides an objective measure of the child's temperament profile • Fosters more effective interactions between parent and child
Child Behavior Checklist Author: TM Achenbach Source: Center for Children, Youth, and Families University of Vermont 1 S Prospect St Burlington, VT 05401	2-3 yr	Observation/ interview	• Provides an overview of the child's behavior • Parent and teacher forms available

Continued.

From Jackson PL, Vessey JA: *Primary care of the child with a chronic condition,* St Louis, 1991, Mosby.

Developmental tools used to assess children with chronic conditions—cont'd

Type of screening tools	Test/source	Age level	Method	Comments
General development—cont'd	Children's Depression Inventory (CDI) Author: M Kovacs Source: *Acta Paedopsychiatr* 1981; 46:305-315 M Kovacs, PhD Assistant Professor of Psychiatry 3811 O'Hara St Pittsburgh, PA 15261	8-13 yr	Paper/pencil inventory	• Used for clinical research in childhood depression • Advisable for individual administration with the psychiatric population
	Denver Developmental Screening Test/Denver II Authors: WK Frankenberg, JB Dodds, et al: *Pediatrics*, 89:91-97, 1992. Source: Denver Developmental Materials, Inc. P.O. Box 6919 Denver, CO 80206-9019 (303) 355-4729	Birth-6 yr	Observation and parental reporting	• Screens for developmental deviations • Minimal training required • Available in Spanish
	Developmental Profile II Authors: GD Alpern, TJ Boll, and MS Shearer Source: Western Psychological Services 12031 Wilshire Blvd Los Angeles, CA 90025	Birth-9½ yr	Interview	• Provides information on physical, self-help, social, academic, and communicative abilities • Requires a qualified practitioner skilled in interviewing

Tool	Age	Method	Comments
McCarthy Scales of Children's Abilities Source: The Psychological Corp 　7500 Old Oak Blvd 　Cleveland, OH 44130	2½-8½ yr	Observation and demonstration by the child	• Measures 6 aspects of children's thinking, motor, and mental abilities • Requires qualified practitioner to administer and evaluate the child
Minnesota Infant Development Inventory Authors: H Ireton and E Thwing Source: Behavior Science Systems 　PO Box 1108 　Minneapolis, MN 55458	Birth-15 mo	Observation/interview	• A developmental guide • Measures the infant's development areas: gross motor, fine motor, language, comprehension and personal-social • Can be done by parent
Minnesota Child Development Inventory Authors: H Ireton and E Thwing Source: Behavior Science Systems 　PO Box 1108 　Minneapolis, MN 55458	1-6 yr	Observation/interview	• Provides a profile of the child's strengths and weaknesses • Can be done by a parent, also available on audiocassette for parents who have difficulty reading
Pediatric Examination of Education Readiness at Middle Childhood Author: MD Levine Source: Educators Publishing 　75 Moulton St 　Cambridge, MA 02138	5-10 yr	Observation/demonstration	• Can be done by parent • Measures school readiness and academic achievement • Allow 1 hr for testing time • Administered by a certified practitioner

Continued.

Developmental tools used to assess children with chronic conditions—cont'd

Type of screening tools	Test/source	Age level	Method	Comments
General development—cont'd	Rapid Developmental Screening Checklist Authors: Committee on Children With Handicaps, American Academy of Pediatrics Source: MJ Giannini, MD Director, Mental Retardation Institute New York Medical College Valhalla, NY 10595	1 mo–5 yr	Checklist	• Requires minimal time allotment • Administered by any adult capable to make required observation
	Riley Motor Problem Inventory (RMPI) Author: GD Riley Source: Western Psychological 12031 Wilshire Blvd. Los Angeles, CA 90025	≥4 yr	Performance tasks by the child	• Provides a quantified system for observation and measurement of neurologic signs that lead to problems in speech, language, learning, and behavior • Needs to be administered by a qualified clinician
	Vineland Adaptive Behavior Scales Authors: SS Sparrow, DA Balla, and DV Cicchetti Source: American Guidance Service Inc. Circle Pines, MN 55014-1796	Birth–adult	Semistructured interview with parent or caregiver	• Assesses adaptive behavior in four sectors: communication, daily living skills, socialization, and motor skills • Used with mentally retarded and handicapped individuals

	Age	Method	Comments
Vineland Social Maturity Scale Author: EA Doll Source: American Guidance Service Inc. Circle Pines, MN 55014-1796	Birth–adult	Interview	• Used to measure normal development or individual difference that may be significant in children with mental deficiencies and emotional disturbances • Assists in planned therapy or specialized individual education
Wheel Guide to Normal Milestones of Development Author: U Hayes Source: *A Developmental Approach to Case Finding*, ed 2, US Dept of Health and Human Services Superintendent of Documents Washington, DC 20402	1–3 yr	Observation	• Assesses basic reflexes and developmental milestones • Reinforces the normal growth and development patterns of children
Vision Allen Picture Card Test of Visual Acuity Source: LADOCA Project and Publishing Foundation E 51st Ave and Lincoln St Denver, CO 80216	3–6 yr	Observation	• Preschooler screening test for visual acuity • Trained volunteers/screeners can conduct the testing
Denver Eye Screening Test (DEST) Source: LADOCA Project and Publishing Foundation E 51st Ave and Lincoln St Denver, CO 80216	3 yr	Observation	• Identifies children with acuity problems • Good for preschool-aged children unable to respond to the Snellen Illiterate E Test

Continued.

Developmental tools used to assess children with chronic conditions—cont'd

Type of screening tools	Test/source	Age level	Method	Comments
Vision—cont'd	Distance Visual Acuity Screening Test for Young Children Source: LB Holt, MD, FICS 195 Professional Bldg 2240 Cloverdale Ave Winston Salem, NC 27103	3-5 yr ≥6 yr	Interview/ observation	• Used in children to measure central visual acuity • Can be administered by any adult, professional, or nonprofessional capable of developing rapport with children
	Picture Card Test (Adaptation of the Preschool Vision Test) Author: HF Allan Source: LADOCA Project and Publishing Foundation E 51st Ave and Lincoln St Denver, CO 80216	≥2½ yr	Interview/ "name the picture"	• Identifies children with acuity problems • Administered by a carefully taught adult who has an interest in working with children
	Snellen Illiterate E Test Author: H Snellen Sources: National Society for Blindness 79 Madison Ave New York, NY 10016 American Association of Ophthalmology 1100 17th St NW Washington, DC 20036	≥3 yr	Observation using 3 persons as a team in screening	• Intended as a screening measure for central acuity of preschool-aged children and of other children who have not learned to read • Administered by a carefully prepared adult

Speech and language	Bankson Language Screening Test (BLST) Author: NW Bankson Source: University Park Press Chamber of Commerce Bldg Baltimore, MD 21201	4-8 yr	Observation	• Identifies children in need of language assistance • Can be administered by a perceptive adult
	The Bzoch-League Receptive Expressive Emergent Language Scale (REEL) Authors: KR Bzoch and R League Source: University Park Press 360 N Charles St Baltimore, MD 21201	Birth-3 yr	Paper-pencil inventory	• Identifies children needing further follow-up in language
	Denver Articulation Screening Exam (DASE) Author: AF Drumwright Reference manual (1971 ed) Manual/workbook WK Frankenburg Source: LADOCA Project and Publishing Foundation Inc E 51st Ave and Lincoln St Denver, CO 80216	2½-6 yr	Observation	• Screening children who may be economically disadvantaged and have a potential with a speech problem (articulation)—pronunciation • Administered by a qualified professional; special training required for the nonprofessional

Continued.

Developmental tools used to assess children with chronic conditions—cont'd

Type of screening tools	Test/source	Age level	Method	Comments
Speech and language—cont'd	Emergent Language Milestone Scale (ELM) (1984) Source: Education Corp PO Box 721 Tulsa, OK 74101	Birth- 36 mo	Interview Observation	• Screening instrument for auditory expressive, auditory receptive, and visual components of language
	Peabody Picture Vocabulary Test, Revised (PPVT-R) Authors: Lloyd M. Dunn Leota M. Dunn Source: American Guidance Service Publishers Bldg Circle Pines, MN 55014	≥2½ yr	"Point to" response test	• Measures hearing vocabulary for standard American English • Used with non–English-speaking students to screen for mental retardation or giftedness • Requires a qualified practitioner to administer
	Physician's Developmental Quick Screen for Speech Disorders (PDQ) Authors: SG Kulig and KA Baker	6 mo- 6 yr	Interview/ demonstration	• Designed to identify children in need of a diagnostic evaluation by a speech pathologist for disorders of language, voice, articulation, and rhythm with speech • Administered by any well-trained paraprofessional or health care professional

	Riley Motor Problems Inventory (RMPI) Author: GD Riley Source: Western Psychological 12031 Wilshire Blvd Los Angeles, CA 90025	≥4 yr	Performance tasks by the child	• Provides a quantified system for observation and measurement of neurologic signs that lead to problems in speech, language, learning, and behavior • Needs to be administered by a qualified clinician
School readiness and academic achievement	Child Behavior Checklist Author: TM Achenbach Source: Center for Children, Youth, and Families University of Vermont 1 S Prospect St Burlington, VT 05401	4-16 yr	Observation/ interview	• Provides an overview of the child's behavior • Parent and teacher forms available
	Peabody Picture Vocabulary Test, Revised (PPVT-R) Authors: LM Dunn and LM Dunn Source: American Guidance Service Publishers Bldg Circle Pines, MN 55014	≥2½ yr	"Point to" response test	• Measures hearing vocabulary for standard American English • Used with non–English-speaking students to screen for mental retardation or giftedness • Requires a qualified practitioner to administer

Continued.

Developmental tools used to assess children with chronic conditions—cont'd

Type of screening tools	Test/source	Age level	Method	Comments
School readiness and academic achievement—cont'd	Peabody Individual Achievement Test (PIAT) Authors: LM Dunn and FC Markwardt, Jr Source: American Guidance Service Publishers Bldg Circle Pines, MN 55014 Authors: LM Dunn	≥5 yr	Interview	• Used to screen for areas of weakness requiring more detailed diagnostic testing in scholastic achievement
	Riley Preschool Developmental Inventory (RPDSI) Author: CMD Riley Source: Western Psychological 12031 Wilshire Blvd Los Angeles, CA 90025	3-5 yr	Observation	• For children who have the tendency for academic problems • Requires a qualified clinician to administer
	The Texas Preschool Screening Inventory Authors: JS Haber and ML Noris	3-6 yr	Observation/demonstration	• Used as a screening tool to identify children with possible learning difficulties
	Wide Range Achievement Test (WRAT) Authors: JF Jastak and S Jastak Source: Jastak Assessment Systems 1526 Gilpin Wilmington, DE 19806	≥5 yr	Observation; paper-pencil subtests	• Used for education placement, measurement of academic achievement, vocational assessment, and job placement training • Large print edition is available

Functional status	Health Interview Survey	6-16 yr	Interview	• Assess functional status
	Source: National Center for Health Statistics B Bloom: *Current Estimates From the* *National Health Interview Survey United* *States, 1981* Vital and Health Statistics, Series 10–No 141 DHHS Pub No (PHS) 83-1569 Washington, DC Public Health Service US Government Printing Office October 1982			

Denver Developmental Screening Test/Denver II

One of the most widely used screening tests for assessing a young child's development is the *Denver Developmental Screening Test* (DDST) which has been substantially revised and renamed the *Denver II*. It is composed of four major categories (personal-social, fine motor–adaptive, language, and gross motor) and is applicable for children from birth through 6 years of age. The age divisions are monthly until 24 months and then every 6 months until 6 years of age. Up to 24 months of age, allowances are made for infants who were born prematurely by subtracting the number of weeks of missed gestation from their present age and testing them at the adjusted age. For example, a 16-week-old infant who was born 4 weeks early is tested at a 12-week adjusted age level.

To determine relative areas of advancement and areas of delay, sufficient items should be administered to establish the basal and ceiling levels in each sector. To identify cautions, all items intersected by the age line are administered. To screen solely for developmental delays, only the items located totally to the *left* of the child's age line are administered. Scoring methods and criteria for referral are under investigation.

Modified from Whaley LF, Wong DL: *Nursing care of infants and children,* ed 5, St Louis, 1994, Mosby.

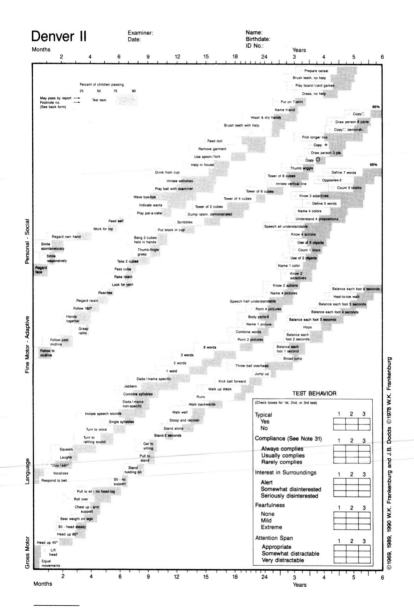

From Frankenburg WK, Dodds, JB: "The Denver II: a major revision and restandardization of the Denver Developmental screening test," *Pediatrics,* 89: 91-97, 1992.

Directions for Administration

1. Try to get child to smile by smiling, talking, or waving. Do not touch him/her.
2. Child must stare at hand several seconds.
3. Parent may help guide toothbrush and put toothpaste on brush.
4. Child does not have to be able to tie shoes or button/zip in the back.
5. Move yarn slowly in an arc from one side to the other, about 8″ above child's face.
6. Pass if child grasps rattle when it is touched to the backs or tips of fingers.
7. Pass if child tries to see where yarn went. Yarn should be dropped quickly from sight from tester's hand without arm movement.
8. Child must transfer cube from hand to hand without help of body, mouth, or table.
9. Pass if child picks up raisin with any part of thumb and finger.
10. Line can vary only 30 degrees or less from tester's line.
11. Make a fist with thumb pointing upward and wiggle only the thumb. Pass if child imitates and does not move any fingers other than the thumb.

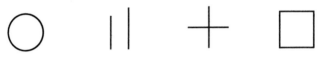

12. Pass any enclosed form. Fail continuous round motions.
13. Which line is longer? (Not bigger.) Turn paper upside down and repeat. (pass 3 of 3 or 5 of 6).
14. Pass any lines crossing near midpoint.
15. Have child copy first. If failed, demonstrate.

When giving items 12, 14, and 15, do not name the forms. Do not demonstrate 12 and 14.

16. When scoring, each pair (2 arms, 2 legs, etc.) counts as one part.
17. Place one curbe in cup and shake gently near child's ear, but out of sight. Repeart for other ear.
18. Point to picture and have child name it. (No credit is given for sounds only.)
    If less than 4 pictures are named correctly, have child point to picture as each is named by tester.

19. Using doll, tell child: Show me the nose, eyes, ears, mouth, hands, feet, tummy, hair. Pass 6 of 8.
20. Using pictures, ask child: Which one flies? . . . says meow? . . . talks? . . . barks? . . . gallops? Pass 2 of 5, 4 of 5.
21. Ask child: Waht do you do when you are cold? . . . tired? . . . hungry? Pass 2 of 3, 3 of 3.
22. Ask child: What do you do with a cup? What is a chair used for? What is a pencil used for?
   Action words must be included in answers.
23. Pass if child correctly places *and* says how many blocks are on paper. (1, 5).
24. Tell child: Put block **on** table: **under** table: **in front of** me, **behind** me. Pass 4 of 4.
   (Do not help child by pointing, moving head or eyes.)
25. Ask child: What is a ball? . . . lake? . . . desk? . . . house? . . . banana? . . . curtain? . . . fence? . . . ceiling? Pass if defined in terms of use, shape, what it is made of, or general category (such as banana is fruit, not just yellow). Pass 5 of 8, 7 of 8.
26. Ask child: If a horse is big, a mouse is ___? If fire is hot, ice is ___? If the sun shines during the day, the moon shines during the ___? Pass 2 of 3.
27. Child may use wall or rail only, not person. May not crawl.
28. Child must throw ball overhand 3 feet to within arm's reach of tester.
29. Child must perform standing braod jump over width of test sheet (8 ½ inches).
30. Tell child to walk forward. heel within 1 inch of toe. Tester may demonstrate.
   Child must walk 4 consecutive steps.
31. If the second year, half of normal children are non-compliant.
OBSERVATIONS:

Cultural Awareness: The Denver Developmental Screening Tests

When administering the DDST, the nurse must consider cultural variations that can erroneously label the child delayed. For example, Southeast Asian children have demonstrated delays in the areas of personal-social development because of lack of familiarity with games such as pat-a-cake and in language because of differences in word usage, such as absence of plurals. The more protective parental attitude of Southeast Asians toward the young child may also prevent early learning of self-help skills. Several of these variations were noted also in native African children. Further research is needed to determine if cultural variations affect screening results with the Denver II.

From Wong DL: *Whaley and Wong's nursing care of infants and children,* ed 5, St Louis, 1995, Mosby.

Denver II Scoring

Interpretation of the Test
(These are suggested guidelines.)

The DENVER II is interpreted as follows:

Normal:

• No Delays and a maximum of 1 Caution.
• Conduct routine rescreeining at next well child visit.

Suspect:

• Two or more Cautions and/or One or more Delays.
• Since communities' and programs' priorities differ in types or severity of problems they seek to identify in screening, it will be necessary to adjust Suspect criteria to most effecienty achieve their goals. Tables of percentages of Cautions and Delays that may be expected for different demographic groups are provided in the DENVER II Technical Manual, pages 20-22.
• Recreen in 1-2 weeks to rule out temporary factors such as fatigue, fear, illness.

From Frankenburg WK, Dodds JB et al: *The Denver II Training Manual,* ed 2, Denver, 1992, Denver Developmental Materials.

Untestable:

- Refusal scores on one or more items completely to the left of the age line or on more than one item intersected by the age line in the 75%-90% area.
- Rescreen in 1-2 weeks.

Referral Considerations

If, upon rescreening, the test result is again Suspect or Untestable, whether or not to refer should be determined by the clinical judgement of the supervising professional based upon:

- Profile of test results (which items are Cautions and Delays)
- Number of Cautions and Delays
- Rate of past development
- Other clinical considerations (clinical history, examination, etc.)
- Availability of referral resources

Monitoring the Screening program is discussed in the *DENVER II Technical Manual,* pages 20-22. The use of such monitoring is strongly recommended to assist the supervising professional in establishing and adjusting referral criteria.

Denver Articulation Screening Examination

Another widely used screening test is the *Denver Articulation Screening Examination* (DASE) (see pp. 676-679). The child repeats each word after the examiner. The examiner circles the underlined sounds that the child pronounces correctly. The total correctly pronounced sounds is the Raw Score.

DENVER ARTICULATION SCREENING EXAMINATION

for children 2½ to 6 years of age

Instructions: Have child repeat each word after you. Circle the underlined sounds that he pronounces correctly. Total correct sounds is the Raw Score. Use charts on reverse side to score results.

NAME

HOSP. NO.

ADDRESS

Date _____ Child's Age: _____ Examiner: _____ Raw Score: _____

Percentile: _____ Intelligibility: _____ Result: _____

1. table	6. zipper	11. sock	16. wagon	21. leaf
2. shirt	7. grapes	12. vacuum	17. gum	22. carrot
3. door	8. flag	13. yarn	18. house	
4. trunk	9. thumb	14. mother	19. pencil	
5. jumping	10. toothbrush	15. twinkle	20. fish	

Intelligibility: (circle one)   1. Easy to understand   3. Not understandable
                                2. Understandable ½ the time. 4. Can't evaluate

Comments:

Date _____ Child's Age: _____ Examiner: _____ Raw Score: _____

Percentile: _____ Intelligibility: _____ Result: _____

1. table	6. zipper	11. sock	16. wagon
2. shirt	7. grapes	12. vacuum	17. gum
3. door	8. flag	13. yarn	18. house
4. trunk	9. thumb	14. mother	19. pencil
5. jumping	10. toothbrush	15. twinkle	20. fish

21. leaf
22. carrot

Intelligibility: (circle one)

1. Easy to understand
2. Understandable ½ the time.

3. Not understandable
4. Can't evaluate

Comments:

Date _____ Child's Age: _____ Examiner: _____ Raw Score: _____

Percentile: _____ Intelligibility: _____ Result: _____

1. table	6. zipper	11. sock	16. wagon
2. shirt	7. grapes	12. vacuum	17. gum
3. door	8. flag	13. yarn	18. house
4. trunk	9. thumb	14. mother	19. pencil
5. jumping	10. toothbrush	15. twinkle	20. fish

21. leaf
22. carrot

Intelligibility: (circle one)

1. Easy to understand
2. Understandable ½ the time.

3. Not understandable
4. Can't evaluate

Comments:

To score DASE words: Note Raw Score for child's performance. Match raw score line (extreme left of chart) with column representing child's age (to the closest previous age group). Where raw score line and age column meet number in that square denotes percentile rank of child's performance when compared to other children that age. Percentiles above heavy line are ABNORMAL percentiles, below heavy line are NORMAL.

Percentile rank

Raw Score	2.5 yr.	3.0	3.5	4.0	4.5	5.0	5.5	6 years
2	1							
3	2							
4	5							
5	9							
6	16							
7	23							
8	31	2						
9	37	4	1					
10	42	6	2					
11	48	7	4					
12	54	9	6	1	1			
13	58	12	9	2	3	1	1	
14	62	17	11	5	4	2	2	
15	68	23	15	9	5	3	2	
16	75	31	19	12	5	4	3	
17	79	38	25	15	6	6	4	
18	83	46	31	19	8	7	4	

University of Colorado Medical Center

19	86	51	38	24	10	9	5	1
20	89	58	45	30	12	11	7	3
21	92	65	52	36	15	15	9	4
22	94	72	58	43	18	19	12	5
23	96	77	63	50	22	24	15	7
24	97	82	70	58	29	29	20	15
25	99	87	78	66	36	34	26	17
26	99	91	84	75	46	43	34	24
27		94	89	82	57	54	44	34
28		96	94	88	70	68	59	47
29		98	98	94	84	84	77	68
30		100	100	100	100	100	100	100

To Score Intelligibility:

	Normal	**Abnormal**
2½ years	Understandable ½ the time, or, "easy"	Not Understandable
3 years and older	Easy to understand	Understandable ½ time Not understandable

Test Results: 1. **Normal** on DASE and Intelligibility = **Normal**

2. **Abnormal** on DASE and/or Intelligibility = **Abnormal**

* If abnormal on initial screening rescreen within 2 weeks. If abnormal again child should be referred for complete speech evaluation.

Growth Measurements: Birth to 18 Years

Height and weight measurements for boys

Age*	Height by percentiles						Weight by percentiles					
	5		50		95		5		50		95	
	cm	inches	cm	inches	cm	inches	kg	lb	kg	lb	kg	lb
Height and weight measurements for boys												
Birth	46.4	18¼	50.5	20	54.4	21½	2.54	5½	3.27	7¼	4.15	9¼
3 months	56.7	22¼	61.1	24	65.4	25¾	4.43	9¾	5.98	13¼	7.37	16¼
6 months	63.4	25	67.8	26¾	72.3	28½	6.20	13¾	7.85	17¼	9.46	20¾
9 months	68.0	26¾	72.3	28½	77.1	30¼	7.52	16½	9.18	20¼	10.93	24
1	71.7	28¼	76.1	30	81.2	32	8.43	18½	10.15	22½	11.99	26½
1½	77.5	30½	82.4	32½	88.1	34¾	9.59	21¼	11.47	25¼	13.44	29½
2†	82.5	32½	86.8	34¼	94.4	37¼	10.49	23¼	12.34	27¼	15.50	34¼
2½†	85.4	33½	90.4	35½	97.8	38½	11.27	24¾	13.52	29¾	16.61	36½
3	89.0	35	94.9	37¼	102.0	40¼	12.05	26½	14.62	32¼	17.77	39¼
3½	92.5	36½	99.1	39	106.1	41¾	12.84	28¼	15.68	34½	18.98	41¾

4	95.8	37¾	102.9	40½	109.9	43¼	13.64	30	16.69	36¾	20.27	44¾
4½	98.9	39	106.6	42	113.5	44¾	14.45	31¾	17.69	39	21.63	47¾
5	102.0	40¼	109.9	43¼	117.0	46	15.27	33¾	18.67	41¼	23.09	51
6	107.7	42½	116.1	45¾	123.5	48½	16.93	37¼	20.69	45½	26.34	58
7	113.0	44½	121.7	48	129.7	51	18.64	41	22.85	50¼	30.12	66½
8	118.1	46½	127.0	50	135.7	53½	20.40	45	25.30	55¾	34.51	76
9	122.9	48½	132.2	52	141.8	55¾	22.25	49	28.13	62	39.58	87¼
10	127.7	50¼	137.5	54¼	148.1	58¼	24.33	53¾	31.44	69¼	45.27	99¾
11	132.6	52¼	143.3	56½	154.9	61	26.80	59	35.30	77¾	51.47	113½
12	137.6	54¼	149.7	59	162.3	64	29.85	65¾	39.78	87¾	58.09	128
13	142.9	56¼	156.5	61½	169.8	66¾	33.64	74¼	44.95	99	65.02	143¼
14	148.8	58½	163.1	64¼	176.7	69½	38.22	84¼	50.77	112	72.13	159
15	155.2	61	169.0	66½	181.9	71½	43.11	95	56.71	125	79.12	174½
16	161.1	63½	173.5	68¼	185.4	73	47.74	105¼	62.10	137	85.62	188¾
17	164.9	65	176.2	69¼	187.3	73¾	51.50	113½	66.31	146¼	91.31	201¼
18	165.7	65¼	176.8	69½	187.6	73¾	53.97	119	68.88	151¾	95.76	211

*Years unless otherwise indicated.

†Height data include some recumbent length measurements, which make values slightly higher than if all measurements had been of stature (standing height).

From Whaley LF, Wong DL: *Nursing care of infants and children,* ed 5, St Louis, 1994, Mosby. As modified from National Center for Health Statistics, Health Resources Administration: Conversion of metric data to approximate inches and pounds by Ross Laboratories, Hyattsville, Md, Department of Health, Education and Welfare.

Height and weight measurements for girls

| | Height by percentiles | | | | | | | | | Weight by percentiles | | | | | | |
| | 5 | | 50 | | 95 | | 5 | | 50 | | 95 | |
Age*	cm	inches	cm	inches	cm	inches	kg	lb	kg	lb	kg	lb
Birth	45.4	17¾	49.9	19¾	52.9	20¾	2.36	5¼	3.23	7	3.81	8½
3 months	55.4	21¾	59.5	23½	63.4	25	4.18	9¼	5.4	12	6.74	14¾
6 months	61.8	24¼	65.9	26	70.2	27¾	5.79	12¾	7.21	16	8.73	19¼
9 months	66.1	26	70.4	27¾	75.0	29½	7.0	15½	8.56	18¾	10.17	22½
1	69.8	27½	74.3	29¼	79.1	31¼	7.84	17¼	9.53	21	11.24	24¾
1½	76.0	30	80.9	31¾	86.1	34	8.92	19¾	10.82	23¾	12.76	28¼
2†	81.6	32¼	86.8	34¼	93.6	36¾	9.95	22	11.8	26	14.15	31¼
2½†	84.6	33¾	90.0	35½	96.6	38	10.8	23¾	13.03	28¾	15.76	34¾
3	88.3	34¾	94.1	37	100.6	39½	11.61	25½	14.1	31	17.22	38
3½	91.7	36	97.9	38½	104.5	41¼	12.37	27¼	15.07	33¼	18.59	41

Age*												
4	95.0	37½	101.6	40	108.3	42¾	13.11	29	15.96	35¼	19.91	44
4½	98.1	38½	105.0	41¼	112.0	44	13.83	30½	16.81	37	21.24	46¾
5	101.1	39¾	108.4	42¾	115.6	45½	14.55	32	17.66	39	22.62	49¾
6	106.6	42	114.6	45	122.7	48¼	16.05	35½	19.52	43	25.75	56¾
7	111.8	44	120.6	47½	129.5	51	17.71	39	21.84	48¼	29.68	65½
8	116.9	46	126.4	49¾	136.2	53½	19.62	43¼	24.84	54¾	34.71	76½
9	122.1	48	132.2	52	142.9	56¼	21.82	48	28.46	62¾	40.64	89½
10	127.5	50¼	138.3	54½	149.5	58¾	24.36	53¾	32.55	71¾	47.17	104
11	133.5	52½	144.8	57	156.2	61½	27.24	60	36.95	81½	54.0	119
12	139.8	55	151.5	59¾	162.7	64	30.52	67¼	41.53	91½	60.81	134
13	145.2	57¼	157.1	61¾	168.1	66¼	34.14	75¼	46.1	101¾	67.3	148¼
14	148.7	58½	160.4	63¼	171.3	67½	37.76	83¼	50.28	110¾	73.08	161
15	150.5	59¼	161.8	63¾	172.8	68	40.99	90¼	53.68	118¼	77.78	171½
16	151.6	59¾	162.4	64	173.3	68¼	43.41	95¾	55.89	123¼	80.99	178½
17	152.7	60	163.1	64¼	173.5	68¼	44.74	98¾	56.69	125	82.46	181¾
18	153.6	60½	163.7	64½	173.6	68¼	45.26	99¾	56.62	124¾	82.47	181¾

*Years unless otherwise indicated.

†Height data include some recumbent length measurements, which make values slightly higher than if all measurements had been of stature (standing height).

Schedule of Clinical Preventive Services

This list of preventive services is not exhaustive. It reflects only those topics reviewed by the U.S. Preventive Services Task Force. Clinicians may wish to add other preventive services on a routine basis, after considering the client's medical history and other individual circumstances. Examples of target conditions not specifically examined by the Task Force include developmental disorders, musculoskeletal malformations, cardiac anomalies, genitourinary disorders, metabolic disorders, speech problems, behavioral disorders, and parent-family dysfunction.

Birth to 18 months—schedule: 2, 4, 6, 15, 18 months[1]

Leading Causes of Death:
Conditions originating in perinatal period
Congenital anomalies
Heart disease
Injuries (non—motor vehicle)
Pneumonia influenza

SCREENING
Height and weight
Hemoglobin and hematocrit[2]
High-risk groups
Hearing[3] (HR1)
Erythrocyte protoporphyrin (HR2)

Remain Alert for:
Ocular misalignment
Tooth decay
Signs of child abuse or neglect

PARENT COUNSELING

Diet
Breast-feeding
Nutrient intake, especially iron-rich foods
Injury Prevention
Child safety seats
Smoke detector

**IMMUNIZATIONS AND
CHEMOPROPHYLAXIS**
Diphtheria-tetanus-pertussis (DTP) vaccine[4]
Oral poliovirus vaccine (OPV)[5]
Measles-mumps-rubella (MMR) vaccine[6]
Haemophilus influenzae type b (Hib)
conjugate vaccine[7]

Hot water heater temperature
Stairway gates, window guards, pool fence
Storage of drugs and toxic chemicals
Syrup of ipecac, poison control telephone
  number

Dental Health
Baby bottle tooth decay

Other Primary Preventive Measures
Effects of passive smoking

High-risk groups
Fluoride supplements (HR3)

FIRST WEEK
Ophthalmic antibiotics[8]
Hemoglobin electrophoresis (HR4)[8]
T4 TSH[7]
Phenylalanine[9]
Hearing (HRI)

HIGH-RISK CATEGORIES

HR1 Infants with a family history of childhood hearing impairment or a personal history of congenital, perinatal infection with herpes, syphilis, rubella, cytomegalovirus, or toxoplasmosis; malformations involving the head or neck (e.g., dysmorphic and syndromal abnormalities, cleft palate, abnormal pinna); birth weight below 1500 g; bacteria, meningitis; hyperbilirubinemia requiring exchange transfusion; or severe perinatal asphyxia (Apgar scores of 0-3, absence of spontaneous respirations for 10 minutes, or hypotonia at 2 hours of age).

HR2 Infants who live in or frequently visit housing built before 1950 that is dilapidated or undergoing renovations who come in contact with other children with known lead toxicity; who live near lead processing plants or whose parents or household members work in a lead-related occupation; or who live near busy highways or hazardous waste sites.

HR3 Infants living in areas with adequate water fluoridation (less than 0.7 parts per million).

HR4 Newborns of Caribbean, Latin American, Asian, Mediterranean, or African descent.

---

[1]Five visits are required for immunizations. Because of lack of data and differing client risk profiles, the scheduling of additional visits and the frequency of the individual preventive services listed in this table are left to clinical discretion (except as indicated in other footnotes). [2]Once during infancy. [3]At age 18-month visit, if not tested earlier. [4]At ages 2, 6, and 15 months. [5]At ages 2, 4, and 15 months. [6]At age 15 months. [7]At age 18 months. [8]At birth. [9]Days 3 to 6 preferred for testing.

From Fisher M, editor: *Guide to clinical preventive services: report of the US Preventive Services Task Force,* Baltimore, 1989, Williams & Wilkins.

Ages 2-6—schedule: see footnote[1]

Leading Causes of Death:
Injuries (nonmotor vehicle)
Motor vehicle crashes
Congenital anomalies
Homicide
Heart disease

SCREENING
Height and weight
Blood pressure
Eye exam for amblyopia and strabismus[2]
Urinalysis for bacteriuria
High-risk groups
Erythrocyte protoporphyrin[3] (HR1)
Tuberculin skin test (PPD) (HR2)
Hearing[4] (HR3)

Remain Alert for:
Vision disorders
Dental decay, malalignment, premature loss
  of teeth, mouth breathing
Signs of child abuse or neglect
Abnormal bereavement

CLIENT AND PARENT COUNSELING

Diet and Exercise
Sweets and between-meal snacks, iron-
  enriched foods, sodium
Caloric balance
Selection of exercise program

Injury Prevention
Safety belts
Smoke detector
Hot water heater temperature
Window guards and pool fence
Bicycle safety helmets
Storage of drugs, toxic chemicals, matches,
  and firearms
Syrup of ipecac, poison control telephone
  number

Dental Health
Tooth brushing and dental visits

IMMUNIZATIONS AND CHEMOPROPHYLAXIS
Diphtheria-tetanus-pertussis (DTP) vaccine[5]
Oral poliovirus vaccine (OPV)[5]
High-risk groups
Fluoride supplements (HR5)

Other Primary Preventive Measures

Effects of passive smoking

High-risk groups

Skin protection from ultraviolet light (HR4)

HIGH-RISK CATEGORIES

HR1 Children who live in or frequently visit housing built before 1950 that is dilapidated or undergoing renovation; who come in contact with other children with known lead toxicity; who live near lead processing plants or whose parents or household members work in a lead-related occupation; or who live near busy highways or hazardous waste sites.

HR2 Household members of persons with tuberculosis or others at risk for close contact with the disease; recent immigrants or refugees from countries in which tuberculosis is common (e.g., countries in Asia, Africa, Central and South America, and the Pacific Islands); residents of homeless shelters; family members of migrant workers; or persons with certain underlying medical disorders.

HR3 Children with a family history of childhood hearing impairment or a personal history of congenital perinatal infection with herpes, syphilis, rubella, cytomegalovirus, or toxoplasmosis malformations involving the head or neck (e.g., dysmorphic and syndromal abnormalities cleft palate, abnormal pima), birth weight below 1500 g, bacterial meningitis; hyperbilirubinemia requiring exchange transfusion or severe perinatal asphyxia (Apgar scores of 0-3 absence of spontaneous respirations for 10 minutes, or hypotonia at 2 hours of age).

HR4 Children with increased exposure to sunlight.

HR5 Children living in areas with inadequate water fluoridation (less than 0.7 parts per million).

---

[1]One visit is required for immunizations. Because of lack of data and differing client risk profiles, the scheduling of additional visits and the frequency of the individual preventive services listed in this table are left to clinical discretion (except as indicated in other footnotes). [2]Ages 3-4. [3]Annually. [4]Before age 3, if not tested earlier. [5]Once between ages 4 and 6.

Ages 7-12—schedule: see footnote[1]

Leading Causes of Death:
Motor vehicle crashes
Injuries (non–motor vehicle)
Congenital anomalies
Leukemia
Homicide
Heart disease

SCREENING
Height and weight
Blood pressure
High-risk groups
Tuberculin skin test (PPD) (HR1)

Remain Alert for:
Vision disorders
Diminished hearing
Dental decay, malalignment, mouth breathing
Signs of child abuse or neglect
Abnormal bereavement

CLIENT AND PARENT COUNSELING

Diet and Exercise
Fat (especially saturated fat), cholesterol, sweets and between-meal snacks, sodium
Caloric balance
Selection of exercise program

Injury Prevention
Safety belts
Smoke detector
Storage of firearms, drugs, toxic chemicals, matches
Bicycle safety helmets

CHEMOPROPHYLAXIS

High-risk groups
Fluoride supplements (HR3)

Dental Health

Regular tooth brushing and dental visits

Other Primary Preventive Measures

High-risk groups

Skin protection from ultraviolet light (HR2)

HIGH RISK CATEGORIES

HR1 Household members of persons with tuberculosis or others at risk for close contact with the disease; recent immigrants or refugees from countries in which tuberculosis is common (e.g., countries in Asia, Africa, Central and South America, and the Pacific Islands); family members of migrant workers, residents of homeless shelters; or persons with certain underlying medical disorders.

HR2 Children with increased exposure to sunlight.

HR3 Children living in areas with inadequate water fluoridation (less than 0.7 parts per million).

---

[1] Because of lack of data and differing client risk profiles, the scheduling of visits and the frequency of the individual preventive services listed in this table are left to clinical discretion.

Ages 13-18—schedule: see footnote[1]

Leading Causes of Death:
Motor vehicle crashes
Homicide
Suicide
Injuries (non–motor vehicle)
Heart disease

SCREENING

History
Dietary intake
Physical activity
Tobacco, alcohol, drug use
Sexual practices

Physical Exam
Height and weight
Blood pressure
High-risk groups
Complete skin exam (HR1)
Clinical testicular exam (HR2)

Laboratory/Diagnostic Procedures
High-risk groups
Rubella antibodies (HR3)
VDRL RPR (HR4)
Chlamydial testing (HR5)
Gonorrhea culture (HR6)

Remain Alert for:
Depressive symptoms
Suicide risk factors (HR11)
Abnormal bereavement
Tooth decay, malalignment, gingivitis
Signs of child abuse and neglect

COUNSELING

Diet and Exercise
Fat (especially saturated fat), cholesterol,
sodium, iron,[3] calcium[3]
Caloric balance
Selection of exercise program

Substance Use
Tobacco: cessation, primary prevention
Alcohol and other drugs: cessation, primary
prevention
Driving, other dangerous activities while
under the influence
Treatment for abuse
High-risk groups
Sharing using unsterilized needle and syringes
(HR12)

Sexual Practices
Sexual development and behavior[4]

IMMUNIZATIONS AND CHEMOPROPHYLAXIS

Tetanus-diphtheria (Td) booster[6]
High-risk groups
Fluoride supplements (HR15)

Sexually transmitted diseases, partner selection, condoms

Unintended pregnancy and contraceptive options

Injury Prevention

Safety belts

Safety helmets

Violent behavior[5]

Firearms[5]

Smoke detector

Dental Health

Regular tooth brushing, flossing, dental visits

Other Primary

Preventive Measures

High-risk groups

Discussion of hemoglobin testing (HR13)

Skin protection from ultraviolet light (HR14)

Counseling and testing for HIV (HR7)

Tuberculin skin test (PPD) (HR8)

Hearing (HR9)

Papanicolaou smear (HR10)[2]

HIGH-RISK CATEGORIES

HR1 Persons with increased recreational or occupational exposure to sunlight, a family or personal history of skin cancer, or clinical evidence of precursor lesions (e.g., dysplastic nevi, certain congenital nevi).

HR2 Males with a history of cryptorchidism, orchiopexy, or testicular atrophy.

HR3 Females of childbearing age lacking evidence of immunity.

[1]One visit is required for immunizations. Because of lack of data and differing client risk profiles, the scheduling of additional visits and the frequency of the individual preventive services listed in this table are left to clinical discretion (except as indicated in other footnotes). [2]Every 1-3 years. [3]For females. [4]Often best performed early in adolescence and with the involvement of parents. [5]Especially for males. [6]Once between ages 14 and 16.

Continued.

Ages 13–18—schedule: see footnote[1]—cont'd

HR4   Persons who engage in sex with multiple partners in areas in which syphilis is prevalent, prostitutes, or contacts of persons with active syphilis.

HR5   Persons who attend clinics for sexually transmitted diseases; attend other high-risk health care facilities (e.g. adolescent and family planning clinics); or have other risk factors for chlamydial infection (e.g., multiple sexual partners or a sexual partner with multiple sexual contacts).

HR6   Persons with multiple sexual partners or a sexual partner with multiple contacts, sexual contacts of persons with culture-proven gonorrhea, or persons with a history of repeated episodes of gonorrhea.

HR7   Persons seeking treatment for sexually transmitted diseases; homosexual and bisexual men; past or present intravenous (IV) drug users; persons with a history of prostitution or multiple sexual partners; women whose past or present sexual partners were HIV-infected bisexual or IV drug users; persons with long-term residence or birth in an area with high prevalence of HIV infection; or persons with a history of transfusion between 1978 and 1985.

HR8   Household members of persons with tuberculosis or others at risk for close contact with the disease; recent immigrants or refugees from countries in which tuberculosis is common (e.g., countries in Asia, Africa, Central and South America, and the Pacific Islands); migrant workers; residents of correctional institutions or homeless shelters; or persons with certain underlying medical disorders.

HR9   Persons exposed regularly to excessive noise in recreational or other settings.

HR10 Females who are sexually active of (if the sexual history is thought to be unreliable) age 18 or older.

HR11 Recent divorce, separation, unemployment, depression, alcohol, or other drug abuse; serious medical illnesses; living alone or recent bereavement.

HR12 Intravenous drug users.

HR13 Persons of Caribbean, Latin American, Asian, Mediterranean, or African descent.

HR14 Persons with increased exposure to sunlight.

HR15 Persons living in areas with inadequate water fluoridation (less than 0.7 parts per million).

Ages 19-39—schedule: every 1-3 years[1]

Leading Causes of Death:
Motor vehicle crashes
Homicide
Suicide
Injuries (non–motor vehicle)
Heart disease

Remain Alert for:
Depressive symptoms
Suicide risk factors (HR17)
Abnormal bereavement
Malignant skin lesions
Tooth decay, gingivitis
Signs of physical abuse

SCREENING

History
Dietary intake
Physical activity
Tobacco/alcohol/drug use
Sexual practices

Physical Exam
Height and weight
Blood pressure
Papanicolaou smear[2]
High-risk groups
Complete oral cavity exam (HR1)
Palpation for thyroid nodules
(HR2)
Clinical breast exam (HR3)
Clinical testicular exam (HR4)
Complete skin exam (HR5)

COUNSELING

Diet and Exercise
Fat (especially saturated fat), cholesterol, complex
carbohydrates, fiber, sodium, iron,[3] calcium[3]
Caloric balance
Selection of exercise program

Substance Use
Tobacco: cessation/primary prevention
Alcohol and other drugs:
Limit alcohol consumption
Driving/other dangerous activities while under
the influence
Treatment for abuse
High-risk groups
Sharing/using unsterilized needles and
syringes (HR18)

IMMUNIZATIONS

Tetanus-diphtheria (Td) booster[5]
High-risk groups
Hepatitis B vaccine (HR24)
Pneumococcal vaccine (HR25)
Influenza vaccine[6] (HR26)
Measles-mumps-rubella vaccine (HR27)

Continued.

[1]The recommended schedule applies only to the periodic visit itself. The frequency of the individual preventive services listed in this table is left to clinical discretion, except as indicated in other footnotes.[2]Every 1-3 years. [3]For women. [4]Especially for young males. [5]Every 10 years. [6]Annually.

Ages 19-39—schedule: every 1-3 years[1]—cont'd

Laboratory/Diagnostic Procedures

Nonfasting total blood cholesterol

High-risk groups

Fasting plasma glucose (HR6)
Rubella antibodies (HR7)
VDRL/RPR (HR8)
Urinalysis for bacteriuria (HR9)
Chlamydial testing (HR10)
Gonorrhea culture (HR11)
Counseling and testing for HIV (HR12)
Hearing (HR13)
Tuberculin skin test (PPD) (HR14)
Electrocardiogram (HR15)
Mammogram (HR3)
Colonoscopy (HR16)

Sexual Practices

Sexually transmitted diseases: partner selection, condoms, and intercourse
Unintended pregnancy and contraceptive options

Injury Prevention

Safety belts
Safety helmets
Violent behavior[4]
Firearms[4]
Smoke detector
Smoking near bedding or upholstery

High-risk groups

Back-conditioning exercises (HR19)
Prevention of childhood injuries (HR20)
Falls in the elderly (HR21)

Dental Health

Regular tooth brushing, flossing, dental visits

Other Primary Preventive Measures

High-risk groups

Discussion of hemoglobin testing (HR22)
Skin protection from ultraviolet light (HR23)

HIGH RISK CATEGORIES

HR1 Persons with exposure to tobacco or excessive amounts of alcohol, or those with suspicious symptoms or lesions deteced through self-examination.

HR2 Persons with a history of upper-body irradiation.

HR3 Women aged 35 and older with a family history of premenopausally diagnosed breast cancer in a first-degree relative.

HR4 Men with a history of cryptorchidism, orchiopexy, or testicular atrophy.

HR5 Persons with family or personal history of skin cancer, increased occupational or recreational exposure to sunlight, or clinical evidence of precursor lesions (e.g., dysplastic nevi, certain congenital nevi).

HR6 The markedly obese, persons with a family hsitory of diabetes, or women with a history of gestational diabetes.

HR7 Women lacking evidence of immunity.

HR8 Prostitutes, persons who engage in sex with multiple partners in areas in which syphilis is prevalent or contacts of persons with active syphilis.

HR9 Persons with diabetes.

HR10 Persons who attend clinics for sexually transmitted diseases; attend other high-risk health care facilities (e.g., adolescent and family planning clinics); or have other risk factors for chlamydial infection (e.g., multiple sexual partners or a sexual partner with multiple sexual contacts, age less than 20).

HR11 Prostitutes, persons with multiple sexual partners or a sexual partner with multiple contacts, sexual contacts of persons with culture-proven gonorrhea, or persons with a history of repeated episodes of gonorrhea.

Continued.

Ages 19-39—schedule: every 1-3 years[1]—cont'd

HR12 Persons seeking treatment for sexually transmitted diseases; homosexual and bisexual men; past or present intravenous (IV) drug users; persons with a history of prostitution or multiple sexual partners; women whose past or present sexual partners were HIV-infected, bisexual, or IV drug users; persons with long-term residence or birth in an area with high prevalence of HIV infection; or persons with a history of transfusion between 1978 and 1985.

HR13 Persons exposed regularly to excessive noise.

HR14 Household members of persons with tuberculosis or others at risk for close contact with the disease (e.g., staff of tuberculosis clinics, shelters for the homeless, nursing homes, substance abuse treatment facilities, dialysis units, correctional institutions); recent immigrants or refugees from countries in which tuberculosis is common; migrant workers; residents of nursing homes, correctional institutions, or homeless shelters; or persons with certain underling medical disorders (e.g., HIV infection).

HR15 Men who would endanger public safety were they to experience sudden cardiac events (e.g., commercial airline pilots).

HR16 Persons with a family history of familiar polyposis coli or cancer family syndrome.

HR17 Recent divorce, separation, unemployment, depression, alcohol or other drug abuse, serious medical illnesses, living alone, or recent bereavement.

HR18 Intravenous drug users.

HR19 Persons at increased risk for low back injury because of past history, body configuration, or type of activities.

HR20 Persons with children in the home or automobile.

HR21 Persons with older adults in the home.

HR22 Young adults of Caribbean, Latin American, Asian, Mediterranean, or African descent.

HR23 Persons with increased exposure to sunlight.

HR24 Homosexually active men, intravenous drug users, recipients of some blood products, or persons in health-related jobs with frequent exposure to blood or blood products.

HR25 Persons with medical conditions that increase the risk of pneumococcal infection (e.g., chronic cardiac or pulmonary disease, sickle cell disease, nephrotic syndrome, Hodgkin's disease, asplenia, diabetes mellitus, alcoholism, cirrhosis, multiple myeloma, renal disease, or conditions associated with immunosuppression).

HR26 Residents of chronic care facilities or persons suffering from chronic cardiopulmonary disorders, metabolic diseases (including diabetes mellitus), hemoglobinopathies, immunosuppression, or renal dysfunction.

HR27 Persons born after 1956 who lack evidence of immunity to measles (receipt of live vaccine on or after first birthday, laboratory evidence of immunity, or a history of physician-diagnosed measles).

Ages 40-64—schedule: every 1-3 years[1]

Leading Causes of Death:

Heart disease
Lung cancer
Cerebrovascular disease
Breast cancer
Colorectal cancer
Obstructive lung disease

SCREENING

History
Dietary intake
Physical activity
Tobacco/alcohol/drug use
Sexual practices

Physical Exam
Height and weight
Blood pressure
Clinical breast exam[2]
High-risk groups
Complete skin exam (HR1)
Complete oral cavity exam (HR2)

Remain Alert for:

Depressive symptoms
Suicide risk factors (HR17)
Abnormal bereavement
Signs of physical abuse or neglect
Malignant skin lesions
Peripheral arterial disease (HR18)
Tooth decay, gingivitis, loose teeth

COUNSELING

Diet and Exercise
Fat (especially saturated fat), cholesterol, complex
   carbohydrates, fiber, sodium, calcium[5]
Caloric balance
Selection of exercise program

Substance Use
Tobacco cessation
Alcohol and other drugs:
   Limiting alcohol consumption
   Driving and other dangerous activities while under
      the influence
   Treatment for abuse

IMMUNIZATIONS

Tetanus-diphtheria (Td) booster[6]
High-risk groups
Hepatitis B vaccine (HR26)
Pneumococcal vaccine (HR27)
Influenza vaccine (HR28)[7]

Palpation for thyroid nodules (HR3)
Auscultation for carotid bruits (HR4)
Laboratory/Diagnostic Procedures
Nonfasting total blood cholesterol
Papanicolaou smear[3]
Mammogram[4]
High-risk groups
Fasting plasma glucose (HR5)
VDRL/RPR (HR6)
Urinalysis for bacteriuria (HR7)
Chlamydial testing (HR8)
Gonorrhea culture (HR9)
Counseling and testing for HIV (HR10)
Tuberculin skin test (PPD) (HR11)
Hearing (HR12)
Electrocardiogram (HR13)
Fecal occult blood sigmoidoscopy (HR14)
Fecal occult blood/colonoscopy (HR15)
Bone mineral content (HR16)

High-risk groups
Sharing/using unsterilized needles and syringes (HR19)
Sexual Practices
Sexually transmitted diseases; partner selection, condoms, anal intercourse
Unintended pregnancy and contraceptive options
Injury Prevention
Safety belts
Safety helmets
Smoke detector
Smoking near bedding or upholstery
High-risk groups
Back-conditioning exercises (HR20)
Prevention of childhood injuries (HR21)
Falls in the elderly (HR22)
Dental Health
Regular tooth brushing, flossing, and dental visits
Other Primary Preventive Measures
High-risk groups
Skin protection from ultraviolet light (HR23)
Discussion of aspirin therapy (HR24)
Discussion of estrogen replacement therapy (HR25)

[1]The recommended schedule applies only to the periodic visit itself. The frequency of the individual preventive services listed in this table is left to clinical discretion, except as indicated in other footnotes. [2]Annually for women. [3]Every 13 years for women. [4]Every 1-2 years for women beginning at age 50 (age 35 for those at increased risk). [5]For women. [6]Every 10 years. [7]Annually.

Continued.

Ages 40-64—schedule: every 1-3 years[1]—cont'd

HIGH RISK CATEGORIES

HR1 Persons with family or personal history of skin cancer, increased occupational or recreational exposure to sunlight, or clinical evidence of precursor lesions (e.g., dysplastic nevi, certain congenital nevi).

HR2 Persons with exposure to tobacco or excessive amounts of alcohol, or those with suspicious symptoms of lesions detected through self-examination.

HR3 Persons with a history of upper-body irradiation.

HR4 Persons with risk factors for cerebrovascular or cardiovascular disease (e.g., hypertension, smoking, CAD, atrial fibrillation, diabetes; or those with neurologic symptoms (e.g., transient ischemic attacks); or a history of cerebrovascular disease.

HR5 The markedly obese, persons with a family history of diabetes, or women with a history of gestational diabetes.

HR6 Prostitutes, persons who engage in sex with multiple partners in areas in which syphilis is prevalent, or contacts of persons with active syphilis.

HR7 Persons with diabetes.

HR8 Persons who attend clinics for sexually transmitted diseases; attend other high-risk health care facilities (e.g., adolescent and family planning clinics); or have other risk factors for chlamydial infection (e.g., mutliple sexual partners or a sexual partner with multiple sexual contacts).

HR9 Prostitutes, persons with multiple sexual partners or a sexual partner with multiple contacts, sexual contacts of persons with culture-proven gonorrhea, or persons with a history of repeated episodes of gonorrhea.

HR10 Persons seeking treatment for sexually transmitted diseases; homosexual and bisexual men; past or present intravenous (IV) drug users; persons with a history of prostitution or multiple sexual partners; women whose past or present sexual partners were HIV-infected, bisexual, or IV drug users; persons with long-term residence or birth in an area with high prevalence of HIV infection; or persons with a history of transfusion between 1978 and 1985.

HR11 Household members of persons with tuberculosis or others at risk for close contact with the disease (e.g., staff of tuberculosis clinics, shelters for the homeless, nursing homes, substance abuse treatment facilities, dialysis units, correctional institutions); recent immigrants or refugees from countries in which tuberculosis is common (e.g., countries in Asia, Africa, Central and South America, and the Pacific Islands); migrant workers; residents of nursing homes, correctional institutions, or homeless shelters; or persons with certain underlying medical disorders (e.g., HIV infection).

HR12 Persons exposed regularly to excessive noise.

HR13 Men with two or more cardiac risk factors (high blood cholesterol, hypertension, cigarette smoking, diabetes mellitus, family history of CAD); men who would endanger public safety were they to experience sudden cardiac events (e.g., commercial airline pilots); or sedentary or high-risk males planning to begin a vigorous exercise program.

HR14 Persons aged 50 and older who have first-degree relatives with colorectal cancer, a personal history of endometrial, ovarian, or breast cancer, or a previous diagnosis of inflammatory bowel disease, adenomatous polyps, or colorectal cancer.

HR15 Persons with a family history of familial polyposis coli or cancer family syndrome.

HR16 Perimenopausal women at increased risk for osteoporosis (e.g., Caucasian race, bilateral oopherectomy before menopause, slender build) and for whom estrogen replacement therapy would otherwise not be recommended.

HR17 Recent divorce, separation, unemployment, depression, alcohol or other drug abuse, serious medical illnesses, living alone, or recent bereavment.

HR18 Persons over age 50, smokers, or persons with diabetes mellitus.

HR19 Intravenous drug users.

HR20 Persons at increased risk for low back injury because of past history, body configuration, or type of activities.

HR21 Persons with children in the home or automobile.

HR22 Persons with older adults in the home.

Continued.

Ages 40-64—schedule: every 1-3 years[1]—cont'd

HR23 Persons with increased exposure to sunlight.

HR24 Men who have risk factors for myocardial infarction (e.g., blood cholesterol, smoking, diabetes mellitus, family history of early-onset CAD) and who lack a history of gastrointestinal or other bleeding problems, and other risk factors for bleeding or cerebral hemorrhage.

HR25 Perimenopausal women at increased risk for osteoporosis (e.g., Caucasian, low bone mineral content, bilateral oopherectomy before menopause or early menopause, slender build) and who are without known contraindications (e.g., history of undiagnosed vaginal bleeding, active liver disease, thromboembolic disorders, hormone-dependent cancer).

HR26 Homosexually active men, intravenous drug users, recipients of some blood products, or persons in health-related jobs with frequent exposure to blood or blood products.

HR27 Persons with medical conditions that increase the risk of pneumococcal infection (e.g., chronic cardiac or pulmonary disease, sickle cell disease, nephrotic syndrome, Hodgkin's disease, asplenia, diabetes mellitus, alcoholism, cirrhosis, multiple myeloma, renal disease, or conditions associated with immunosuppression).

HR28 Residents of chronic care facilities and persons suffering from chronic cardiopulmonary disorders, metabolic diseases (including diabetes mellitus, hemoglobinopathies, immunosuppression, or renal dysfunction)

Ages 65 and over—schedule: every year[1]

Leading Causes of Death:

Heart disease
Cerebrovascular disease
Obstructive lung disease
Pneumonia/influenza
Lung cancer
Colorectal cancer

SCREENING

History

Prior symptoms of transient ischemic
  attack
Dietary intake
Physical activity
Tobacco/alcohol/drug use
Functional status at home

Remain Alert for:

Depression symptoms
Suicide risk factors (HR11)
Abnormal bereavement
Changes in cognitive function
Medications that increase risk of falls
Signs of physical abuse or neglect
Malignant skin lesions
Peripheral arterial disease
Tooth decay, gingivitis, loose teeth

COUNSELING

Diet and Exercise

Fat (especially saturated fat), cholesterol, complex
  carbohydrates, fiber, sodium, calcium[4]
Caloric balance
Selection of exercise program

IMMUNIZATIONS

Tetanus-diphtheria (Td) booster[6]
Influenza vaccine[2]
Pneumococcal vaccine
High-risk groups
Hepatitis B vaccine (HR16)

---

[1]The recommended schedule applies only to the periodic visit itself. The frequency of the individual preventive services listed in this table is left to clinical discretion, except as indicated in other footnotes. [2]Annually. [3]Every 1-2 years for women until age 75, unless pathology detected. [4]For women. [5]Every 1-3 years. [6]Every 10 years.

Continued.

Ages 65 and over—schedule: every year[1]—cont'd

Physical Exam
Height and weight
Blood pressure
Visual acuity
Hearing and hearing aids
Clinical breast exam[2]
High-risk groups
Auscultation for carotid bruits (HR1)
Complete skin exam (HR2)
Complete oral cavity exam (HR3)
Palpation of thyroid nodules (HR4)
Laboratory/Diagnostic Procedures
Nonfasting total blood cholesterol
Dipstick urinalysis
Mammogram[3]
Tyroid function tests[4]
High-risk groups
Fasting plasma glucose (HR5)
Tuberculin skin test (PPD) (HR6)
Electrocardiogram (HR7)
Papanicolaou smear[5] (HR8)
Fecal occult blood sigmoidoscopy (HR9)
Fecal occult blood colonoscopy (HR10)

Substance Use
Tobacco cessation
Alcohol and other drugs:
    Limiting alcohol consumption
    Driving other dangerous activities while under the influence
    Treatment for abuse
Injury Prevention
Prevention of falls
Safety belts
Smoke detector
Smoking near bedding or upholstery
Hot water heater temperature
Safety helmets
High-risk groups
Prevention of childhood injuries (HR12)
Dental Health
Regular dental visits, tooth brushing, flossing
Other Primary Preventive Measures
Glaucoma testing by eye specialist
High-risk groups
Discussion of estrogen replacement therapy (HR13)
Discussion of aspirin therapy (HR14)
Skin protection from ultraviolet light (HR15)

HIGH RISK CATEGORIES

HR1 Persons with risk factors for cerebrovascular or cardiovascular disease (e.g., hypertension, smoking, CAD, atrial fibrillation, diabetes) or those with neurologic symptoms (e.g., transient ischemic attacks) or a history of cerebrovascular disease.

HR2 Persons with a family or personal history of skin cancer or clinical evidence of precursor lesions (e.g., dysplastic nevi, certain congenital nevi) or those with increased occupational or recreational exposure to sunlight.

HR3 Persons with exposure to tobacco or excessive amounts of alcohol, or those with suspicious symptoms or lesions detected through self-examination.

HR4 Persons with a history of upper-body irradiation.

HR5 The markedly obese, persons with a family history of diabetes, or women with a history of gestational diabetes.

HR6 Household members of persons with tuberculosis or others at risk for close contact with the disease (e.g., staff of tuberculosis clinics, shelters for the homeless, nursing homes, substance abuse treatment facilities, dialysis units, correctional institutions); recent immigrants or refugees from countries in which tuberculosis is common (e.g., countries in Asia, Africa, Central and South America, and the Pacific Islands); migrant workers, residents of nursing homes, correctional institutions, or homeless shelters; or persons with certain underlying medical disorders (e.g., HIV infection).

HR7 Men with two or more cardiac risk factors (high blood cholesterol, hypertension, cigarette smoking, diabetes mellitus, family history of CAD); men who would endanger public safety were they to experience sudden cardiac events (e.g., commercial airline pilots); or sedentary or high-risk males planning to begin a vigorous exercise program.

HR8 Women who have not had previous documented screening in which smears have been consistently negative.

HR9 Persons who have first-degree relatives with colorectal cancer; a personal history of endometrial, ovarian, or breast cancer; or a previous diagnosis of inflammatory bowel disease, adenomatous polyps, or colorectal cancer.

HR10 Persons with a family history of familial polyposis coli or cancer family syndrome.

HR11 Recent divorce, separation, unemployment, depression, alcohol or other drug abuse, serious medical illnesses, living alone, or recent bereavement.

Continued.

Ages 65 and over—schedule: every year[1]—cont'd

HR12 Persons with children in the home or automobile.

HR13 Women at increased risk for osteoporoisis (e.g., Caucasian, low bone mineral content, bilateral oophorectomy before menopause or early menopause, slender build) and who are without known contraindications (e.g., history of undiagnosed vaginal bleeding, active liver disease, thromboembolic disorders, hormone-dependent cancer).

HR14 Men who have risk factors for myocardial infarction (e.g., blood cholesterol, smoking, diabetes mellitus, family history of early-onset CAD) and who lack a history of gastrointestinal or other bleeding problems, and other risk factors for bleeding or cerebral hemorrhage.

HR15 Persons with increased exposure to sunlight.

HR16 Homosexually, active men, intravenous drug users, recipients of some blood products, or persons in health-related job with frequent exposure to blood or blood products.

Pregnant women[1]

Prenatal visit	Follow-up visits
Remain Alert for: Signs of physical abuse	**Remain Alert for:** Signs of physical abuse Schedule: See footnote[2]
SCREENING History Generic and obstetric history Dietary intake Tobacco alcohol drug use Risk factors for intrauterine growth retardation and low birthweight Prior genital herpetic lesions **Laboratory/Diagnostic** Procedures Blood pressure Hemoglobin and hematocrit ABO Rh typing Rh(D) and other antibody screen VDRL RPR Hepatitis B surface antigen (HBsAg) Urinalysis for bacteriuria	**SCREENING** Blood pressure Urinalysis for bacteriuria **Screening Tests at Specific Gestational Ages** *14-16 Weeks:* Maternal serum alpha-fetoprotein (MSAFP) Ultrasound cephalometry (HR8) *24-28 Weeks:* 50 g oral glucose tolerance test Rh(d) antibody (HR9) Gonorrhea culture (HR10) VDRL/RPR (HR11) Hepatitis B surface antigen (HBsAg) (HR12) Counseling and testing for HIV 13) *36 Weeks:* Ultrasound exam (HR14)
COUNSELING Nutrition Tobacco use Alcohol and other drug use Safety belts *High-risk groups* Discuss amniocentesis (HR5) Discuss risks of HIV infection (HR4)	**COUNSELING** Nutrition Safety belts Discuss meaning of upcoming tests *High-risk groups* Tobacco use (HR6) Alcohol and other drug use (HR7)

[1]See earlier for other preventive services for women. [2]Beause of lack of data and differing patient risk profiles, the scheduling of visits and the frequency of the individual preventive services listed in this table are left to clinical discretion, except for those indicated at specific gestational ages.

Continued.

Pregnant women[1]—cont'd

Gonorrhea culture
High-risk groups
Hemoglobin electrophoresis
   (HR1)
Rubella antibodies (HR2)
Chlamydial testing (HR3)
Counseling and testing for HIV
   (HR4)

HIGH RISK CATEGORIES

HR1 Black women.

HR2 Women lacking evidence of immunity (proof of vaccination after the first birthday or laboratory evidence of immunity).

HR3 Women who attend clinics for sexually transmitted diseases, attend other high-risk health care facilities (e.g., adolescent and family planning clinics) or have other risk factors for chlamydial infection (e.g., multiple sexual partner or a sexual partner with multiple sexual contacts)

HR4 Women seeking treatment for sexually transmitted diseases, past or present intravenous (IV) drug users; women with a history of prostitution or multiple sexual partners; women whose past or present sexual partners were HIV-infected, bisexual, or IV drug users; women with long-term residence or birth in an area with high prevalence of HIV infection in women; or women with a history of transfusion between 1978 and 1985.

HR5 Women aged 35 and older.

HR6 Women who continue to smoke during pregnancy.

HR7 Women with excessive alcohol consumption during pregnancy.

HR8 Women with uncertain menstrual histories or risk factors for intrauterine growth retardation (e.g., hypertension, renal disease, short maternal stature, low prepregnancy weight, failure to gain weight during pregnancy, smoking, alcohol and other drug abuse, and history of a previous fetal death or growth-retarded baby).

HR9 Unsensitized Rh-negative women.

HR10 Women with multiple sexual partners or a sexual partner with multiple contacts, or sexual contracts of persons with culture-proven gonorrhea.

HR11 Women who engage in sex with multiple partners in areas in which syphilis is prevalent or contacts of persons with active syphilis.

HR12 Women who engage in high-risk behavior (e.g., intravenous drug use) or in whom exposure to hepatitis B during pregnancy is suspected.

HR13 Women at high risk (see HR4) who have a nonreactive HIV test at the first prenatal visit.

HR14 Women with risk factors for intrauterine growth retardation (see HR8).

Sleep Interview

General Data

1. Statement of the sleep problem by client, bed partner, or family: obtain a quantifiable answer about sleep, such as never sleeps, dozes off for an hour several times a night, or has trouble sleeping 5 nights out of 7, every other night, or on weekends only
2. Initiation of sleep problem: when possible, elicit cause
3. Factors that make it worse or better
4. Previous occurrences to client or to other family member or friend
5. Modifications that need to be made for daytime activities or travel
6. Memories of frightening or upsetting incidences during sleep, such as sudden illness or death of a loved one or damage from storm, fire, or robbery
7. Occurrences of accidents or "near misses" as a result of sleep problems *(very important)*

Insomnia Data

(Remember that a complaint of insomnia may be caused by sleep apnea or other difficulties with sleep.)

1. Time person gets into bed and time person falls asleep
2. Number and times of awakenings at night
3. Interval before returning to sleep after each awakening
4. Time of final awakening, time of arising from bed, and what wakes the person up, such as noises, alarm clock, or treatment
5. Daytime naps: number, when, and how long
6. Dozing off briefly (same question as napping, but some persons answer this question differently)
7. Lying down to rest on couch or "resting eyes for a moment" (this counts as napping because person may be falling asleep)
8. Practices used to assist with sleep: type and regularity of use
9. Changes in sleep patterns because of sleep deficit
10. Places where sleep occurs more readily, such as somewhere else in the house or on vacation
11. Concerns that delay getting into bed or falling asleep
12. Amount of and recent changes in caffeine intake (coffee, tea, colas, other cafeinated beverages, caffeinated gum) and alcohol

---

From Phipps WJ, Sands J, Lehman MK, Cassmeyer V: *Medical-surgical nursing: concepts and clinical practice,* ed 5, St Louis, 1995, Mosby.

13. Types of weekly excercise and recreational activities
14. Measures of coping with concerns
15. Recent illness or loss of relatives, friends, or pets
16. Activities of others in house or neighborhood that affect sleep, such as child who returns home late, spouse who leaves home early in morning, noise from a neighbor or dog, and noise from a nearby highway or airport

Sleep Apnea Data

1. Description or reenactment by bed partner of the person's breathing pattern, including sound and volume of snoring, length of time that no air passes, and how the person starts to breathe again
2. Description by bed partner of differences in client's breathing while on back, each side, and stomach and of changes in client's skin color while asleep
3. Presence of morning headaches
4. Difficulty in awakening for the day
5. Number of pillows used; preference of sleeping in a certain chair
6. Degree of sleepiness during day; falling asleep at a movie, during a conversation, or while driving

Narcolepsy-Related Data

1. Presence of sudden irresistible urges to sleep; falling asleep and then awakening a few minutes later feeling refreshed
2. Experiences of a sudden loss of muscle tone, leading to drooping of the head or slumping to the floor, that occur during episodes of strong emotions (surprise, laughter, anger)
3. Experiences on awakening of feeling paralyzed until touched by another
4. Presence of visual, auditory, or tactile hallucinations at time of sleep initiation or awakening
5. Family history of unusual experiences in sleep

Sleep Schedule Data

1. Working hours
2. Experience of going to bed later each night
3. Daily schedule activities, flexibility
4. Changes in sleep schedule as a result of changes in life schedule, such as retirement or hospitalization
5. Interruption of sleep because of family activities
6. Practice of sleeping through the day or staying up at night because of a specific purpose, such as fear that a calamity will befall during the night

Other Sleep-Related Events

1. Uncomfortable feelings in legs when ready to fall asleep: location, type of sensations, duration, actions that make it better or worse, attempted remedies, and effect on sleep
2. Reports from bed partner of client kicking or moving legs in sleep
3. Bed-wetting: frequency, time of occurrence, actions that make it better or worse, and reports of any nights of dryness
4. Dreams: upsetting recurring dreams, frightening nightmares, or sleep terrors
5. Sleepwalking: initiation, frequency, ability to be awakened easily or guided back to bed, experience of injury while sleepwalking, actions that make it better or worse, and steps taken to keep the person safe
6. Teeth grinding during sleep
7. Dysfunctions associated with sleep, such as chest pain, shortness of breath, hearburn/ulcer pain, morning headache, asthmatic attacks, frequent awakenings to urinate, hot flashes in menopausal wormen, coughing, chocking ad gagging, and arthritic or other neuromuscular pain

External Factors Regulating Sleep

Sunrise, sunset, and length of day
Ambient temperature
Physical activity and rest
Timing and composition of meals
Timing of social/environmental cues, such as increased morning traffic noise

Modified from Association of Sleep Disorder Centers and the Association for the Psychophysiological Study of Sleep, *Sleep* 2(1):21, 1979. In Phipps WJ, Sands J, Lehman MK, Cassmeyer V: *Medical-surgical nursing: concepts and clinical practice,* ed 5, St Louis, 1995, Mosby.

Classification of Sleep and Arousal Disorders

Disorders of Initiating and Maintaining Sleep (DIMS)

1. Psychophysiologic: transient and situational, persistent
2. Associated with:
   a. Psychiatric disorders: symptom and personality disorders, affective disorders, other functional psychoses

From Phipps WJ, Sands J, Lehman MK, Cassmeyer V: *Medical-surgical nursing: concepts and clinical practice,* ed 5, St Louis, 1995, Mosby.

b. Use of drugs and alcohol: tolerance to or withdrawal from central nervous system (CNS) depressants, sustained use of CNS stimulants, sustained use or withdrawal for other drugs, chronic alcoholism

c. Slee-induced respiratory impairment: sleep apnea DIMS syndrome, alveolar hypoventilation DIMS syndrome

d. Sleep-related (nocturnal) myoclonus DIMS syndrome and/or "restless legs"

e. Other medical, toxic, and environmental conditions

f. Child-onset DIMS

g. Other DIMS conditions: repeated REM interruptions, atypical polysomnographic features

h. No DIMS abnormality: "short sleeper," subjective DIMS complaints without objective findings

Disorders of Excessive Somnolence (DOES)

1. Psychophysiologic: transient and situational, persistent
2. Associated with:
   a. Psychiatric disorders: symptom and personality disorders, affective disorders, other functional psychoses
   b. Use of drugs and alcohol: tolerance to or withdrawal from CNS stimulants, sustained use of CNS depressants
   c. Sleep-induced respiratory impairment: sleep apnea DOES syndrome, alveolar hypoventilation DOES syndrom
   d. Sleep-related (nocturnal) myoclonus DOES syndrom and/or "restless legs"
   e. Other medical, toxic, and environmental conditions
   f. Other DOES conditions
   g. Intermittent DOES (periodic) syndroms: Kleine-Levin syndrome, menstrual-associated syndrome
   h. Insufficient sleep
   i. Sleep drunkeness

3. Narcolepsy
4. Idiopathic CNS hypersomnolence
5. No DOES abnormality: "short sleeper," subjective DOES complaints without objective findings

Disorders of the Sleep-Wake Schedule

1. Transient: time-zone (jet lag) syndrome, work shift change in conventional sleep-wake schedule
2. Persistent: frequently changing sleep-wake schedule, delayed sleep phase syndrome, advanced sleep phase syndrome, non-24-hour sleep-wake syndrome, irregular sleep-wake pattern

Dysfunctions Associated with Sleep, Sleep Stages, or Partial Arousals—Parasomnias or Disorders of Arousal

1. Sleepwalking (somnambulism)
2. Sleep teror (pavor noctumus, incubus)
3. Sleep-related enuresis
4. Other dysfunctions
   a. Dream anxiety attaks (nightmares)
   b. Familial sleep paralysis
   c. Impaired sleep-related penile tumescence
   d. Sleep-related epileptic seizures, bruxism, head banging (jactatio capitis nocturnal), painful erections, cluster headaches and chronic paroxysmal hemicrania, abnormal swallowing syndrome, asthma, cardiovascular symptoms, gastroesophagel reflux, hemolysis (paroxysmal nocturnal hemoglobinuria)
   e. Asymptomatic polysomnographic findings

Parasomnias or Disorders of Arousal

Type of Dysfunction	Comments
Sleepwalking	Walking while asleep
Sleep terror	Panic attack while asleep
Sleep-related enuresis	Bed-wetting; event begins in stage III/IV sleep, and enuresis occurs as sleep lightens
Dream anxiety attacks	Nightmares; REM phenomenon
Sleep-related epileptic seizures	Seizures occur more often during sleep; explains why sleep encouraged during short routine electroencephalograms (EEGs)
Sleep-related bruxism	Teeth grinding; dental assistance may be needed to preserve teeth
Sleep-related head banging (jactatio capitis nocturna)	Rhythmic head rocking and banging common in young children under age 5 years; occurs in stage I/II sleep
Familial sleep paralysis	Inability to move muscles when first awakening
Sleep-related cluster headaches	Associated with REM and relieved by indomethacin
Sleep-related abnormal swallowing syndrome	Inadequate swallowing of saliva during sleep

From Phipps WJ, Sands J, Lehman MK, Cassmeyer V: *Medical-surgical nursing: concepts and clinical practice,* ed 5, St Louis, 1995, Mosby.

Type of Dysfunction	Comments
Sleep-related asthma	Early morning increase in bronchoconstriction; 46% of asthmatic attacks occur during last third of night
Sleep-related cardiovascular symptoms	Include paroxysmal nocturnal dyspnea, myocardial infarction (peak incidence 4 AM to 6 AM), nocturnal angina, and premature ventricular contrictions (more common in REM sleep)
Sleep-related gastroesophageal reflux	Caused more by posture than sleep
Sleep-related hemolysis	Probably related to combinatio of respiratory acidosis, change in acid-base balance, and renal clearance of defective red blood cells
Morning headaches	May be related to sleeping longer on weekends and delayin usual morning dose of caffeine
Impairment in penile erections	Changes in normal incidence of erections; painful erections

Warning Signs that May Indicate the Presence of Childhood Cancer

Cancer is a leading cause of death in children less than 15 years old, second only to accidents. In this age-group, one out of every five deaths is caused by cancer. In the United States each year 12.5:100,000 children develop cancer.

General

- Documented weight loss without explanation; failure to thrive
- Persistent poor appetite
- Easy tiring or lack of energy

Modified from the Cancer Association of Greater New Orleans, Inc., 211 Camp St., Room 600, New Orleans, LA 70130. From Hancock LA: The preschool period. In Edelman CL, Mandle CL, editors: *Health promotion throughout the lifespan*, ed 3, St Louis, 1994, Mosby.

Leukemia or Lymphomas—"Liquid Tumors"

(Cancer of the blood, blood-making system, lymph nodes)

- Persistent fever (more than 2 weeks)
- Bruising without injury and purple or red patches appearing on the skin

Cancer Prevention Tips

- On a daily basis, choose foods high in dietary fiber (fruits, vegetables, and whole-grain breads and cereals).
- Choose foods low in dietary fat.
- If you drink alcoholic beverages, do so only in moderation.
- Avoid unnecessary x-rays.
- Know and follow health and safety rules of your workplace.
- Avoid too much sunlight: wear protective clothing; use effective sunscreens.
- Take estrogens only as long as necessary.
- Above all, don't smoke.

From U.S. Department of Health and Human Services: *Nutrition and cancer prevention: the good news,* NIH Pub No. 87-2878, December, 1986.

Dietary Recommendations for Cancer Prevention

1. Reduce the amount of saturated and unsaturated fats in the diet from 40% to 30% of total daily caloric intake.
2. Increase the amount of fiber in the diet by eating fresh fruits, vegetables (including cruciferous vegetables—cabbage, broccoli, brussel sprouts, kohlrabi, cauliflower), and whole grain breads/cereals.
3. Foods rich in vitamin C—citrus fruits, strawberries, currants, cabbage, tomatoes, walnuts, and rosehips.
4. Foods rich in vitamin A—peaches, cantaloupe, apricots, and the dark green and yellow vegetables (carrots, spinach, squash, asparagus, sweet potatoes).
5. Foods rich in vitamin E—vegetable oils (soybean, corn, cotton-seed, sunflower seed), alfalfa, and lettuce leaves.

From Otto SE: *Oncology nursing,* ed 2, St Louis, 1994, Mosby.

Summary of American Cancer Society Recommendations For the Early Detection of Cancer in Asymptomatic People

Test or procedure	Population		
	Sex	**Age**	**Frequency**
Sigmoidoscopy, preferably flexible	M/F	50 and over	Every 3-5 years
Fecal occult blood test	M/F	50 and over	Every year
Digital rectal examination	M/F	40 and over	Every year
Prostate examination*	M	50 and over	Every year
Pap test	F	All women who are, or who have been, sexually active, or have reached age 18, should have an annual Pap test and pelvic examination. After a woman has had three or more consecutive satisfactory normal annual examinations, the Pap test may be performed less frequently at the discretion of her physician.	
Pelvic examination	F	18-40	Every 1-3 years with Pap test
		Over 40	Every year
Endometrial tissue sample	F	At menopause if at high risk†	At menopause and thereafter at the discretion of the physician
Breast self-examination	F	20 and over	Every month
Clinical breast examination	F	20-40	Every 3 years
		Over 40	Every year
Mammography‡	F	40-49	Every 1-2 years
		50 and over	Every year
Health counseling and cancer checkup§	M/F	Over 20	Every 3 years
	M/F	Over 40	Every year

*Annual digital rectal examination and prostate-specific antigen should be performed on men 50 years and older. If either is abnormal, further evaluation should be considered.

†History of infertility, obesity, failure to ovulate, abnormal uterine bleeding, or unopposed estrogen or tamoxifen therapy.

‡Screening mammography should begin by age 40.

§To include examination for cancers of the thyroid, testicles, prostate, ovaries, lymph nodes, oral region, and skin.

Prevention, Screening, and Early Detection of Cancer

The number of people who develop cancer is on the rise—it is estimated that one in three Americans will have some type of cancer. Some of these cancers can be cured in the early stages, but not when the disease is too advanced. Early detection and treatment are the keys to curing cancer; preventing cancer in the first place is even better.

General Prevention Guidelines

There is much you can do to help prevent cancer. Smoking has been scientifically proven to cause cancer, so if you smoke, stop. What you eat can also have an effect on whether you develop cancer. The following are dietary recommendations for preventing cancer:

Reduce the amount of fat in your diet to 30% of your total daily calorie intake.
Limit the amount of alcohol you drink to one or two drinks a day.
Limit the amount of charbroiled, smoked, and salted foods you eat.
Maintain your ideal weight.
Eat foods high in:
Vitamin A—apricots, peaches, carrots, spinach, asparagus, squash, and sweet potatoes.
Vitamin C—oranges, lemons, grapefruit, strawberries, tomatoes, cabbage, and walnuts
Vitamin E—lettuce, alfalfa, and vegetable oils
Fiber—fresh vegetables and fruits, whole grain breads and cereals, nuts, beans, and peas

Prevention, Screening, and Early Detection Guidelines for Common Cancers

Breast cancer. Reduce the amount of fat in your diet. Any one or a combination of these signs may be a warning signal for cancer: a lump in the breast; dimpling of the skin; a sinking in of the nipple, or discharge from the nipple; swelling in the breast; or a change in the size or shape of the breast. Early detection includes breast self-examination once a month; a yearly breast examination by a health care provider; a baseline mammogram between the ages of 35 and 39; and a yearly mammogram after age 40. If you have a family history of breast cancer, you should start having mammograms at age 30.*

---

*American Cancer Society guidelines; National Cancer Institue recommends baseline mammogram at or about age 50 for women not at risk.

Cervical cancer. Avoid sex at an early age (especially before age 18), and don't have numerous partners. Use *condoms,* and practice good perineal hygiene. Cancer warning signs include abnormal vaginal bleeding and spotting after having sex. Early detection involves an annual Pap smear for women over age 18. After at least three normal examinations, the test can be done less often.

Colon/rectal cancer. Follow the dietary guidelines listed above. Have colorectal polyps removed. Cancer warning signs include rectal bleeding, a change in stools, pain in the abdomen, and pressure on the rectum. Early detection includes an annual digital rectal examination starting at age 40; an annual stool blood test starting at age 50; and an annual inspection of the colon with a special instrument (sigmoidoscopy) starting at age 50.

Endometrial cancer. Follow the dietary guidelines listed above. Discuss with your doctor the benefits and risks of estrogen therapy if you are past menopause. Cancer warning signs include abnormal vaginal bleeding and pain or a mass in the abdomen. Early detection includes pelvic examinations and endometrial biopsy at menopause and in high-risk women.

Head and neck cancer. Follow the dietary guidelines listed above. Avoid tobacco in all forms. Practice good oral hygiene. Cancer warning signs include difficulty chewing; a persistent sore throat; hoarseness; a color change in the mouth; earache; a lump in the neck; loss of sense of smell; and difficulty breathing. Early detection includes monthly oral self-examination and an annual physical exam.

Lung cancer. Do not smoke. Follow guidelines at work to reduce exposure to cancer-causing substances. Warning signs include a persistent cough or cold; pain in the chest; wheezing; difficulty breathing; and a change in the volume or odor of phlegm. No tests exist for early detection.

Prostate cancer. There are no prevention guidelines for prostate cancer. Warning signs include difficulty urinating, painful and frequent urination, and blood in the urine. Early detection includes an annual digital rectal exam starting at age 40; measurement of PSA is controversial.

Skin cancer. Use a sunscreen with a sun protection factor (SPF) of at least 15 (the SPF is shown on the bottle), and wear protective clothing when in the sun. Avoid tanning booths. Cancer warning signs include a change in a wart or mole, and a sore that does not heal. Early detection includes an annual physical examination, monthly self-examination of the skin, and paying particular attention to moles, warts, and birthmarks.

Testicular cancer. No prevention guidelines exist for testicular cancer. Cancer warning signs include swelling, a lump, or a heavy feeling in the testicle. Early detection includes an annual physical exam and monthly testicular self-exam.

Testicular Self-Examination

1. The best chance for early detection of testicular cancer is a simple, 3-minute, monthly self-examination.
2. The best time is after a warm bath or shower, when the scrotal skin is most relaxed.
3. Roll each testicle gently between the thumb and fingers of both hands. (See Fig. A.)
4. If any hard lumps or nodules are found, contact a doctor promptly.
5. The first sign of testicular cancer is usually a slight enlargement of one of the testes and a change in its consistency. (See Fig. B.)
6. Pain may be absent.

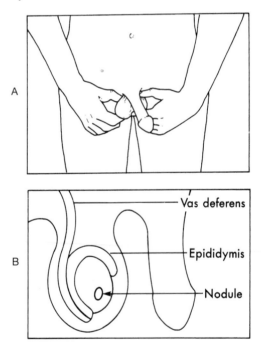

7. There may be a dull ache in the lower abdomen and groin as well as a sensation of dragging and heaviness.

Modified from American Cancer Society: *For men only,* American Cancer Society, 1990.

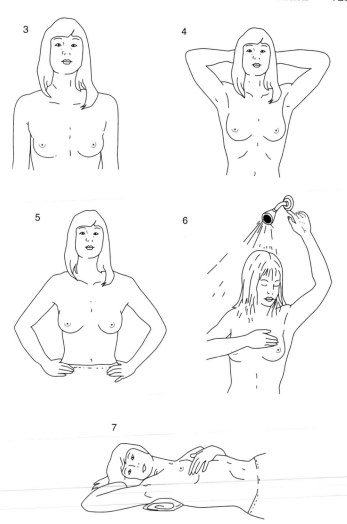

Figures 3 to 8

Breast Self-Examination

How to Perform Breast Self-Examination (BSE)

1. Undress and stand in front of a mirror with your arms at your sides (Figure 3). Look for any changes in the shape or size of your breasts or for anything unusual, such as discharge from the nipples or puckering or dimpling of the skin.

From American Cancer Society, 1988.

2. Raise your arms above and behind your head, and press your hands together (Figure 4). Look for the same things as in step 1.

3. Place the palms of your hands firmly on your hips (Figure 5); look again for any changes.

4. Raise your left arm over your head. Examine your left breast by firmly pressing the fingers of your right hand down and around in a circular motion until you have examined every part of the breast (Figure 6). Be sure to include the area between your breast and armpit and the armpit itself. You are feeling for any lump or mass under the skin. If you find a lump, notify your doctor.

5. Repeat step 4 on your right breast. (You may also perform step 4 in the shower.)

6. Lie down. Flatten your right breast by placing a pillow under your right shoulder (Figure 7). If your breasts are large, use your right hand to hold your right breast while you do the exam with your left hand.

7. Use the sensitive pads of the middle three fingers on your left hand. Feel for lumps using a rubbing motion.

8. Press firmly enough to feel different breast tissues.

9. Completely feel all of the breast and chest area to cover breast tissue that extends toward the shoulder. Allow enough time for a complete exam. Women with small breasts will need at least 2 minutes to examine each breast. Larger breasts will take longer.

10. Use the same pattern to feel every part of the breast tissue. Choose the method easiest for you. The diagrams show the three patterns preferred by women and their doctors: the circular, clock or oval pattern, *A;* the vertical strip, *B;* and the wedge, *C.* (See Figure 8.)

11. After you have completely examined your right breast, examine your left breast using the same method. Compare what you have felt in one breast with the other.

Your monthly BSE should be carried out when your breasts are likely to be the least lumpy. If you have a regular menstrual cycle, you should examine your breasts at the end of your menstrual period. If you do not have menstrual periods, BSE should be done on the same day of every month.

If you notice any changes, see your doctor without delay.

Take the opportunity whenever you see your doctor to discuss how you do BSE and what you feel when you do self-exams. Ask if you are doing BSE correctly and for comments to improve your BSE skills.

Remember, the best means of controlling breast cancer is by finding it early. Talk with your doctor. As partners, you will want to share information and you'll want to request advice on where to go

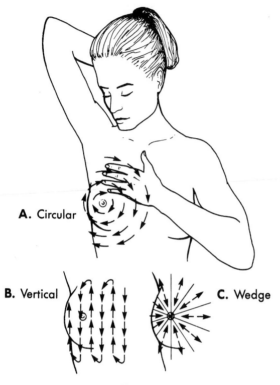

Figure 8
A, Circular pattern, **B,** vertical pattern, **C,** wedge pattern.

to have a mammogram and how often you need to have the exams done.

Fibrocystic Changes of the Breast

What are Fibrocystic Changes? Does This Mean I Have Breast Cancer?

Fibrocystic changes are the most common cause of breast lumps in women 30 to 50 years of age. These changes may also be referred to as fibrocystic disease, cystic disease, chronic cystic mastitis, or mammary dysplasia. This condition is not cancerous. At least 50% of women in their reproductive years have lumpy breasts as a result of this noncancerous condition.

How Are Breast Changes Diagnosed?

Usually fibrocystic changes can be diagnosed by physical examination or mammography, an x-ray of the breast. Fibrocystic changes may also be found with a biopsy, in which a small amount of tissue or fluid is removed from the breast and examined in the laboratory. Fortunately, only about 5% of women who require biopsies for a fibrocystic condition have the type of changes that would be considered a risk factor for cancer.

What Causes Fibrocystic Changes?

Fibrocystic changes occur because of the way breast tissue responds to monthly changes in the levels of estrogen and progesterone, two female hormones produced by the ovaries during a woman's reproductive years. Each month during the menstrual cycle, breast tissue alternately swells and returns to normal. Hormonal stimulation of breast tissue causes the blood vessels to swell, the milk glands and ducts to enlarge, and the breasts to retain water. The breasts frequently feel swollen, painful, tender, and lumpy at this time. After menstruation, the swelling decreases and the breasts feel less tender and lumpy; that's why the best time to examine your breasts for unusual or sudden changes is right after your menstrual period ends.

How Do Fibrocystic Changes Feel? What Should I Look For?

Repeated hormone stimulation from monthly changes causes breast tissue to become firmer, and pockets of fluid, called cysts, may form in obstructed or enlarged milk ducts. The breast tissue may feel like an irregularly shaped area of thicker tissue with a lumpy or ridgelike surface. Fibrocystic tissue may also feel like tiny beads scattered throughout the breast.

Fibrocystic changes usually are found in both breasts, most often in the upper outer quadrant and the underside of the breast, where a ridge may sometimes be felt. In premenopausal women with a fibrocystic condition, lumpy areas in the breast may increase in size, and the woman may feel discomfort ranging from a feeling of fullness or heaviness to a dull ache, extreme sensitivity to touch, or a burning sensation. For some women the pain is so severe that it precludes exercise or even lying on the abdomen. The condition tends to subside after menopause (change of life).

How Do I Tell Fibrocystic Changes from a "Lump" in My Breast?

Confusion arises because not all women with lumps have fibrocystic changes. The breast is naturally a lumpy gland. The lumpy consistency arises from the milk glands and ducts and the fibrous tissue that separates and supports them. Practicing breast self-examination (BSE) regularly helps a woman distinguish between normal lumps and ones that must be evaluated by a physician.

How Is a Fibrocystic Condition Treated?

Treatment of a fibrocystic condition may require surgical removal (biopsy) of lumps that fail to disappear after brief observation or after attempts to remove fluid by a physician. For painful breasts a physician may recommend aspirin or other pain relievers. Also, applying warmth to the breasts (such as with a heating pad), wearing a good support bra, and avoiding caffeine in coffee, tea, chocolate, and soft drinks may help decrease water retention. *Patients with cystic breasts should not have caffeine.* Occasionally a physician may prescribe medications such as vitamin E, danazol, or tamoxifen to help relieve the symptoms.

What Is a Mammogram?

A mammogram is a low-dose x-ray examination that can detect lumps infinitely smaller than fingers can feel, and with minimal risk. It is recommended that women between the ages of 35 and 39 who have no symptoms of breast cancer have a mammogram as a baseline for comparison; women ages 40 to 49 should have a mammogram every 1 or 2 years; and women age 50 or over should have a mammogram yearly.

Six Warning Signs of Kidney Disease

1. Burning or difficulty during urination
2. More frequent urination, particularly at night
3. Passage of bloody-appearing urine
4. Puffiness around eyes, swelling of hands and feet, especially in children
5. Pain in small of back just below the ribs (not aggravated by movement)
6. High blood pressure

From National Kidney Foundation: *Six warning signs of kidney disease,* New York, 1991, The Foundation.

Warning Signals of Stroke

The warning signals of a stroke are as follows:

- Sudden weakness or numbness of the face, arm, or leg on one side of the body
- Sudden dimness or loss of vision, particularly in only one eye
- Loss of speech, or trouble talking or understanding speech
- Sudden, severe headaches with no known cause
- Unexplained dizziness, unsteadiness, or sudden falls, especially along with any of the previous symptoms

If you notice one or more of these signs, don't wait. See a doctor right away.

About 10% of strokes are preceded by "little" strokes (transient ischemic attacks [TIAs]). However, of those who've had one or more TIA, about 36% will later have a stroke. In fact, a person who's had one or more TIA is 9.5 times more likely to have a stroke than someone of the same age and sex who hasn't. Thus TIAs are extremely important stroke warning signs.

TIAs are more useful for predicting *if* a stroke will occur than *when* one will happen. They can occur days, weeks, or even months before a major stroke. In about 50% of the cases, the stroke occurs within 1 year of the TIA; in about 20% of the cases, it occurs within 1 month.

TIAs occur when a blood clot temporarily clogs an artery and part of the brain doesn't get the blood it needs. The symptoms occur rapidly and last a relatively short time. More than 75% of TIAs last less than 5 minutes. The average is about a minute, although some last several hours. By definition, TIAs can last up to, but not over, 24 hours, although this is very unusual. Unlike stroke, when a TIA is over, people return to normal.

The usual TIA symptoms are very similar to those of stroke. They are as follows:

1. Temporary weakness, clumsiness, or loss of feeling in an arm, leg, or the side of the face on one side of the body (or some combination thereof)
2. Temporary dimness or loss of vision, particularly in one eye (also often in combination with other symptoms)

Heart and Stroke Facts, Dallas, 1994, American Heart Association.

3. Temporary loss of speech or difficulty in speaking, or difficulty in understanding speech, particularly with a right-side weakness. Sometimes dizziness, double vision, and staggering also occur. The short duration of these symptoms and lack of permanent damage is the main distinction between TIA and stroke.

Although TIAs signal only about 10% of strokes, they're very strong predictors of stroke risk. Don't ignore them! *Get medical attention immediately.* A doctor should determine if a TIA or stroke has occurred, or if it is another medical problem with similar symptoms (seizure, fainting, migraine, or general medical or cardiac condition). Prompt medical or surgical attention to these symptoms could prevent a fatal or disabling stroke from occurring.

Factors to Consider When Assessing Coping in Stroke Clients

What losses has the client experienced as a result of the stroke?
Has the client experienced other recent losses in his life?
How do the client and family appraise their situation (primary, secondary)?
Does the client have deficits that interfere with appraisal of her situation?
What adaptive tasks does the client have to accomplish?
What goals do the client and family have?
Are goals of the client and family consistent with one another?
How did the client cope before the stroke?
How did the family cope before the stroke?
Are the client's coping strategies enabling him to manage his stressors effectively?
Are the family's coping strategies effective?
What are the sources of hope for the client and family?

Background/Personal
What was the client's premorbid lifestyle?
What strengths do the client and family exhibit?
What weaknesses do the client and family exhibit?
What are the client's and family's values and beliefs?
What is the control orientation of the client and family?

From Bronstein KS, Popovich J, Stewart-Amidei CM: *Promoting stroke recovery: a research-based approach for nurses,* St Louis, 1991, Mosby.

What are the client's demographic characteristics (age, sex, cultural background, education level, employment status, socioeconomic status, and occupation)?

What is the likelihood that the client will resume prestroke roles in family, school, and employment?

Illness-Related Factors

Was the stroke onset sudden or gradual?

How recently did the stroke occur?

In what part of the brain is the lesion located?

How extensive is the stroke lesion?

What was the cause of the stroke?

Is the client at high risk for recurrence?

Does the client have concomitant acute or chronic illnesses?

What cognitive/perceptual deficits are present that may impair coping?

What are the type and severity of the client's functional limitations?

Environmental Factors

Does/will the client receive rehabilitative care?

What is the extent and level of social support from family and friends?

What material resources are available (money, equipment, place for discharge)?

Will the client require a caregiver? If so, who?

Other Behavioral-Perceptual Consequences of Stroke

Abulia: Extreme apathy seen after anterior cerebral artery stroke.

Agitated confusional state: Hyperactivity, restlessness, and easy distractibility associated with stroke to the inferior branch of the right MCA, the mirror area for Wernicke's aphasia in the left hemisphere.

Allesthesia: Perception that stimuli delivered to the affected side were delivered to the unaffected side.

Anton's syndrome: Also called cortical blindness, this is a form of neglect in which the client denies blindness.

Aprosodia: Lack of awareness of affective quality of speech; emotional aspect.

Autotopagnosia: An agnosia for body part recognition.

From Bronstein KS, Popovich J, Stewart-Amidei CM: *Promoting stroke recovery: a research-based approach for nurses,* St Louis, 1991, Mosby.

Figure ground deficit: The inability to distinguish the foreground from the background.

Form constancy deficit: The inability to recognize subtle variations in form (e.g., the difference between a water pitcher and a urinal).

Hemiakinesia: Failure to move the affected limb because of hemiinattention.

Impulsivity: The tendency to act quickly without forethought and without concern for safety, seen commonly in right brain–injured clients.

Motor impersistence: Failure to persist at motor tasks, such as eye closure.

Multiinfarct dementia: Stepwise deterioration in higher mental capacities as the result of multiple small strokes over time.

Right-left disorientation: The inability to discriminate between right and left.

Simultanagnosia: A rare spatial analysis deficit in which the client is unable to make meaning of an image in its entirety and sees and understands only a small fraction at a time. The client literally cannot see the forest for the trees.

Topographic disorientation: Difficulty understanding and remembering relationships of places to one another; gets lost easily.

Tests of Specific Disabilities That Commonly Follow Stroke

Hemianopia (loss of part of visual field)

Sitting opposite client, simultaneously hold up two pens of different colors 30 cm in front of patient and 30 cm apart; clients with hemianopia will be unable to see one of the pens or may turn head toward hemianopic side in an effort to see.

Proprioception (awareness of body in space)

The wrist of the affected arm is held between the thumb and forefinger of the examiner; client's hand is raised and lowered and client, with closed eyes, is asked the position of the hand; this exercise can also be done with fingers to determine even more specific loss of proprioception.

Sensation (feeling generated by sensory receptors)

With client's eyes closed the examiner strokes the back of the unaffected hand and then the affected hand and in both cases asks the client to describe the sensation. The affected side may have varying degrees of loss of sensation, or total loss of feeling.

Balance (bodily poise)

Client asked to sit on side of bed with feet off floor and maintain balance and sit unaided for 1 minute; it is usually readily apparent if individual has a problem maintaining balance.

Arm function (range of motion and control)

Client asked to lift affected arm to shoulder height and press against examiner's upheld hand:

>   Complete paralysis = inability to move arm
>   Severe weakness = can move arm but not lift up or push
>   Moderate weakness = able to lift arm but unable to push
>   Slight weakness = able to do task requested but cannot push as hard as with unaffected arm
>   No weakness = no difference in abilities of either arm

Data summarized from Anderson R: *The aftermath of stroke: the experience of patients and their families,* Cambridge, 1992, Cambridge University Press. In Ebersole P, Hess P: *Toward healthy aging: human needs and nursing response,* ed 4, St Louis, 1994, Mosby.

Cardiovascular Disease Risk Factors

Many deaths from cardiovascular disease are preventable. In addition, for people who already have been diagnosed with cardiovascular disease, the risk of death and further complications can be reduced. Research has uncovered several factors that contribute to heart attacks and strokes. The more risk factors a person has, the greater the chance of developing cardiovascular disease. Although some risk factors cannot be changed, you can modify others with your doctor's help, and still others can be eliminated altogether. The following checklists can help you determine your risk.

Major Risk Factors that Cannot be Changed

Heredity. A tendency toward heart disease runs in families. If one or both parents had cardiovascular disease, one's chances of developing it are higher.

Race. For reasons presently unknown, blacks have a much greater risk of developing high blood pressure than whites; twice as many have moderately high blood pressure, and three times as many have extremely high blood pressure. As a result, their risk of heart disease is greater.

Sex. Men have a higher risk of heart attack and stroke than women. During the childbearing years, women produce hormones that keep blood cholesterol levels low. Male hormones have the opposite effect—they raise blood cholesterol. However, women lose this protection after menopause or surgical removal of the ovaries, and women over age 55 have a 10 times greater risk than younger women. In recent years, however, more women under age 40 have developed coronary artery disease and high blood pressure. This probably results from the use of oral contraceptives and increased smoking.

Age. Fifty-five percent of heart attacks occur in people age 65 or older.

Major Risk Factors that can be Changed

Smoking. Smokers have more than twice as many heart attacks as nonsmokers. Sudden cardiac death occurs two to four times more frequently in smokers. Peripheral vascular disease (narrowing of the blood vessels in the arms and legs) is almost exclusively a disease of smokers. When people stop smoking, the risk of heart disease drops rapidly, and 10 years after quitting, their risk of death from cardiovascular disease is about the same as for people who never smoked.

High blood pressure. High blood pressure makes the heart work harder, causing it to enlarge and become weaker over time. This can lead to stroke, heart attack, kidney failure, and congestive heart failure. For some people, high blood pressure can be controlled by a low-salt diet, weight reduction, and regular exercise. Other people also require medication to lower their blood pressure.

Blood cholesterol levels. A cholesterol level between 200 and 240 mg/dl increases the risk of heart disease. A cholesterol level greater than 240 mg/dl doubles the risk of coronary artery disease. The American Heart Association Diet, which is low in cholesterol and other fats, is recommended for anyone with a level of 200 or higher. Medication may also be necessary.

Other Risk Factors

Diabetes. Diabetes increases the risk of heart attack because it raises blood cholesterol levels. In addition, people who develop diabetes in midlife are often overweight, which is an additional risk factor.

Obesity. Excess weight forces the heart to work harder. People who are overweight are more prone to high blood pressure and high blood cholesterol levels. Obesity is defined as 30% or more over your ideal weight.

Physical inactivity. Researchers have found that people who seldom exercise do not recover as well from heart attacks. Although it is not clear if lack of exercise alone is a risk factor for developing heart disease, in combination with other risk factors, such as overweight, the risk is higher.

Stress. Excessive emotional stress over a prolonged period appears to increase the risk of heart disease. Stress can increase other existing risk factors, such as overeating, smoking, and high blood pressure.

Oral contraceptives. Birth control pills can worsen other risk factors. They raise blood cholesterol levels and increase blood pressure, so women who already have these problems should not take oral contraceptives. Smokers who take "the pill" run the risk of developing dangerous blood clots (thrombosis).

Alcohol. Heavy drinking can cause high blood pressure and lead to heart failure. Alcohol should be consumed only in moderate amounts—2 ounces of liquor a day or less.

Failure to Thrive—Nonorganic

The Child with Nonorganic Failure to Thrive
Description

A group of clinical diagnoses, usually in infants and toddlers, with the principal characteristic of inadequate weight gain

Organic: failure to grow or gain weight as a result of organic causes, usually gastrointestinal or neurologic

Nonorganic: failure to grow or gain weight as a result of psychosocial factors; 50% caused by emotional, environmental, or maternal deprivation

Clinical manifestations

Static: weight that is 20% or more below the ideal weight for an infant's height

Dynamic: decreased weight velocity crossing at least two standard percentiles and discrepant from normal linear growth

Associated manifestations

Developmental retardation—social, motor, adaptive, and language

Apathy

Poor hygiene

Withdrawing behavior

Feeding or eating disorders, such as vomiting, anorexia, voracious appetite, pica

Demonstrates no fear of strangers (at age when stranger anxiety is normal)

Often avoids eye-to-eye contact

Exhibits a wide-eyed gaze and tends to continually scan the environment

Stiff and unyielding or flaccid and unresponsive

Diagnostic evaluation

Organic failure to thrive determined by specific laboratory studies

Nonorganic failure to thrive determined by

Physical examination

Growth as plotted on growth charts

Feeding history

Developmental assessment

Observation of

Johnson S: *Nursing assessment and stragegies for the family at risk: high-risk parenting,* ed 2, Philadelphia, 1986, JB Lippincott.

General treatment
Maternal-infant interactions, especially during feeding
Feeding trial away from caregiver
Approach-withdrawal behavior
Radiologic bone survey
Psychosocial family evaluation

Objectives of therapeutic management

Determine the cause of failure to thrive
Facilitate growth and development
Structure the environment for positive psychosocial interactions

Characteristics of Failure-to-Thrive Family

Infant Characteristics

The most commonly identified physical and behavioral characteristics of failure-to-thrive infants include

* Failure to grow and gain weight
* Developmental slowness
* Gastrointestinal difficulties and feeding problems
* Unusual watchfulness
* Minimal smiling
* Decreased vocalizations
* Lack of cuddliness
* Position of tonic immobility
* Sleep disturbances
* Lack of interest in environmental stimuli or toys

Characteristics of the Failure-to-Thrive Family
Infant characteristics

Physical characteristics—failure to grow and gain weight
Behavioral characteristics—developmental slowness

Characteristics of mothers

Low self-esteem and feelings of inadequacy
Desire to be taken care of
Literal concrete thinking patterns
Use of denial, isolation, and projection defense mechanisms
Predisposition to acting out rather than thinking

Johnson S: *Nursing assessment and strategies for the family at risk: high-risk parenting,* ed 2, Philadelphia, 1986, JB Lippincott.

Inaccessibility and suspicion of helping persons
Difficulty in accurately perceiving the infant's needs

Characteristics of fathers

Ineffectual in child-rearing behaviors
Often absent from home

Characteristics of siblings

Poor physical health

Family stability and socioeconomic characteristics

Marital problems
Low socioeconomic class

Other family difficulties

Guilt
Grief
Child abuse

Nutritional Guidelines
Form for Assessing Eating Habits and Nutritional State

Record all foods and drinks that you had during the day and during the night.

			Day of week				
(Circle	Mon	Tues	Wed	Thurs	Fri	Sat	Sun)

Breakfast
   Foods/amount (cup, tbsp)   Drinks/amounts (cup, glass)

Lunch
   Foods/amounts (cup, tbsp)   Drinks/amounts (cup, glass)

Dinner
   Foods/amounts (cup, tbsp)   Drinks/amounts (cup, glass)

Snacks
   Time   Foods or drinks   Amount (cup, glass, tbsp, or pieces)

Do you take vitamin or mineral supplements?
If yes, please list kind and how many per day.
                        Yes _____   No _____

Do you take any other nutritional supplement? (e.g., yeast, protein bran)
If yes, please list and describe
                        Yes _____   No _____

From Murray RB, Zentner JP: *Nursing assessment and health promotion,* ed 5, Norwalk, Conn., 1993, Appleton & Lange.

Clinical Signs of Nutritional Status

Body area	Signs of good nutrition	Signs of poor nutrition
General appearance	Alert, responsive	Listless, apathetic, cachectic
Weight	Normal for height, age, body build	Overweight or underweight (special concern for underweight)
Posture	Erect, arms and legs straight	Sagging shoulders, sunken chest, humped back
Muscles	Well developed, firm, good tone, some fat under skin	Flaccid, poor tone, undeveloped, tender, "wasted" appearance, cannot walk properly
Nervous control	Good attention span, not irritable or restless, normal reflexes, psychologic stability	Inattentive, irritable, confused, burning and tingling of hands and feet (paresthesia), loss of position and vibratory sense, weakness and tenderness of muscles (may result in inability to walk), decrease or loss of ankle and knee reflexes
Gastrointestinal function	Good appetite and digestion, normal regular elimination, no palpable (perceptible to touch) organs or masses	Anorexia, indigestion, constipation or diarrhea, liver or spleen enlargement
Cardiovascular function	Normal heart rate and rhythm, no murmurs, normal blood pressure for age	Rapid heart rate (above 100 beats/minute tachycardia), enlarged heart, abnormal rhythm, elevated blood pressure
General vitality	Endurance, energetic, sleeps well, vigorous	Easily fatigued, no energy, falls asleep easily, looks tired, apathetic
Hair	Shiny, lustrous, firm, not easily plucked, healthy scalp	Stringy, dull, brittle, dry, thin and sparse, depigmented, can be easily plucked

Continued.

Williams SR: Nutritional guidance in prenatal care. In Worthington-Roberts BS, Vermeersch J, Williams SR: *Nutrition in pregnancy and lactation*, St Louis, 1993, Mosby.

Clinical signs of nutritional status—cont'd

Body area	Signs of good nutrition	Signs of poor nutrition
Skin (general)	Smooth, slightly moist, good color	Rough, dry, scaly, pale, pigmented, irritated, bruises, petechiae
Face and neck	Skin color uniform, smooth, pink, healthy appearance, not swollen	Greasy, discolored, scaly, swollen, skin dark over cheeks and under eyes, lumpiness or flakiness of skin around nose and mouth
Lips	Smooth, good color, moist, not chapped or swollen	Dry, scaly, swollen, redness and swelling (cheilosis), or angular lesions at corners of the mouth or fissures or scars (stomatitis)
Mouth, oral membranes	Reddish pink mucous membranes in oral cavity	Swollen, boggy oral mucous membranes
Gums	Good pink color, healthy, red, no swelling or bleeding	Spongy, bleed easily, marginal redness, inflamed, gums receding
Tongue	Good pink color or deep reddish in appearance, not swollen or smooth, surface papillae present, no lesion	Swelling, scarlet and raw, magenta color, beefy (glossitis), hyperemic and hypertrophic papillae, atrophic papillae
Teeth	No cavities, no pain, bright straight, no crowding, well-shaped jaw, clean, no discoloration	Unfilled caries, absent teeth, worn surfaces mottled (fluorosis), malpositioned
Eyes	Bright, clear, shiny, no sores at corner of eyelids, membranes moist and healthy pink color, no prominent blood vessels or mount of tissue or sclera, no fatigue circles beneath	Eye membranes pale (pale conjunctivae), redness or membrane (conjunctival injection), dryness of infection Bitot's spots, redness and fissuring of eyelid corners (angular palpebritis), dryness of eye membrane (conjunctival xerosis), dull appearance of cornea (corneal xerosis), soft cornea (keraomalacia)
Neck (glands)	No enlargement	Thyroid enlarged
Nails	Firm, pink	Spoon-shaped (koilonychia), brittle, ridged
Legs, feet	No tenderness, weakness, or swelling, good color	Edema, tender calf, tingling weakness
Skeleton	No malformations	Bowlegs, knock-knees, chest deformity at diaphragm, beaded ribs, prominent scapulas

The Basic Food Groups

Food group	Main nutrients	Daily amounts
Vegetables	Vitamin A Vitamin C (ascorbic acid) Folate Magnesium Fiber	3-5 servings 1 serving equals: ⅓ cup raw or cooked vegetables 1 cup raw leafy vegetables Include: 1 dark green or deep yellow vegetable or fruit rich in vitamin A, at least every other day
Fruits	Vitamin C Fiber	2-4 servings 1 serving equals: ¼ cup dried fruit ½ cup cooked fruit ¾ cup juice 1 whole piece of fruit 1 melon wedge
Breads, cereals, and other grains	Thiamin Niacin Riboflavin Iron Protein	6-11 servings of whole-grain, enriched, or restored 1 serving equals: 1 slice bread 1 oz (1 cup) ready-to-eat cereal, flake or puff varieties ½–¾ cup cooked cereal ½–¾ cup cooked pasta (macaroni, spaghetti, noodles) Crackers: 5 saltines, 2 squares graham crackers, etc.

Continued.

Source: U.S. Department of Agriculture, Home and Garden Bulletin #23 2-1, April, 1986; and USDA Food Pyramid, no. HG249, August 1992. From Stanhope M, Lancaster J: *Community health nursing: process and practice for promoting health*, ed 3, St Louis, 1996, Mosby.

The basic food groups—cont'd

Food group	Main nutrients	Daily amounts
Meats Beef, veal, lamb, pork, poultry, fish, eggs	Protein Iron Thiamin	2 or more servings 1 serving equals:2-3 oz lean, boneless, cooked meat, poultry, or fish 2 eggs 1-1½ cup cooked dry beans or peas 4 tbsp peanut butter ½-1 cup nuts
Alternatives: dry beans and peas, nuts, peanut butter	Niacin Riboflavin	
Milk	Calcium Protein Riboflavin Potassium Zinc	Children under 9: 2-3 cups Children 9 to 12: 3 or more cups Teenagers: 4 or more cups Adults: 2 or more cups Pregnant women: 3 or more cups Nursing mothers: 4 or more cups (1 cup = 8 oz fluid milk or designated milk equivalent) 1 serving equals: 1 cup milk, skim milk, buttermilk ¼ cup dry skimmed powdered milk ½ cup evaporated milk 1½ oz cheese 2 oz processed cheese 1 cup yogurt 2 cups cottage cheese 1 cup custard/pudding 1½ cups ice cream 1 cup ice milk
Fats, sweets, and alcoholic beverages		Avoid

Promotion of Good Dietary Habits: Foods for Everyday Use

	Milk and milk products	Protein foods	Breads, cereals, and whole grains	Vitamin C-rich fruits/vegetables	Dark green and yellow fruits and vegetables	Other fruits and vegetables
First year of life						
Number of servings	24-32 oz	7 mo: 1-3 T	4-6 mo: 4-6 T	4-6 mo: 2-4 T	4-6 mo: 2-4 T	4-6 mo: 2-4 T
	Encourage breast milk or iron-fortified formula, sufficient for the first 4 to 6 months of life. Solid foods by 4 to 6 months. Offer single foods in small amounts. No solids, sugar, or honey in bottles. No Koolaid, sodas, or empty-calorie snacks. Always hold your baby when giving bottle. Use iron-fortified cereals.					
Toddler/preschool: 1 to 5 years						
Number of servings	3	2	4	1-2	1-2	1-2
	Use fresh milk, either whole or 2% lowfat. Continue introduction of a variety of foods. Have regular meals, at least two snacks per day. Be aware of appetite changes. Parents should not be anxious. Don't force-feed. Make snacks part of the food groups.					
Children and teenagers						
Number of servings	4-5	3	4	2	1-2	2
	Have regular meals. Serve small portions. Offer finger foods frequently. Relax; don't bribe or reward with food. Don't force your child to eat. Keep the TV off when eating. Eat with the rest of the family. Encourage exercise. Avoid fatty foods.					

Continued.

Modified from Gutierrez Y, May K: Nutrition and the family. In Gilliss C and others, editors: *Toward a science of family nursing*, Reading, Mass, 1989, Addison-Wesley.

Promotion of good dietary habits: foods for everyday use—cont'd

	Milk and milk products	Protein foods	Breads, cereals, and whole grains	Vitamin C–rich fruits/vegetables	Dark green and yellow fruits and vegetables	Other fruits and vegetables
Young adults, men and women						
Number of servings	2	2	4	2	1-2	2
	Have regular meals. Encourage exercise. Particular attention to calcium and iron-rich foods. Avoid fried foods, salty snacks, sodas, alcohol, cookies, cakes, or other high-sugar snacks. Use cooking methods such as broiling, baking, roasting.					
Pregnant and lactating women						
Number of servings	4-5	4	4	2	2	2
	Have small, frequent meals. Use iron and folacin supplements. Avoid alcohol, fried foods, empty calorie snacks. Particular attention to foods from milk group for calcium, vitamin C and A foods. Whole grains for fiber. Protein foods for iron.					
Elderly						
Number of servings	2	3	4	2	2	2
	Have small, frequent meals. Liquids are important even if not thirsty. Use whole grains to avoid constipation. Socializing with groups will help to increase activity and increase motivation to eat with company. May need vitamin and mineral supplements, especially calcium in the order of 1200 mg per day. Avoid alcohol. Nutrient-drug interactions can be minimized by eating a balanced diet and carefully following the instructions for use.					

Suggestions for People Eating Alone

Set an attractive table—make meals an event.

Eat by a window or any pleasant setting.

Watch TV or listen to radio.

Eat outdoors when weather allows.

Treat yourself to a meal out every now and then.

Invite guests often—a potluck or meal exchange is a good idea.

Participate in Senior Nutrition Programs in your area. Call your area's agency on aging for locations.

Modified from *A guide for food and nutrition in later years,* Berkeley, Calif, 1980, Society for Nutrition Education.

Development of Feeding Skills

Age	Oral and neuromuscular development	Feeding behavior
Birth	Rooting reflex Sucking reflex Swallowing reflex Extrusion reflex	Turns mouth toward nipple or any object brushing cheek Initial swallowing involves the posterior of the tongue, by 9-12 week anterior portion is increasingly involved, which facilitates ingestion of semisolid food Pushes food out when placed on tongue; strong the first 9 wk By 6-10 wk recognizes the position in which he is fed and begins mouthing and sucking when placed in this position
3-6 mo	Beginning coordination between eyes and body movements Learning to reach mouth with hands at 4 mo Extrusion reflex present until 4 mo Able to grasp objects voluntarily at 5 mo Sucking reflex becomes voluntary, and lateral motions of the jaw begin	Explores world with eyes, fingers, hands, and mouth; starts reaching for objects at 4 mo but overshoots; hands get in the way during feeding Finger sucking; by 6 mo all objects go into mouth May continue to push out food placed on tongue Grasps objects in mittenlike fashion Can approximate lips to rim of cup by 5 mo; chewing action begins; by 6 mo begins drinking from cup
6-12 mo	Eyes and hands working together Sits erect with support at 6 mo Sits erect without support at 9 mo Development of grasp (finger to thumb opposition) Relates to objects at 10 mo	Brings hand to mouth; at 7 mo able to feed self biscuit Bangs cup and objects on table at 7 mo Holds own bottle at 9-12 mo Pincer approach to food Pokes at food with index finger at 10 mo Reaches for food and utensils including those beyond reach; pushes plate around with spoon

Age	Skill	Description
1-3 yr	Development of manual dexterity	Insists on holding spoon not to put in mouth but to return to plate or cup
		Increased desire to feed self:
		15 mo: begins to use spoon but turns it before reaching mouth; may hold cup; likely to tilt cup rather than head, causing spilling
		18 mo: eats with spoon, spills frequently, turns spoon in mouth; holds glass with both hands
		2 yr: inserts spoon correctly, occasionally with one hand; holds glass; plays with food; distinguishes between food and inedible materials
		2-3 yr: self-feeding complete with occasional spilling; uses fork; pours from pitcher; obtains drink of water from faucet

From Scipien GM et al: *Pediatric nursing care,* St Louis, 1990, Mosby.

Developmental Milestones Associated with Feeding

Age (months)	Development
Birth	Has sucking, rooting, and swallowing reflexes
	Feels hunger and indicates desire for food by crying; expresses satiety by falling asleep
1	Has strong extrusion reflex
3-4	Extrusion reflex is fading
	Begins to develop hand-eye coordination
4-5	Can approximate lips to the rim of a cup
5-6	Can use fingers to feed self a cracker
6-7	Chews and bites
	May hold own bottle, but may not drink from it (prefers for it to be held)
7-9	Refuses food by keeping lips closed; has taste preferences
	Holds a spoon and plays with it during feeding
	May drink from a straw
	Drinks from a cup with assistance
9-12	Picks up small morsels of food (finger foods) and feeds self
	Holds own bottle and drinks from it
	Drinks from a household cup without assistance but spills some
	Uses a spoon with much spilling
12-18	Drools less
	Drinks well from a household cup, but may drop it when finished
	Holds cup with both hands
24	Can use a straw
	Chews food with mouth closed and shifts food in mouth
	Distinguishes between finger and spoon foods
	Holds small glass in one hand; replaces glass without dropping
36	Spills small amount from spoon
	Begins to use fork; holds it in fist
	Uses adult pattern of chewing, which involves rotary action of jaw
48	Rarely spills when using spoon
	Serves self finger foods
	Eats with fork held with fingers
54	Uses fork in preference to spoon
72	Spreads with knife
84	Cuts tender food with knife

From Wong D, Whaley L: *Clinical manual of pediatric nursing,* ed 3, St Louis, 1990, Mosby.

Nutrition Education and Counseling Screening Alerts

If older individuals indicate that the following questions listed on the Checklist, Level I and II Screens are descriptive of their condition or life situation, nutrition education interventions may help them solve their nutritional problems and improve their nutritional status.

Determine Your Nutritional Health Checklist Alerts

I have an illness or condition that made me change the kind or amount of food I eat.

I eat fewer than two meals per day.

I eat few fruits or vegetables, or milk products.

I have 3 or more drinks of beer, liquor, or wine almost every day.

I have tooth or mouth problems that make it hard for me to eat.

Without wanting to, I have lost or gained 10 pounds in the last 6 months.

Level I Screen Alerts

Has lost or gained 10 pounds or more in the past 6 months.

Body mass index <22.

Body mass index >27.

Has poor appetite.

Is on a special diet.

Eats vegetables two or fewer times daily.

Eats milk or milk products once or not at all daily.

Eats fruit or drinks fruit juice once or not at all daily.

Eats breads, cereals, pasta, rice, or other grains five or fewer times daily.

Has difficulty chewing or swallowing.

Has more than one alcoholic drink per day (if woman); more than two drinks per day (if man).

Has pain in mouth, teeth, or gums.

Lives on an income of less than $6000 per year (per individual in the household).

Is unable or prefers not to spend money on food (<$25-30 per person spent on food each week).

Usually or always needs assistance with preparing food, shopping for food or other necessities.

From *Nutrition interventions manual for professional caring for older americans,* 1992, American Academy of Family Physicians, American Dietetic Association, National Council on the Aging, Nutrition screening initiative, Washington, DC.

Level II Screen Alerts

Has lost or gained 10 pounds or more in the past 6 months.

Body mass index <22.

Body mass index >27.

Has poor appetite.

Is on a special diet.

Eats vegetables two or fewer times daily.

Eats milk or milk products once or not at all daily.

Eats fruit or drinks fruit juice once or not at all daily.

Eats breads, cereals, pasta, rice, or other grains five or fewer times daily.

Has difficulty chewing or swallowing.

Has more than one alcoholic drink per day (if woman); more than two drinks per day (if man).

Has pain in mouth, teeth, or gums.

Lives on an income of less than $6000 per year (per individual in the household).

Is unable or prefers not to spend money on food (<$25-30 per person spent on food each week).

Usually or always needs assistance with preparing food, shopping for food or other necessities.

Three or more prescription drugs, OTC medications, or vitamin/ mineral supplements daily.

Skin changes (dry, loose nonspecific lesions, edema).

Nutrition Education and Counseling Interventions

Screening alerts	Older adults, family, friends	Social service professionals	Dietitians, health professionals/nurses	Physicians
Doesn't eat enough (skips meals, eats few meals daily, doesn't spend enough money on food)	✓ Eat at least 3 meals daily ✓ Eat in social settings ✓ Eat small, frequent meals and snacks ✓ Cook large meals in advance and freeze leftovers ✓ Buy read-to-eat foods ✓ Eat out at senior centers, inexpensive restaurants (ask about discount)	✓ All prior interventions ✓ Bring easily prepared foods (soups, mixes) ✓ Call older adults to encourage eating ✓ Identify social isolation and encourage socialization ✓ Eat with the person	✓ All prior interventions ✓ Arrange eating clubs ✓ Give large print/colorful schedules with times for meals and snacks and suggested foods to eat ✓ Rearrange kitchen to simplify cooking	✓ All prior interventions ✓ Screen for protein-energy malnutrition, deficiency diseases ✓ Make referral to dietitian
Doesn't eat food from all groups (vegetables, fruits, grains, dairy, meat)	✓ Use milk and cheese in soups and casseroles ✓ Chop vegetables in blender and add to soups and casseroles ✓ Eat canned fruits for desserts and snacks ✓ Eat puddings made with milk, ice cream, frozen yogurt, cocoa with milk	✓ All prior interventions ✓ Encourage older adults to attend adult education classes on nutrition, cooking, dining out ✓ Determine if money is an issue	✓ All prior interventions ✓ Identify reason for avoiding food group(s) (afraid of adverse GI problems, dislike taste, hard to prepare, etc.) and recommend diet modifications/substitutions accordingly	✓ All prior interventions ✓ Screen for deficiency diseases ✓ Advise if eating habits could make existing health conditions worse ✓ Make referral to dietitian

Continued.

From *Nutrition interventions manual for professional caring for older Americans*, 1992, American Dietetic Association, American Academy of Family Physicians, National Council on the Aging. Nutrition screening initiative, Washington, DC.

Nutrition education and counseling interventions—cont'd

Screening alerts	Older adults, family, friends	Social service professionals	Dietitians, health professionals/nurses	Physicians
Inadequate/unbalanced diet	✓ Eat-well-balanced diet: ■ 3-5 servings vegetables ■ 2-4 servings fruits ■ 6-11 servings breads, cereals, rice, pasta ■ 2-3 servings milk ■ 2-3 servings poultry, fish, meats, eggs ✓ Consume sugars, salt, and fat in moderation	✓ All prior interventions ✓ Determine whether older adult has difficulty understanding/reading English so that recommendations can be made in appropriate language	✓ Adjust therapeutic diet ✓ Suggest alternatives or use food/nutritional supplements ✓ All prior interventions ✓ Do complete nutrition assessment ✓ Check functional status ✓ Determine if food texture/consistency should be modified ✓ Consider vitamin/mineral supplements	✓ All prior interventions ✓ Screen for deficiency diseases ✓ To encourage compliance, reinforce recommendations of dietitian ✓ Seek nutrition support interventions
Special diet (due to illness or self-imposed)	✓ Ask doctor or dietitian before eating any special diet that hasn't been prescribed ✓ Ask doctor or dietitian if special diet is needed due to change in health	✓ All prior interventions ✓ Weigh older adults weekly and monitor for other changes in health ✓ Assist in selecting, preparing, and eating	✓ All prior interventions ✓ Review diet/disease status to identify deficiencies/excesses and to prescribe appropriate diet, medical nutritionals	✓ All prior interventions ✓ Screen for deficiency diseases ✓ Advise if eating habits could make existing health conditions worse

		special or modified foods (pureed, thickened)	✔ Recommended that food texture/consistency be modified as needed ✔ Adjust therapeutic diet	✔ Make referral to dietitian ✔ See medications use and nutrition support interventions
Overweight or underweight	✔ Ask doctor whether current body weight is healthy ✔ Contact dietitian to modify diet to achieve healthy body weight ✔ Eat more protein foods if underweight and fewer fatty foods (especially sweets) if overweight	✔ All prior interventions ✔ Weigh older adults weekly ✔ Encourage appropriate eating patterns and food selection	✔ All prior interventions ✔ Screen for nutrient deficiencies/excesses ✔ Recommend nutritional supplements, hypercaloric diet for weight gain ✔ Recommend low-fat/hypocaloric diet for weight loss ✔ Encourage physical activity	✔ All prior interventions ✔ Screen for protein-energy malnutrition, physical (cancer, diabetes, HIV, etc.) and psychiatric (depression, dementia, etc.) causes for weight change ✔ See nutrition support interventions ✔ Make referral to dietitian
Consumes alcohol regularly	✔ Complete questionnaire on alcohol use (CAGE, HEAT, MAST) ✔ Limit number of daily drinks to one or none if woman, 2 or fewer if man	✔ All prior interventions ✔ Monitor alcohol intake for pattern of alcohol use	✔ All prior interventions ✔ Monitor diet of home and hospitalized older adults with alcohol-related problems for adequate protein, complex carbohydrates,	✔ All prior interventions ✔ Screen for blood alcohol levels, anemia, malnutrition, weight loss, cardiac arrhythmias, GI bleeding, trauma, hypertension,

Continued.

Nutrition education and counseling interventions—cont'd

Screening alerts	Older adults, family, friends	Social service professionals	Dietitians, health professionals/nurses	Physicians
	✔ Contact counseling center if concerned about alcohol use/abuse		micronutrients, and fluids ✔ Provide alcohol counseling ✔ Make referral to dietitian	heart failure, edema, mental changes, chronic fatigue, seizures, etc.

Food Sources of Calcium (RDAs for Adults: 800 mg)

	Quantity	Calcium (mg)
Bread, cereal, rice, pasta		
Bran muffin, homemade	1 muffin	54
Bread, whole wheat	1 slice	18
Corn muffin, from mix	1 muffin	96
Cream of wheat (cooked)	¾ cup	38
Pasta, enriched (cooked)	1 cup	16
Rice, enriched	1 cup	21
Wheat flakes	1 cup	43
Vegetables		
Artichoke (boiled)	1 med	47
Asparagus (boiled)	½ cup (6 spears)	22
Avocado (raw)	1 med	19
Broccoli (raw)	½ cup	21
Brussels sprouts (boiled)	½ cup (4 sprouts)	28
Carrots (raw)	1 med	19
Collards (boiled)	1 cup	148
Corn, yellow (boiled)	½ cup	2
Kale (chopped)	½ cup	47
Peas, green (boiled)	½ cup	19
Potato (baked, with skin)	1 med	115
Tomato (raw)	1 med	8
Fruits		
Apricots (raw)	3 med	15
Banana (raw)	1 med	7
Cantaloupe (raw)	½ cup	8
Figs (dried)	10 figs	269
Orange juice (fresh)	8 fl oz	27
Orange, navel (raw)	1 med	56
Papaya (raw)	1 med	72
Raspberries (raw)	½ cup	14
Strawberries (raw)	½ cup	11
Tangerine (raw)	1 med	12
Meat, poultry, fish, dry beans, eggs, nuts		
Almonds (roasted)	1 oz	148
Beef liver (fried)	3.5 oz	11
Cashews (roasted)	1 oz	13
Chicken, dark (roasted, without skin)	3.5 oz	179
Chicken, light (roasted, without skin)	3.5 oz	216
Egg, whole	1 large	90
Ham (canned)	3.5 oz	6
Kidney beans (boiled)	1 cup	50
Lentils (boiled)	1 cup	37

From Williams SR: *Nutrition and diet therapy,* ed 7, St Louis, 1993, Mosby.

Food sources of calcium (RDAs for adults: 800 mg)—cont'd

	Quantity	Calcium (mg)
Meat, poultry, fish, dry beans, eggs, nuts—cont'd		
Lima beans (boiled)	1 cup	32
Peanuts (roasted)	1 oz	15
Soybeans (boiled)	1 cup	175
Milk, dairy products		
Milk, skim	8 fl oz	302
Milk, whole	8 fl oz	290
Yogurt, whole	8 fl oz	355
Fats, oils		
This food group is not an important source of calcium.		
Sugar		
Brown sugar	1 cup	123
Molasses, barbados	1 tbsp	49

Optimal Calcium Requirements

Group	Optimal daily intake (in mg of calcium)
Infant	
Birth-6 months	400
6 months-1 year	600
Children	
1-5 years	800
6-10 years	800-1200
Adolescents/young adults	
11-24 years	1200-1500
Men	
25-65 years	1000
Over 65 years	1500
Women	
25-50 years	1000
Over 50 years (postmenopausal)	
On estrogens	1000
Not on estrogens	1500
Over 65 years	1500
Pregnant and nursing	1200-1500

From NIH Consensus Development Conference, 1994.

Foods High in Potassium

Apricots (dried or fresh)
Bananas
Broccoli
Brussels sprouts
Cantaloupe
Collard greens
Dandelion greens
Dates
Figs
Grapefruit juice
Lentils
Lima beans

Navy beans
Nectarines
Orange juice
Peas
Potatoes—sweet and white
Prunes
Prune juice
Raisins
Squash (acorn and butternut)
Tomatoes
Tomato juice

From Lexington-Fayette County Health Department, Division of Nutrition and Health Education, Lexington, KY, 1984.

Food Sources of Potassium (Estimated Safe and Adequate Daily Intake for Adults: 1875-5625 mg)

	Quantity	Potassium (mg)
Bread, cereal, rice, pasta		
Bran flakes	¾ cup	184
Bran muffin, homemade	1 muffin	99
Bread, whole wheat	1 slice	44
Oatmeal (cooked)	¾ cup	99
Pasta, enriched (cooked)	1 cup	85
Rice, white, enriched	1 cup	57
Wheat flakes	1 cup	110
Wheat germ, toasted	¼ cup (1 oz)	268
Vegetables		
Artichoke (boiled)	1 med	316
Asparagus (boiled)	½ cup (6 spears)	279
Avocado (raw)	1 med	1097
Broccoli (raw)	½ cup, chopped	143
Brussels sprouts (boiled)	½ cup (4 sprouts)	247
Carrot (raw)	1 med	233
Corn, yellow (boiled)	½ cup	204
Mushrooms (boiled)	½ cup, pieces	277

Continued.

From Williams SR: *Nutrition and diet therapy,* ed 7. St Louis, 1993, Mosby.

Food Sources of Potassium (Estimated Safe and Adequate Daily Intake for Adults: 1875-5625 mg)—cont'd

	Quantity	Potassium (mg)
Vegetables—cont'd		
Potato (baked, with skin)	1 med	844
Spinach (boiled)	1 med	397
Sweet potato (baked)	½ cup	419
Tomato (raw)	1 med	254
Fruits		
Apple, (raw, with skin)	1 med	159
Banana	1 med	451
Cantaloupe	1 cup, pieces	494
Dates (dried)	10 dates	541
Figs (dried)	10 figs	1332
Orange juice (fresh)	8 fl oz	486
Orange, navel	1 med	250
Prunes (dried)	10 prunes	626
Prune juice (canned)	8 fl oz	706
Raisins, seedless	⅔ cup	751
Meat, poultry, fish, dry beans, eggs, nuts		
Almonds (dry roasted)	1 oz (22 nuts)	219
Beef liver (fried)	3.5 oz	364
Beef top round, lean (broiled)	3.5 oz	442
Black-eyed peas (boiled)	1 cup	476
Chicken, dark (roasted, without skin)	3.5 oz	240
Chicken, light (roasted, without skin)	3.5 oz	247
Clams (steamed)	3 oz (9 small)	534
Crab, blue (steamed)	3 oz	275
Egg, whole	1 large	65
Ground beef, regular (broiled)	3.5 oz	292
Halibut (baked)	3 oz	490
Ham, canned (lean)	3.5 oz	364
Lentils (boiled)	1 cup	731
Lima beans (boiled)	1 cup	955
Lobster (steamed)	3 oz	299
Mackerel (baked)	3 oz	341
Oysters (steamed)	3 oz (12 med)	389
Peanut butter, creamy	1 tbsp	110
Peanuts (dry roasted)	1 oz	184
Pinto beans (boiled)	1 cup	800
Salmon (baked)	3 oz	319
Sirloin steak, lean (broiled)	3.5 oz	403
Soybeans (boiled)	1 cup	886

Food Sources of Potassium (Estimated Safe and Adequate Daily Intake for Adults: 1875-5625 mg)—cont'd

	Quantity	Potassium (mg)
Meat, poultry, fish, dry beans, eggs, nuts—cont'd		
Trout, rainbow (baked)	3 oz	539
Tuna, light, canned in water (with salt)	3 oz	267
Milk, dairy products		
Cottage cheese, creamed	1 cup	177
Milk, skim	8 fl oz	406
Milk, whole	8 fl oz	368
Yogurt, whole	8 fl oz	351
Fats, oils		
This food group is not an important source of potassium.		
Sugar		
Molasses, black	1 tbsp	585
Sugar, brown	1 cup	499

High-Fiber Foods

	Serving	Calories	Grams of fiber
Breads and cereals			
Air-popped popcorn	1 cup	25	1.0
All Bran	1/3 cup	70	8.5
All Bran-Extra Fiber	1/2 cup	60	13.0
All-Bran, Fruit & Almonds	2/3 cup	100	10.0
100% bran	1/2 cup	75	8.4
Bran Buds	1/3 cup	75	7.9
Bran Chex	2/3 cup	90	4.6
Bran Flakes	3/4 cup	90	4.0
Corn Bran	2/3 cup	100	5.4
Cracklin' Oat Bran	1/3 cup	110	4.3
Fiber-One	1/2 cup	60	12.0
Grapenuts	1/4 cup	100	1.4
Whole-wheat bread	1 slice	60	1.4
Whole-wheat spaghetti	1 cup	120	3.9

Continued.

From Lanza E, Butrum R: A critical review of food fiber analysis and data, *J Am Dietetic Assoc* 86(6), 1986.

High-fiber foods—cont'd

	Serving	Calories	Grams of fiber
Legumes, cooked			
Kidney beans	½ cup	110	7.3
Lima beans	½ cup	130	4.5
Navy beans	½ cup	110	6.0
Vegetables, cooked			
Beans, green	½ cup	15	1.6
Broccoli	½ cup	20	2.2
Brussels sprouts	½ cup	30	2.3
Cabbage, red and white	½ cup	15	1.4
Carrots	½ cup	25	2.3
Cauliflower	½ cup	15	1.1
Corn	½ cup	70	2.9
Green peas	½ cup	55	3.6
Kale	½ cup	20	1.4
Parsnip	½ cup	50	2.7
Potato, with skin	1 medium	95	2.5
Fruits			
Apple	1 medium	80	3.5
Apricot, fresh	3 medium	50	1.8
Apricot, dried	5 halves	40	1.4
Banana	1 medium	105	2.4
Blueberries	½ cup	40	2.0
Cantaloupe	¼ melon	50	1.0
Cherries	10	50	1.2
Dates, dried	3	70	1.9
Dried prunes	3	60	3.0
Grapefruit	½	40	1.6
Orange	1 medium	60	2.6
Peach	1 medium	35	1.9
Pineapple	½ cup	40	1.1
Raisins	¼ cup	110	3.1
Strawberries	1 cup	45	3.0

Relationship Between Fiber and Various Health Problems

Problem	Effect of fiber	Possible mode of action	Future research needs
Diabetes mellitus	Reduces fasting blood sugar levels Reduces glycosuria Reduces insulin requirements Increases insulin sensitivity	Slows carbohydrate absorption by: Delaying gastric emptying time Forming gels with pectin or guar gum in the intestine, thus impeding carbohydrate absorption "Protecting" carbohydrates from enzymatic activity with a fibrous coat Allow "protected" carbohydrates to escape into large colon where they are digested by bacteria	Influence of short-chain fatty acid production or metabolism of glucose and fats in the liver Exact mechanisms by which fiber influences glucose metabolism
	Inhibits postprandial (after meals) hyperglycemia	Alters gut hormones (for example, glucagon) to enhance glucose metabolism in the liver	
Obesity	Increases satiety rate	Prolongs chewing and swallowing movements	Cause of increased satiety rate reported by subjects

Continued.

From Williams SR: Nutrition and diet therapy, ed 7, St Louis, 1993, Mosby.

Relationship between fiber and various health problems—cont'd

Problem	Effect of fiber	Possible mode of action	Future research needs
Obesity—cont'd	Reduces nutrient bioavailability	Increases fecal fat content	Effect of nutrient binding on nutritional status
	Reduces energy density	Inhibits absorption of carbohydrates in high-fiber foods	Studies based on food composition and kcaloric density instead of fiber content alone
		Decreases transit time	Effects of different types of fiber on gastric, small intestine, and colonic emptying time
	Alters hormonal response	Alters action of insulin, gut glucagon, and other intestinal hormones	
	Alters thermogenesis		
Coronary heart disease	Inhibits recirculation of bile acids	Alters bacterial metabolism of bile acids	Influence of fiber on cholesterol content of specific lipoprotein fractions
		Alters bacterial flora, resulting in a change in metabolic activity	Influence on production of short-chain fatty acids
		Forms gels that bind bile acids	Role of dietary fiber as an independent variable in reducing risk of heart disease
		Alters the function of pancreatic and intestinal enzymes	
	Reduces triglyceride and cholesterol levels*	Reduces insulin levels†	Relationship between lipoprotein turnover and glucose turnover/sensitivity to insulin

Health problem		Effect of fiber	Research needs
Colon cancer	Reduces incidence of disease‡	Binds cholesterol, preventing absorption Slows fat absorption by forming gel matrices in the intestine Bile acids or their bacterial metabolites may affect the structure of the colon, its cell turnover rate, and function	Effect of higher concentration of bile salts on colon function Testing of current hypotheses regarding the effects of dietary factors on the structure of the colon and cell turnover rate
Other gastrointestinal disorders Diverticular disease Constipation Hiatal hernia Hemorrhoids	Reduces pressure from within the intestinal lumen Increases diameter of the intestinal lumen, thus allowing intestinal tract to contract more, propelling contents more rapidly and inhibiting segmentation§	Decreases transit time Increases water absorption resulting in a larger, softer stool	

*This effect is based on epidemiologic studies, usually observed in combination with reduced fat intake.

†Insulin is required for fat synthesis.

‡Preventive effect of fiber is assumed from epidemiologic studies that associate low-fiber, high-fat diets with an *increased* incidence of disease.

§Segmentation increases pressure and weakness along the walls of the intestinal tract.

Tips for a Low-Sodium Diet

Low sodium	High sodium
Use these foods:	**Avoid these foods:**
Fresh or frozen meats—chicken, turkey, fish, veal and *lean* beef, pork and lamb (limit to three ounce servings), eggs	Bacon, sausage, luncheon meats (bologna, salami, etc.), hotdogs, chipped or corned beef, canned beef (Spam), canned fish (tuna, sardines, anchovies), pot pies, TV dinners, breaded meats, ham
Dried beans (pinto, navy, others)	
Peanut butter	
Swiss,* Mozzarella,* Ricotta cheese,* and low-sodium cheese	Packaged mixes (Hamburger Helper, macaroni and cheese, etc.), canned dinners (Spaghetti O's, Ravioli, etc.)
Dry curd, unsalted cottage cheese	
Milk, yogurt, tofu	
Fresh and frozen vegetables (if you use regular, canned vegetables, drain the liquid off and rinse the vegetables with water)	Foods from "fast food" restaurants
	American and processed cheeses, cheddar, colby, blue cheese, Roquefort cheese, cottage cheese and any cheese not listed on the left, cheese spreads and cheese sauces
Low-sodium soups (or homemade soups that are prepared without sodium)	
Fresh, frozen, or canned fruits	Canned vegetables (unless *low sodium*), sauerkraut, pickles, pickle relish, olives, "pickled" products, canned soups, dehydrated soups, tomato juice and tomato sauce (with salt)
Fruit juices	
Fresh vegetables	
Unsalted popcorn	
Crackers with unsalted tops	
Allspice, basil, bay leaves, chives, cinnamon, dill, onion powder, garlic powder, nutmeg, paprika, parsley, pepper, sage, thyme, lemon juice, vinegar	Potato chips, pretzels, and other salted chips
	Chip dip
	Salted nuts
	Crackers with salted tops
	Mustard, ketchup, chili sauce, barbeque sauce, soy sauce, meat tenderizers, Worchestershire sauce, steak sauce, salad dressings, onion salt, garlic salt, celery salt, lemon pepper, MSG
	Avoid: salt

*Limit to 1 oz only 3 times a week.

Modified from Lexington-Fayette County Health Department, Division of Nutrition and Health Education, Lexington, KY, 1984.

Over-the-Counter (OTC) Drugs

Some drugs contain large amounts of sodium. Make it a practice to read carefully the labels on all over-the-counter drugs. Look at the ingredient list and warning statement to see if sodium is in the product. A statement of sodium content must appear on labels of antacids containing 5 milligrams or more per dosage unit (tablet, teaspoon). Some companies are now producing low-sodium over-the-counter products. If in doubt, ask your physician or pharmacist if the drug is appropriate for your use.

From American Heart Association: *Salt, sodium and blood pressure,* Dallas, Tex, 1979, National Center.

Food Sources of Sodium (Estimated Safe and Adequate Daily Intakes for Adults: 1100-3300 mg)

	Quantity	Sodium (mg)
Bread, cereal, rice, pasta		
Bran flakes	¾ cup	264
Bran muffin, homemade	1 muffin	168
Bread, whole wheat	1 slice	159
Corn flakes	1 cup	310
Wheat flakes	1 cup	270
Vegetables		
Artichoke (boiled)	1 med	79
Broccoli (boiled)	½ cup	12
Brussels sprouts (boiled)	½ cup	17
Carrot (raw)	1 med	25
Potato (baked, with skin)	1 med	16
Spinach (boiled)	½ cup	63
Tomato (raw)	1 med	10

Fruits

This food group is not an important source of sodium.

Meat, poultry, fish, dry beans, eggs, nuts		
Almonds (roasted, unsalted)	1 oz (22 nuts)	3
Bacon (broiled/fried)	3 med pieces	303
Beef liver (fried)	3.5 oz	106
Beef top round, lean (broiled)	3.5 oz	61
Black-eyed peas (boiled)	1 cup	6
Chicken, dark (roasted, without skin)	3.5 oz	93
Chicken, light (roasted, without skin)	3.5 oz	77
Clams (steamed)	3 oz	237
Crab, blue (steamed)	3 oz (9 small)	95
Egg, whole	1 large	69
Ground beef, regular (broiled)	3.5 oz	83
Halibut (baked)	3 oz	59
Ham, canned (lean)	3.5 oz	1255
Lentils (boiled)	1 cup	4
Lobster (steamed)	3 oz	323
Mackerel (baked)	3 oz	71
Oysters (steamed)	3 oz (12 med)	190
Peanut butter, creamy (unsalted)	1 tbsp	3
Peanut butter, creamy (with salt)	1 tbsp	131
Shrimp (steamed)	3 oz (15 large)	190

From Williams SR: *Nutrition and diet therapy*, ed 7, St Louis, 1993, Mosby.

Food Sources of Sodium (Estimated Safe and Adequate Daily Intakes for Adults: 1100-3300 mg)

	Quantity	Sodium (mg)
Meat, poultry, fish, dry beans, eggs, nuts—cont'd		
Sirloin steak, lean (broiled)	3.5 oz	66
Soybeans (boiled)	1 cup	1
Tuna, light, canned in water (with salt)	3 oz	303
Milk, dairy products		
Cheddar cheese	1 oz	176
Cottage cheese, creamed	1 cup	850
Milk, skim	8 fl oz	126
Milk, whole	8 fl oz	119
Swiss cheese	1 oz	74
Yogurt, whole	8 fl oz	105
Fats, oils, sugar		
Butter (salted)	1 tbsp	123
Butter (unsalted)	1 tbsp	2
Margarine, stick, corn oil (salted)	1 tbsp	132
Margarine, stick, corn oil (unsalted)	1 tbsp	3
Molasses, black	1 tbsp	19
Sugar, brown	1 cup	44

Salt-Free Seasoning Guide

Fish	Beef	Poultry and veal	Gravies and sauces
Breaded, battered fillets Dry mustard and onion; oregano, basil, and garlic; thyme Broiled steaks or fillets Chili or curry powder; tarragon Fillets in butter sauce Thyme and chervil; dill; fennel Fish soup Italian seasoning; bay leaf, thyme, and tarragon Fish cakes Tarragon and savory; dry mustard and white pepper; red pepper and oregano	Swiss steak Rosemary and black pepper; bay leaf and thyme; clove Roast beef Basil and oregano; bay leaf; nutmeg; tarragon and marjoram Beef stew Chili powder; bay leaf and tarragon; caraway; marjoram Meatballs Garlic and thyme; basil, oregano, and onion; thyme and garlic; black pepper and dry mustard Beef stroganoff Red pepper, onion, and garlic; nutmeg and onion; curry powder	Fried chicken Basil, oregano, and garlic; onion and dill; sesame seed and nutmeg Roast chicken or turkey Ginger and garlic; onion, thyme, and tarragon Chicken croquettes Dill; curry; chili and cumin; tarragon and oregano Veal patties Italian seasoning; tarragon; dill, onion, and sesame seed Barbecue chicken Garlic and dry mustard; clove, allspice, and dry mustard; basil, garlic, and oregano	Barbecue Bay leaf, thyme, and red pepper; cinnamon, ginger, allspice, dry mustard, and red pepper; chili powder Brown Chervil and onion; onion, bay leaf, and thyme; onion and nutmeg; tarragon Chicken Dry mustard; ginger and garlic; marjoram, thyme, and bay leaf Cream White pepper and dry mustard; curry powder; dill, onion, and paprika; tarragon and thyme

Soups	Salads	Pasta, beans, and rice	Vegetables
Chicken Thyme and savory; ginger; clove, white pepper, and allspice	Chicken Curry or chili powder; Italian seasoning; thyme and tarragon	Baked beans Dry mustard; chili powder; clove and onion; ginger and dry mustard	Asparagus Ginger; sesame seed; basil and onion
Clam chowder Basil and oregano; nutmeg and white pepper; thyme and garlic powder	Coleslaw Dill; caraway; poppy; dry mustard and ginger	Rice and vegetables Curry; thyme, onion, and paprika; rosemary and garlic; ginger, onion, and garlic	Broccoli Italian seasoning; marjoram and basil; nutmeg and onion; sesame seed
Mushroom Ginger; oregano; thyme and tarragon; bay leaf and black pepper; chili powder	Fish or seafood Dill; tarragon, ginger, dry mustard, and red pepper; ginger, onion, and garlic	Spanish rice Cumin, oregano, and basil; Italian seasoning	Cabbage Caraway; onion and nutmeg; allspice and clove
Onion Curry and caraway; marjoram and garlic; cloves	Macaroni Dill; basil, thyme, and oregano; dry mustard and garlic	Spaghetti Italian seasoning and nutmeg; oregano, basil, and nutmeg; red pepper and tarragon	Carrots Ginger; nutmeg; onion and dill
Tomato Bay leaf and thyme; Italian seasoning; oregano and onion; nutmeg	Potato Chili powder; curry; dry mustard and onion	Rice pilaf Dill; thyme; savory and black pepper	Cauliflower Dry mustard; basil; paprika and onion
Vegetable Italian seasoning; paprika and caraway; rosemary and thyme; fennel and thyme			Tomatoes Oregano; chili powder; dill and onion
			Spinach Savory and thyme; nutmeg; garlic and onion

From Williams SR: *Nutrition and diet therapy*, ed 7, St Louis, 1993, Mosby.

Food Sources High in Iron

If your blood iron levels are low, eat the foods listed below. (Try to eat two of these foods every day.)

* Cream of Wheat	Whole wheat breads and cereals
* Total cereal	Brown rice
* Product 19 cereal	Dried apricots
* Bran flakes	Raisins
Oatmeal	Prunes
* Liver	Molasses
Veal	Walnuts
* Collard greens	Almonds
Mustard greens	
Spinach	* Pork-n-beans
* Chili with beans	* Lima beans

*Especially good sources.

Cooking in cast iron pots increases the iron in your food.

To increase iron absorption, drink orange juice or another food high in vitamin C along with these high-iron foods.

Modified from Lexington-Fayette County Health Department, Division of Nutrition and Health Education, Lexington, KY, 1984.

Food Sources of Iron (RDAs for Adult Women, 15 mg; for Adult Men, 10 mg)

	Quantity	Iron (mg)
Bread, cereal, rice, pasta		
Bran flakes	¾ cup	4.50
Bran muffin, homemade	1 muffin	1.26
Bread, whole wheat	1 slice	0.86
Cream of wheat, regular (cooked)	¾ cup	7.70
Oatmeal (cooked)	¾ cup	1.19
Pasta, enriched (cooked)	1 cup	2.40
Rice, white, enriched (cooked)	1 cup	1.80
Wheat flakes	1 cup	4.45
Vegetables		
Artichoke (boiled)	1 med	1.62
Avocado (raw)	1 med	2.04
Broccoli (boiled)	½ cup	0.89
Brussels sprouts (boiled)	½ cup	0.94
Peas, green (boiled)	½ cup	1.24

From Williams SR: *Nutrition and diet therapy,* ed 7, St Louis, 1993, Mosby.

Food sources of iron (RDAs for adult women, 15 mg; for adult men, 10 mg)

	Quantity	Iron (mg)
Vegetables—cont'd		
Potato (baked, with skin)	1 med	2.75
Spinach (boiled)	½ cup	3.21
Fruits		
Dates (dried)	10 dates	0.96
Figs (dried)	10 figs	4.18
Prune juice (canned)	8 fl oz	3.03
Prunes (dried)	10 prunes	2.08
Raisins, seedless	⅔ cup	2.08
Meat, poultry, fish, dry beans, eggs, nuts		
Almonds (roasted)	1 oz (22 nuts)	1.08
Beef liver (fried)	3.5 oz	6.28
Beef top round, lean (broiled)	3.5 oz	2.88
Black-eyed peas (boiled)	1 cup	4.29
Cashews (roasted)	1 oz	1.70
Chicken, dark (roasted, without skin)	3.5 oz	1.33
Chicken, light (roasted, without skin)	3.5 oz	1.06
Chick-peas (boiled)	1 cup	4.74
Clams (steamed)	3 oz (9 small)	23.76
Crab, blue (steamed)	3 oz	0.77
Egg, whole	1 large	1.04
Ground beef, regular (broiled)	3.5 oz	2.44
Halibut (baked)	3 oz	0.91
Ham, canned (lean)	3.5 oz	0.94
Lentils (boiled)	1 cup	6.59
Lima beans (boiled)	1 cup	4.50
Mackerel (baked)	3 oz	1.33
Oysters (steamed)	3 oz (12 med)	11.39
Pinto beans (boiled)	1 cup	4.47
Shrimp (steamed)	3 oz (15 large)	2.62
Sirloin steak, lean (broiled)	3.5 oz	3.36
Sole (baked)	3.5 oz	1.40
Soybeans (boiled)	1 cup	8.84
Trout, rainbow (baked)	3 oz	2.07
Tuna, light, canned in water	3 oz	2.72
Milk, dairy products		
Cheddar cheese	1 oz	0.19
Cottage cheese, creamed	1 cup	0.29
Milk, skim	8 fl oz	0.10

Continued.

Food sources of iron (RDAs for adult women, 15 mg; for adult men, 10 mg)—cont'd

	Quantity	Iron (mg)
Milk, dairy products—cont'd		
Milk, whole	8 fl oz	0.12
Yogurt, whole	8 fl oz	0.11
Fats, oils		
This food group is not an important source of iron.		
Sugar		
Molasses, black	1 tbsp	3.20
Sugar, brown	1 cup	4.90

Low-Gluten Diet for Children with Celiac Disease

Dietary principles

- Kcalories—high, usually about 20% above normal requirement, to compensate for fecal loss
- Protein—high, usually 6 to 8 g/kg body weight
- Fat—low, but not fat-free, because of impaired absorption
- Carbohydrates—simple, easily digested sugars (fruits, vegetables) should provide about one half of the kcalories
- Feedings—small, frequent feedings during ill periods; afternoon snack for older children
- Texture—smooth, soft, avoiding irritating roughage initially, using strained foods longer than usual for age, adding whole foods as tolerated and according to age of child
- Vitamins—supplements of B vitamins, vitamins A and B in water-miscible forms, and vitamin C
- Minerals—iron supplements if anemia is present

Food groups	Foods included—low gluten	Foods excluded—high gluten
Milk	Milk (plain or flavored with chocolate or cocoa) Buttermilk	Malted milk; preparations such as Cocomalt, Hemo, Postum, Nestles chocolate
Meat or substitute	Lean meat, trimmed well of fat Eggs, cheese Poultry, fish Creamy peanut butter (if tolerated)	Fat meats (sausage, pork) Luncheon meats, corned beef, frankfurters, all common prepared meat products with any possible wheat filler

Continued.

From Williams SR: *Nutrition and diet therapy,* ed 7, St Louis, 1993, Mosby.

Low-gluten diet for children with celiac disease—cont'd

Food groups	Foods included—low gluten	Foods excluded—high gluten
Meat or substitute—cont'd		Duck, goose Smoked salmon Meat prepared with bread, crackers, or flour
Fruits and juices	All cooked and canned fruits and juices Frozen or fresh fruits as tolerated, avoiding skins and seeds	Prunes, plums (unless tolerated)
Vegetables	All cooked, frozen, canned as tolerated (prepared *without* wheat, rye, oat, or barley products); raw as tolerated	Any causing individual discomfort All prepared with wheat, rye, oat, or barley products
Cereals	Corn or rice	Wheat, rye, oat, barley; any product containing these cereals
Breads, flours, cereal products	Breads, pancakes, or waffles made with suggested flours (cornmeal, cornstarch; rice, soybean, lima bean, potato, buckwheat)	All bread or cracker products made with gluten; wheat, rye, oat, barley; macaroni, noodles, spaghetti; any sauces, soups, or gravies prepared with gluten flour, wheat, oat, or barley
Soups	Broth, bouillon (no fat or cream; no thickening with wheat, rye, oat, or barley products); soups and sauces may be thickened with cornstarch	All soups containing wheat, rye, oat, or barley products

Caffeine Content of Beverages and Foods

Item	Milligrams caffeine	
	Average	Range
Coffee (5 oz cup)		
Brewed, drip method	115	60-180
Brewed, percolator	80	40-170
Instant	65	30-120
Decaffeinated, brewed	3	2-5
Decaffeinated, instant	2	1-5
Tea (5 oz cup)		
Brewed, major U.S. brands	40	20-90
Brewed, imported brands	60	25-110
Instant	30	25-50
Iced (12 oz glass)	70	67-76
Cocoa beverage (5 oz cup)	4	2-20
Chocolate milk beverage (8 oz)	5	2-7
Milk chocolate (1 oz)	6	1-15
Dark chocolate, semisweet (1 oz)	20	5-35
Baker's chocolate (1 oz)	26	26
Chocolate-flavored syrup (1 oz)	4	4

Source: FDA, Food Additive Chemistry Evaluation Branch, based on evaluations of existing literature on caffeine levels, 1988. From DDHS Pub #88-2221, FDA, Rockville, Md.

Caffeine Content of Soft Drinks

Item	Caffeine (mg per 6 oz serving)
Regular	
Cola, Pepper	15-23
Decaffeinated cola, Pepper	0-0.09
Cherry Cola	18-23
Lemon-Lime (clear)	0
Orange	0
Other citrus	0-32
Root beer	0
Ginger ale	0
Tonic water	0

Continued.

Source: National Soft Drink Association, Washington, DC, 1988. Amount of fruit juices added varies from 10% to 25%. From DHHS Pub #88-2221, FDA, Rockville, MD.

Caffeine content of soft drinks—cont'd

Item	Caffeine (mg per 6 oz serving)
Regular—cont'd	
Other regular	0-22
Juice added	less than 0.24
Diet drinks	
Diet cola, Pepper	0.3
Decaffeinated diet cola, Pepper	0-0.1
Diet Cherry Cola	0-23
Diet Lemon-Lime	0
Diet root beer	0
Other diets	0-35
Club soda, seltzer, sparkling water	0
Diet juice added	less than 0.24

Caffeine Content of Drugs

Caffeine is an ingredient in many prescription and nonprescription drug products. It is often used in alertness or stay-awake tablets, headache and pain relief remedies, cold products, and diuretics. When caffeine is an ingredient, it is listed on the product label. Some drugs that contain caffeine are listed in the following table.

Drug	Caffeine (mg per tablet or capsule)
Prescription drugs	
Cafergot (migraine headaches)	100
Norgesic Forte (muscle relaxant)	60
Norgesic (muscle relaxant)	30
Fiorinal (tension headache)	40
Fioricet (headache pain relief)	40
Darvon compound (pain relief)	32.4
Synalgos-DC (pain relief)	30
Synalgos-DC-A (pain relief)	30
Nonprescription drugs	
Alertness tablets	
No Doz	100
Vivarin	200

Source: FDA's Center for Drugs and Biologics, 1988. From DHHS Pub #88-2221, FDA, Rockville, MD.

Caffeine content of drugs—cont'd

Drug	Caffeine (mg per tablet or capsule)
Nonprescription drugs—cont'd	
Pain relief	
Anacin, Maximum Strength Anacin	32
Vanquish	33
Excedrin	65
Midol	32.4
Diuretics	
Aqua-Ban	100
Cold/allergy remedies	
Coryban-D capsules	30

Facts about Cholesterol

Types of cholesterol

LDL "bad cholesterol"

Clogs blood vessels

HDL "good cholesterol"

Cleans blood vessels

What is cholesterol and why should it be of concern?

Cholesterol is a soft, fatlike substance found in the bloodstream. It comes from the *animal source* foods you eat and the cholesterol your body makes.

Too much cholesterol can clog the blood vessels and lead to strokes and heart attacks.

Source: National Cholesterol Education Program, National Heart, Lung, and Blood Institute: *The detection, evaluation, and treatment of high blood cholesterol in adults,* National Institutes of Health, Public Health Service, US Department of Health and Human Services, 1987.

*To convert mg/dl cholesterol to mmol/L, divide cholesterol by 38.7 or multiply by 0.02586.

Continued.

Modified from Lexington-Fayette County Health Department, Division of Nutrition and Health Education, Lexington, KY, and Kentucky Department of Human Resources, Frankfort, KY, 1984.

Types of cholesterol—cont'd

Classification based on total cholesterol	Classification based on LDL cholesterol
<200 mg/dl (<5.17 mmol/L*) Desirable blood cholesterol	<130 mg/dl (<3.36 mmol/L) Desirable LDL cholesterol
200 mg/dl to 239 mg/dl (5.17 mmol/L to 6.18 mmol/L) Borderline-high blood cholesterol	130 mg/dl to 159 mg/dl (3.36 mmol/L to 4.11 mmol/L) Borderline-high-risk LDL cholesterol
≥240 mg/dl (≥6.21 mmol/L) High blood cholesterol	≥160 mg/dl (≥4.13 mmol/L) High-risk LDL cholesterol

To prevent or decrease high cholesterol in the blood, what can one eat?

Increase fiber:

1. Whole wheat bread
2. Hot cereals (oatmeal)

Increase exercise:

1. Walking three times per week if doctor approves

Follow these suggestions:

1. Limit intake of meats, poltry, and seafood to no more than 5-7 oz per day.
2. Use fish, chicken, or turkey in most of your main meals, limiting "red" meats to 3-4 servings per week.
3. Use "low-meat" dishes or vegetable protein dishes such as dried beans or peas for regular entrees.
4. Use low-fat dairy products—2 cups skim milk daily.
5. Limit egg yolks to 2 a week including those in cooking. (1 egg = 274 mg cholesterol)
6. Limit added fat to 5-8 teaspoons daily. Use soft margarines, vegetable oils (olive oil, too) in cooking.

For cholesterol control

Foods to eat	Foods to limit
Egg whites	Egg yolks
Skim milk and low-fat cheeses	Liver
mozzarella, gouda, ricotta,	Heart
farmer's and low-fat cottage	Kidney and other organ meats
cheese	Whole milk
Liquid vegetable oil	Cheese
Olive oil	Oysters
Fish, chicken, turkey (no skin)	Shrimp
Fruits, vegetables and whole	Crabs
grain foods	Lobster
	Butter
	Cream
	Red meat

	Low cholesterol		High cholesterol
Substitute:	Skim milk	for	Whole milk
	Liquid corn oil	for	Butter
	Margarine		
	Safflower oil	for	Vegetable shortening
	Corn oil		

Other tips: Use smaller portions of red meats!

Use less animal food, more plant food.

Switch to whole grains; (i.e., whole wheat bread, wheat or oats cereals, brown rice.)

Cholesterol: The Numbers

- For total cholesterol levels, you do not need to fast.
- For triglycerides, you do need to fast.

Cholesterol level	Classification (adults over age 20)
Total cholesterol level	
Less than 200 mg/dl	Desirable
200-239 mg/dl	Borderline-high
Greater than 240 mg/dl	High

From Quinnipiack Valley Health Dept., Conn.

Cholesterol: the numbers—cont'd

Cholesterol level	Classification (adults over age 20)
LDL ("bad") cholesterol level	
Less than 130 mg/dl	Desirable
130-159 mg/dl	Borderline-high
Greater than 160 mg/dl	High
HDL ("good") cholesterol level	
Average for men is 45 mg/dl	
Average for women is 55 mg/dl	
Below 35 mg/dl is a cause for concern	
Triglyceride levels	
Less than 250 mg/dl	Desirable
250-500 mg/dl	Borderline-high
Greater than 500 mg/dl	High

Total cholesterol = LDL + HDL + (Triglycerides ÷ 5)
(formula for calculating VLDL)

LDL/HDL ratio—less than 3:1 is desirable
(mg-dl-milligrams per deciliter of blood)

Diet and Cancer

- Reduce intake of dietary fat from 40% to 30% of total calories.
- Increase the intake of fresh fruits and vegetables.
- Increase the intake of whole grain breads and cereals.
- Drink alcoholic beverages in moderation, if at all.
- Avoid obesity by regulating total caloric intake.
- Increase intake of foods rich in vitamins A and C.
- Increase intake of cabbage family (cruciferous) vegetables.
- Choose lean meats or legumes as protein sources.
- Trim off excess fat from meats.
- Limit intake of butter, cream, margarine, shortening, and coconut oil, and foods made with such products.
- Broil, bake, or boil rather than fry foods.
- Moderate intake of eggs and organ meats.
- Substitute skim or low-fat milk for whole milk.

Modified from Darnell LS: Nutrition and cancer prevention, *Fam Comm Health* 10(3), 1987.

Diet Guidelines for a Healthy Heart

These guidelines offer a brief summary of three diets for a healthy heart. If your doctor has prescribed one of these diets for you, you need more complete information. The American Heart Association has free pamphlets available that explain the low-cholesterol and low-sodium diets in detail.

Reading Labels

Labels on packaged foods make it easier to select healthier products, but you must understand how to interpret them. If the product makes any nutritional claim, the label lists two categories of information. **"Nutritional Information per Serving"** lists the amount of calories, protein, carbohydrates, fat, and sodium (salt) in one serving. It also tells you how much is considered *one* serving, which can be confusing. For example, one normal serving of milk is 1 cup, or 8 ounces. If you pour milk into a tall drinking glass, however, you may have 10 to 16 ounces.

The second category is **"Percentage of U.S. Recommended Daily Allowances (U.S. RDA)"** for protein, vitamins, and minerals in each serving. Remember that these numbers are percentages, so if the label on a milk carton says "Protein 20," this means that 1 cup provides 20% of the protein you need each day.

Packaged foods that don't claim to provide nutrition don't have these labels, but they do list the ingredients. The largest quantity is listed first and the smallest amount last. For example, a jar of sweet pickles lists the ingredients as "Cucumbers, water, corn syrup, vinegar, peppers, salt, natural and artificial flavors, preservatives, and artificial coloring." This tells you cucumbers are the main ingredient, water the next highest ingredient, and so forth.

Of course, fresh meats, fish and seafood, fruits, and vegetables do not carry labels. You need to learn which ones are the best for your diet and which ones to avoid.

Low-Cholesterol Diet

The average American consumes a large amount of cholesterol every day: men about 500 milligrams (mg) and women about 320 mg. A low-cholesterol diet limits cholesterol intake to less than 300 mg a day. To manage this, only 30% (or less) of the total calories you eat every day should come from fat. In addition, most of this fat should come from **polyunsaturated fat,** the "good" fat that helps lower blood cholesterol.

How can you tell the difference between "good" and "bad" fat? Polyunsaturated oil is usually liquid and comes from vegetables such as corn, cottonseed, soybean, sunflower, and safflower. Peanut, canola, and olive oil are **monounsaturated fats** that are neutral and do not add cholesterol. The "bad" fats are **saturated fats,** which harden at room temperature and are found in meat, dairy products made from whole milk or cream, solid and hydrogenated shortening, coconut oil, palm oil, and cocoa butter.

Here are some tips for avoiding too much saturated fat:

1. Eat less meat. Adults need about 5-7 ounces of meat, poultry, fish, or seafood a day.
2. Avoid "prime grade" or heavily marbled meats, corned beef, pastrami, regular ground beef, frankfurters, sausage, bacon, lunch meat, goose, duck, or organ meats. Select very lean cuts of meat. Trim skin off chicken and turkey.
3. Avoid fried meat, chicken, fish, or seafood. Use a rack to drain off fat when broiling, baking, or roasting.
4. Eat no more than two whole eggs (yolks and whites) per week. (Egg whites are allowed because they contain little cholesterol.)
5. Avoid dairy products containing more than 1% milk fat, such as butter, sour cream, cream cheese, creamed cottage cheese, and most natural and processed cheeses. Select milk products that contain only up to 1% milk fat. Use polyunsaturated margarine.
6. Avoid packaged foods or bakery items that contain egg yolks, whole milk, saturated fats, cream sauces, or butter. Select only those that have a low-cholesterol rating.
7. Avoid cashews, coconut, pistachios, and macadamia nuts. Most other types of vegetables, fruits, nuts, and seeds are low in cholesterol.

Low-Sodium Diet

The average American consumes about 1 to 2 teaspoons of salt every day, 6 to 18 grams, and most of this salt is added at the table. Your body needs only about 0.5 gram of salt a day. Since most foods that come from animals (meat, poultry, fish, eggs, milk) are naturally high in sodium, your body's requirements are easily met without adding salt to your food.

What is the difference between salt and sodium? Sodium keeps the right amount of water in your body, so some is necessary for good health. However, too much sodium causes water retention, which raises your blood pressure.

It may take a little time to get used to a low-sodium diet, particularly if you are accustomed to eating highly salted foods. Start by eliminating salt from the table. Use spices and herbs that contain no sodium to add flavor, and try some of the new salt substitutes that contain no sodium.

Many packaged and processed foods are now marketed as low sodium, including cheeses, luncheon meats, canned and packaged food, and even snacks such as potato chips. However, beware if the package reads "reduced sodium"; the sodium content may still be too high. If you are not sure of a product, read the ingredients carefully and look for the words "salt, sodium, soda, baking powder, monosodium glutamate (MSG), and disodium phosphate." If you are still in doubt, don't eat it.

Here are some tips for eliminating the "hidden" sodium from your diet:

1. Avoid cured or smoked meat, poultry, or fish. These include ham, bacon, corned beef, regular luncheon meats, sausage, commercially frozen fish, canned fish packed in oil or brine, and canned shellfish.
2. Avoid frozen, canned, and dehydrated main-dish foods such as pizza, TV dinners, spaghetti, chili, stews, and soups.
3. Avoid canned vegetables and vegetable juices.
4. Avoid cheese, buttermilk, and cocoa mixes.
5. Avoid commercial sauces (catsup, chili sauce, steak sauce, soy sauce), mayonnaise, salad dressing, olives, pickles, meat tenderizers, and seasoning salts.

Low-Calorie Diet

Losing weight (or keeping weight off) is an important part of controlling blood pressure and reducing blood cholesterol levels. Your doctor, a dietitian, or a nutritionist can advise you about calories, because this depends on your how active you are, your height, and your physical condition.

The low-cholesterol diet is an excellent basis for a weight loss program. Fats are high in calories, and the low-cholesterol diet is essentially a low-fat diet. For example, 1 cup of whole milk contains 150 calories, but the same amount of skim milk has only 86 calories. Also, because it emphasizes fresh fruits and vegetables and discourages processed foods, the low-cholesterol diet is nutritionally well balanced.

Weight loss should be gradual. Remember: it probably took you several years to put the pounds on, so expect it to take several months to lose them.

Here are some other tips for helping you lose weight:

1. Divide your daily calorie allowance into several small meals a day, instead of eating one or two large meals.

2. For between-meal snacks, choose high-fiber, low-calorie foods such as apples or celery. High-fiber foods make your stomach feel full quicker.

3. For between-meal hunger pangs, fool your stomach with a glass of ice water, hot tea, or calorie-free soda.

4. If you eat when you're bored, busy yourself to take your mind off food. Change your activity—do something you enjoy, take a walk, or take a shower.

5. If you eat when you are "blue," try the "buddy system" with a dieting friend. Agree to call each other for help whenever you're tempted to indulge.

6. Regular exercise that burns calories (walking, jogging, swimming, etc.) is the magic ingredient in many people's exercise programs. Check with your doctor first about the safest program for you.

7. "Too good to be true" weight loss programs are just that—they are either worthless or dangerous. Follow a diet that has been medically recommended and skip the "fad" diets.

Cultural and Regional Foods

Name of food	Culture/region	Type of food	Description
Adobo	Filipino	Meat	Meat with soy sauce
Ajinomoto	Japanese	Grain	Wheat germ
Anadama	New England	Grain	Cornmeal-molasses yeast bread
Arroz blanco	Puerto Rican	Grain	Enriched white rice
Bacalao	Puerto Rican	Meat	Salted codfish
Bagels	Jewish	Grain	Bread dough, doughnut-shaped, boiled in water and baked
Baklava	Greek	Dessert	Layered pastry made with honey
Bok choy	Oriental	Vegetable	Green leafy, stalk-like vegetable
Brioche	French	Grain	Egg-rich cake bread, used as sweet roll or shell for entrees
Bulgur	Middle Eastern	Grain	Granular wheat product with nutlike flavor
Burrito	Mexican	Combination	Sandwich; tortilla filled with beef-bean mixture and fried or baked
Café con leche	Latin American	Beverage	Coffee with milk
Cape Cod turkey	New England	Meat	Codfish balls
Challah	Jewish	Grain	Sabbath or holiday twisted eggbread
Chayote	Mexican	Vegetable	Squashlike vegetable
Chitterlings	Southern U.S.	Meat	Intestine of young pigs, soaked, boiled, and fried
Chorizo	Mexican	Meat	Sausage
Cilantro	Mexican	Seasoning	Coriander, similar to parsley
Crackling	Southern U.S.	Snack	Crispy pieces of fried pork fat

Continued.

From Burtis G, Davis J, Martin S: *Applied nutrition and diet therapy,* Philadelphia, 1988, Saunders.

Cultural and regional foods—cont'd

Name of food	Culture/region	Type of food	Description
Croissants	French	Grain	Buttery, flaky, crescent-shaped rolls
Crumpets	English	Grain	Muffinlike produce cooked on griddle then toasted
Cush	Montana	Grain	Cornbread mixed with butter and water and fried
Dandelion greens	Southern U.S.	Vegetable	Leaves from dandelion plant
Dolmathes	Greek	Combination	Grape leaves stuffed with beef
Enchiladas	Mexican	Combination	Tortilla filled with meat and cheese
Escargots	French	Meat	Snails
Falafel	Jewish	Meat	Mashed chick peas mixed with spices and fried
Fatback	Southern U.S.	Fat	Fat from loin of pig
Feijoada	Brazilian	Meat	Black beans with meat
Feta	Greek	Milk	Soft, salty white cheese from sheep's or goat's milk
Finnan haddie	Scottish	Milk	Salted, smoked haddock
Frijoles fritos	Mexican	Meat	Refried pinto beans
Gazpacho	Spanish	Soup	Cold soup with chopped tomatoes, green peppers, and cucumbers
Gefilte fish	Jewish	Meat	Seasoned fish ground and shaped into balls
Goulash	Hungarian	Meat	Stew seasoned with paprika
Grits	Southern U.S.	Grain	Hulled and coarsely ground corn
Guava	Cuban	Fruit	Small, yellow or red sweet tropical fruit
Gumbo	Creole	Combination	Well-seasoned okra stew with meat or seafood
Hangtown fry	California	Meat	Fried oysters and eggs
Hoe cake	Southeast U.S.	Grain	Thin corn cake
Hog maw	Southern U.S.	Meat	Stomach of pig
Hoppin' John	Southern U.S.	Combination	Blackeyed peas and rice
Hush puppies	Southern U.S.	Grain	Fried cornbread

Food	Origin	Category	Description
Jalapeños	Latin American	Vegetable	Hot peppers
Jambalaya	Creole	Combination	Well-seasoned combination of seafoods, tomatoes, and rice
Kale	Southern U.S.	Vegetable	Dark green leafy vegetable, similar to spinach
Kasha	Jewish	Grain	Coarsely ground buckwheat, toasted before cooking in liquid
Kelp	Oriental	Vegetable	Seaweed
Kibbeh	Middle East	Meat	Fresh raw lamb, ground and seasoned, similar to meat loaf
Keilbasa	Polish	Meat	Sausage
Kimchi	Korean	Vegetable	Peppery fermented combination of pickled cabbage, turnips, radishes, and other vegetables
Kuchen	German	Dessert	Yeast cake
Latkas	Jewish	Grain	Pancakes, sometimes from potatoes
Lard	—	Fat	Shortening-like product from pork
Limpa	Swedish	Grain	Rye bread
Lox	Jewish	Meat	Smoked salmon
Matsoh	Jewish	Grain	Unleavened bread
Menudo	Mexican	Meat	Stew made with tripe (cow's stomach)
Minestrone	Italian	Soup	Vegetable soup
Miso	Oriental	Meat	Fermented soybean paste
Moussaka	Greek	Combination	Meat and eggplant casserole
Mush	Soutwest U.S.	Grain	Cooked cereal, usually cornmeal
Pan Dowdy	New England	Dessert	Dumplings and fruit
Papaya	—	Fruit	Large, yellow melonlike tropical fruit
Pasta	Italian	Grain	Macaroni, spaghetti, and noodles in various shapes made from wheat
Pepperoni	Italian	Meat	Hot sausage
Phyllo	Greek	Grain	Paper-thin pastry for making meat, vegetables, cheese and egg dishes, and sweet pastries

Continued.

Cultural and regional foods—cont'd

Name of food	Culture/region	Type of food	Description
Pilaf	Middle Eastern	Grain	Rice enriched with fat and sometimes vegetables, bits of meat, and spices
Poi	Polynesian	Vegetable	Root vegetable, especially taro, cooked and grounded, mixed with water, and sometimes fermented
Polenta	Italian	Grain	Cornmeal or cornmeal mush
Polk	Southern U.S.	Vegetable	Dark green leafy vegetable
Potato knishes	Jewish	Vegetable	Potato pancakes
Pot liquor (likker)	Southern U.S.	Vegetable	Liquid from cooking green vegetables or bones
Prosciutto	Italian	Meat	Ready-to-eat, cured, smoked ham
Prickly pear	Native American	Fruit	Fruit of cactus
Pumpernickel	—	Grain	Yeast bread with wheat, corn, rye, and potatoes
Ratatouille	French	Vegetable	Well-seasoned casserole of eggplant, zucchini, tomato, and green pepper
Red-eye gravy	Southern U.S.	Gravy	Fried ham gravy
Sake	Oriental	Beverage	Rice wine
Salt pork	Southern U.S.	Fat	Salted pork fat from the belly
Sancocho	Puerto Rican	Combination	Soup with meat and viandas
Sashimi	Japanese	Meat	Raw fish
Sauerbrauten	German	Meat	Pot roast in spicy, aromatic, sweet-and-sour marinade
Scones	English	Grain	Round, flat, unleavened sweetened bread
Scrapple	Pennsylvania Dutch	Combination	Solid mush from cornmeal and the by-products of hog butchering

Shoofly pie	Pennsylvania Dutch	Dessert	Molasses pie
Shoyu	Japanese	Seasoning	Soy sauce
Sofrito	Puerto Rican	Seasoning	Specially seasoned tomato sauce
Sopapillos	Mexican	Grain	Rich fried bread
Spaetzle	German	Grain	Small dumplings
Spoonbread	Virginia	Grain	Baked dish with cornmeal
Spumoni	Italian	Dessert	Fruited ice cream
Stollen	German	Dessert	Christmas fruitcake
Stricle sheets	Pennsylvania Dutch	Dessert	Coffee cake
Strudel	German	Dessert	Light pastry, filled with fruit or cheese
Tacos	Mexican	Combination	Fried tortillas, filled wth meat, vegetables, and hot sauce
Tamales	Mexican	Grain	Pancakelike leathery bread
Tempura	Japanese	Combination	Deep-fried seafood or vegetables
Teriyaki sauce	Hawaiian	Accessory	Sweetened soy sauce
Tofu	Oriental	Meat	Soybean curd
Trotters	Southern U.S.	Meat	Pig's feet
Viandas	Puerto Rican	Vegetable	Starchy tropical vegetables, including plantain, green bananas, and sweet potatoes

Food Restrictions of Various Religions

Religious group and food restrictions	Clinical implications with institutional situations or with modified diets
Catholics	
Abstinence from meat, meat soups, or gravy on Ash Wednesday and Fridays during Lent.	Fish or other meat substitutes are generally offered on these days.
Mormons	
No alcoholic beverages. No stimulants.	Substitutes should be given to patients for regular coffee, tea, and most carbonated beverages, especially if the patient is on a liquid diet.
Moslems	
No pork or pork products. No animal shortenings. Only kosher meats allowed. Regular gelatin, marshmallow, and other confections containing gelatin are not allowed. No alcoholic products or beverages (including extracts such as vanilla or lemon). Fasting is common (mandatory for 1 month each year). Recommended foods: honey, milk, dates, meat, seafood, and vegetable and olive oil.	Hospitalized patients may need assistance in selecting from hospital menus to see that the vegetables are not cooked with any animal shortenings or pork seasonings. Although institutional meats are not normally kosher, they may be purchased. Assist patients in selecting from the hospital menu to be certain they receive adequate food considering these restrictions. Fasting can be precarious with some medical problems, especially diabetes and hypoglycemia. Some of these foods may be contraindicated on a special diet (honey on a diabetic diet) and should be noted.

Seventh-Day Adventists

Optional vegetarianism: (1) strict vegetarianism, (2) lacto-ovo-vegetarianism, (3) no pork or pork products, shellfish, or blood.

No alcoholic beverages.
No beverage containing caffeine.
Snacking between meals is discouraged (mealtimes are at intervals of 5 to 6 hours).

If sodium is restricted, the use of soy-based meat analogs should be noted because they are high in sodium. Strict vegetarians need assistance to select a well-balanced menu from the regular hospital diet. Assist patients in choosing from hospital menu to receive foods not seasoned with pork.

Substitutes should be made for the regular coffee, tea, and some carbonated beverages ordinarily given, especially if the patient is on a liquid diet. Some diabetic, hypoglycemic, and ulcer-type diets require more frequent feedings.

From Burtis G, Davis J, Martin S: *Applied nutrition and diet therapy*, Philadelphia, 1988, Saunders.

Nutritional Analysis of Fast Foods

Food Name	Portion	Wt. gm	Kcal Kc	Prot gm	Carb gm	Fat gm	Chol mg	Sod mg
Arby's-Beef and Cheese Sandwich	Item	176	402	32.2	27.1	18	77	1634
Arby's-Chicken Breast Sandwich	Item	184	493	23	47.9	25	91	1019
Arby's-Club Sandwich	Item	252	560	30	43	30	100	1610
Arby's-Ham and Cheese Sandwich	Item	146	353	20.7	33.4	15.5	58	772
Arby's-Roast Beef Sandwich	Item	139	346	21.5	33.5	13.8	52	792
Arby's-Super Roast Beef Beef Sandwich	Item	234	501	25.1	50.4	22.1	40	798
Arby's-Turkey Deluxe	Item	236	510	28	46	24	70	1220
Arby's-Soup-Boston Clam Chowder	Serving	227	207	10	18	11	28	1157
Arby's-Soup-Cream of Broccoli	Serving	227	180	9	19	8	3	1113
Arby's-Soup-French Onion	Serving	227	67	2	7	3	0	1248
Arby's Soup-Lumberjack Mixed Vegetable	Serving	227	89	2	13	4	41075	
Arby's-Soup-Old Fashioned Chicken Noodle	Serving	227	99	6	15	2	25	929
Arby's-Soup-Pilgrim Clam Chowder	Serving	227	193	10	18	11	28	1157
Arby's-Soup-Roast Beef and Vegetable	Serving	227	96	5	14	3	10	996
Arby's-Soup-Split Pea and Ham	Serving	227	200	8	21	10	30	1029
Arby's-Soup-Tomato Florentine	Serving	227	84	3	15	2	2	910
Arby's-Soup-Wisconsin Cheese	Serving	227	287	9	19	19	31	1129
Beef Burger-Fast Food	Ounce	28.3	72.3	4.99	7.26	2.58	—	54.7
Bun-Hamburger/Hotdog-Fast Food	Ounce	28.3	97.8	2.66	16.3	2.41	—	22.1
Burger King-Bacon Double Cheese Deluxe	Serving	195	592	33	28	39	111	804
Burger King-Barbecue Bacon Double Cheese	Serving	174	536	32	31	31	105	795
Burger King-BK Broiler	Item	168	379	24	31	18	53	764
Burger King-BK Broiler Sauce	Serving	14	90	0	0	10	7	95
Burger King-Chicken Tenders	Piece	90	39.3	2.67	2.33	2.17	7.67	90.2

Food	Unit							
Burger King-Croissant-Egg and Cheese	Item	127	369	12.8	24.3	24.7	216	551
Burger King-Croissant-Egg/Cheese/Ham	Item	152	475	18.9	24.2	33.6	213	1080
Burger King-Double Cheeseburger	Item	172	483	30	29	27	100	851
Burger King-Fish Tenders	Serving	99	267	12	18	16	28	870
Burger King-Mushroom Swiss Double Cheese	Item	176	473	31	27	27	95	746
Burger King-Ranch Dip Sauce	Serving	28	171	0	2	18	0	208
Burger King-Sweet & Sour Sauce	Serving	28	45	0	11	0	0	52
Burger King-Tartar Dip Sauce	Serving	28	174	0	3	18	16	302
Burger King-Tater Tenders	Serving	71	213	2	25	12	3	318
Cheese Burger-Fast Food	Ounce	28.3	78	5.61	6.55	3.26	12.3	198
Chicken-Breast and Wing-Breaded-Fried	Serving	163	494	35.7	19.6	29.5	149	975
Chicken-Breast-Fast Food	Ounce	28.3	73.1	7.65	2.61	3.57	23.6	142
Chicken-Drumstick & Thigh-Breaded-Fried	Serving	148	430	30.1	15.7	26.7	165	756
Chicken-Drumstick-Fast Food	Ounce	28.3	59	7.03	4.2	1.56	25.6	133
Chicken-Fried-Fast Food-Various Portions	Ounce	28.3	82.2	4.71	5.67	4.51	25.4	153
Chicken-Meat-Shaped-Fried-Fast Food	Ounce	28.3	81.6	4.85	4.65	4.85	—	141
Chicken-Shoulder-Fast Food	Ounce	28.3	92.4	5.33	3.18	6.49	—	150
Chicken-Thigh-Fast Food	Ounce	28.3	104	7.26	2.75	7.14	26.2	139
Chicken-Wing-Fast Food	Ounce	28.3	91.9	7.85	2.78	5.47	—	198
Coleslaw-Fast Food	Ounce	28.3	23.8	0.68	2.75	1.13	1.07	76.5
Double Cheese Burger-Fast Food	Ounce	28.3	66.3	4.2	6.63	2.55	16.6	49.9
Fast Food-Pizza with Cheese	Ounce	28.4	63.2	3.46	9.23	1.45	4.25	151
Fast Food-Pizza with Pepperoni	Ounce	28.4	72.3	4.04	7.93	2.78	5.67	107

Continued.

From Williams SR: *Nutrition and diet therapy*, ed 7, St Louis, 1993, Mosby.

Nutritional analysis of fast foods—cont'd

Food Name	Portion	Wt. gm	Kcal Kc	Prot gm	Carb gm	Fat gm	Chol mg	Sod mg
Fish Cake-Fried-with Bun-Fast Food	Ounce	28.3	84.5	2.72	7.63	4.79	19.7	167
Frankfurter-Coney Dog-Fast Food	Ounce	28.3	69.2	3.12	6.95	3.2	14.7	242
Frankfurter-Hot Dog-Fast Food	Ounce	28.3	77.7	3.12	7.37	3.97	14.7	219
Hamburger-Double Patty-Everything On It	Ounce	28.4	67.8	4.3	5.05	3.33	15.3	99.2
Hardee-Bacon and Egg Buscuit	Serving	124	410	15	35	24	155	990
Hardee-Bacon Egg and Cheese Biscuit	Serving	137	460	17	35	28	165	1220
Hardee-Big Country Breakfast-Country Ham	Serving	254	670	29	52	38	345	2870
Hardee-Big Country Breakfast-Sausage	Serving	274	850	33	51	57	340	1980
Hardee-Big Country Breakfast-with Bacon	Serving	217	660	24	51	40	305	1540
Hardee-Big Country Breakfast-with Ham	Serving	251	620	28	51	33	325	1780
Hardee-Big Roast Beef Sandwich	Serving	134	300	18	32	11	45	880
Hardee-Big Twin Hamburger	Serving	173	450	23	34	25	55	580
Hardee-Biscuit N Gravy	Serving	221	440	9	45	24	15	1250
Hardee-Chicken N Pasta Salad	Serving	414	230	27	23	3	55	380
Hardee-Crispy Curls	Serving	85	300	4	36	16	0	840
Hardee-Grilled Chicken Sandwich	Serving	192	310	24	34	9	60	890
Hardee-Ham & Egg Biscuit	Serving	138	370	15	35	19	160	1050
Hardee-Ham Egg & Cheese Biscuit	Serving	151	420	18	35	23	170	1270
Hardee-Mushroom N Swiss Hamburger	Serving	186	490	30	33	27	70	940
Hardee-Regular Roast Beef Sandwich	Serving	114	260	15	31	9	35	730
Hardee-The Lean One Sandwich	Item	220	420	27	37	18	85	760
Hardee-Three Pancakes	Serving	137	280	8	56	2	15	890
KFC-Chicken Hot Wings	Piece	119	62.6	3.66	2.99	3.99	24.6	113
KFC-Chicken Sandwich	Serving	16	482	21	39	27	47	1060

Food	Unit							
KFC-Crispy Chicken-Breast	Piece	135	342	33	12	20	114	790
KFC-Crispy Chicken-Drumstick	Piece	69	204	14	6	14	71	324
KFC-Crispy Chicken-Thigh	Piece	119	406	20	14	30	129	688
KFC-Crispy Chicken-Wing	Piece	65	254	12	9	19	67	422
Long John Silver-Battered Shrimp-9 Piece	Piece	357	95.4	2.66	9.76	4.99	13.9	163
Long John Silver-Breaded Shrimp	Piece	420	51	1.19	6.19	2.43	5.95	85.2
Long John Silver-Catfish Fillet	Serving	373	860	28	90	42	65	990
Long John Silver-Chicken Plank-4 Piece	Serving	415	940	39	94	44	70	1660
Long John Silver-Chicken-Light Herb	Serving	498	630	35	85	17	85	2170
Long John Silver-Clam Chowder with Cod	Serving	198	140	11	10	6	20	590
Long John Silver-Clam Dinner	Serving	363	980	21	122	45	15	1200
Long John Silver-Cole Slaw	Serving	98	140	1	20	6	15	260
Long John Silver-Fish & Chicken Entree	Serving	398	870	35	91	40	70	1520
Long John Silver-Fish & More Entree	Serving	381	800	31	88	37	70	1390
Long John Silver-Fish and Fries-3 Piece	Serving	358	810	42	77	38	85	1630
Long John Silver-Fish Sandwich Platter	Serving	379	870	26	108	38	55	1110
Long John Silver-Fries	Serving	85	220	3	30	10	5	60
Long John Silver-Garden Salad	Serving	246	170	9	13	9	5	380
Long John Silver-Gumbo-Cod & Shrimp Bobs	Serving	198	120	9	4	8	25	740
Long John Silver-Homestyle Fish Sandwich	Serving	196	510	22	58	22	45	780
Long John Silver-Homestyle Fish-3 Piece	Serving	456	960	43	97	44	100	1890
Long John Silver-Homestyle Fish-6 Piece	Serving	513	1260	49	124	64	130	1590
Long John Silver-Hush puppies	Piece	24	70	2	10	2	5	25
Long John Silver-Light Fish-Lemon	Serving	291	320	24	49	4	75	900
Long John Silver-Light Fish-Paprika	Serving	284	300	24	45	2	70	650
Long John Silver-Mixed Vegetables	Serving	113	60	2	9	2	0	330
Long John Silver-Ocean Chef Salad	Serving	321	250	24	19	9	80	1340

Continued.

Nutritional analysis of fast foods—cont'd

Food Name	Portion	Wt. gm	Kcal Kc	Prot gm	Carb gm	Fat gm	Chol mg	Sod mg
Long John Silver-Rice Pilaf	Serving	142	210	5	43	2	0	570
Long John Silver-Seafood Platter	Serving	400	970	30	109	46	70	1540
Long John Silver-Seafood Salad	Serving	337	270	16	36	7	90	670
Long John Silver-Seafood Salad-Scoop	Serving	142	210	14	26	5	90	570
Long John Silver-Shrimp & Fish Dinner	Serving	348	770	25	85	37	80	1250
Long John Silver-Shrimp Fish & Chicken	Serving	380	840	31	89	40	80	1450
Long John Silver-Shrimp Scampi	Serving	529	610	25	87	18	220	2120
McDonalds-Apple Bran Muffin	Serving	85	190	5	46	0	0	230
McDonalds-Apple Danish	Slice	115	390	5.8	51.2	17.9	25.7	370
McDonalds-Apple Pie	Serving	83	260	2.2	30	14.8	0	240
McDonalds-Bacon and Egg Biscuit	Serving	156	440	17.5	33.3	26.4	253	1230
McDonalds-Bacon Bits	Serving	3	16	1.3	0.1	1.19	0	95
McDonalds-Barbeque (Barbecue) Sauce	Serving	32	50	0.3	12.1	0.5	0	340
McDonalds-Biscuit with Spread	Serving	75	260	4.6	31.9	12.7	1	730
McDonalds-Chef Salad	Serving	283	230	20.5	7.5	13.3	128	490
McDonalds-Chicken McNuggets-6 Piece	Serving	113	290	19	16.5	16.3	65	520
McDonalds-Chocolate Milkshake-Lowfat	Serving	293	320	11.6	66	17	10	240
McDonalds-Chunky Chicken Salad	Serving	250	140	23.1	5.3	3.4	78	230
McDonalds-Cinnamon and Raisin Danish	Item	110	440	6.4	57.5	21	34.7	430
McDonalds-Cookie-Chocolaty	Serving	56	330	4.2	41.9	15.6	4	280
McDonalds-Cookie-McDonaldLand	Serving	56	290	4.2	47.1	9.2	0	300
McDonalds-Croutons	Serving	11	50	1.39	6.8	2.17	0	140
McDonalds-English Muffin	Serving	59	170	5.4	26.7	4.6	9	270
McDonalds-French Fries-Large	Serving	122	400	5.61	45.9	21.6	16	200

McDonalds-French Fries-Medium	Serving	97	320	4.44	36.3	17.1	12	150
McDonalds-French Fries-Regular Order	Serving	68	220	3.13	25.6	12	9	110
McDonalds-Garden Salad	Serving	213	110	7.1	6.2	6.6	83	160
McDonalds-Hashbrown Potato	Serving	55	130	1.4	14.9	7.3	9	330
McDonalds-Honey Sauce	Serving	14	45	0	11.5	0	0	0
McDonalds-Hot Cakes with Syrup	Serving	176	410	8.2	74.4	9.2	21	640
McDonalds-Hot Caramel Sundae	Serving	174	270	6.6	59.3	2.8	13	180
McDonalds-Hot Fudge Sundae	Serving	169	240	7.3	50.5	3.2	6	170
McDonalds-Hot Mustard Sauce	Serving	30	70	0.5	8.2	3.6	5	250
McDonalds-Iced Cheese Danish	Serving	110	390	7.4	42.3	21.8	47	420
McDonalds-McChicken Sandwich	Serving	190	490	19.2	39.8	28.6	42.6	780
McDonalds-McDLT Hamburger	Item	234	580	26.3	36	36.8	109	990
McDonalds-McLean Deluxe Hamburger	Serving	206	320	33	35	10	60	670
McDonalds-Milkshake-Chocolate-Lowfat	Serving	293	320	12	66	2	10	240
McDonalds-Milkshake-Strawbery-Lowfat	Serving	293	320	11	67	1	10	170
McDonalds-Milkshake-Vanilla-Lowfat	Serving	293	290	11	60	1	10	170
McDonalds-Pork Sausage	Serving	48	180	8.4	0	16.3	48	350
McDonalds-Raspberry Danish	Item	117	410	6.1	61.5	15.9	26	310
McDonalds-Salad Dressing-Peppercorn	Ounce	28.4	160	0	2	18	14	170
McDonalds-Salad Dressing-Red French	Ounce	28.4	80	0	10	4	0	220
McDonalds-Sausage and Egg Biscuit	Item	180	520	19.9	32.6	34.5	275	1250
McDonalds-Sausage Biscuit	Item	123	440	13	31.9	29	49	1080
McDonalds-Sausage McMuffin	Item	117	370	16.5	27.3	21.9	64	830
McDonalds-Sausage McMuffin with Egg	Item	167	440	22.6	27.9	26.8	263	980
McDonalds-Scrambled Eggs	Serving	98	140	12.4	1.2	9.8	399	290
McDonalds-Side Salad	Serving	115	60	3.7	3.3	3.3	41	85

Continued.

Nutritional analysis of fast foods—cont'd

Food Name	Portion	Wt, gm	Kcal Kc	Prot gm	Carb gm	Fat gm	Chol mg	Sod mg
McDonalds-Strawberry Milkshake-Lowfat	Serving	293	320	10.7	67	1.3	10	170
McDonalds-Strawberry Sundae	Serving	171	210	5.7	49.2	1.1	5	95
McDonalds-Sweet and Sour Sauce	Serving	32	60	0.2	13.8	0.2	0	190
McDonalds-Vanilla Milkshake-Lowfat	Serving	293	290	10.8	60	1.3	10	170
McDonalds-Vanilla-Frozen Yogurt	Serving	80	100	4	22	0.75	3	80
Pizza-Beef/Chicken/Onion	Ounce	28.3	72.6	5.53	7.23	2.38	—	267
Pizza-Beef/Onion	Ounce	28.3	72.9	4.34	7.88	2.66	—	132
Pizza-Chicken Curry/Peas	Ounce	28.3	81.6	3.74	9.41	3.23	—	146
Pizza-Chicken/Mushroom/Tomato	Ounce	28.3	60.7	4.9	7.31	1.3	—	167
Pizza-Chicken/Pineapple	Ounce	28.3	80.5	4.22	6.32	4.25	—	267
Pizza-Combination Supreme	Ounce	28.3	50.5	4.14	7.09	0.625	5.66	165
Pizza-Curry Beef/Peas	Ounce	28.3	70.6	4.51	7.31	2.58	8.33	130
Pizza-Onion/Tomato/Green Pepper/Mushroom	Ounce	28.3	45.4	3.49	6.58	0.567	—	136
Pizza-Pepperoni/Beef/Salami/Mushroom/Etc	Ounce	28.3	83.3	5.07	4.56	4.96	—	367
Pizza-Shrimp/Cucumber	Ounce	28.3	68.6	4.45	6.83	2.61	—	143
Pizza-Shrimp/Squid/Mushroom	Ounce	28.3	70.3	4.96	7.43	2.3	—	160
Potatoes-French Fried-Fast Food	Ounce	28.3	91.3	1.08	10.3	5.07	2.76	17
Potatoes-Mashed-Fast Food	Ounce	28.3	26.4	0.624	5.44	0.227	0.544	82.2
RAX-Grilled Chicken Sandwich	Item	190	440	24	36	19	87.9	1050
Salad-Fast Food	Ounce	28.3	33.5	0.454	3.29	2.04	—	128
Spaghetti-Vegetables/Sauce/Cheese	Ounce	28.3	28.3	3.8	3.01	0.113	—	83.6
Subway Sandwich-Ham and Cheese-on Wheat	Item	194	673	39	86	22	73	2508
Subway-BMT Sandwich-on Honey Wheat Roll	Item	220	1011	45	88	57	133	3199
Subway-BMT Sandwich-on Italian Roll	Item	213	982	44	83	55	133	3139

Subway-Club Sandwich on Honey Wheat	Item	220	722	47	89	23	84	2777
Subway-Club Sandwich-on Italian Roll	Item	213	693	46	83	22	84	2717
Subway-Cold Cut Combo Sandwich-Italian	Item	184	853	46	83	40	166	2218
Subway-Cold Cut Combo Sandwich-on Wheat	Item	191	883	48	88	41	166	2278
Subway-Ham & Cheese Sandwich-on Italian	Item	184	643	38	81	18	73	1710
Subway-Meatball Sandwich-on Italian Roll	Item	215	918	42	96	44	88	2022
Subway-Meatball-on Honey Wheat Roll	Item	224	947	44	101	45	88	2082
Subway-Roast Beef Sandwich-Italian Roll	Item	184	689	42	84	23	83.3	2288
Subway-Roast Beef Sandwich-on Wheat Roll	Item	189	717	41	89	24	75	2348
Subway-Salad Dressing-Buttermilk Ranch	Serving	56.7	348	1	2	37	6	492
Subway-Salad Dressing-Lite Italian	Serving	56.7	23	1	4	1	0	952
Subway-Seafood/Crab Sandwich-on Italian	Item	210	986	29	94	57	56	1967
Subway-Seafood/Crab Sandwich-on Wheat	Item	219	1015	31	100	58	56	2027
Subway-Spicy Italian Sandwich-on Italian	Item	213	1043	42	83	63	137	2282
Subway-Steak & Cheese Sandwich-Italian	Item	213	765	43	83	32	82	1556
Subway-Turkey Breast Sandwich-Wheat Roll	Item	192	674	42	88	20	67	2520
Taco Bell-Double Beef Burrito Supreme	Item	255	457	23.6	41.7	21.8	56.8	1053
Taco Bell-Enchirito	Item	213	382	19.8	30.9	19.7	54.2	1243
Taco Bell-Mexican Pizza	Serving	223	575	21.3	39.7	36.8	52	1031
Taco Bell-Nachos	Serving	106	346	7.49	37.5	18.5	8.82	399
Taco Bell-Nachos Bellgrande	Serving	287	649	21.6	60.6	35.3	36.3	997
Taco Bell-Pintos & Cheese	Serving	128	190	8.97	19	8.72	16.2	642
Taco Bell-Soft Taco	Serving	92.1	228	11.8	17.9	11.8	31.8	516
Taco Bell-Taco Bellgrande	Item	163	355	18.3	17.7	23.1	55.9	472
Taco Bell-Taco Light	Item	170	410	19	18.1	28.8	55.6	594
Taco Bell-Taco Salad with Salsa/No Shell	Serving	530	520	30.6	30	31.4	79.8	1431

Continued.

Nutritional analysis of fast foods—cont'd

Food Name	Portion	Wt. gm	Kcal Kc	Prot gm	Carb gm	Fat gm	Chol mg	Sod mg
Taco Bell-Taco Salad with Salsa/Shell	Serving	595	941	36	63.1	61.3	80.4	1662
Taco Bell-Taco Salad-No Salsa-No Shell	Serving	530	502	29.5	26.3	31.3	79.8	1056
Wendys-Bacon and Cheese Potato	Serving	347	450	15	57	18	10	1125
Wendys-Big Classic-Quarter Pound Burger	Serving	277	570	27	46	33	85	1075
Wendys-Broccoli and Cheese Potato	Serving	377	400	9	59	16	0	470
Wendys-Cheese Potato	Serving	348	470	13	57	21	0	580
Wendys-Cheese Sauce	Serving	56	40	1	5	2	0	300
Wendys-Cheese Tortellini/Spaghetti Sauce	Serving	112	120	4	24	1	5	280
Wendys-Chicken Club Sandwich	Serving	231	500	30	42	24	75	950
Wendys-Chicken Salad	Serving	56	120	7	4	8	0	215
Wendys-Chili	Serving	255	220	21	23	7	45	750
Wendys-French Fries-Regular Size	Serving	134	440	5	53	23	25	265
Wendys-Kidsmeal Hamburger	Serving	104	260	14	30	9	35	545
Wendys-Refried Beans	Serving	56	70	4	10	3	0	215
Wendys-Seafood Salad	Serving	56	110	4	7	7	0	455
Wendys-Single CheeseBurger/Everything	Serving	252	490	29	35	27	90	1155
Wendys-Single Hamburger/Everything	Serving	234	420	25	35	21	70	865
Wendys-Spanish Rice	Serving	56	70	2	13	1	0	440
Wendys-Taco Salad with Taco Chips	Serving	791	660	40	46	37	35	1110
Wendys-Tuna Salad	Serving	56	100	8	4	6	0	290

Labeling: What's Old and What's New

What's old?	What's new?	Terms with legal definitions		
		What's old?		What's new?
Label information	**Label information**	**Terms with legal definitions**		**Terms with legal definitions**
Serving size (set by manufacturer)	Serving size (set by federal government)	Low kcalorie		Kcalorie free
		Reduced kcalorie		Sugar free
Servings per container	Servings per container	Diet		Sodium free (salt free)
Kcalories (total per serving)	Kcalories (total per serving)	Low sodium		Low sodium
	Kcalories from fat (total per serving)	Sodium free		Very low sodium
		Very low sodium		Low kcalorie
Protein, carbohydrate, fat (g per serving)	Protein, carbohydrate, fat (g per serving)	Reduced sodium		High
	Saturated fat (g per serving)			Source of
	Cholesterol (mg per serving)			Reduced
	Complex carbohydrates (g per serving)			Light
				Less
	Sugars (g per serving)			More
	Dietary fiber (g per serving)			Fat free
				Low fat
				Reduced fat

Continued.

From Williams SR: *Nutrition and diet therapy*, ed 7, St Louis, 1993, Mosby.

Labeling: what's old and what's new—cont'd

What's old?	What's new?	What's old?	What's new?
Sodium (mg per serving)	Sodium (mg per serving)		Low in saturated fat Reduced saturated fat Cholesterol free Low in cholesterol Reduced cholesterol Fresh Freshly
Percentage of USRDA for: Protein, vitamin A, vitamin C, Thiamine, riboflavin, niacin, cal- cium, and iron	Vitamin A (µg per serving) Vitamin C (mg per serving) Calcium (mg per serving) Iron (mg per serving) Percentage of daily recommended amount for: Total fat, saturated fat, unsatu- rated fat, cholesterol, total carbo- hydrates, complex carbohydrates, sugars, dietary fiber, sodium, po- tassium, vitamin A, vitamin C, calcium, and iron		

Definitions of FDA Food Labeling Terms

High (rich in, excellent source): contains ≥20% of recommended daily intake for the nutrient

Good source: contains 10%-19% of the daily value/serving for a desirable nutrient

More (fortified, enriched, added): contains ≥10% of daily value for protein, vitamins, minerals, dietary fiber, or dietary potassium than the reference food; may not be used as a claim on meat or poultry items

Low (little, few, low source): foods that can be eaten in reasonable amount without exceeding dietary guidelines

Low calorie: ≤40 kcal/serving

Low fat: ≤3 g/serving; low saturated fat: ≤1 g/serving and <15% of calories from saturated fat

Low cholesterol: ≤20 mg/serving

Low sodium: ≤140 mg/serving; very low sodium: ≤35 mg/serving

Free (without, no, zero): contains very small or insignificant amounts of one or more of the following—fat, saturated fat, cholesterol, sodium, sodium/salt, sugars, or calories

Light/lite: one-third fewer calories or 50% less fat; also may be used to describe texture or color (must be specified on label)

Reduced, less, fewer: food has been changed to contain at least 25% less of a nutrient or calories than the reference food

Lean: <10 g fat, <4 g saturated fat, <95 mg cholesterol/serving per 100 g of meats, poultry, seafood, or game meats

Extra lean: <5 g fat, <2 g saturated fat, <95 mg cholesterol per 100 g of meats, poultry, seafood, or game meats

Fresh: raw or unprocessed food never frozen, heated, or preserved (milk and bread excepted)

Fresh frozen: allowed on foods that have been quickly frozen while fresh

---

Modified from American Dietetic Association: *Understanding food labels* [pamphlet], Chicago, 1993, The Association. In Phipps WJ et al: *Medical-surgical nursing: concepts and clinical practice,* ed 5, St Louis, 1995, Mosby.

Selected Examples of Bacterial Foodborne Disease

Foodborne disease	Causative organisms (genus and species)	Food source	Symptoms and course
Bacterial food infections			
Salmonellosis	Salmonella S. typhi S. paratyphi	Milk, custards, egg dishes, salad dressings, sandwich fillings, polluted shellfish	Mild to severe diarrhea, cramps, vomiting. Appears 12-24 hours or more after eating; lasts 1-7 days.
Shigellosis	Shigella S. dysenteriea	Milk and milk products, seafood, salads	Mild diarrhea to fatal dysentery (especially in young children). Appears 7-36 hours after eating; lasts 3-14 days.
Listeriosis	Listeria L. monocytogenes	Soft cheese, poultry, seafood, raw milk, meat products (paté)	Severe diarrhea, fever, headache, pneumonia, meningitis, endocarditis. Symptoms begin after 3-21 days.
Bacterial food poisoning			
(enterotoxins) (Staphylococcal	Staphylococcus S. aureus	Custards, cream fillings, processed meats, ham, cheese, ice cream, potato salad, sauces, casseroles	Severe abdominal pain, cramps, vomiting, diarrhea, perspiration, headache, fever, prostration. Appears suddenly 1-6 hours after eating; symptoms subside generally within 24 hours.

Bacterial food poisoning—cont'd

Clostridial Perfringens enteritis	Clostridium *C. perfringens*	Cooked meats, meat dishes held at warm or room termperature	Mild diarrhea, vomiting. Appears 8-24 hours after eating; lasts a day or less
Botulism	*C. botulinum*	Improperly homecanned foods; smoked and salted fish, ham, sausage, shellfish	Symptoms range from mild discomfort to death within 24 hours; initial nausea, vomiting, weakness, dizziness, progressing to motor and sometimes fatal breathing paralysis.

From Williams SR: *Nutrition and diet therapy,* ed 7, St Louis, 1993, Mosby.

Food Safety

Food contaminated with bacteria, viruses, or parasites can cause illness. The following tips are designed to help you guard against contaminated food. **Wash hands with soap before and after handling food.** Most food contamination happens at home.

Commercially Packaged Food

The U.S. government has strict standards aimed at protecting the consumer from improperly canned and packaged foods. Even so, contaminated foods occasionally find their way to the grocery shelves. Observe the following guidelines and remember: **If in doubt, throw it out! Do not even taste a small amount.**

- Do not buy containers that appear to have been opened or have broken seals on jar lids.
- Do not buy or use cans that have bulging ends, leaks, or rust.
- Do not use food that shows spoilage, such as mold, an off-color, or an off-odor. A can that spurts liquid when opened is unsafe.
- Be sure to refrigerate a jar after opening it if the label so instructs.

Home Canned Foods

Home canning requires following very precise methods of preparing the food, using the proper kind of jars, and sealing the jars carefully. Nonacid foods are especially susceptible to the bacteria responsible for botulism. (Note: Nonacid foods include all vegetables, tomatoes, meat, poultry, and fish.) Pressure canning using 10 pounds of pressure at 240° F is the only method recommended for nonacid foods. The botulism bacteria does not cause an odor, a change in color or texture, or the formation of gas. **Never taste home-canned nonacid food before first cooking!** To cook nonacid home-canned foods, vigorously boil in an uncovered pot (vegetables for 3 to 5 minutes, meat, poultry, and fish for 10 minutes).

Meat and Poultry

Salmonella and other bacteria may be present in raw meat and poultry. Any kitchen equipment that comes in contact with raw meat or poultry should be washed thoroughly before it is used with other foods.

- Use hot water and detergent to wash utensils that have touched raw meat or poultry before using the equipment with other food.

- When cutting raw meat or poultry, use a nonporous cutting board (plastic, marble, or glass) and wash it immediately.
- Keep meat refrigerated at 35° to 40° F. Ground meats are very perishable and should be cooked (or frozen) within 24 hours after purchase. Roasts will keep for 3 or 4 days without freezing. Poultry should be eaten within 2 days. Before cooking, check the odor of meats and poultry. Do not risk it if there is an unpleasant smell. Wash hands between handling raw meat and other foods, and **cook** all meat.

Pork

Pork may contain a parasite that causes trichinosis. The only way to destroy the parasite is to cook pork thoroughly until the meat is white or grayish all the way through or registers 137° F on a meat thermometer.

Eggs

Eggs may be infected with *Salmonella* or other bacteria. Never use an egg that has an unpleasant odor or that has a cracked shell. Eat only eggs that have been cooked. Refrigerate eggs and prepared food that contain eggs (mayonnaise and other salad dressings) until ready to serve.

Milk and Dairy Products

Milk and other dairy products made from raw (unpasteurized) milk have caused tuberculosis. Buy only pasteurized dairy products.

Fish and Shellfish

Because of environmental pollution, hepatitis has been caused by eating raw oysters, and several types of bacterial food poisoning can occur from eating raw shellfish or fish. Avoid eating any uncooked fish and shellfish.

Travel outside the United States

Travelers to developing countries should not drink local water or eat uncooked vegetables. Fruits that require peeling are safe, but peel them yourself. Do not eat food from street vendors.

Acquired Immune Deficiency Syndrome
Facts About AIDS

Risk Factors for HIV Infection
Male patients

- History of homosexuality or bisexuality
- History of sexual intercourse with many different partners
- History of IV drug use
- History of sexual relations with prostitutes
- History of hemophilia
- History of sexual relations with a partner who later developed AIDS or AIDS-related complex (ARC)
- History of multiple blood transfusions (1978-1985)
- History of prostitution

Female patients

- History of sexual relations with a bisexual man
- History of sexual relations with an IV drug user
- History of sexual relations with a hemophiliac
- History of sexual relations with a partner who later developed AIDS or ARC
- History of sexual intercourse with many different partners
- History of prostitution
- History of IV drug use
- History of multiple blood transfusions (1978-1985)
- History of artificial insemination (1978-1985)

How AIDS is Transmitted

- Spread by sharing needles to inject IV drugs
- Spread during anal sex, sexual intercourse, and possibly oral sex with someone who has AIDS or is carrying the AIDS virus

Symptoms of the AIDS Patient

- Early influenza-like symptoms (swollen lymph glands, night sweats, diarrhea) with recurrent respiratory and digestive infections
- Recurrence of fungus infections
- Development of purplish skin lesions (Kaposi's sarcoma)
- Spread of Kaposi's resulting in bleeding from vital organs

From Valdiserri R: The immediate challenge of health planning for AIDS: an organizational model, *Fam Comm Health* 10(4), 1988.

- Development of non-Hodgkins lymphoma
- Recurrent infections becoming more severe
- Forgetfulness, impaired speech, tremors, seizures

Consequences of the Disease
- You can give AIDS to your sexual partner(s) or someone you share a needle with.
- AIDS cannot be cured. Most people die from the disease.
- A mother with AIDS can give it to her baby in the womb.

Lifestyle Recommendations

In 1985 the Public Health Service published several life style recommendations designed to reduce the risk of contracting AIDS. The recommendations were as follows:

1. Do not have sexual contact with persons known to have or suspected of having AIDS.
2. Do not have sex with multiple partners.
3. Do not use IV drugs.
4. Do not have sex with people who are known to inject drugs.
5. Do not use inhalant nitrites. They may play a role in regard to Kaposi's sarcoma.
6. Avoid anal intercourse.
7. Protect yourself and your partner during sexual intercourse by using condoms, avoiding oral-genital contact and open mouth kissing, and avoiding contact with body fluids (semen, blood, urine, and feces).

From Miller D: *Dimensions of community health,* ed 2, Dubuque, Iowa, 1988, William C Brown.

Guidelines for Safer Sex

Five Steps to a Healthier and Safer Sex Life
1. Use a condom every time.
   - Condoms offer the best protection against sexually transmitted infections (STIs) for people having sexual intercourse.

From Planned Parenthood Federation of America, Inc: *Sexually transmitted infections: the facts,* New York, 1995, The Federation.

> **Condoms Work!** In a 1987-1991 study of couples in which one partner had HIV, all 123 couples who used condoms every time for four years prevented transmission of HIV. In 122 couples who did not use condoms every time, 12 partners became infected.
>
> A similar 1993 study showed that using condoms every time prevented HIV transmission for all but two of 171 women with male partners with HIV. However, eight out of 55 women whose partners didn't use condoms every time became infected.

2. Talk with your partners before the heat of passion, *and use a condom every time.*
   - Partners should care about each other and be interested in one another's pleasure, comfort, and health.
   - Be open. Let your partner know your health concerns and sexual health history, and encourage your partner to be open, too.
   - Be direct. Talk about your sexual needs and expectations.
   - Be persistent. Don't let your partner remain silent on these issues.
3. Keep medically fit, *and use a condom every time.*
   - Have a checkup for STIs every year.
   - Protect your immune system. Eat well, get enough rest, and limit your use of alcohol, tobacco, and other drugs.
4. If you think you or your partner has an STI, do the following:
   - See a clinician for testing, diagnosis, and treatment.
   - Find out if your partner(s) needs to be examined and treated too.
   - Use all the medication that is prescribed since symptoms often disappear before an infection is cured.
   - Do not take anyone else's medicine, and do not share your own.
   - Do not have sex until your infection is under control, *then use a condom every time.*
5. Stay in charge, and use a condom every time.
   - Alcohol and other drugs weaken good judgment and self-control. Don't let them jeopardize your self-control.

How to Use Condoms*

Don't tear the condom while unwrapping it. Don't use one that's brittle, stiff, or sticky.

---

*From Planned Parenthood Federation of America, Inc: *Sex—safer and satisfying: A guide for the sexually active,* New York, 1996, The Federation.

Use plenty of water-based lubricant. It helps prevent rips and tears, and it increases sensitivity. Oil-based lubricants destroy latex condoms.

Use a condom only once. Have a good supply on hand.

Practice makes perfect.

- Put a drop or two of lubricant inside the condom.
- Place the rolled condom over the tip of the hard penis.
- Leave a half-inch space at the tip to collect semen.
- If uncircumcised, pull back the foreskin before rolling on the condom.
- Pinch the air out of the tip with one hand. Friction against air bubbles causes most condom breaks.
- Unroll the condom over the penis with the other hand.
- Unroll it all the way down to the base of the penis.
- Smooth out any air bubbles.
- Lubricate the outside of the condom.

Enjoy.

- Pull out before the penis softens.
- Don't spill the semen. Hold the condom against the base of the penis while pulling out.

HIV Risk Comparisons

Here are some common sex behaviors grouped according to relative risk for the transmission of HIV:

Very Low Risk

No reported cases due to the following behaviors:

- Masturbation/mutual masturbation
- Touching/massage
- Erotic massage/body rubbing
- Kissing/deep kissing
- Oral sex on a man with a condom
- Oral sex on a woman with a dental dam, plastic wrap, or cut-open condom

(Don't worry about getting vaginal secretions, menstrual flow, urine, or semen on unbroken skin away from the vulva.)

From Planned Parenthood Federation of America, Inc: *The Condom,* New York, 1995, The Federation.

Low Risk

Rare reported cases due to the following behaviors:

- Oral sex
- Vaginal intercourse with a condom or vaginal pouch
- Anal intercourse with a condom or vaginal pouch

(Try not to get semen or blood into the mouth or on broken skin.)

High Risk

Millions of reported cases due to the following behaviors:

- Vaginal intercourse without a condom
- Anal intercourse without a condom

Some of the Drugs that Encourage Taking Risks with Sex

- Alcohol
- Poppers
- Cocaine
- Ecstasy
- Speed
- Marijuana
- Crack cocaine

Some of the Feelings that Encourage Taking Risks with Sex

- Desire to be swept away
- Fear of losing a partner
- Insecurity
- Embarrassment
- Anger
- Shame
- Low self-esteem
- Need to be loved

Practicing Safer Sex

What Does It Mean to Practice "Safer Sex"?

The term "safer sex" refers to the practice of protecting yourself against sexually transmitted diseases (STDs), sometimes referred to as venereal disease (VD). There are at least 50 different kinds of STDs, some of them even life-threatening. You can catch an STD by having sex with someone who is infected.

What If I Have Sex without Actually Having Intercourse?

You can still get an STD without having vaginal intercourse or penetration. STDs are spread by having vaginal, oral, or anal sex with an infected person. STD-causing germs can pass from one person to another through body fluids such as semen, vaginal fluid, saliva, and blood; genital warts and herpes are STDs that are spread by direct contact with a wart or blister.

No One I Date Looks to Me As If They Could Have an STD. They Look Really Healthy.

You can't tell if a person has an STD just by appearance. In fact, some people with STDs have no signs at all and may not even know they are infected. Still, some signs to look for in your partner are a heavy discharge, rash, sore, or redness near your partner's sex organs. If you see any of these, don't have sex or be sure to use a condom.

How Can I Tell If I Might Have an STD?

You may have an STD if you experience the following: burning or pain when urinating; sores, bumps, or blisters near the genitals or mouth; swelling around the genitals; fever, chills, night sweats, or swollen glands; or tiredness, vomiting, diarrhea, or sore muscles. In addition, you may have any of the following: an unusual discharge or smell from the vagina; burning and itching around the vagina; pain in the lower abdomen; vaginal pain during sex; or vaginal bleeding between periods. *But don't forget, you may not have any warning signs at all. Regular medical checkups are essential to your health. If you have sex with more than one partner, routine cultures and blood tests may be needed.*

I Think I Have an STD! What Should I Do?

Get help right away. If you don't, you may pass the STD to your partner or, if you're pregnant, to your baby. In fact, without treatment an STD may make it impossible for you to have a baby at all. You may also develop brain damage, blindness, cancer, heart disease, or arthritis. In some cases you can even die. So go to a doctor or clinic right away.

If your health care provider determines that you do have an STD, tell your partner or partners to get tested too. Take all of your medication; don't stop just because all your symptoms go away. Do not have sex until you have received full treatment. The disease could still be present in your body. Finally, keep all your appointments, and always use a condom and spermicide when you have sex.

What Are the Signs of STDs?

There are many different kinds of STDs, and some of them have similar symptoms. You should never attempt to make a diagnosis on your own. The nurse can give you a list with general descriptions of a few of the most common STDs.

How Can I Reduce My Chances of Contracting an STD?

Remember, the more sexual partners you have, the greater your risk. Naturally, the best way to reduce your risk is by not having sex or by having sex with one mutually faithful, uninfected partner, or by using a latex condom and spermicide with nonoxynol 9 during sex. Some STDs may be avoided by placing spermicide in the vagina before having sex, because it kills sperm and some STD germs. It helps to urinate and wash after sex (but do not douche, because douching may actually force germs higher up into the body). Avoid having sex with someone who uses intravenous drugs or engages in anal sex. Don't engage in oral, anal, or vaginal sex with an infected person. If you think you may be at risk for AIDS or an STD, seek medical help immediately. Use a new condom each time you have sexual intercourse. *Recent research indicates that the prevention of HIV transmission and developing AIDS is not 100% effective when using condoms as a barrier against this infection.*

What If the Condom Breaks? What Should We Do?

If a condom breaks, do not douche. Insert more spermicide into the vagina right away. Men should wash their genitals immediately. Go to a doctor or clinic for an STD examination as soon as possible.

Center for Disease Control Classification System for HIV-Infected Clients

Group	Classification and description
I	Acute HIV infection: Clients with transient signs and symptoms of HIV infection.
II	Asymptomatic HIV infection: Clients without previous signs or symptoms leading to classification in Group III or IV.
III	Persistent generalized lymphadenopathy (PGL): Clients with lymph nodes >1 cm in diameter that persisted for longer than 3 months at two or more extrainguinal sites.
IV	Other HIV disease: *Subgroup A (constitutional disease):* clients with one or more of the following: fever for longer than 1 month, involuntary weight loss>10%, diarrhea for longer than 1 month. *Subgroup B (neurological disease):* clients with dementia, myelopathy, or peripheral neuropathy. *Subgroup C (secondary infectious disease):* clients diagnosed with infectious disease from the following categories: *Category C-1:* 1 of 12 specified diseases listed in the CDC surveillance definition of AIDS-*Pneumocystis carinii* pneumonia, chronic cryptosporidosis, toxoplasmosis, extraintestinal strongyloidiasis, isosporiasis, candidiasis (esophageal, bronchial, or pulmonary), cryptococcosis, histoplasmosis, mycobacterial infection with *Mycobacterium avium* complex or *M. kansasii,* cytomegalovirus infection, chronic mucocutaneous or disseminated herpes simplex virus infection, and progressive multifocal leukoencephalopathy. *Category C-2:* symptomatic or invasive disease with oral, hairy leukoplakia, multidermatomal herpes zoster, recurrennt *Salmonella* bacteremia, nocardiosis, tuberculosis, or oral candidiasis. *Subgroup D (secondary cancers):* clients diagnosed with cancers known to be associated with HIV infection: Kaposi's sarcoma, non-Hodgkin's lymphoma (small, noncleaved lymphoma or immunoblastic sarcoma), or primary lymphoma of the brain. *Subgroup E (other conditions in HIV infection):* clients exhibiting clinical findings which may be due to HIV disease: chronic lymphoid interstitial pneumonitis, constitutional symptoms not meeting Subgroup IV-A, clients with infectious diseases not meeting Subgroup IV-C, and clients with neoplasms not meeting subgroup IV-D.

Adapted from Centers for Disease Control: Classification system for human T-lyphotropic virus type III/lymphadenopathy-associated virus infections, *MMWR* 35:334, 1986 and Raiten, DJ: Nutrition and HIV infection: a review and evaluation of the extant knowledge of the relationship between nutrition and HIV infection, *Nutr Clin Prac*6(3):1S, 1991. In Williams SR: *Nutrition and diet therapy,*ed 7. St Louis, 1993, Mosby.

Medical Treatment of HIV-Infected Clients

Evaluation for antiretroviral therapy and prophylaxis for *Pneumocystis carinii* pneumonia by monitoring T-helper lymphocyte count and clinical status.

T-cell count <500 is an indication for zidovudine

T-cell count <200 is an indication for PCP prophylaxis

History of tuberculin reactivity, TB exposure, or chest x-ray compatible with old TB should lead to evaluation for prophylaxis

Education to improve general health knowledge and to avoid possible sources of infection.

Discussion of applicable research protocols.

Regular follow-ups to alert physician to earliest signs of AIDS-related complications.

Consideration of antiretroviral therapy failure in client on prolonged treatment who develops new or recurrent symptoms and to rule out AIDS-related complications.

Adapted from Gold, JWM: HIV-1 infection: diagnosis and management, *Med Clin North Am* 76(1):1, 1992. In Williams SR: *Nutrition and diet therapy,* ed 7, St Louis, 1993, Mosby.

Toxicities of Dideoxynucleoside Drugs

AZT (azidothymidine, zidovudine, 3′-azido-2′,3′-dideoxythymidline)

Bone marrow suppression; anemia with increased mean corpuscular volume; leukopenia and thrombocytopenia often dose-limiting

Nausea and vomiting

Headache

Malaise, fatigue, fever

Myalgias

Seizures (rare, but reported to be fatal)

Confusion, tremulousness

Encephalopathy resembling Wernicke's encephalopathy

Bluish pigmentation of finger and toenails

Hepatic transaminase elevation

Stevens-Johnson syndrome

Adapted from Pluda JM, et al: Hematologic effects of AIDS therapies, *Hematol Oncol Clin North Am* 5(2):229, 1991. In Williams SR: *Nutrition and diet therapy,* ed 7, St Louis, 1993, Mosby.

ddl (dideoxyinosine, 2′,3′-dideoxyinosine)
Painful peripheral neuropathy
Sporadic pancreatitis (may be fatal)
Hyperamylasemia, hypertriglyceridemia
Headache
Insomnia, restlessness
Hepatic transaminase elevations (occasional hepatitis)
Hyperuricemia (with high doses)

ddC (dideoxycytidine, 2′,3′-dideoxycytidine)
Painful peripheral neuropathy
Aphthous stomatitis
Maculopapular rash (occasionally pseudovesicular)
Fevers
Arthralgias, edema
Thrombocytopenia

d4T (2′,3′-dideoxythymidinene, 2′,3′-dideoxy-2′,3′-didehydrothymidine)
Painful peripheral neuropathy
Anemia
Hepatic transaminase elevations

The ABCDs of Nutrition Assessment in AIDS

Biochemical Indices
- Serum proteins: albumin, prealbumin, transferrin
- Liver function test (evaluate liver function)
- Blood urea nitrogen, serum electrolytes (evaluate renal function)
- Urinary urea nitrogen excretion over 24 hours (nitrogen balance)
- Creatinine height index
- Complete blood count (evaluate for anemia)
- Fasting glucose (evaluate for hyperglycemia or hypoglycemia)

Clinical Observations
- General signs of nutritional status
- Drug effects

From Williams SR: *Nutrition and diet therapy,* ed 7, St Louis, 1993, Mosby.

Diet Evaluation

- Usual intake, current intake, restrictions, modifications (use both 24-hour recall and food diaries)
- Nutrition supplements, vitamin-mineral supplements
- Food allergies, intolerances
- Activity level (general kcal expended per day)
- Support system (care givers to help with nutrition care plan)

Environmental, Behavioral, and Psychologic Assessment

- Living situation, personal support
- Food environment, types of meals, eating assistance needed

Financial Assessment

- Medical insurance
- Income, financial support through care givers
- Current medical and other expenses
- Ability to afford food, enteral supplements, added vitamins-minerals

Planning Nutrition Care for Clients with AIDS

Type of problem	Possible causes	Patient care plan considerations
Food intake	Anorexia	Patient, caregiver roles
	Drug, food interaction	Motivation, patient decision-making
	HIV, other infection	Education, counseling
	Taste alteration	Resource materials
	Food intolerances, allergies	Nutrition supplements
	Lack of access or ability to prepare food	Vitamin, mineral supplements
	Depression	Drug or food reactions
		Special enteral or parenteral nutrition support
		Monitoring, adjustments as needed
Nutrient absorption	HIV related infections or cancers	Treatment of underlying disease or disorder
	Diminished gastric HCl secretion	Pancreatic enzymes supplement
	Altered mucosal absorbing surface	Drug or nutrient reactions
	Organ involvement: liver, pancreas, gallbladder, kidney	Special enteral-parenteral nutrition support, appropriate formula design
	Drug or nutrient interaction	Monitoring, adjustments as needed

Continued.

Adapted from Newman CF: *Practical guide for improving nutritional status in HIV-related disease,* University of California, Davis Medical School Fifth Annual Conference on Clinical Nutrition, Nutrition in the Treatment of Serious Medical Problems, Feb 28-29, 1992. In Williams SR: *Nutrition and diet therapy,* ed 7, St Louis, 1993, Mosby.

Planning nutrition care for clients with AIDS—cont'd

Type of problem	Possible causes	Patient care plan considerations
Altered metabolism, excretion	HIV infection Associated infections, diseases Drug or nutrient interactions Altered hormonal function Organ dysfunction	Review of drug dosage, schedule Modification of diet, meal pattern Treatment of infection, symptoms Review of diet nutrients, increase or decrease Special enteral-parenteral nutrition support, appropriate formula design Monitoring, adjustments as needed

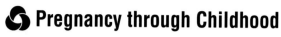 Pregnancy through Childhood

Prenatal, postnatal, and maternal-child care are important components of public/community health nursing. Through education, the nurse can promote and improve the health of pregnant women and infants. The tools on the following pages will assist in this endeavor.

Normal Discomforts Experienced during Pregnancy

Discomfort	Known or probable cause	Nursing suggestions for relief
Backache	Changes in posture, such as increased lumbar curve Excessive bending and lifting	Practice good posture Perform pelvic rocking Wear comfortable, low-heeled shoes Squat to lift Avoid prolonged sitting Sleep on firm mattress
Constipation	Pressure of enlarged uterus Slowed peristalsis caused by progesterone Side effect of iron supplement	Increase fluid intake, especially juices Eat high-fiber foods Exercise Drink warm liquids in morning Only if other methods fail, use mild laxative, stool softener, or glycerine suppository
Fatigue	Decreased metabolic rate in early pregnancy	Get full night's sleep Nap or rest during day Share work load when possible "Usually better after first trimester"
Hemorrhoids	Constipation Pressure of enlarged uterus	Relieve constipation with measures just listed Take sitz baths Use ice pack or witch hazel for local relief Reinsert hemorrhoid; do perineal tightening exercises Local preparation for analgesia

Discomfort	Cause	Prevention/Treatment
Leg cramps	Pressure of large uterus on blood vessels Fatigue or chilling Lack of calcium Sudden stretching or overextension of the foot Excessive phosphorus in diet	Take calcium supplement Practice gentle, steady stretch to relieve cramp Never massage cramping muscle Avoid toe-pointing when exercising
Leukorrhea (increased vaginal discharge)	Increased vascularity of cervix and vagina	Wear cotton crotch panties Wash genital area more frequently If infection develops, have physician treat Do not douche
Nausea and vomiting (may occur any time of day)	Increase in estrogen and progesterone levels Change (especially lowering) of blood glucose level	Eat small, frequent meals Eat dry cracker before getting up in morning Snack at bedtime Usually stops after first trimester
Urinary frequency (day and night)	Pressure of uterus on bladder in first and third trimesters Nocturia caused by increased venous return from extremities when lying down	(Explanation of why frequency is occurring) If interfering with sleep, reduce fluids in evening Rest during day
Varicosities	Increased vascularity of pelvic organs Venous return slowed by pressure of uterus Familial tendency Progesterone effect in smooth muscles	Avoid knee socks and tight elastic on underwear Elevate feet for 10 to 15 minutes several times a day Avoid long periods of standing Avoid crossing legs when sitting Wear support stockings

From Edelman CL, Mandle CL: *Health promotion throughout the lifespan*, ed 2, St Louis, 1994, Mosby.

Prenatal High-Risk Factors

Factor	Maternal implication	Fetal/neonatal implication
Social-personal		
Low income level or educational level	Poor antenatal care	Low birth weight
	Poor nutrition	Intrauterine growth retardation (IUGR)
	↑ risk of preeclampsia	
Poor diet	Inadequate nutrition	Fetal malnutrition
	↑ risk of anemia	Prematurity
	↑ risk of preeclampsia	
Living at high altitude	↑ hemoglobin	Prematurity
		IUGR
Multiparity >3	↑ risk of antepartum or postpartum hemorrhage	Anemia
		Fetal death
Weight <100 lb	Poor nutrition	IUGR
	Cephalopelvic disproportion	Hypoxia associated with difficult labor and birth
	Prolonged labor	
Weight >200 lb	↑ risk of hypertension	↓ fetal nutrition
	↑ risk of cephalopelvic disproportion	
Age <16	Poor nutrition	Low birth weight
	Poor antenatal care	↑ fetal demise
	↑ risk of preeclampsia	
	↑ risk of cephalopelvic disproportion	

Factor	Maternal Implications	Fetal/Neonatal Implications
Age >35	↑ risk of preeclampsia ↑ risk of cesarean birth	↑ risk of congenital anomalies ↑ chromosomal aberrations
Smoking one pack/day or more	↑ risk of hypertension ↑ risk of cancer	↓ placental perfusion → ↓ O_2 and nutrients available Low birth weight IUGR Preterm birth
Use of addicting drugs	↑ risk of poor nutrition ↑ risk of infection with IV drugs	↑ risk of congenital anomalies ↑ risk of low birth weight Neonatal withdrawal Lower serum bilirubin
Excessive alcohol consumption	↑ risk of poor nutrition Possible hepatic effects with long-term consumption	↑ risk of fetal alcohol syndrome
Preexisting medical disorders Diabetes mellitus	↑ risk of preeclampsia, hypertension Episodes of hypoglycemia and hyperglycemia ↑ risk of cesarean birth	Low birth weight Macrosomia Neonatal hypoglycemia ↑ risk of congenital anomalies ↑ risk of respiratory distress syndrome

Continued.

Data from Garn SM et al: Maternal hematologic levels and pregnancy outcomes, *Semin Perinatol* 5(April):155, 1981.From Olds S. London M, Ladewig P: *Maternal-newborn nursing,* ed 4, Reading, 1992, Addison-Wesley.

Prenatal high-risk factors—cont'd

Factor	Maternal implication	Fetal/neonatal implication
Cardiac disease	Cardiac decompensation Further strain on mother's body ↑ maternal death rate	↑ risk of fetal demise ↑ perinatal mortality
Anemia: <9 g/dl hemoglobin (white) <29% hematocrit (white) <8.2 g/dl hemoglobin (black) <26% hematocrit (black)	Iron deficiency anemia Low energy level ↓ oxygen-carrying capacity	Fetal death Prematurity Low birth weight
Hypertension	↑ vasospasm ↑ risk of CNS irritability → convulsions ↑ risk of CVA ↑ risk of renal damage	↓ placental perfusion → low birth weight Preterm birth
Thyroid disorder Hypothyroidism	↑ infertility ↓ basal metabolic rate, goiter, myxedema	↑ spontaneous abortion ↑ risk of congenital goiter Mental retardation → cretinism
Hyperthyroidism	↑ risk of postpartum hemorrhage ↑ risk of preeclampsia Danger of thyroid storm	↑ incidence of congenital anomalies ↑ incidence of preterm birth ↑ tendency to thyrotoxicosis

Renal disease (moderate to severe)	↑ risk of renal failure	↑ risk of IUGR ↑ risk of preterm birth
DES exposure	↑ infertility, spontaneous abortion ↑ cervical incompetence	↑ spontaneous abortion ↑ risk of preterm birth
Obstetric considerations		
Previous pregnancy Stillborn	↑ emotional/psychologic distress	↑ risk of IUGR ↑ risk of preterm birth
Habitual abortion	↑ emotional/psychologic distress ↑ possibility of diagnostic workup	↑ risk of abortion
Cesarean birth	↑ probability of repeat cesarean birth	↑ risk of preterm birth ↑ risk of respiratory distress
Rh or blood group sensitization	↑ financial expenditure for testing	Hydrops fetalis Icterus gravis Neonatal anemia Kernicterus Hypoglycemia
Large baby	↑ risk of cesarean birth ↑ risk of gestational diabetes	Birth injury Hypoglycemia

Continued.

Prenatal high-risk factors—cont'd

Factor	Maternal implication	Fetal/neonatal implication
Current pregnancy		
Rubella (first trimester)		Congenital heart disease
		Cataracts
		Nerve deafness
		Bone lesions
		Prolonged virus shedding
Rubella (second trimester)		Hepatitis
		Thrombocytopenia
Cytomegalovirus		IUGR
		Encephalopathy
Herpesvirus type 2	Severe discomfort	Neonatal herpesvirus type 2
	Concern about possibility of cesarean birth, fetal infection	Secondary hepatitis with jaundice
		Neurologic abnormalities
Syphilis	↑ incidence of abortion	↑ fetal demise
		Congenital syphilis
	↑ risk of hemorrhage	Fetal or neonatal anemia
Abruptio placenta and placenta previa	Bed rest	Intrauterine hemorrhage
	Extended hospitalization	↑ fetal demise

Preeclampsia/eclampsia (PIH)	See hypertension	↓ placental perfusion → low birth weight
Multiple gestation	↑ risk of postpartum hemorrhage	↑ risk of preterm birth ↑ risk of fetal demise
Elevated hematocrit >41% (white) >38% (black)	Increased viscosity of blood	Fetal death rate five times the normal rate
Spontaneous premature rupture of membranes	↑ uterine infection	↑ risk of preterm birth ↑ fetal demise

Risk Factors Affecting Pregnancy

Physiologic Factors

Maternal age

Parity

Late or no prenatal care

Maternal health status (conditions occurring before or during pregnancy)

    Neuromuscular disorders

    Seizures or other neurologic disorders

    Mental illness

    Cardiovascular disease, history of rheumatic heart disease

    Respiratory disease (chronic conditions, severe infections)

    Gastrointestinal disorders, liver or gallbladder disease

    Urinary tract disorders (renal disease, repeated urinary tract infections, anomalies)

    Metabolic disorders (e.g., diabetes mellitus and thyroid, pituitary and adrenal disorders)

    Blood disorders (e.g., anemias, hemoglobinopathies)

    Major anomalies of the reproductive tract

    Poor nutritional status (obesity, underweight, eating disorders, poor-quality nutrition, weight losses between visits)

    Severe skin diseases

    Malignancy

    Infections (sexually transmitted diseases and other infections)

Pregnancy-related risk factors

    Grand multiparity

    Previous pregnancy loss

    History of previous prenatal risks

    Risk of inherited disorders

    Risk of neural tube defects

    Multiple fetuses

    Vaginal bleeding

    Isoimmunization

    Lack of immunization to diseases such as rubella and hepatitis B (at-risk groups)

    Premature labor

        Risk of spontaneous abortion (first and second trimesters)

        Risk of premature delivery (second and third trimesters)

    Premature rupture of membranes

From Sherwen L, Scoloveno M, Weingarter: *Nursing care of the childbearing family,* ed 2. Norwalk, Conn., 1995, Appleton & Lange.

Ectopic pregnancy (first trimester)

Hydatidiform mole (first and second trimesters)

Preeclampsia/eclampsia (second and third trimesters, first trimester with hydatidiform mole)

Gestational diabetes

Disproportionate uterine growth, oligohydraminios, polyhyramnios

Abnormal fetal growth

Abnormal results of tests for fetal well-being

Abnormalities of placenta formation or function (infarction, previa, abruptio, infections)

Psychosocial Factors

Unwanted pregnancy

Previous obstetric loss

Real or potential high-risk condition

No previous contact with young children

Severe career–parenting conflict

Client raised with no maternal role model or with poor maternal role model

Resentment/rejection of fetus

Inability to attach to fetus

Lack of support from significant others, persistent feelings of isolation

Severe social problems affecting self and others

    Turbulent marriage

    Pending divorce

    Problems with children already in family

    Crises/catastrophe in family system

    Client, expectant father, or family member incarcerated

Abuse (current or past, physical or emotional)

Pregnancy resulting from rape (by husband or other)

Other

Socioeconomic Factors

Inability to provide basic needs for self and family

Perceived financial stress, complicated by pregnancy

Poor housing/lack of housing (homelessness)

Unemployment, threatened loss of income from usual source of support

Lifestyle Factors

Smoking

Alcohol use

Use of drugs that could affect fetus or pregnancy

Hazardous, stressful, or strenuous occupation

Number of sexual partners; sexual partners with high-risk behavior (e.g., IV users)

Environmental Factors

Potentially hazardous home environment (e.g., lack of plumbing; no potable water source; lack of heat, electricity, or other utilities; exposure to chemicals such as lead; unsafe housing structure; infestations of rodents and vermin)

Potentially hazardous work environment (e.g., exposure to teratogens or carcinogens in the workplace; occupation that requires strenuous physical activity, balance, or other)

Potentially hazardous recreational environment (e.g., swimming in polluted waters, exposure to teratogens during recreational activities)

Assessment Focus at First Prenatal Visit and Return Visits

Focus during First Prenatal Visit

Existence of pregnancy

Past and present maternal health status through health history, physical examination, and laboratory data

Risk factors for childbearing and early parenting, including physical, psychologic, and sociologic factors

Signs and symptoms of pregnancy

Well-being of embryo or fetus

Psychosocial adaptation to pregnancy

Cultural, socioeconomic, or other factors that influence health care practices

Client/family strengths and resources

Client/family educational needs

Focus during Return Visits

Maternal health status through updated health history, physical examination, and laboratory testing as indicated

Risk factors (new or ongoing)

Progress of pregnancy

Fetal well-being

From Sherwen L, Scoloveno M, Weingarter: *Nursing care of the childbearing family,* ed 2, Norwalk, Conn., 1995, Appleton & Lange.

Progression of psychosocial adaptation to pregnancy

Cultural, socioeconomic, or other factors that influence health care practices as pregnancy progresses

Client/family strengths and resources

Client/family educational needs

Nursing Strategies for Working with Childbearing Clients Experiencing Crisis and Grief

- Anticipate the potential for crisis and grief. For example, clients who receive news of a high-risk condition, particularly a condition requiring a change in lifestyle or having long-term implications, may be expected to experience crisis.
- Assess the event itself and its implications for the client's health and well-being.
- Assess the responses of the client and family in light of their religious and cultural backgrounds.
- Provide an atmosphere of privacy and confidentiality to encourage the client to express her feelings.
- Allow adequate time to discuss the high-risk condition and the family's feelings. Listen carefully, but do not make unrealistic promises, such as "Everything will turn out fine." Having another nurse temporarily "cover" other clients can allow the staff nurse the opportunity to talk uninterrupted with a client in crisis.
- Help clients identify physical, emotional, and behavioral responses related to crisis and grief. Reassure clients when responses are normal. Promptly enlist the assistance of mental health resources if a client's responses pose a threat to the health or safety of herself or others.
- Ensure that the client receives support in coping with crisis and grief. Assist the client in identifying sources of support within her own network of family and friends. Offer to speak with significant others if the client so desires. Provide the client with referrals, for example, for appropriate support groups, for telephone "hot line" assistance, for relevant counseling, or for appropriate financial aid services. Make certain that a plan for follow-up of the client experiencing crisis and grief is implemented (e.g., telephone contact at intervals or home visits if appropriate).

From Sherwen L, Scoloveno M, Weingarter: *Nursing care of the childbearing family,* ed 2, Norwalk, Conn., 1995, Appleton & Lange.

- Communicate with other health care providers directly involved in the family's care so that a consistent and supportive approach may be implemented.
- Provide a mechanism to deal with tension on the part of health care providers, such as interdisciplinary staff conferences, so that staff members can discuss their own feelings related to working with clients in crisis and grief.

Family System Changes during the Childbearing Cycle

Family system component	Change during childbearing
Structure	First pregnancy involves shift from a stable dyad to a volatile triangle. Subsequent pregnancies involve development of several complex, shifting triangular structures. Family members must occasionally cope with being the "isolate" in a triangle. Stress and tension may increase. Additional subsystems must be established: mother–child; father–child; sibling; grandparent–grandchild
Power	Patterns often alter; egalitarian power patterns often become more "traditional," with father as decision maker. Fetus and newborn may become very powerful in family system, producing major changes in parents' behavior and family patterns.
Boundaries	Mother's boundary incorporates another human within, the embryo/fetus. Becomes a "protective container" for fetus, progressively closing in and focusing her attention inward. Father's boundary must expand to give support and become empathetic with mother. Family boundary must become highly permeable to selected input, for example, health care and education.
Affect or feelings	Stress arising from structural change may alter feeling tone in family system. Danger signs are perception of hidden anger and hostility; pervasive depression; and apathy, unresponsiveness, or "flat" emotion.

From Sherwen L, Scoloveno M, Weingarter: *Nursing care of the childbearing family,* ed 2, Norwalk, Conn., 1995, Appleton & Lange.

Family system changes during the childbearing cycle—cont'd

Family system component	Change during childbearing
Intergenerational patterns and roles	Parents' parents must "move up" a generation to become grandparents. Each member of the family system (both nuclear and extended) must assume new roles, whether it is a first or subsequent pregnancy.
Communication patterns	Family members must learn to communicate as a triangle. One member needs to learn to be a temporary outsider or "isolate" left out of communications, because only two people can communicate at one time.
Cultural background and rituals	Family members from different cultural backgrounds may have different values concerning pregnancy and childbearing, may perceive new roles differently, and may have different practices and rituals for this event. Differences can produce family conflict and stress.

Parenting Tasks for Developmental Landmarks in Infancy

Age (months)	Landmark	Parenting task
1	Lifts head when prone	Place infant in prone position and dangle colorful object above head
2	Social smile	Promote by talking to infant and allowing opportunity to smile
4	Squeals	Encourage and praise for doing
5	Rolls from back to front	Place infant in protected area (crib, playpen) and encourage to move by placing toy out of reach

Continued.

From Edelman CL, Mandle CL: *Health promotion throughout the lifespan,* ed 3, St Louis, 1994, Mosby.

Parenting tasks for developmental landmarks in infancy—cont'd

Age (months)	Landmark	Parenting task
8-9	Uses pincer grasp to feed self cracker	Make finger foods available
10	Pulls self to standing position	Provide safe environment: place chair or object of appropriate height in reach
11-12	Initiates vocalization	Talk to infant frequently and include in family gatherings
12-15	Walks	Encourage and provide clutter-free, safe walkway; praise for attempts
15	Drinks from cup	Supply cup with appropriate drink; do not scold for clumsiness in handling cup or spills
18	Mimics household chores	Give rag to help with dusting, allow to fold clothes, and so on

Normal Sleep Patterns for Infants

Age (months)	Hours in 24-hour period
2-3	Low:10 Average: 16½ High: 23 (Two to four naps)
3-4	Low: 8-10 nightly High: 11-12 nightly (Two or three naps daily)
6-12	11-12 nightly (Two or three naps daily)
12-18	8-12 nightly (One or two naps daily)

From Edelman CL, Mandle CL: *Health promotion throughout the lifespan,* ed 3, St Louis, 1994, Mosby.

Visual Development Milestones during Infancy

Age (months)	Milestones
1-3	Stares at objects
	Follows light with eyes
	Looks toward sound
3-5	Fixates on objects 3 feet away
	Accommodation begins to develop
	Follows moving objects well
	Looks at and grabs objects
	Visual acuity is 20/200
5-7	Developing hand-eye coordination
	Ultimate color of iris is established
	Eye movements coordinated and mature
	Searches for fallen objects
7-12	Depth perception begins to develop
	Demonstrates interest in small objects
	Reaches for unseen object
	Visual acuity is 20/100
12-18	Looks at pictures with interest
	Able to identify forms
	Convergence becomes well established

Modified from Chinn PL: *Child health maintenance: concepts in family-centered care,* ed 2, St Louis, 1979, Mosby. From Edelman CL, Mandle CL: *Health promotion throughout the lifespan,* ed 3 St Louis, 1994, Mosby.

Progressive Auditory Development
of Infants during Infancy

Age (months)	Development
1-2	Startled by sounds (Moro reflex)
	Quiets when hears voice
	Turns head toward familiar sound
3-5	Searches for sound in room
	Stops sucking to listen
	Locates sound below ear
6-8	Reacts to changes in music volume
	Recognizes familiar sounds
9-12	Listens to talking
	Responds to simple commands
	Begins to differentiate between words
12-18	Begins to show voluntary control over responses to sound
	Begins to develop gross discrimination by learning to distinguish between sounds

Modified from Chinn PL: *Child health maintenance: concepts in family-centered care,* ed 2, St Louis, 1979, Mosby. In Edelman CL, Mandle CL: *Health promotion throughout the lifespan,* ed 3, St Louis, 1994, Mosby.

Nutritional Inadequacies during Infancy

Nutrient	Requirement	Excess	Deficiency	Sources
Water	Age 3 mo: 140-165 ml/kg 6 mo: 130-155 ml/kg 9 mo: 125-145 ml/kg 12 mo: 115-135 ml/kg	Abdominal pain, headache, water intoxication	Thirst, dehydration	Breast or formula milk
Protein	Age 6 mo: 2.2 g/kg 12 mo: 2 g/kg	Dehydration	Reduction in growth rates	Egg yolk, breast or formula milk
Fat	30%-50% of total calorie intake	Obesity, atherosclerosis, hyperlipidemia (lipemia) later in life	Dry, thickened skin; weight loss	Breast or formula milk
Carbohydrate	50-100 g/day	Obesity, dental caries, diarrhea	Ketosis, weight loss	Milk, prepared baby foods
Vitamins	5000 IU/day	Anorexia, irritability	Impaired vision; dry, scaly skin; failure to thrive	Milk, yellow vegetables
A (retinol) D	400 IU/day	Anorexia, weight loss, calcification of soft tissue	Poor bone and teeth development	Milk, sunlight (30 min/ day)

Continued.

Data from Chow MP, et al: *Handbook of pediatric primary care*, New York, 1984, Wiley; and Pipes PL: *Nutrition in infancy and childhood*, ed 4, St Louis, 1989, Mosby. In Edelman CL, Mandle CL: *Health promotion throughout the lifespan*, ed 3, St Louis, 1994, Mosby.

Nutritional inadequacies during infancy—cont'd

Nutrient	Requirement	Excess	Deficiency	Sources
C (ascorbid acid)	35 mg/day	Unknown	Coagulation problems	Citrus fruits, vegetables
B₁ (thiamine)	0.5 mg/1000 kcal	Unknown	Fatigue, insomnia	Pork, liver, wheat germ, grain, cereals, milk
B₂ (riboflavin)	0.6 mg/1000 kcal	Unknown	Skin and visual problems	Leafy vegetables, dairy products
B₆ (pyridoxine)	0.3-0.6 mg/day	Unknown	Irritability, seizures, anemia	Bananas, brewer's yeast, liver
B₁₂ (cobalamin)	0.3-1.0 mg/day	Unknown	Dyspepsia, sore tongue, fatigue	Lean meat, eggs, fish, milk
Niacin	8 mg/1000 kcal	Unknown	Pellagra, skin problems, diarrhea	Dairy products, meats, peanut butter
Minerals	360-800 mg/day	Unknown	Bone and teeth problems, growth retardation	Milk, dairy products
Calcium				
Iron	10-15 mg/day	Cardiovascular collapse	Anemia	Enriched cereals, liver, beef
Potassium	6 mEq/day	Heart block	Muscle weakness, fatigue	Meats, fish, whole-grain cereals
Sodium	6 mEq/day	Edema	Dehydration, muscle cramps, nausea and vomiting	Table salt, milk, cheese, preservatives

Development of Feeding Skills

Age	Oral and neuromuscular development	Feeding behavior
Birth	Rooting reflex	Turns mouth toward nipple or any object brushing cheek
	Swallowing reflex	Initial swallowing involves the posterior of the tongue; by 9-12 weeks anterior portion is increasingly involved, which facilitates ingestion of semisolid food
	Extrusion reflex	Pushes food out when placed on tongue; strong the first 9 weeks
	Sucking reflex	By 6-10 weeks recognizes the feeding position and begins mouthing and sucking when placed in this position
3-6 months	Beginning coordination between eyes and body movements	Explores world with eyes, fingers, hands, and mouth; starts reaching for objects at 4 months but overshoots; hands get in the way during feeding
	Learning to reach mouth with hands at 4 months	Finger sucking; by 6 months all objects go into the mouth
		Sucking reflex becomes voluntary, and lateral motions of the jaw begin
	Extrusion reflex present until 4 months	May continue to push out food placed on tongue
	Able to grasp objects voluntarily at 5 months	Grasps objects in mitten-like fashion

Continued.

From Scipien GM et al: *Comprehensive pediatric nursing*, ed 2, New York, 1979, McGraw-Hill, p 163. Used with permission.

Development of feeding skills—cont'd

Age	Oral and neuromuscular development	Feeding behavior
6-12 months	Eyes and hands working together	Can approximate lips to rim of cup by 5 months; chewing action begins; by 6 months begins drinking from cup Brings hand to mouth; at 7 months able to feed self biscuit Bangs cup and objects on table at 7 months
	Sits erect with support at 6 months Sits erect without support at 9 months Development of grasp (finger-to-thumb opposition)	Holds own bottle at 9-12 months Pincer approach to food Pokes at food with index finger at 10 months
	Relates to objects at 10 months	Reaches for food and utensils, including those beyond reach; pushes plate around with spoon Insists on holding spoon, not to put in mouth, but to return to plate or cup Increased desire to feed self
1-3 years	Development of manual dexterity	*15 months:* begins to use spoon but turns it before reaching mouth; may hold cup, likely to tilt cup rather than head, causing spilling *18 months:* eats with spoon, spills frequently, turns spoon in mouth; holds glass with both hands *2 years:* inserts spoon correctly, occasionally with one hand; holds glass; plays with food; distinguishes between food and inedible materials *2-3 years:* self-feeding complete with occasional spilling; uses fork; pours from pitcher; obtains drink of water from faucet

Feeding for the First 12 Months of Life

Month

1	2	3	4	5	6	7	8	9	10	11	12

Breast milk: nutritionally sound; believed to provide immunity; facilitates a close mother-baby relationship; decreases allergies; decreases incidence of dental caries and malocclusion

Formula: 24-32 oz/24 hr; well tolerated when breast milk is not available

Iron fortified rice cereal: source of calories, iron, and fiber; avoid wheat products first 12 months of life

Strained vegetables: source of calories, fiber, iron, vitamins A and B, and minerals; introduce yellow vegetables before green

Strained fruits: source of calories, iron, fiber, vitamin C, and minerals; will offset constipating effect of cereals

Plain lowfat yogurt: excellent source of calcium, phosphorus, vitamin B, and protein

Meats: source of protein, calories, iron, and vitamins

Finger foods: assist in teething and fine motor coordination

From Ingalls JA, Salerno MC: *Ingalls and Salerno's maternal and child health nursing*, ed 8, St Louis, 1995, Mosby.

Infant State-Related Behavior Chart

Behavior/description of behavior	Infant state consideration	Implications for caregiving
Alertness		
Widening and brightening of the eyes. Infants focus attention on stimuli, whether visual, auditory, or objects to be sucked	From drowsy or active alert to quiet alert	Infant state and timing are important. When trying to alert infants, try to do the following: 1. Unwrap infant (arms out at least). 2. Place infant in upright position. 3. Talk to infant, putting variation in your pitch and tempo. 4. Show your face to infant. 5. Elicit the rooting, sucking, or grasp reflexes.
Visual response		
Newborns have pupillary responses to differences in brightness. Infants can focus on objects or faces about 7-8 inches away. Newborns have preferences for more complex patterns, human faces, and moving objects.	Quiet alert	Newborn's visual alertness provides opportunities for eye-to-eye contact with caregivers, an important source of beginning caregiver–infant interaction.
Auditory response		
Reaction to a variety of sounds, especially in the human voice range. Infants can hear sounds and locate the general direction of the sound (if the source is constant).	Drowsy, quiet alert, active alert	Enhances communication between infants and caregivers. Crying infants can often be consoled by voice.

Irritability

How easily infants are upset by loud noises, handling by caregivers, temperature changes, removal of blankets or clothes, etc.

From deep sleep, light sleep, drowsy, quiet alert, or active alert to fussing or crying

Irritable infants need more-frequent consoling and more-subdued external environments. Parents can be helped to cope with more-irritable infants.

Readability

The cues infants give through motor behavior and activity, looking, listening, and behavior patterns.

All states

Parents need to learn that newborns' behaviors are part of their individual temperaments and not reflections on their parenting abilities. By observing and understanding an infant's characteristic pattern, parents can respond more appropriately.

Smile

Ranging from a faint grimace to a full-fledged smile; reflexive.

Drowsy, active alert, quiet alert, light sleep

Initial smile in the neonatal period is the forerunner of the social smile at 3 to 4 weeks of age. Important for caregivers to respond to it.

Continued.

Modified from Barnard KE et al: Infant state-related behavior chart. In *Early parent-infant relationships*, White Plains, N.Y., 1978 March of Dimes Birth Defects Foundation. In Bobak IM, Lowdermilk DL, Jensen MD: *Maternity nursing*, ed 4, St Louis, 1995, Mosby.

In Bobak IM, Lowermilk DL, Jensen MD: *Maternity nursing*, ed 4, St Louis, 1995, Mosby.

Infant State-Related Behavior Chart—cont'd

Behavior/description of behavior	Infant state consideration	Implications for caregiving
Habituation		
The ability to lessen one's response to repeated stimuli, seen where the Moro response is repeatedly elicited. If a noise is continually repeated, infants will usually cease to respond.	Deep sleep, light sleep, also seen in drowsy	Because of this ability, families can carry out normal activities without disturbing infants. Infants who have more difficulty with this will probably not sleep well in active environments.
Cuddliness		
Infants' response to being held. Infants nestle and work themselves into the contours of caregivers' bodies.	Primarily in awake states	Cuddliness is usually rewarding behavior for the caregivers. If infants do not nestle and mold, show the caregivers how to position infants to maximize this response.
Consolability		
Measured when infants have been crying for at least 15 seconds. The ability of infants to bring themselves or to be brought by others to a lower state.	From crying to active alert, quiet alert, drowsy, or sleep states	Crying is the infant behavior that presents the greatest challenge to caregivers. Parents' success or failure in consoling their infants has a significant impact on their feelings of competence as parents.
Self-consoling		
Maneuvers used by infants to console themselves and move to a lower state: 1. Hand-to-mouth movement 2. Sucking on fingers, fist, or tongue 3. Paying attention to voices or faces 4. Changes in position	From crying to active alert, quiet alert, drowsy, or sleep states	If caregivers are aware of these behaviors, they may allow infants the opportunity to gain control of themselves. This does not imply that newborns should be left to cry. Once newborns are crying and do not initiate self-consoling activities, they may need attention from caregivers.

Consoling by caregivers

After crying for longer than 15 seconds, the care-givers may try to:
1. Show face to infant.
2. Talk to infant in a steady, soft voice.
3. Hold both infant's arms close to body.
4. Swaddle infant.
5. Pick up infant.
6. Rock infant.
7. Give infant a pacifier or feed.

From crying to active alert, quiet alert, drowsy, or sleep states

Often parental initial reaction is to pick up infants or feed them when they cry. Parents could be taught to try other soothing maneuvers, after ascertaining that the diaper is clean and dry.

Motor behavior and activity

Spontaneous movements of extremities and body when stimulated vs. when left alone. Smooth, rhythmical movements vs. jerky ones.

Quiet alert, active alert

Smooth, nonjerky movements with periods of inactivity seem most natural. Some parents see jerky movements and startles as negative response to their caregiving and are frightened.

Common Concerns and Problems of the First Year

Problem or concern	Assessment	Nursing intervention
Burping	Swallowed air bubbles trapped in stomach; occurs more frequently in bottle-fed infants who cry during feeding.	Burp frequently during feeding (i.e., before, during, and after, or after every 1 ounce of formula or every 4-5 minutes at breast). Use upright position to burp (gently rub infant's back while baby sits on parent's knee and rests forward against parent's arm). Try to burp every 10-15 minutes while awake if not successful burping during and after feeding. Sit upright in infant seat for 30-45 minutes after feeding if awake or position with head elevated and on right side if sleeping.
Colic	Unexplained bouts of crying frequently occurring at same time of day (usually busiest) and often accompanied by abdominal distention, spasms, drawing up legs to stomach and/or passing gas. May be caused by feeding problems, maternal anxiety, allergy, and is aggravated by tension in household. Can last 3 months. Also see section on Crying.	Review basic infant needs with parents (i.e., is infant hungry, wet, does infant have air bubble, is infant in uncomfortable position). Review feeding method, technique and burping, review maternal diet for offending foods if breast-fed. Record time when colic episodes occur. Soothe and comfort before "attack." Swaddle infant (i.e., wrap warmly and in an encompassing manner). Walk, rock, and hold infant over shoulder. Try a monotonous soothing noise (music, ticking clock) or activity (ride in a car).

Crying	Periodic crying for unexplained reason; ascertain if a pattern exists for crying spells; may be related to colic; obtain a detailed history of time and length of spell; feeding frequency, method, technique and burping; stool patterns; meeting contact and sucking needs; parental handling of crying and feelings regarding crying; other household factors (e.g., siblings, relative advice, parental support of each other, presence of other symptoms and/or allergies).	Change infant position from stomach to side to back to sitting position. Rest infant on abdomen on warm hard surface (e.g., parent knee, warmed crib surface). Change household routine if indicated, create a quiet environment. Try pacifier or sugar water; if bottle fed, try soy formula. Reassure parents that infant is not ill, that they are providing good care, and that colic will definitely go away. Provide support to parents, giving them an opportunity to discuss feelings. Explain theories about origin and cycle of colic. See previous section on colic. Reinforce that babies cry for a reason. Best to respond to crying vs. letting baby cry it out. Crying is a release and/or exercise for infant. One or two periods a day of 5-10 minutes is normal for most infants. Assist parents to develop positive, relaxed approach. Reassure and support parents in this time of stress. Suggest parents alternate infant care and meeting infant demands.

Continued.

From Stanhope M, and Lancaster J: *Community health nursing: process and practice for promoting health*, ed 3, St Louis, 1992, Mosby. Developed by Nancy Dickenson Hazard.

Common concerns and problems of the first year—cont'd

Problem or concern	Assessment	Nursing intervention
Constipation	Consistency of stool that is hard, pebbly, rocklike. Not related to frequency, straining, grunting or number of days between stools. Ascertain color, consistency, frequency, and presence of blood or mucus. Review infant diet and verify parent perception of constipation and expectation of normal stool patterns.	Discuss normal elimination/stool patterns for type of feeding method (i.e., breast fed stools vs. bottle fed stools). Reassure that straining, grunting, and infrequent number are normal. Reinforce that each infant has individual stool pattern and educate parents regarding what constipation actually is (i.e., consistency). Discuss parents attitude regarding toilet habits and expectations about stool patterns. If constipated, increase liquids in diet; may offer water between meals. If introduced to solids too early or in too large a quantity, discontinue use until constipation clears, then begin again with smaller amounts. Karo syrup, 1 tsp/3 oz of water may be given several times a day. If appropriate for feeding stage, add prunes (up to 3 tbsp) or prune juice to diet.
Flatus	Air in stomach or intestines causing abdominal distress, distension, and discomfort; frequently expelled through anus. May be caused by excess swallowing of air, overfeeding, underfeeding, or allergy. Ascer-	Burp frequently during and after feedings (see first section of this table). Calm infant when crying and burp after crying. Place on left side to ease expelling of gas.

	tain details regarding feeding (e.g., frequency and size of nipple, type of bottle used, breast feeding technique, maternal diet, use of pacifier, propping of bottle, burping).	If allergies are suspected, try soy formula or elimination diet. Reassure parents.
Hiccoughs	Sudden sharp involuntary spasms of diaphragm usually occur following a meal.	Reassure parents that infant will cry if truly distressed. Offer infant something to suck (e.g., pacifier, breast, bottle with warm water).
Pacifier	Infants demonstrate a need for non–nutritional sucking.	Assist parents to understand aspects of positive and negative use of pacifier. Positive use: indicated immediately after birth before newborn can manipulate thumb into mouth; assists in developing sucking function; contributes to establishment of breast feeding; good means of satisfying sucking need especially for bottle-fed infants who need extra sucking time; does not usually become a habit unless child sucks beyond infancy; most infants substitute thumb for pacifier around 3-4 months. Parents should look for clues to eliminate pacifier use at this time and provide stimulation suitable for the age. Negative use: pacifiers do not replace parent holding the baby; stimulation, or needs satisfaction; pacifiers should not be used constantly, especially before tending to infants needs; parents should be encouraged to discontinue use by age 5 months since continued use may become hard to overcome.

Continued.

Common concerns and problems of the first year—cont'd

Problem or concern	Assessment	Nursing intervention
Pacifier—cont'd		If thumb is substituted, it generally is used less frequently than pacifier.
Spoiling	Ascertain parent definition of spoiling. Generally it is the result of basic needs not being met in early infancy leading to a demanding, undisciplined child because the need for gratification continues beyond normal time; overgratification usually occurs then. It generally is believed that infants cannot be spoiled under 6 months of age.	Parents require counseling and education that reinforces the following: Early infant needs must be gratified. A child cannot handle frustrations well until the age of 8-9 months, and is unable to delay gratification of needs until this age. A gradual and gentle approach to limits and delaying gratification is best. A relaxed, positive approach is helpful. Parents often find support groups helpful in dealing with this problem.
Biting	In first year, it is frequently related to teething. It is particularly a problem for breast-feeding mothers. In toddlers it is related to normal aggressive impulses.	If related to teething, see section on teething later in this table for alleviation of discomfort. Breast-feeding mothers should remove infant from breast at every occurrence and may accompany with a "no"; should also allow time to lapse before finishing feeding.

Separation anxiety	Occurs at 9-10 months as infant is learning to differentiate self from mother. Can occur again in toddlerhood as child is learning to distance and separate self from mother in attempt to establish autonomy.	Reassure mother that this is a normal developmental process. Advise parents, especially mother, to do the following: • Play "peek-a-boo" games. • Allow sufficient time (30-45 minutes) for child to acquaint himself or herself with new person (e.g., visitor, babysitter). • Avoid "sneaking out." Tell child firmly that "mommy leaves, mommy comes back." Reinforce this with "peek-a-boo" or "hide and seek" games. • Avoid making major changes in child's or household routines during this period (e.g., mother returning to work; changing child's room, changing regular babysitter or day care situation).
Stranger anxiety	Begins at 6-8 months and gradually diminishes by 18 months. Process of child development.	See preceding section on separation anxiety. Advise parents, particularly mother, to hold infant in presence of strangers. If infant is to be left, mother should spend a short time with stranger.
Infant sleep patterns	Some infants have difficulty releasing into sleep or awaken easily. Separation anxiety, teething, and illness are among the common causes. Ascertain history of problem to include how long infant sleeps, what the feeding schedule is, bedtime and household routines, the presence of illness or teething, and how the problem is handled.	Counseling should be directed toward education of the parents; infants need gratification and normal sleep patterns, emphasizing the following: • Differences in temperament and incidence of sleep problems can be related. • Infants generally sleep through the night by age 3 months.

Continued.

Common concerns and problems of the first year—cont'd

Problem or concern	Assessment	Nursing intervention
Infant sleep patterns—cont'd		• Infant may need help getting to sleep by rocking, holding, pacifier, walking, etc. • Environment and atmosphere conducive to sleep (e.g., quiet and dim) should be provided. • If sleep problem is related to a physical problem, measures to remedy this should be implemented.
Teething	Eruption of primary or deciduous teeth starting at about 6 months, usually with lower incisors; will continue every 2 months for first 2 years. Signs which maybe included, but are not always present: red, swollen gums, irritability, crying and rubbing gums. Since other events in infant development are occurring simultaneously, nurse must help parents distinguish between these and teething as follows: • Drooling, which normally occurs at 3 to 4 months and has little to do with teething, although it may persist throughout teething. • Fever does not usually accompany teething; must be assessed separately because maternal antibody protection is diminishing and presence of fever is suspect for infectious process. • Separation anxiety, sleep disturbances, or fussiness from other causes are all common development	Recommend to parents hard, clean objects for baby to chew on (e.g., rubber teething rings, beads, hard rubber toys, a cool spoon, teething biscuits, or pretzels). Parents should avoid use of teething toys or rings filled with liquid because plastic covers are easily broken and liquid can be ingested.

Diaper rashes	symptoms associated with the infant age group, as is reaching for and mouthing objects.	Preventive measures to keep the diaper area clean, dry, and aerated including the following:
	Rashes of various types occurring in diaper area. Persistent rashes which do not respond to home management, or which continue to occur despite preventive measures, should be referred to the appropriate care provider for medical evaluation.	• Diapers should be changed frequently.

Preventive measures to keep the diaper area clean, dry, and aerated including the following:

- Diapers should be changed frequently.
- Cleanse with water (and mild soap after bowel movement) at each changing; dry area well.
- Thick diapers and/or absorbent pads are recommended; plastic or rubber pants are not.
- A *thin* film of lubrication, such as A and D ointment or petroleum jelly, may be used.
- Remove diapers for short periods every day.

Wash diapers well as follows:

1. Soak soiled diapers in Borateen or borax solution (½ cup to 1 gallon of water).
2. Prerinse before washing.
3. Wash in full cycle with mild soap, such as Ivory, Dreft, or Lux.
4. Avoid softeners and strong detergents.
5. Rinse diapers 2 to 3 times, and ¼ to ½ cup vinegar may be added to final rinse.
6. Dry in sun if possible. Home management of diaper rash includes the following:
   - Follow preventive measures with an emphasis on leaving diaper off more frequently, changing when wet, and cleaning area thoroughly during changes.

Continued.

Common concerns and problems of the first year—cont'd

Problem or concern	Assessment	Nursing intervention
Diaper rashes—cont'd		• Zinc oxide ointment often is helpful in checking early nonfungal rashes. • Cornstarch is never recommended for rashes or their prevention. • Seek medical help if rash worsens or does not improve.
Cradle cap	Form of seborrheic dermatitis in neonate characterized by scalping, flaking of scalp skin especially over anterior fontanelle. May persist beyond neonatal age into infancy.	Preventive measures include the following: • Teach parents how to shampoo infant head and recommend shampooing every other day. • Reassure that vigorous scrubbing will not injure fontanelle or skull. Home management for mild cases: • Shampoo head daily with warm water and soap, using firm pressure on scalp. • Loosen cap by applying mineral or baby oil to scalp 15 to 20 minutes before shampooing. Remove with shampoo. • Comb scalp with fine comb to loosen and dislodge scaly cap. • Severe cases will require medical attention, and are generally managed with antiseborrheic shampoos.

Problems related to feeding

Parental concerns about overfeeding or underfeeding

Some parents find it difficult to determine the appropriate amount of milk and/or solid food to give an infant. Ascertain parents' understanding, knowledge, and perceptions through the following:
- Diet history
- Height and weight measurement and charting on growth curve
- Elimination habits and description

Assist parents in constructing a workable feeding schedule.

Discuss normal feeding pattern for breast and bottle fed infants.

Discuss infants needs for non-nutrient sucking.

Convey that infants will eat more than they need or require if food is offered at each cry.

Offer water between feedings to postpone next feeding to a reasonable time.

Suggest a schedule of solid food introduction.

Reassure parents that if infant is gaining weight, he or she is not underfed.

Explain growth and appetite spurts.

Refusal of solids

Infant may refuse new foods for a number of reasons (e.g., temperature, texture, manner presented by person feeding, or too-early introduction). Ascertain through diet history which foods accepted, and likes and dislikes and parental feelings and perception regarding solid foods.

Discuss normal feeding patterns for age.

Review the following indications for starting or not starting solid foods:
- No need for solid foods before 4 to 6 months.
- Digestion begins with salivation around 4 months.
- Feeding of solid foods is not necessarily related to sleeping through the night.
- Tongue thrusting of solid food is normal and not a refusal.

Continued.

Common concerns and problems of the first year—cont'd

Problem or concern	Assessment	Nursing intervention
Refusal of solids—cont'd		Discuss ways to encourage solid food acceptance. Some examples follow: • Allow infant to feed self. • Avoid forcing infant to eat since this will only increase resistance. • Solids may be stopped for a while, offering only ones that infant likes. • Offer solid foods before milk when infant is hungriest. • Offer food in a calm, positive manner.
Refusal of food and variations in appetite	Once solid foods have been introduced and established, infants and especially toddlers will go through periods of refusal, pickiness, and preference. Obtain a diet history as reviewed in the preceding section of this table (Refusal of solids).	See preceding section of this table (Refusal of solids). Discuss the following with parents: • Refusal may be due to loss of interest in food when more active or due to a form of negativism and a means to control. • Avoid use of food as a substitute for attention or stimulation. • Some degree of refusal and variation in appetite is normal for age. Try the following approaches: • Offer small amounts of food frequently. • Emphasize favorite foods as much as possible. • Use as few non-nutritive foods as possible.

- Allow the child to feed self if he desires and provide finger foods.
- Be patient as child tries to master use of utensils.
- Eating should be an enjoyable and sociable time. If hunger does not permit infant to wait until family dinner time, feed before and offer nibbles during family meal.
- Give older infant and toddler a place, chair, utensils, and plate at the table.

Reinforce the following with parents:
- Correct preparation of formula.
- Use of appropriate size nipple and nipple hole.
- Regular and frequent burping is needed.
- Place infant in an upright position for 30 minutes after feeding.
- Correct position of infant during feeding.

Determine the need to change the method of feeding or formula.

Assist parents to make decision to wean. The criteria include the following:
- Should be discussed and decided by both parents.
- If breast feeding, it is helpful to mother to assess every 3 months whether or not to continue nursing.

Spitting up

Regurgitation commonly following a feeding; usually related to air swallowed with food, inability to relax esophageal sphincter, possible overfeeding, or allergy to milk. Ascertain nature of regurgitation (e.g., frequency, amount, color, consistency) as well as diet history and data regarding weight gain. Regurgitation is frequently outgrown by the time the infant is sitting well in upright position.

Weaning

A transition of feeding methods. May be from bottle to cup or from breast to bottle and/or cup. Weaning from breast is difficult if parents (especially mother) have ambivalent feelings or if infant refuses alternative methods. Ascertain who wants baby weaned and why as well as schedule of feedings.

Continued.

Common concerns and problems of the first year—cont'd

Problem or concern	Assessment	Nursing intervention
Weaning—cont'd	Weaning from bottle should be attempted gradually when child is ready, usually around 1 year. Ascertain who wants child weaned, what has been tried, feeding schedule and number of bottles, and ability to use cup.	• Positive attitude toward weaning is essential, especially for breast-feeding mothers. • Weaning at times of separation anxiety is not advised, especially in breast-fed infants. • If possible, an infant should be weaned from breast to cup. This avoids having to wean from bottle later one. Active weaning for breast feeding mothers includes: • Start by substituting a bottle or cup for the breast at one feeding and allow 5-6 days before substituting second breast feeding. • If resistance is encountered, try giving water or juice in a bottle or cup before weaning starts, using nipple similar to breast or pacifier if one is used, heating milk before offering, and having someone other than mother offer the bottle or cup. Keep to a schedule and be firm, positive, and patient.

Active weaning to cup—continue preceding steps with the following additions:

- Reinforce idea of accomplishment in using a cup to child.
- May give child one bottle a day, but should contain only water to avoid incidence of dental caries.
- Avoid forcing child to wean; forcing the use of a cup may increase the need to suck.
- A calm, relaxed, positive approach is essential.

Infant Stimulation Guide

Infant Stimulation
Birth to 1 month
Babies like to
  Suck
  Listen to repeated soft sounds
  Stare at movement and light
  Be *held* and *rocked*
Give your baby
  Your *talking* and *singing*
  Lamps throwing light patterns
  Your *arms*
  Rocking

1 month
Babies like to
  Listen to your voice
  Look up and to the side
  Hold things placed in their hands
Give your baby
  A lullaby *record*
  A *mobile* overhead
  Pictures on the walls
  Your *face* near his
  A *change in scenery* and *position*

2 months
Babies like to
  Listen to musical sounds
  Focus (especially on their hands)
  Reach and *bat* nearby objects
  Smile
Give your baby
  A *music box* or a soft *musical toy*
  A soft security *cuddle toy* tied to crib
  Your *smile*
  Play time with you

3 months
Babies like to
  Reach and *feel* with open hands

From Stanhope M, Lancaster J: *Community health nursing: promoting health of aggregates, families, and individuals,* ed 4, 1996, Mosby.

Grasp crudely with two hands
Wave their fists and *watch* them
Give your baby
  Musical records
  Rattles
  Dangling toys
  Textured toys

4 months
Babies like to
  Grasp things and *let go*
  Kick
  Laugh at unexpected sights and sounds
  Make *consonant sounds*
Give your baby
  Bells
  A *crib gym*
  More *dangling toys*
  Space to kick and move

5 months
Babies like to
  Shake, feel, and *bang* things
  Sit with support
  Play peek-a-boo
  Roll over
Give your baby
  A *high chair* with a rubber *suction toy*
  A *play pen*
  A *kicking toy*
  Toys that make noise

6 months
Babies like to
  Shake, bang, and *throw things down*
  Gum objects
  Recognize familiar *faces*
Give your baby
  Many *household objects*
  Tin *cups, spoons,* and pot *lids*
  Wire *whisks*
  A *clutch ball* and *squeaky toys*
  A *teether* and *gumming toys*
  Bouncing, swinging seat

7 months

Babies like to

Sit alone

Use their *fingers* and *thumb*

Notice *cause* and *effect*

Bite on their *first tooth*

Give your baby

Bath tub toys

More *"things"*

String

More *squeaky toys*

Finger foods

8 months

Babies like to

Pivot on their stomachs

Throw, wave, and *bang* toys together

Look for toys they have

Make *vowel sounds*

Give your baby

Space to pivot and creep

2 *toys* at once to *bang together*

Big *soft blocks*

A *Jack-in-the-box*

Nested plastic *cups*

Your *conversation*

9 months

Babies like to

Pull themselves up

Creep

Place things generally where they're wanted

Say "da-da"

Play pat-a-cake

Give your baby

A *safe corner* of the room to *explore*

Toys tied to the *high chair*

A metal *mirror*

Jack-in-the-box

10 months

Babies like to

Poke and *prod* with
   their forefingers

Put things in other things
Imitate sounds
Give your baby
A big *pegboard*
Some *cloth books*
Motion toys
Textured toys

11 months to 1 year
Babies like to
Use their *fingers*
Lower themselves from standing
Drink from a cup
Mark on paper
Give your baby
Pyramid disks
A large *crayon*
A baking *tin* with *clothespins*
Personal *drinking cup*
More *picture books*

Tips for a Baby's Safety

Nursery Equipment Safety Checklist

From the beginning of a child's life, products such as cribs, crib gyms, playpens, high chairs, gates, and other equipment intended for a child must be selected with safety in mind. Parents and caretakers of babies and young children need to be aware of the many potential hazards in their environment—hazards occurring through misuse of products or those involved with products that have not been well designed for use by children.

This checklist is a safety guide to help you when buying new or second-hand nursery equipment. It also can be used when you are checking over nursery equipment now in use in your home or in other facilities that care for infants and young children.

Ask yourself: does the equipment have the safety features in this checklist? If it does not, can missing or unsafe parts be easily replaced with the proper parts? Can breaks or cracks be repaired to give more safety? Can I fix the older equipment without creating a "new" hazard?

Modified from U.S. Consumer Product Safety Commission: *Nursery equipment safety checklist,* Washington, D.C., September, 1985. The Commission.

If most of your answers are "NO," the equipment might be too old, or overused and beyond help. If the equipment can be repaired, do the repairs *before* you allow any child to use it.

The Consumer Product Safety Commission's concern is that the children in your care have a safe environment in which to grow.

Carrier Seats

	Yes	No
1. Carrier seat has a wide sturdy base for stability.	☐	☐
2. Carrier has non–skid feet to prevent slipping.		
3. Supporting devices are locked securely.	☐	☐
4. Carrier set has crotch and waist straps.	☐	☐
5. Buckle or strap is easy to use.	☐	☐

The commission recommends that you never use the carrier as a car seat.

Changing Tables

	Yes	No
1. Table has safety straps to prevent falls.	☐	☐
2. Table has drawers or shelves that are easily accessible without leaving the baby unattended.	☐	☐

The commission recommends that you do not leave the baby on the table unattended and always use the straps to prevent the baby from falling.

Cribs

	Yes	No
1. Slats are spaced no more than 2⅜ inches apart.	☐	☐
2. No slats are missing or cracked.	☐	☐
3. Mattress fits snugly—less than two fingers width between edge of mattress and crib side.	☐	☐
4. Mattress support is securely attached to the head and footboards.	☐	☐
5. Corner posts are no higher than ⅝ of an inch to prevent entanglement of clothing or cords around the neck.	☐	☐
6. There are no cutouts in the head and footboards which allow head entrapment.	☐	☐
7. Drop-side latches cannot be released easily by an infant.	☐	☐
8. Drop-side latches securely hold sides in raised position.	☐	☐

9. All screws or bolts which secure components
   of crib are present and tight.   ☐   ☐

The commission recommends that you do not place crib near draperies or blinds where child could become entangled and strangle on the cords. When the child reaches 35 inches in height or can climb or fall over the sides, the crib should be replaced with a bed.

Crib Toys

	Yes	No

1. Crib toys have no strings longer than 12 inches
   to prevent entanglement.   ☐   ☐
2. Crib gyms or cribmobiles suspended over the crib
   are securely fastened to the crib to prevent it from
   being pulled into the crib.   ☐   ☐
3. Components of toys are not small enough
   to be a choking hazard.   ☐   ☐

The commission recommends that you avoid hanging toys across the crib or on crib corner posts with strings long enough to result in strangulation. Remove crib gyms when child is able to pull or push up on hands and knees.

Gates and Enclosures

	Yes	No

1. Openings in the gate are too small to entrap a
   child's head.   ☐   ☐
2. Gate has a pressure bar or other fastener that will
   resist forces exerted by a child.   ☐   ☐

The commission recommends that, in order to avoid head entrapment, do not use accordion-style gates or expandable enclosures with *large* y-shaped openings along the top edge, or diamond-shaped openings within.

High Chairs

	Yes	No

1. High chair has waist and crotch straps that
   are independent of the tray. Tray locks securely. ☐   ☐
2. High chair has a wide base for stability.   ☐   ☐
3. High chair has caps or plugs on tubing that
   are firmly attached and cannot be pulled off
   and choke a child.   ☐   ☐

4. If it is a folding high chair, it has an effective
locking device to keep the chair from collapsing.   ☐   ☐

5. High chair has caps or plugs on tubing that are
firmly attached and cannot be pulled off and
choke a child   ☐   ☐

6. If it is a folding high chair, it has an effective
locking device to keep the chair from collapsing.   ☐   ☐

The commission recommends that you keep high chair away from
the table, counter, wall, or other surface so that a child can't push off
from it.

Hook-On Chairs

	Yes	No

1. Chair has a restraint system to secure the child.   ☐   ☐

2. Chair has a clamp that locks onto the table for
added security.   ☐   ☐

3. Hook-on chair has caps or plugs on tubing
which cannot be pulled off and choke a child.   ☐   ☐

4. Hook-on chair has a warning that you should
never place the chair where the child can push
off with feet.   ☐   ☐

The commission recommends that you don't leave a child
unattended in a hook-on chair.

Pacifiers

	Yes	No

1. Pacifier has no ribbon, string, cord, or yarn attached.   ☐   ☐

2. Shield is large and firm enough so it cannot
fit in child's mouth.   ☐   ☐

3. Guard or shield has ventilation holes so the baby can
breathe if the shield does get into the mouth.   ☐   ☐

4. Pacifier nipple has no holes or tears that might cause
it to break off in baby's mouth.   ☐   ☐

The commission recommends that, in order to prevent strangulation, you should never put a pacifier or other items on a string around
a baby's neck.

Playpens

	Yes	No

1. Drop-side mesh playpen or mesh crib has warning
label about never leaving a side in the down position.   ☐   ☐

2. Playpen mesh has small weave (less than ¼ inch openings).   ☐ ☐
3. Mesh has not tears, holes, or loose threads.   ☐ ☐
4. Mesh is securely attached to top rail and floorplate.   ☐ ☐
5. Top rail cover has no tears or holes.   ☐ ☐
6. Wooden playpen has slats spaced no more than 2⅜ inches apart.   ☐ ☐
7. If staples are used in construction, they are firmly installed and none are missing or loose.   ☐ ☐

The commission recommends that you never leave an infant in a mesh playpen or crib with the drop-side down. Even a very young infant can roll into the space between the mattress and loose mesh side and suffocate.

Rattles, Squeeze Toys, Teethers

	Yes	No
1. Rattles, squeeze toys, and teethers are too large to lodge in a baby's throat.	☐	☐
2. Rattles are of sturdy construction so they will not break apart in use.	☐	☐
3. Squeeze toys do not contain a squeaker that could detach and choke a baby.	☐	☐

The commission recommends that you take rattles, squeeze toys, teethers, and other toys out of the crib or playpen when the baby sleeps to prevent suffocation.

Strollers

	Yes	No
1. Stroller has a wide base to prevent tipping.	☐	☐
2. Seat belt and crotch strap are securely attached to frame.	☐	☐
3. Seat belt buckle is easy to fasten and unfasten.	☐	☐
4. Brakes securely lock the wheel(s).	☐	☐
5. Shopping basket is low on the back and located directly over or in front of rear wheels.	☐	☐

The commission recommends that you always secure the seat belts; never leave a child unattended in a stroller. Keep children's hands away from pinching areas when stroller is being folded or unfolded.

Toy Chests

	Yes	No
1. Toy chest has no lid latch which could entrap child within the chest.	☐	☐
2. Toy chest has a spring-loaded lid support that will support the lid in any position and will not require periodic adjustment.	☐	☐
3. Chest has holes or spaces in front or sides, or under the lid for ventilation should a child get inside.	☐	☐

The commission recommends that if you already own a toy chest or trunk with a freely falling lid, *remove the lid* to avoid a head injury to a small child, or install a spring-loaded lid support.

Walkers

	Yes	No
1. Walker has a wide wheel base for stability.	☐	☐
2. Walker has covers over coil springs to avoid finger pinching.	☐	☐
3. Seat is securely attached to frame of walker.	☐	☐
4. There are no X-frames that could pinch or amputate fingers.	☐	☐

The commission recommends that you place gates or guards at top of all stairways, or keep stairway doors closed to prevent falls. Do not use walkers as baby sitters.

Protocol for Postpartum Home Visit

Previsit Interventions

1. Contact family to arrange details for home visit.
   a. Identify self, credentials, and agency role.
   b. Review purpose of home visit follow-up.
   c. Schedule convenient time for visit.
   d. Confirm address and route to family home.
2. Review and clarify appropriate data.
   a. All available assessment data for mother and infant (i.e., referral forms, hospital discharge summaries, family identified learning needs).
   b. Review records of any previous nursing contacts.

From Bobak IM, Lowdermilk DL, Jensen MD: *Maternity nursing,* ed 4, St Louis, 1995, Mosby.

    c. Contact other professional caregivers as necessary to clarify data (i.e., obstetrician, nurse-midwife, pediatrician, referring nurse).
3. Identify community resources and teaching materials appropriate to meet needs already identified.
4. Plan the visit and prepare bag with equipment, supplies, and materials necessary for the assessments of mother and infant, actual care anticipated for mother and infant, and teaching.

In-Home Interventions: Establishing a Relationship

1. Reintroduce self and establish purpose of postpartum follow-up visit for mother, infant, and family; offer family opportunity to clarify their expectations of contact.
2. Spend brief time socially interacting with family to become acquainted and establish trusting relationship.

In-Home Interventions: Working with Family

1. Conduct systematic assessment of mother and newborn to determine physiologic adjustment and any existing complications.
2. Throughout visit, collect data to assess the emotional adjustment of individual family members to newborn and lifestyle changes. Note evidence of family-newborn bonding and sibling rivalry; note relationships among mother, father, children, and grandparents.
3. Determine adequacy of support system.
    a. To what extent does someone help with cooking, cleaning, and other home management tasks?
    b. To what extent is help being provided in caring for the newborn and any other children?
    c. Are support persons encouraging the new mother to care for herself and get adequate rest?
    d. Who is providing helpful information? Emotional support?
4. Throughout the visit, observe home environment for adequacy of resources.
    a. Space: privacy, safe play of children, sleeping.
    b. Overall cleanliness and state of repair.
    c. Number of steps new mother must climb.
    d. Adequacy of cooking arrangements.
    e. Adequacy of refrigeration and other food storage areas.
    f. Adequacy of bathing, toileting, and laundry facilities.
    g. Arrangements in home for newborn: sleeping, bathing, formula preparation (if needed), layette items, and diapers.
5. Throughout the visit, observe home environment for overall state of repair and existence of safety hazards.

a. Storage of medications, household cleaners, and other substances hazardous to children.
b. Presence of peeling paint on furniture, walls, or pipes.
c. Factors that contribute to falls, such as dim lighting, broken steps, scatter rugs.
d. Presence of vermin.
e. Use of crib or playpen that fails to meet safety guidelines.
f. Existence of emergency plan in case of fire; fire alarm or extinguisher.

6. Provide care to mother and/or newborn as prescribed by their respective primary care provider or in accord with agency protocol.
7. Provide teaching on basis of previously identified needs.
8. Refer family to appropriate community agencies or resources, such as warm lines and support groups.
9. Ascertain that woman knows potential problems to watch for and whom to call if they occur.
10. Ensure that used disposable items have been handled appropriately and that reusable items are cleaned and repacked appropriately in the nurse's bag.

In-Home Interventions: Ending the Visit*

1. Summarize the activities and main points of the visit.
2. Clarify future expectations, including schedule of next visit.
3. Review teaching plan, and provide major points in writing.
4. Provide information about reaching the nurse or agency if needed before the next scheduled visit.

Postvisit Interventions

1. Document the visit thoroughly, using the necessary agency forms to serve as a legal record of the visit and to allow third-party reimbursement, as possible.
2. Initiate the plan of care on which the next encounter with the client/family will be based.
3. Communicate appropriately (by telephone, letter, progress notes, or referral form) with primary care provider, other health professionals, or referral agencies on behalf of client/family.

---

*If this is the nurse's final planned encounter with the woman/family, it is important to recognize that both the women and nurse may have feelings evoked by ending a meaningful relationship and by saying goodbye. Such feelings as anger, denial, and sadness are normal in this situation. Freely expressing these feelings at the end of the relationship is encouraged. Often patients are encouraged to do so if the nurse shares such feelings first.

INDEX

892